Instructional
Course Lectures
Spine
Volume 2

Edited by
Christopher M. Bono, MD
Chief, Orthopedic Spine Service
Brigham and Women's Hospital
Assistant Professor
Department of Orthopedic Surgery
Harvard Medical School
Boston, Massachusetts

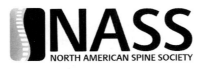

Developed with support from
North American Spine Society

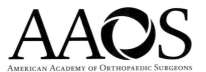

Published by the
American Academy
of Orthopaedic Surgeons
6300 North River Road
Rosemont, IL 60018

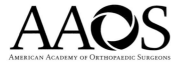

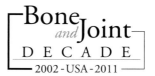

Editorial Board

Contributors

William A. Abdu, MD, MS
Associate Professor of Orthopaedic Surgery
Dartmouth-Hitchcock Medical Center
Lebanon, New Hampshire

Todd J. Albert, MD
Professor and Chairman
Department of Orthopaedic Surgery
The Rothman Institute
Thomas Jefferson University Hospital
Philadelphia, Pennsylvania

D. Greg Anderson, MD
Associate Professor
Department of Orthopaedic Surgery
Thomas Jefferson University
Philadelphia, Pennsylvania

David T. Anderson, MD
Resident Physician
Department of Orthopaedic Surgery
Thomas Jefferson University Hospital
Philadelphia, Pennsylvania

Paul A. Anderson, MD
Associate Professor
Department of Orthopedics and Rehabilitation
University of Wisconsin
Madison, Wisconsin

Mark Bernhardt, MD
Clinical Professor
University of Missouri at Kansas City School
  of Medicine
Dickson-Diveley Midwest Orthopaedic Clinic
St. Luke's Hospital and Children's Mercy Hospital
Kansas City, Missouri

Randal R. Betz, MD
Chief of Staff
Shriners Hospitals for Children
Philadelphia, Pennsylvania

Oheneba Boachie-Adjei, MD
Associate Clinical Professor
Department of Orthopaedic Surgery
Weill Medical College of Cornell University
New York, New York

Christopher M. Bono, MD
Chief, Orthopedic Spine Service
Brigham and Women's Hospital
Assistant Professor
Department of Orthopedic Surgery
Harvard Medical School
Boston, Massachusetts

Keith H. Bridwell, MD
Asa C. and Dorothy W. Jones Professor
Chief, Orthopaedic Spine Surgery
Department of Orthopaedic Surgery
Washington University
St. Louis, Missouri

Darrel S. Brodke, MD
Department of Orthopaedics
University of Utah
Salt Lake City, Utah

Andrew K. Brown, MD
Orthopaedic Spine Research
The Rothman Institute
Philadelphia, Pennsylvania

Douglas C. Burton, MD
Marc and Elinor Asher Spine Research Professor
Department of Orthopedic Surgery
University of Kansas School of Medicine
Kansas City, Kansas

Jens R. Chapman, MD
Professor
Director, Spine Service
Hansjoerg Wyss Endowed Chair
Department of Orthopaedics and Sports Medicine
University of Washington
Seattle, Washington

Charles H. Crawford III, MD
Administrative Chief Resident
Department of Orthopaedic Surgery
University of Louisville
Louisville, Kentucky

Bradford L. Currier, MD
Professor
Department of Orthopaedic Surgery
Mayo Clinic
Mayo Foundation
Rochester, Minnesota

Scott D. Daffner, MD
Assistant Professor
Department of Orthopaedics
West Virginia University School of Medicine
Morgantown, West Virginia

Michael D. Daubs, MD, FACS
Instructor
Department of Orthopaedic Surgery
Washington University
St. Louis, Missouri

Clinton J. Devin, MD
Fondren Orthopedic Group
Houston, Texas

Mohammad Diab, MD
Associate Professor
Department of Orthopaedic Surgery
University of California, San Francisco
San Francisco, California

William F. Donaldson, MD
Associate Professor
Chief of the Division of Spinal Surgery
Department of Orthopaedic Surgery
University of Pittsburgh Medical Center
Pittsburgh, Pennsylvania

Jason C. Eck, DO, MS
Resident
Department of Orthopaedic Surgery
Memorial Hospital
York, Pennsylvania

Frank J. Eismont, MD
Vice Chairman
Professor
Department of Orthopedics and Rehabilitation
University of Miami School of Medicine
Miami, Florida

Michael T. Espiritu, MD
Clinical Instructor
Department of Orthopaedics
University of Pittsburgh Medical Center
Pittsburgh, Pennsylvania

Ernest M. Found, MD
Associate Professor
University of Iowa Hospitals and Clinics
Department of Orthopaedic Surgery
Iowa City, Iowa

Charley Gates, MD
Resident Physician
Department of Orthopaedic Surgery
University of Pittsburgh Medical Center
Pittsburgh, Pennsylvania

Alexander J. Ghanayem, MD
Professor
Department of Orthopaedic Surgery and Rehabilitation
Chief, Division of Spine Surgery
Department of Orthopaedic Surgery and Rehabilitation
Loyola University Medical Center
Maywood, Illinois

John A. Glaser, MD
Professor, Orthopaedic Surgery
Medical University of South Carolina
Charleston, South Carolina

Steven D. Glassman, MD
Associate Professor of Orthopaedic Surgery
Orthopaedic Department
University of Louisville
Louisville, Kentucky

Eric Harris, MD
Spine Fellow
Department of Orthopaedic Surgery
The Rothman Institute
Thomas Jefferson University Hospital
Philadelphia, Pennsylvania

Mitchel B. Harris, MD, FACS
Chief, Orthopedic Trauma Service
Brigham and Women's Hospital
Associate Professor
Department of Orthopedic Surgery
Harvard Medical School
Boston, Massachusetts

Robert A. Hart, MD, MA
Associate Professor
Department of Orthopaedics and Rehabilitation
Oregon Health and Sciences University
Portland, Oregon

Harry N. Herkowitz, MD
Chairman, Department of Orthopaedic Surgery
Director, Fellowship in Spinal Surgery
William Beaumont Hospital
Royal Oak, Michigan

Alan S. Hilibrand, MD
Professor
Department of Orthopaedic Surgery
The Rothman Institute
Thomas Jefferson University Hospital
Philadelphia, Pennsylvania

Justin B. Hohl, MD
Resident
Department of Orthopaedic Surgery
University of Pittsburgh Medical Center
Pittsburgh, Pennsylvania

Serena S. Hu, MD
Professor and Vice Chair
Chief, Spine Surgery
Department of Orthopaedic Surgery
University of California, San Francisco
San Francisco, California

James D. Kang, MD
Professor of Orthopaedics and Neurosurgery
Department of Orthopaedics and Neurosurgery
University of Pittsburgh Medical Center
Pittsburgh, Pennsylvania

Yongjung J. Kim, MD
Visiting Scholar
Department of Orthopaedic Surgery
Washington University
St. Louis, Missouri

Mark A. Knaub, MD
Fellow, Spinal Surgery
Department of Orthopaedic Surgery
William Beaumont Hospital
Royal Oak, Michigan

James Lawrence, MD
Spine Fellow
Department of Orthopaedic Surgery
The Rothman Institute
Thomas Jefferson University Hospital
Philadelphia, Pennsylvania

Lawrence G. Lenke, MD
The Jerome J. Gilden Professor of Orthopaedic Surgery
Professor of Neurologic Surgery
Department of Orthopaedic Surgery
Washington University School of Medicine
St. Louis, Missouri

Thomas G. Lowe, MD
Clinical Professor
University of Colorado Health Sciences Center
Orthopaedic Spine Surgery
Woodridge Orthopaedic and Spine Center PC
Wheat Ridge, Colorado

Neil A. Manson, MD, FRCSC
Spine Fellow
Midwest Orthopaedics at Rush
Rush University Medical Center
Chicago, Illinois

Satyajit V. Marawar, MD
Fellow
Department of Orthopaedic Surgery
Medical College of Wisconsin
Milwaukee, Wisconsin

Gregory S. McDowell, MD
Cofounder, Northern Rockies Regional Spine
  Injury Center
Orthopaedic Surgeons PSC
Billings, Montana

Robert A. McGuire Jr, MD
Professor and Chairman
Department of Orthopedics and Rehabilitation
University of Mississippi Medical Center
Jackson, Mississippi

Peter O. Newton, MD
Chief of Scoliosis Service and Orthopedic Research
Children's Hospital, San Diego
Associate Clinical Professor
University of California, San Diego
San Diego, California

Gbolahan O. Okubadejo, MD
Fellow
Department of Orthopaedic Surgery
University of Pittsburgh Medical Center
Pittsburgh, Pennsylvania

Stefan Parent, MD, PhD
Pediatric Orthopedic Spine Fellow
Department of Pediatric Orthopedics
Children's Hospital at San Diego
San Diego, California

Frank M. Phillips, MD
Professor, Orthopaedic Surgery
Rush University Medical Center
Chicago, Illinois

Peter D. Pizzutillo, MD
Director, Orthopaedic Surgery
St. Christopher's Hospital for Children
Philadelphia, Pennsylvania

Kornelis A. Poelstra, MD, PhD
Assistant Professor of Orthopaedics
Department of Orthopaedics
University of Maryland, Shock Trauma
Baltimore, Maryland

Michael A. Prendergast, BA
Department of Orthopaedics
Robert Wood Johnson Medical School
New Brunswick, New Jersey

Raj D. Rao, MD
Professor of Orthopaedic Surgery
Director, Spine Surgery
Department of Orthopaedic Surgery
Medical College of Wisconsin
Milwaukee, Wisconsin

John M. Rhee, MD
Assistant Professor
Department of Orthopaedic Surgery
Emory Spine Center
Emory University School of Medicine
Atlanta, Georgia

K. Daniel Riew, MD
Professor
Chief, Cervical Spine Surgery
Department of Orthopaedic Surgery
Washington University School of Medicine
St. Louis, Missouri

Jeffrey A. Rihn, MD
Assistant Professor of Spine Surgery
Department of Orthopaedic Surgery
Thomas Jefferson University
The Rothman Institute
Philadelphia, Pennsylvania

Stephen M. Ritter, MD
Department of Orthopedics
University of Utah
Salt Lake City, Utah

Rick C. Sasso, MD
Associate Professor
Clinical Orthopaedic Surgery
Indiana University School of Medicine
Indiana Spine Group
Indianapolis, Indiana

Michael K. Schaufele, MD
Assistant Professor
Departments of Orthopedics and
    Rehabilitative Medicine
Emory University
Atlanta, Georgia

James D. Schwender, MD
Spine Surgeon
Twin Cities Spine Center
Minneapolis, Minnesota

Lewis L. Shi, MD
Department of Orthopedics
Brigham and Women's Hospital
Boston, Massachusetts

Gordon H. Stock, MD
Orthopaedic Research Fellow
Department of Orthopaedics
Thomas Jefferson University
The Rothman Institute
Philadelphia, Pennsylvania

Clifford B. Tribus, MD
Associate Professor
Department of Orthopaedics and
    Rehabilitative Medicine
University of Wisconsin, Madison
Madison, Wisconsin

Alexander R. Vaccaro, MD, PhD
Professor
Department of Orthopaedic Surgery
Thomas Jefferson University
The Rothman Institute
Philadelphia, Pennsylvania

Jeffrey C. Wang, MD
Associate Professor of Orthopaedic Surgery
    and Neurosurgery
University of California Los Angeles
    Comprehensive Spine Center
Department of Orthopaedic Surgery
University of California Los Angeles School of Medicine
Los Angeles, California

Dennis R. Wenger, MD
Director, Pediatric Orthopedic Training Program
Pediatric Orthopedic and Scoliosis Center
Children's Hospital, San Diego
University of California, San Diego
Department of Orthopaedics
San Diego, California

F. Todd Wetzel, MD
Associate Professor and Chair, Division of Surgery
University of Chicago-Weiss, Orthopaedic Surgery
University of Chicago Spine Center
Chicago, Illinois

Douglas S. Won, MD
Fellow in Spinal Surgery
Department of Orthopaedic Surgery
William Beaumont Hospital
Royal Oak, Michigan

Thomas A. Zdeblick, MD
Professor and Chair
Department of Orthopaedics
University of Wisconsin
Madison, Wisconsin

Preface

Although the field of orthopaedics shares credit for advancements in spinal care with other subspecialties such as neurosurgery, physical medicine, rehabilitation, and radiology, the American Academy of Orthopaedic Surgeons (AAOS) and its respective publications deserve recognition as a reliable source of accurate information and educational material on spinal disorders for practitioners across multiple disciplines. This volume is the second edition in the *Instructional Course Lectures* (ICL) specialty series dedicated to the spine. The esteemed Howard An, MD, from Rush Medical College served as the editor of the first ICL Spine volume published in 2003. It was my distinct honor to be asked to serve as the book editor for *Instructional Course Lectures Spine 2*. Assuredly, Dr. An's work has served as an excellent template.

It is the editor's privilege and challenge to choose from the scores of superb instructional course chapters on the spine that have been published over the past 5 years. In an attempt to provide a well-balanced view of contemporary spine surgery, the selected chapters have been organized into 10 sections. Although I could take credit for this organization, even a quick perusal of the individual chapters reveals natural groupings of like-themed topics. It was my more simple responsibility to choose the section titles—Spinal Trauma, Pediatric Spinal Deformity, Adolescent Idiopathic Scoliosis, Adult Spinal Deformity, Low Back Pain and Radiculopathy, Degenerative Lumbar Stenosis, The Geriatric Spine, Advanced Surgical Techniques, Degenerative Cervical Disorders, and Complications of Cervical Spine Surgery. The chapters by themselves are excellent, but grouped together their impact is more potent. The reader is provided with a comprehensive review of spinal disorders and treatments that are framed by the relevant perspectives presented in commentaries by established leaders in the field of spine surgery. I am indebted to each of the section editors for their contribution to this publication.

The first section, Spinal Trauma, was reviewed by Mitchel B. Harris, MD, an associate professor of orthopedic surgery at Harvard Medical School and the chief of the orthopedic trauma service at Brigham and Women's Hospital. Dr. Harris has established himself as a nationally and internationally recognized expert in the field of spinal trauma. In addition to his insight as a co-author of three of the four chapters in this section, Dr. Harris' commentary relates the information in the chapters to trends and shifts in spinal trauma, both past and current, and helps balance the zeal for recent advancements in the field with foundational basics on which the care of the acutely injured patient is rooted.

Daniel J. Hedequist, MD is a well-respected and renowned pediatric orthopaedic surgeon at Children's Hospital in Boston, Massachusetts and is an assistant professor of orthopedics at Harvard Medical School. I was fortunate that Dr. Hedequist accepted the invitation to provide a commentary for the section on pediatric spinal deformity. With the focus of the four chapters in this section on kyphotic deformity in children, Dr. Hedequist highlights the critical information detailed in the chapters, including an understanding of normal alignment, implementation of nonsurgical care, and the application of surgical treatment. Paraphrasing Dr. Hedequist's statements, the four chapters in this section provide the necessary principles to guide decision-making in treating patients with pediatric kyphosis.

Evidenced by its name, the exact causes of adolescent idiopathic scoliosis remain elusive. However, a laudable amount of energy and research continues to be devoted to a better understanding of this disorder, as highlighted by Jeffrey S. Shilt, MD. Dr. Shilt is the medical director of pediatric orthopaedics at St. Alphonsus Regional Medical Center in Boise, Idaho. His commentary reflects his experience as a pediatric spine surgeon and describes how the currently available data and recommendations can be applied in practice. The shifts in care trends that have occurred in recent years are outlined, along with a forecast concerning the impact of future developments.

There are few more experienced surgeons in the field of adult spinal deformity than Serena Hu, MD, a professor and vice chair of the department of orthopaedic surgery at the University of California, San Francisco. Dr. Hu has published countless articles on adult spinal deformity and is an internationally renowned figure in this field. The expertise and perspectives provided in the commentary on adult spine deformity are invaluable.

In my role as the section editor for Low Back Pain and Radiculopathy, my commentary attempts to poise the reader for a current and relevant incorporation of the information presented and to provide a brief summary of the core substance of each chapter. Since the publication of these chapters in the period from 2004 to 2008, there have been paradigmatic shifts in the perception of the proper treatment of nonspecific low back pain and the role of fusion. The chapter by Rhee and associates on radiculopathy and herniated disks is perhaps the best single work I have read on the topic; anyone who treats patients with this condition should closely study this informative chapter.

Jeffrey S. Fischgrund, MD is an authority on degenerative lumbar stenosis. He first authored one of the most widely quoted studies regarding the role of instrumentation and fusion in the setting of spinal stenosis with degenerative spondylolisthesis and has since not tired in his research efforts to better understand this and related issues. A practicing orthopaedic spine surgeon at the William Beaumont Hospital in Royal Oak, Michigan, Dr. Fischgrund is the Editor-in-Chief of the *Journal of the American Academy of Orthopaedic Surgeons* (JAAOS). With these credentials, I was honored that he was willing to serve as section editor for this ICL volume. In his commentary, the reader will find not only a highlight of the content of the chapters but a distillation of the "important message" in each. Dr. Fischgrund's commentary reflects the zeal of a true academic balanced with the sage temperance of an experienced clinician.

Although relatively short with only two chapters, the section on the geriatric spine edited by Raj Rao, MD has a great impact. Dr. Rao is a professor of orthopaedic surgery and director of spine surgery at the Medical College of Wisconsin in Milwaukee. In his commentary, he asks important and challenging questions such as, "Do we need to think differently when dealing with older patients?" As the population of the United States becomes increasingly older and more active, the demand of these patients to maintain a high quality of life becomes greater. The unique challenges of providing appropriate surgical care for older patients are underscored by Dr. Rao in his commentary.

Spine surgeons are continually bombarded with a myriad of new techniques, implants, and other technologies that are purported to improve the efficiency, expediency, and results of surgical procedures for the spine. Traveling through this sea of "advancements" requires not only a degree in navigation (so to speak) but a functioning crystal ball to foresee which claims are true and which are false. In the section dedicated to advanced surgical techniques, John Rhee, MD, serves as the captain of our vessel. Dr. Rhee is an assistant professor of orthopaedic surgery at Emory University and a practicing member of the Emory Spine Center in Atlanta, Georgia. In his careful review of the chapters, Dr. Rhee makes a concerted effort to recognize the potential use of new advancements while not discarding more traditional techniques. For example, Dr. Rhee acknowledges that image guidance may one day evolve to a level of universal acceptance but points out that intraoperative fluoroscopy remains the current modality of choice in most cases. With similar intent, Dr. Rhee emphasizes that the traditional bone grafting technique for occipitocervical fusion should not be overlooked when using the latest plate-rod-screw fixation constructs.

Jonathan N. Grauer, MD, an associate professor of orthopaedic surgery and co-director of the orthopaedic spine service at Yale University, and his co-editor, Shawn Hermenau, MD, provide a succinct review of the three chapters in the section about degenerative cervical disorders. The section editors acknowledge that the first chapter in the section is a primer on the topic, which reviews nearly all facets of the varying entities within this group of degenerative disorders. Although the chapter on cervical disk replacement could have easily been placed in the Advanced Surgical Techniques section, its inclusion in a discussion of cervical disk disease was perhaps more appropriate. Above all, the section editors emphasize the paramount value of adhering to sound treatment principles and, when indicated, obtaining the anticipated surgical goals of decompression and stabilization.

To deny the existence of surgical complications implies either untruthfulness or that one is not really a surgeon. All spine surgeons will benefit from the information presented in the section, Complications of Cervical Spine Surgery, and from the commentary provided by Alexander R. Vaccaro, MD, PhD, and his co-editor Jeffrey Rihn, MD. Dr. Vaccaro is professor of orthopaedic and neurological surgery at Thomas Jefferson University Hospital in Philadelphia, Pennsylvania and is also the co-director of the Delaware Valley Regional Spinal Cord Injury Center. Dr. Rihn is an assistant professor of spine surgery at Thomas Jefferson University. The complications discussed in this section range from the inevitable, such as dysphagia following anterior approaches, to the potentially catastrophic, such as vertebral artery injury. In addition to a summary of the information in each chapter, Drs. Vaccaro and Rihn judiciously interject their own invaluable experience in preventing and dealing with these unwelcome events.

Like any publication, there are many layers and pieces that are adjoined to create a final product. It is with some guilt that my name will appear as editor of this volume when in truth unending credit should be given to the original authors of these classic lectures, the section editors for their expertise and viewpoint, and the AAOS staff, including Marilyn Fox, PhD; Lisa Claxton Moore; and notably Kathleen Anderson, who did a superb job of guiding this project to completion. Gratitude also is owed to the great people of the North American Spine Society who supported my nomination for this endeavor. The AAOS should be congratulated for all of its efforts in providing educational material for orthopaedic surgeons and particularly for the publication of this critical ICL volume dedicated to spinal care. It should, in my opinion, be considered essential reading for all spine practitioners across all disciplines.

Christopher M. Bono, MD

Contents

Section 9 Degenerative Cervical Disorders

Section 10 Complications of Cervical Spine Surgery

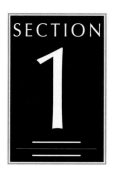

SECTION 1

Spinal Trauma

Spinal Trauma

As Eismont and associates aptly state in their abstract, "cervical spine injuries are frequently encountered in any practice treating patients in the emergency department or outpatient trauma victims." The authors emphasize the principles of immediate cervical immobilization and transportation to an appropriate treatment facility. After a comprehensive physical examination, the needed radiographic studies are determined by the examination results and the clinical setting. If spinal shock is identified during the initial examination, the examiner is precluded from determining the extent of the neural injuries.

At the time of the original publication of the chapter by Eismont and associates in 2004, the use of plain radiographs was supported. Currently, however, in most trauma centers the management algorithm has eliminated the use of plain radiographs, replacing them with multidetector CT scans with sagittal and coronal reconstructions. If the patient's condition is too unstable to allow CT imaging, the classic trauma series consisting of chest, AP pelvis, and lateral cervical spine radiographs should be obtained in the trauma bay, concomitant with active resuscitation. A single lateral cervical spine radiograph can quickly reveal unstable injuries such as facet dislocations, burst fractures with significant malalignment, and occipital-cervical dissociations. This information will allow urgent intervention and/or stabilization. MRI scans have become increasingly integrated into the early spinal trauma evaluation, particularly when a spinal cord injury (SCI) or root injury is identified or an unstable soft-tissue injury is suspected.

This chapter provides a detailed analysis of the most commonly encountered cervical spine injuries. The authors use the Allen-Ferguson mechanistic classification system as an organizational framework for the chapter along with the common division of upper cervical injuries (occiput to C2) and subaxial injuries (C3 to C7). The authors appropriately emphasize the importance of associated soft-tissue injuries in cervical spinal trauma. In the upper cervical spine, the soft-tissue structures requiring specific scrutiny include the tectorial membrane, which spans the occipitocervical junction; the transverse ligament, which provides stability across the C1-2 junction; and the C2-3 intervertebral disk, which is commonly disrupted in patients with a hangman's fracture.

As a result of its initial publication in 2004, the chapter includes considerable discussion and support for halo immobilization for upper cervical injuries. Although this apparatus is still commonly used in younger trauma patients, its use in geriatric trauma patients has steadily declined in popularity. With increasingly more sophisticated methods of internal fixation being developed and championed, treatment options now usually involve either nonsurgical treatment with a rigid cervical orthosis or surgical stabilization. The use of halo immobilization has declined over the past 6 years. The section on upper cervical injury is worthy of close review because of the technical pearls shared by these experienced and expert spinal surgeons.

The section on subaxial injuries is an excellent review of the Allen-Ferguson mechanistic classification system. Although newer cervical spine injury classification systems have been published, they have not yet reached the popularity of this classic schema. The authors again stress the necessity to fully assess the degree of associated soft-tissue injury in the subaxial spine. The importance of thoroughly understanding the injury is highlighted by the frequent references to the use of CT and MRI scanning. The controversy regarding the timing of MRI in an injury involving jumped facets also is discussed.

The section on SCIs provides an excellent overview of primary and secondary injury mechanisms. Additionally, it covers the contemporary approaches to minimizing the injury as well as attempts to "reverse the paralysis." Six years after the original publication of the chapter by Eismont and associates, it is still believed that early spinal cord decompression is safe and offers some optimism for potential recovery after SCI. Conversely, the initial optimism associated with the administration of high-dose steroids within the first 3 to 8 hours after SCI has waned. It has, in fact, been reclassified as a treatment option but is no longer a standard or guideline.[1] Many emergency departments no longer routinely administer the Bracken protocol and will discontinue it on patients who are transferred from an outside institution during its administration.

The remaining chapters in this section provide a comprehensive description of the importance of accurately assessing a thoracolumbar spinal injury, classifying it for ease and accuracy of communication, and determining if surgery is required. If surgery is needed, information is presented on using an anterior, posterior, or combined approach.

There are many similarities in the diagnostic workups of spinal injuries. The importance of a comprehensive examination with attention to neurologic function cannot be overstated. However, as is appropriately pointed out in the initial paragraph of the chapter by Rihn and associates, assessing airway, breathing capacity, and circulatory status takes priority in the initial treatment of any spinal column injury, with or without an associated SCI. Evaluation with plain radiographs has generally been replaced by evaluation with multidetector CT scans because of the speed of acquisition and sensitivity for injuries.[2] In the polytrauma patient, the advantages of CT scanning are further substantiated by the versatility of surveillance CT scans of the chest, abdomen, and pelvis (CAP CT) to simultaneously assess for solid and hollow organ injuries. If a significant spinal injury is identified on the CAP CT scan, a dedicated spinal CT scan often is necessary to improve the image accuracy needed for preoperative planning. Adherence to the Advanced Trauma Life Support protocol remains the mainstay of the initial evaluation because of the significant percentage of associated injuries in patients with SCIs. MRI has proven to be quite helpful in assessing the posterior ligaments of the thoracolumbar spine, a major determinant of mechanical stability in this region.

A new system called the Thoracolumbar Injury Classification System[3] is gaining popularity because of its ease of use and its uniqueness in incorporating the neurologic status of the injured patient. This system also places significant importance on the integrity of the posterior ligamentous complex. It is simple and useful because it is a scoring system rather than a mechanistic, morphologic, or hybrid classification system. Points are awarded for morphology of the fracture, neurology, and the integrity of the posterior ligamentous complex. When the points are added with a few additional modifiers, a sum is determined. This number will help direct the surgeon toward surgical or nonsurgical treatment. As this scoring system gains popularity, it is quite likely that future modifications will emerge.

Numerous studies have supported the benefits of nonsurgical management of thoracolumbar injuries. The chapter by Harris and associates documents the expansive literature describing this treatment approach while acknowledging that some injuries will benefit from surgical intervention.

The final chapter in this section, written by five seasoned spine surgeons with strong interest in the management of spinal trauma, outlines the indications for surgical stabilization. The goals of surgical management are clearly defined—reduction of the deformity in association with restoration of stability, decompression of the spinal canal if there is a neurologic deficit, and early mobilization. These goals are consistent regardless of the surgical plan. The anterior approach has shown more consistent and complete canal decompression and a higher likelihood of functional bladder recovery, whereas the posterior approach offers the advantages of greater biomechanical strength and more capacity for deformity correction.

0Mitchel B. Harris, MD, FACS
Chief, Orthopedic Trauma Service
Brigham and Women's Hospital
Associate Professor
Department of Orthopedic Surgery
Harvard Medical School
Boston, Massachusetts

References

1. Hugenholtz H: Methylprednisolone for acute spinal cord injury: Not a standard of care. *CMAJ* 2003;168:1145-1146.

2. Berry GE, Adams S, Harris MB, et al: Are plain radiographs of the spine necessary during evaluation after blunt trauma? Accuracy of screening torso computed tomography in thoracic/lumbar spine fracture diagnosis. *J Trauma* 2005;59:1410-1413.

3. Vaccaro AR, Zeiller SC, Hulbert RJ, et al: The thoracolumbar injury severity score: A proposed treatment algorithm. *J Spinal Disord Tech* 2005;18:209-215.

Dr. Harris or an immediate family member has received research or institutional support from AO, DePuy, Medtronic Sofamor Danek, Synthes, and OMeGA.

1

Cervical Spine and Spinal Cord Injuries: Recognition and Treatment

Frank J. Eismont, MD
Bradford L. Currier, MD
Robert A. McGuire Jr, MD

Abstract

Cervical spine injuries are frequently encountered in any practice treating patients in the emergency department or outpatient trauma victims. When upper or lower cervical spine injuries are suspected, immediate immobilization, physical and neurologic examination, and radiographic evaluation are imperative. For spinal cord injuries, knowledge of microscopic and cellular pathology helps to determine appropriate management.

Cervical spine injuries can be grouped into upper (occiput to C2) and lower (C3 to T1) cervical spine injuries. This categorization is appropriate based on the most frequent mechanism of injury, clinical presentation, and treatment options. For those patients who also have a neurologic deficit as a result of their injuries, a review of the underlying pathology, recommended treatment, and research options may allow neurologic improvement in the future.

Initial Treatment

The treatment of individuals with suspected cervical spine injury consists of immediate immobilization using an extrication collar and transportation to a treatment facility.[1] Physical examination and radiographic evaluation can then be performed to make the appropriate diagnosis and determine appropriate treatment. If the injury is unstable, skeletal traction using Gardner-Wells tongs should be used. A detailed neurologic examination should be performed including a thorough motor, sensory, and reflex examination.[2] The presence of spinal shock may make it impossible initially to determine the extent of the neural injury. Once spinal shock has resolved (in 24 to 48 hours), the deficit can be more accurately assessed.

Radiographic evaluation initially consists of AP and lateral cervical radiographs. The cervicothoracic junction must always be seen. The AP and lateral views will reveal abnormalities in approximately 88% of cases. Malalignment of the vertebral elements is most accurately determined from these radiographs. CT scans will better delineate bony ab-

normalities such as sagittal fractures in the vertebral body, injury to the posterior elements, and retropulsion of bone into the spinal canal. CT scans will also reveal previously unrecognized fractures in approximately 10% of patients with injuries. MRI scans can be used to evaluate soft-tissue injuries such as spinal cord or nerve root injuries, disruption of the posterior ligaments, and injury to the disk and annular structures.[3,4]

Upper Cervical Spine Injuries
Jefferson Fractures

Jefferson fractures are defined as axial load injuries with one or two fractures of both the anterior and posterior arch of C1. The C1 posterior arch fractures almost always occur through the vertebral artery groove. Because of the wedge configuration of the C1 lateral masses, any axial load that produces a fracture tends to drive the lateral masses of C1 apart. The transverse ligament is the primary soft-tissue structure joining the lateral masses together and as the energy of the initial injury increases, failure of the transverse ligament will occur eventually; it may fail within

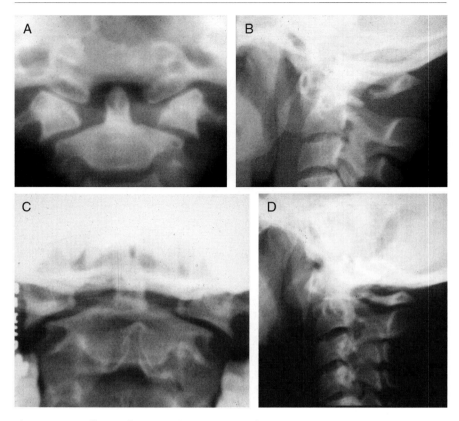

Figure 1 C1 Jefferson fracture. The overhang of the C1 lateral mass on C2 measures approximately 14 mm and the transverse ligament is disrupted. This patient was treated in a halo vest for 3 months. **A** and **B,** Radiographs taken immediately after injury. **C** and **D,** Radiographs taken 3 years later. The patient had regained full function and had no pain.

the ligament or via bone avulsion at its bony junction on the inner aspect of the lateral mass of C1. Total overhang is achieved by adding the overhang of the lateral masses of C1 to those of C2. If the total overhang is less than 5.7 mm, then the ligament will usually be intact. If the overhang is more than 6.9 mm, the ligament has most likely failed. If the total overhang is more than 5.7 mm but less than 6.9 mm, the status of the ligament is uncertain. These measurements were determined in an in-vitro study using cadaver spines and directly observing the ligament.[5]

Optimal treatment of Jefferson fractures usually requires application of a halo vest. This is true whether or not the transverse ligament is intact. Two excellent reviews of this treatment have been published.[6,7] After 3 months of immobilization, a CT scan of C1 would help verify that the fractures have healed. If the fractures have healed, the halo vest is disconnected and lateral flexion-extension radiographs of the cervical spine are obtained. If there is no movement between C1 and C2 regardless of the atlanto-dens interval or if the atlanto-dens interval is less than 3.5 mm on both flexion and extension radiographs, then it is determined that there is no C1-2 instability. Provided the fractures have healed and also provided that there is no C1-2 insta-

bility after removal of the halo vest, the patient is started on isometric exercises and active range-of-motion exercises (Figure 1). If the atlanto-dens interval is more than 3.5 mm with movement present, then a posterior C1-2 fusion would be recommended. In most cases at this point, the C1 posterior laminar fracture (fractures) are healed and a standard posterior C1-2 fusion would then be performed.

For those patients with Jefferson fractures in whom the halo vest is contraindicated, surgery can be performed in the acute stage. McGuire and Harkey[8] describe reducing the C1 fractures with traction and placing C1-2 transarticular screws to hold the lateral masses reduced. They would also perform an onlay bone graft posteriorly from C1 to C2 and supplement this with a C1-2 joint fusion bilaterally. Another early surgical option would be to immediately perform a posterior occiput to C2 fusion, but the disadvantage is that the patient would lose 50% of rotational and 50% of flexion-extension movement.

Some authors have described initial treatment of significantly displaced Jefferson fractures with traction and later application of a halo vest.[7] Because the length of time in traction may be as long as 3 to 5 weeks, this technique is not popular.

There is a subgroup of patients with "stable" Jefferson fractures in whom the total overhang from side to side is less than 6.9 mm, implying that the transverse ligament is intact. A review by Lee and associates[9] showed that the average amount of overhang was 1.8 mm with a range of zero to 7 mm. These patients were treated in a rigid cervical collar for 10 to 12 weeks and no instability was noted in any of the 12 patients.

For those patients with united Jefferson fractures, treatment is based on the degree of instability and pain. In the study by Segal and associates,[6] there were nonunions in 3 of 18 patients, and 2 of the 3 patients with nonunions had significant pain. Symptomatic patients were treated with posterior fusion, which resulted in resolution of their symptoms.

A recent report[10] describes patients with Jefferson fractures having injuries to C9-12 and significant problems with dysphagia. It is likely that these cranial nerves were injured as they left the base of the skull at the time of the original displacement of the bone. This situation should be kept in mind during early evaluation and treatment of these patients.

A completely different fracture involving the atlas is the isolated posterior C1 arch fracture. This injury is thought to be the result of hyperextension with the posterior arch of C1 abutting against the occiput. This is a stable injury, and a soft collar for comfort is adequate treatment.[7]

Hangman's Fracture of the Pedicles of C2

A useful classification system for these injuries divides them into type I, minimally displaced fractures of the pedicles with less than 3 mm of translation and little or no angulation of C2 in relation to the adjacent cervical spine; type II, displacement of 3.0 mm or more and a significant angulation (usually more than 11°); type IIa, more severe injury of the C2-3 disk and instability in traction; and type III, associated facet dislocation at C2-3 in addition to the C2 pedicle fractures.

The majority of these injuries will heal with immobilization (Fig-

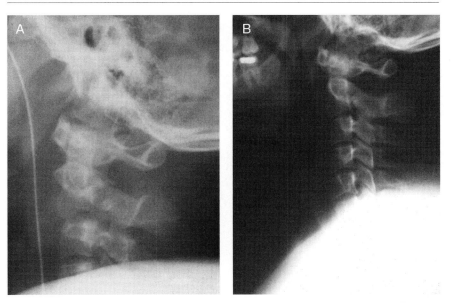

Figure 2 C2 hangman's fracture that occurred after a motor vehicle accident. There is minimal displacement and minimal angulation (type 1 injury). The patient was treated in a rigid collar for 8 weeks. **A,** Radiograph immediately after injury. **B,** Radiograph taken 6 months after injury showing complete healing and stability.

ure 2). Type I injuries are treated with a rigid cervical collar. Type II and IIa injuries are all treated with halo vest immobilization. For patients with type IIa injuries, it is very important that initial treatment with traction is contraindicated because the anterior longitudinal ligament is disrupted and severe overdistraction may result, which could be neurologically perilous for the patient. Type III fractures have to be treated surgically to reduce the C2-3 facet dislocation and, because this is a strictly ligamentous injury at this level, it should be accompanied by a posterior C2-3 fusion. The C2 pedicle fractures can then be treated the same as any other type II hangman's fracture by using a halo vest or pedicle screws to reattach the posterior elements of C2 to the anterior elements. If C2 pedicle screws are to be considered, it is extremely important to determine the exact course of the vertebral arteries using a combination of CT scans and CT recon-

structions. Magnetic resonance arteriography can also be used to evaluate the status of the vertebral arteries. If one vertebral artery is occluded, a screw on that side would not be contraindicated. A screw on the opposite side would be contraindicated because occlusion of both vertebral arteries would likely be fatal.

In a review of 123 patients with hangman's fractures, union was obtained in 116 of 123 patients. In those patients who had symptomatic nonunions, an anterior C2-3 fusion was performed with good final results.[11]

Atypical fracture patterns can occur with any of these types of hangman's fractures. These are so termed because the fracture is not limited to the pedicle but rather a portion of the posterior vertebral body breaks off and remains attached to the lamina and pedicle on that side.[12] In contrast to most of the hangman's fractures, which enlarge the spinal canal, the spinal canal in these atypical cases does not enlarge. If there is significant displacement and if the patient has a congenitally small spinal canal at the C2 level, then the patient is at greater risk for paralysis than those patients who have only the standard hangman's fracture. This atypical hangman's fracture occurs most commonly in patients with type II and IIa injuries. The standard treatment of these patients would be halo vest immobilization.

When evaluating whether hangman's fractures have adequately healed, the fracture line at the pedicle very often remains persistent. Healing is confirmed when there is no abnormal motion of C2 on C3 on flexion-extension radiographs and the posterior elements of C2 move in a normal fashion with the anterior elements of C2.

Occipitocervical Instability
Although these injuries are relatively uncommon in the hospital, they are found in approximately 6% of patients fatally injured in motor vehicle accidents.[13-15] These patients rarely survive the initial injury; however, there are reviews describing the clinical course in the survivors.[16,17] If the patient has any degree of movement in the arms or legs following this injury, there is a significant potential for having improved neurologic function. At this level of injury at the pyramidal decussation, it is also possible to have Bell's cruciate paralysis, which involves weakness of one arm and the contralateral leg. It is also possible to have involvement of both arms with relative sparing of the legs, or involvement of both legs with relative sparing of the arms.[18] When the arms are more affected than the legs, the condition can be initially mistaken for a central cord syndrome.

Radiographic findings in these patients will almost always reveal a very large degree of soft-tissue swelling, often 20 or 30 mm of swelling in front of C3. The best guide for isolating the injury to the occipitocervical junction is an abnormality in Wackenheim's line. Normally, this line should come from the posterior aspect of the sela turcica and proceed down through the basion and be tangential to the posterior aspect of the odontoid. If the patient has been placed in traction, then overdistraction at occiput C1 may be seen. The normal distance from the basion to the tip of the odontoid should be 5 mm or less. The use of Power's ratio,[19] which measures the distance from the anterior arch of C1 to the opisthion and the distance from the basion to the posterior arch of C1, is helpful; the ratio should equal 1. If the ratio is less than 1, there is anterior subluxation of the head on the cervical spine. It is not generally stated as such, but if it is significantly greater than 1, then this also means that there is a disturbance in the occiput to C1 relationship and that there may be a posterior occipitocervical dislocation. A third type of occipitocervical instability shows that the occiput is still directly above the cervical spine, but occipitocervical distraction is present.[20]

These patients should be placed in a halo vest as soon as their injury is recognized. Traction in these patients is dangerous and can cause significant occipitocervical distraction. A posterior occipitocervical fusion should be performed as soon as the patient is medically stable. Very often these patients will also have associated bony and ligamentous injuries of C1 and C2 and a fusion to C2 is usually necessary[21] (Figure 3).

Anderson and Montesano[22] have classified patients with occipital condyle fractures into three groups. Type 1 patients have impacted occipital condyle fractures that are stable. Type 2 patients have a basilar skull fracture and occipital condyle fracture that is stable. Type 3 patients have associated avulsion of the alar ligaments and are likely unstable. Type 3 patients will require the same type of treatment as described previously for occipitocervical instability.

Odontoid Fractures
Odontoid fractures were originally classified by Anderson and D'Alonzo.[23] Type I involves a small avulsion chip off the superior lateral aspect of the odontoid. Type II involves a fracture of the odontoid at the odontoid neck. Type III involves a fracture extending down into the body of C2. Type I fractures have traditionally been regarded as benign, but the chance that this could be a component of a significant occipitocervical dislocation must be recognized. Because the type II fracture occurs at the neck of the odontoid, the fracture involves a greater than normal proportion of cortical bone to cancellous bone and the cross-sectional area is small. Because of this combination of small appositional fracture surface as well as a greater proportion of cortical compared with cancellous bone, these particular fractures are less likely to heal despite appropriate immobilization. Type III fractures, because they extend into the body of C2, involve a significantly greater proportion of cancellous bone. In addition, the cross-sectional surface area is significantly greater. Because of those factors, healing of a type III odontoid fracture is more likely than that of a type II odontoid fracture.

Prospective evaluation of 144 patients has shown that 68% of patients with type II fractures heal with halo vest immobilization and that 81% of patients with type III odontoid fractures heal with halo immobilization. Ninety-six percent of type II fractures healed with posterior fusion using bone grafts and wires.[24]

Other factors that predispose to nonunion include those fractures displaced 4 mm or more, patient age of 40 years or older, those fractures that involve a posterior displacement of the odontoid in relationship to the body of C2,[25] and patients with a history of tobacco use.

The effectiveness of treating type II "stable" odontoid fractures in a collar was evaluated; 47% of these patients developed nonunion in contrast to 26% who developed nonunion after being treated in a halo vest.[26]

The decision for surgery versus halo vest treatment should be made on an individual basis after discussing the options with the patient. Those patients with type II odontoid fractures and extra risk factors for nonunion should be counselled that the chance of having a nonunion is greater than 33%. On the other hand, those patients who have a nondisplaced fracture, especially a type III fracture in a young patient, would have a very good chance of healing in a halo vest alone.

In patients with odontoid fractures, the attending physician should always be aware of acute respiratory compromise. In a recent study, 13 of 32 posteriorly displaced odontoid fractures were found to develop significant respiratory compromise, whereas only 3 of 123 other C2 fractures developed respiratory compromise.[27]

Surgery is indicated in those patients who specifically prefer surgery, in those patients who have a very high risk of nonunion, and in those patients who cannot be re-

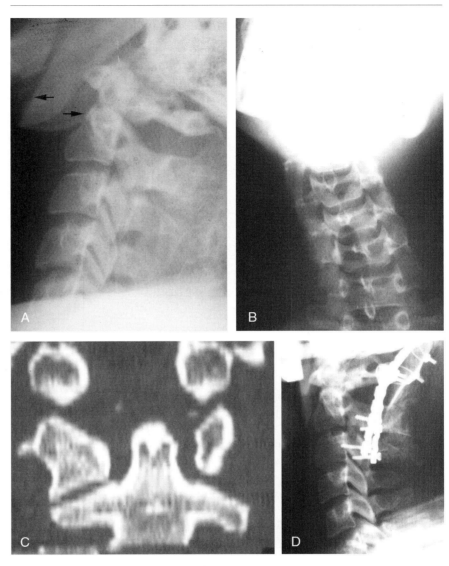

Figure 3 Radiographs and CT of a patient who was involved in a motor vehicle accident and who reported severe upper neck pain. **A,** Lateral radiograph showing severe prevertebral soft-tissue swelling (*arrows*). **B,** AP radiograph showing a severe deformity of the upper cervical spine. **C,** CT scan showing the asymmetry of the occipito-cervical articulations and the wide gap that exists in this joint. **D,** After immediate immobilization in a halo vest and occipito-cervical fusion with plates, screws, cables, and autogenous bone graft (C1-2 transarticular screws could not be used because of vertebral artery anomalies), complete healing and normal neurologic function were achieved. (Reproduced with permission from Eismont FJ, Frazier DD: Craniocervical trauma, in Levine AM, Eismont FJ, Garfin SR, Zigler JE (eds): *Spine Trauma*. Philadelphia, PA, WB Saunders, 1998, pp 205-206.)

duced in a halo vest (Figure 4). The next decision is to determine the type of surgery.

For the technique of posterior fusion using autogenous bone graft combined with wires, Brooks and Jenkins[28] described a 6.6% nonunion rate. A more current method of fixation would involve use of cables instead of solid wires for this procedure.

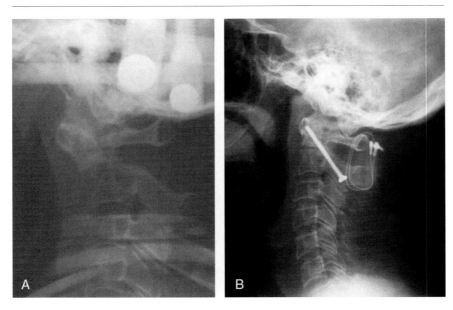

Figure 4 Radiographs of a patient who was involved in a motor vehicle accident and who sustained multiple trauma and a type II odontoid fracture. **A,** Lateral radiograph in halo vest shows the best reduction that was possible with initial traction followed by manipulation in a halo vest. **B,** Postoperative radiograph. Reduction was performed under general anesthesia. Fixation included one C1-2 transarticular screw and two sublaminar cables and posterior bone graft. The second transarticular screw could not be used because of vertebral artery location. Postoperatively the patient's halo vest was removed and treatment was with a rigid cervical collar. At 6 months, the patient had complete healing and no neck symptoms, with a normal neurologic status.

The advantage of this technique is that the risk is relatively low and the results are good. This is less acceptable for those patients who have a posteriorly displaced odontoid fracture because, as the posterior cables are tightened, further posterior displacement of the odontoid will often occur.

Indications for posterior C1-2 transarticular screws include those patients who have a type II odontoid fracture that is posteriorly displaced as discussed previously, those patients who have a type II odontoid fracture and a fracture of the C1 posterior arch, and those patients who have previously had a nonunion of a Brooks C1-2 fusion. Prior to performing any C1-2 transarticular fusion, appropriate reconstructed CT scans must be used to

ensure that the course of the vertebral artery is such that screws can be placed from posterior through the pedicles of C2 and into the lateral masses of C1 without endangering the vertebral arteries. In most series, it has been found that 15% of patients have a vertebral artery course, which prevents safe placement of bilateral C1-2 transarticular screws. In a European series of 161 patients with a follow-up of 24 months, the fusion rate using C1-2 transarticular screws was 99.4% and there were no vertebral artery injuries. In addition, 5.9% of patients had screw complications, many of whom required revision surgery for screw removal or revision.[29] Even though there were no vertebral artery injuries in this series, there have been other instances of patients dying during or

immediately following this procedure. If there is any difficulty with placing one C1-2 transarticular screw in terms of any aberrant bleeding, then no attempt should be made to place a second C1-2 transarticular screw. It has also been shown that C1-2 transarticular screws, as they penetrate the anterior aspect of C1, may endanger the internal carotid artery that lies directly anterior to the lateral mass of C1. In most cases, it is located in the midportion of the lateral mass. This can be seen preoperatively on a CT scan with contrast.[30]

The third surgical option is placement of an anterior odontoid screw. This is ideal in patients with good bone who can be completely reduced. It is also important to use biplanar fluoroscopy during the procedure. Preservation of C1-2 motion is a consideration, but thorough evaluation has shown that, even in patients with anterior odontoid screws, there is often a marked reduction in C1-2 rotation on final follow-up evaluation.[31]

Contraindications for anterior odontoid screw fixation include those patients with an anteriorly displaced odontoid, osteopenia (all elderly patients), a barrel chest (in whom anatomy prevents proper angulation of the drill and screw), and nonunion of an old odontoid fracture. In a series of 46 patients treated with anterior odontoid screw fixation (36 type II odontoid fractures), there were three patients with nonunions, two patients with malunions, and one patient with a misplaced screw requiring revision. This represents a 13% failure rate.[32] Another series of 18 patients (all type II odontoid fractures) shows that 3 patients (17%) developed nonunions and required revisions.[33]

Lower Cervical Spine Injuries (C3 to T1)

When evaluating lower cervical spine injuries, the Allen-Ferguson classification determines the mechanism of injury.[34] Fractures are divided into the vertical compression category, which has three subtypes; the compressive-flexion category, which has five subtypes; the distractive-flexion category, which has four subtypes; and compressive extension, distractive extension, and lateral flexion categories. The first three mechanisms are by far the most commonly seen in subaxial cervical injuries, and each of these three will be discussed in detail.

Vertical Compression Injuries

The subaxial burst fracture occurs as a result of vertical compressive forces, which cause a comminuted vertebral body fracture that may be associated with retropulsion of bone into the spinal canal. Vertical compression injuries can be divided into three stages. Stage 1 is a fracture of the superior or inferior end plate with a cupping deformity of the vertebral body and no ligament failure (Figure 5). Stage 2 is a fracture of both end plates with cupping deformity and minimal posterior displacement. Stage 3 is described as a stage 2 injury with fragmentation and significant posterior displacement of the vertebral body into the spinal canal.

Subaxial burst fractures can be treated nonsurgically or surgically.[35] Nonsurgical treatment should be considered if patients are neurologically intact, have no posterior element structural damage, and have normal sagittal alignment. A cervical orthosis or halo immobilization can be used to maintain stability. In patients with a neurologic deficit, posterior bone or soft-tissue instability, or significant kyphosis, surgical treatment is consid-

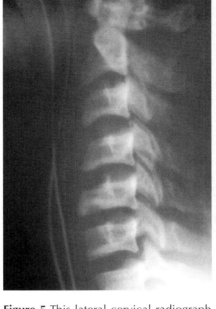

Figure 5 This lateral cervical radiograph reveals the loss of C5 vertebral height associated with vertical compression injuries.

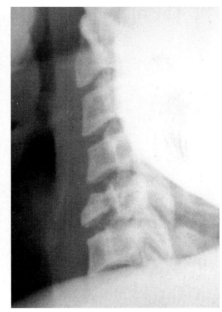

Figure 6 The severe fragmentation noted in this lateral radiograph indicates the loss of axial support from the anterior column with resulting vertebral instability in the compression and flexion type of injury.

ered to be the best treatment. The use of Gardner-Wells tongs to reduce the fracture initially can result in realignment and indirect decompression of the canal through ligamentotaxis.[36] Surgical intervention allows decompression of the neural elements and spinal stabilization, allowing early mobilization of the patient. Anterior corpectomy and fusion with instrumentation, and posterior decompression and fusion with instrumentation are treatment options. It is quite uncommon for patients with a true vertical compression injury to require both anterior and posterior procedures. In patients with an unstable spine and anterior spinal cord compression, posterior wiring and fusion alone is not an acceptable option.

Compressive-Flexion (Flexion-Axial Load) Injuries

This "teardrop fracture" is the result of flexion and axial load forces (Figure 6). Stage 1 is described as a

blunting of the anterior and superior margin, causing a rounded contour of the vertebral body with intact ligaments. Stage 2 is identified as obliquity and height loss of the anterior vertebral body. Stage 3 is an oblique fracture through the anterior vertebral body. Stage 4 progresses to mild displacement (3 mm or less) of the inferior and posterior vertebral body into the canal. Stage 5 is the oblique fracture through the vertebral body with significant displacement of the inferior and posterior vertebral body into the spinal canal posteriorly (more than 3 mm) and with ligamentous disruption posteriorly.[34] In addition, stages 4 and 5 will also usually have a midsagittal vertebral body fracture, which is clearly seen on CT scan (Figure 7). Schneider and Kahn[37] originally described this fracture and its association with the anterior cord syn-

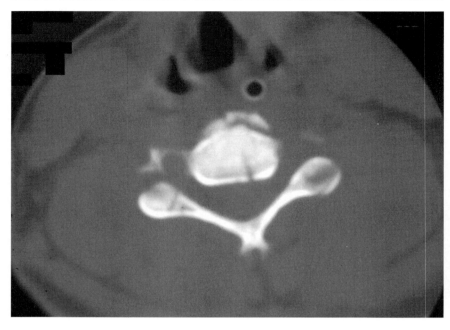

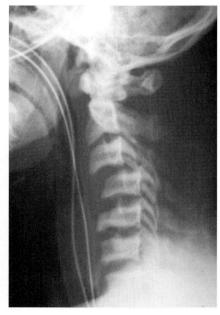

Figure 7 This CT scan reveals the fracture in the sagittal plane of the vertebral body that is usually seen with severe stage 4 and stage 5 flexion-axial load injuries to the spine.

Figure 8 This lateral cervical radiograph reveals bilateral facet dislocation as a result of complete soft-tissue disruption posteriorly and illustrates the significant canal compromise these injuries produce.

drome resulting in loss of motor and sensory function distal to the injury, but sparing the dorsal column of the spinal cord with its proprioception and deep pressure sensation. Nonsurgical treatment can be considered in the compressive flexion injuries stages 1 through 3 if there is less than 11° of angulation and no neural deficit. A rigid cervical orthosis or halo should be used in the treatment of these patients.

When considering surgical treatment of this injury, if the posterior elements are disrupted, lateral mass plates and screws can be used to provide stability for the posterior structures. For stages 4 and 5 with retropulsion of bone into the spinal canal, anterior corpectomy with reconstruction of the vertebral body and anterior plate stabilization should be considered. Fisher and associates[38] compared halo treatment to anterior decompression and plate stabilization in 45 patients, with 24 being

treated in a halo and 21 being treated surgically; clinical outcomes were similar. However, those patients treated with a halo developed 11.4° of kyphosis, whereas those treated with internal fixation only developed 3.5° of kyphosis. There were five failures with the halo treatment with four patients requiring surgery.

Distractive-Flexion Injuries

This group of subaxial cervical injuries consists of fractures and soft-tissue injuries to the posterior column of the spine.[39,40] These injuries occur as a disruption of the spinal integrity caused by flexion and distraction forces (Figure 8). Stage 1 is a failure of the posterior ligamentous complex. Stage 2 is a unilateral facet dislocation with 25% subluxation. Stage 3 is a bilateral facet dislocation with 50% subluxation. Stage 4 is a full vertebral body dislocation. The most common levels of involvement are C5-6 and C6-7. These injuries

can be further subdivided into soft-tissue injuries only and those involving combinations of fractures and soft-tissue injuries.[34]

Diagnosis of the type and stage of injury can usually be made on the initial plain radiographs. Primary attention should be given to assessment of facet position and the degree of subluxation on the lateral radiograph. The bony injury and alignment can best be assessed with CT sagittal reconstruction, which will clearly define fractures (including facet fractures) and document facet subluxation or dislocation. MRI is especially useful for assessing injuries of the posterior ligaments such as tears of the interspinous ligament and ligamentum flavum. MRI can also assess the degree of injury to the intervertebral disk, which occurs in up to 70% of patients with facet dislocations[3] (Figure 9).

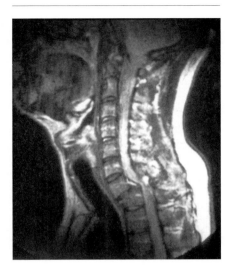

Figure 9 This MRI scan provides excellent detail of the soft tissues in cervical spine injuries. In this particular case, disk material is noted posterior to the C7 vertebral body.

Patients with distractive-flexion injuries can also have associated facet fractures. Although both superior and inferior facet fractures may occur, the most common is a fracture of the superior facet alone. CT is the best test to diagnose this injury. It is important to understand that the facet capsules may be intact in these bony facet injuries. Unilateral facet fractures most commonly occur as a result of flexion and rotation. Lateral mass fracture separation injuries can also occur as a result of unilateral pedicle and laminar fractures, resulting in complete dissociation of the lateral mass and gross instability.

Neurologic deficit in these injuries is highly dependent on the spinal canal size.[41] Patients with spinal canal diameters greater than 17 mm have a better prognosis than those with canal diameters less than 17 mm. Stage 3 and 4 injuries have more potential for spinal cord injury because of increased spinal canal narrowing.

The timing of obtaining the MRI scan is controversial in patients with facet dislocation. One recommendation is that those patients who are awake, alert, and cooperative with evidence of facet dislocation on plain radiographs may undergo reduction immediately using tongs and traction. If the patient's neurologic status changes during the reduction maneuver, the procedure should be halted and an MRI scan obtained at that time. Vaccaro and associates[3] found postreduction disk material to be present in 50% of those individuals who had undergone reduction while awake, and they found no change in the neurologic status of these patients during or following the reduction. If the patient is obtunded or noncooperative, consideration should be given to performing MRI before reduction is attempted. Another recommendation is to perform MRI before attempting reduction in patients who are neurologically normal or nearly normal, and to perform reduction before MRI scan in those patients with American Spinal Injury Association (ASIA) A, B, or C level of paralysis.[42]

Definitive surgical treatment in individuals with ligamentous injury should be designed to reestablish spinal stability and allow rapid mobilization. If the posterior bony elements are intact, the triple wire technique provides excellent stability. If the posterior bony elements are fractured, the use of lateral mass plates and screws can be used. A third recommendation is that if an anterior disk herniation is present, an awake controlled reduction should be performed if possible. If this is not possible, then an anterior cervical diskectomy should be performed, followed by reduction of the subluxation and stabilization of the anterior column with bone grafting and cervical plating. The use of bracing and halos alone in patients with ligamentous disruption often fails because the soft tissues do not heal sufficiently to provide adequate restraint and further subluxation often occurs. Fractures of the facet joints are also often difficult to immobilize with bracing and halos even after adequate initial reduction, and surgery should be considered for those patients with a neural deficit or progressive loss of reduction.

Spinal Cord Injuries
More than 10,000 new spinal cord injuries occur each year in the United States.[43] The lifetime direct medical cost per patient ranges between $326,000 and $1.3 million and the direct national cost is more than $7 billion per year.[44,45] The financial impact is staggering if loss of income and productivity are added, but the greatest toll cannot be measured in dollars and cents. Most spinal cord injuries affect young, active adults and have a devastating impact on the patient, the family, and society in general. Current treatment strategies and an overview of promising research programs designed to reverse paralysis are discussed.

Pathophysiology
The rationale for different treatment regimens is based on the pathophysiology of spinal cord injury. There are two interrelated phases of functional changes that accompany a spinal cord injury.[46,47] The primary injury results from the initial contusion and compression of the cord, which damages neuronal cells, axonal membranes, and blood vessels. The primary injury initiates an autodestructive biochemical cascade called the secondary injury. This phase, lasting hours to days, causes the zone of injury to expand.

Several different mechanisms have

been postulated to explain secondary injury, and these events probably work in synergy.[46-48] Vascular events occurring at the time of injury include reduced blood flow, loss of autoregulation, neurogenic shock, hemorrhage into the cord, loss of microcirculation, vasospasm, and thrombosis. Electrolyte shifts include increased intracellular calcium, increased extracellular potassium, and increased sodium permeability. Neurotransmitters accumulate, including extracellular glutamate, which can lead to excitotoxic cell injury. Additional mechanisms include release of arachidonic acid and endogenous opioids, free radical formation, lipid peroxidation, inflammation leading to edema, and loss of energy metabolism. All of these events lead to secondary cell death from either normal cell necrosis or apoptosis (programmed cell death).[49] The loss of neuronal and glial cells leads to cavitation or cyst formation within the substance of the cord, causing the familiar changes seen on MRI (Figure 10). The injury disrupts the normal anatomy and physiology of the cord.

The main components of normal gray matter include neuronal cell bodies and the supporting glial cells including astrocytes, oligodendrocytes, and microglial cells (Figure 11). The white matter is primarily composed of axons, traveling up and down the cord, wrapped in white insulating myelin (Figure 11). The myelinating cells in the central nervous system (CNS) are oligodendrocytes, which have important distinctions from the Schwann's cells that myelinate axons in the peripheral nervous system.

The injury severs some axons and renders others useless by destroying their myelin sheaths. Typically, the distal portion of a severed axon de-

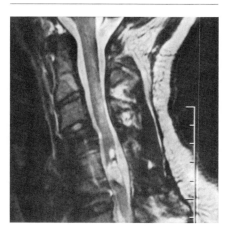

Figure 10 Sagittal MRI scan of the cervical spine of a 23-year-old patient with complete tetraplegia sustained 5 years earlier shows a cavitary defect in the spinal cord at the C5-6 levels. The patient underwent an anterior and posterior C4-6 decompression and fusion shortly after injury. The MRI appearance of the cyst has been stable for 4 years.

generates and the proximal portion develops growth cones. Normally, sprouts extend only about 1 mm before their growth is aborted and the sprouts are resorbed. Some axons may escape injury altogether and, depending on their numbers, may permit some useful function.

At the edge of the injury area, activated astrocytes proliferate and encapsulate the lesion, leading to a glial scar[50] (Figure 12). The scar inhibits the regrowth of CNS axons, and it is one of the primary targets of regeneration strategies. The scar is a physical barrier blocking the advancement of the growth cone, and it is also a chemical inhibitor of axonal outgrowth.

Neuroprotective Strategies

Knowledge of the pathophysiology of acute spinal cord injury has led to numerous approaches designed to lessen the deleterious effects of the secondary injury cascade. The well-publicized effects of methylpred-

nisolone are discussed in a later section. Other agents that have been shown to be effective in experimental spinal cord injury models include opiate receptor blockers including naloxone and nalmefine, thyrotropin-releasing hormone and excitatory neurotransmitter receptor blockers including blockers of the N-methyl-D-aspartate subtype of glutamate receptors.[51]

Spinal cord cooling has shown promise in the treatment of spinal cord injuries but logistical problems have limited enthusiasm for the modality.[52,53] Spinal cord injury research is advancing rapidly, and new strategies will undoubtedly emerge in the near future.

Regeneration

CNS regeneration does not occur following injury in mammals because of the lack of conducive environment in the CNS and the limited regenerative capacity of the neurons.[54] Experimental regeneration in the CNS was first described in 1908.[54,55] Pioneering studies in the early 1980s renewed interest in the field when it was demonstrated that regeneration was possible using peripheral nerve grafts as bridges.[56-58]

Barriers to Regeneration

The native environment in the CNS prohibits axonal regeneration. This phenomenon was demonstrated in landmark studies, and it has been shown that by using an antibody against myelin-associated inhibitors of neurite growth a degree of axonal regeneration could be achieved.[59,60] Recently, a gene has been identified that encodes proteins that inhibit neurite outgrowth.[61,62] The gene, *Nogo*, has been found to be oligodendrocyte-specific, and therefore absent from the Schwann cells

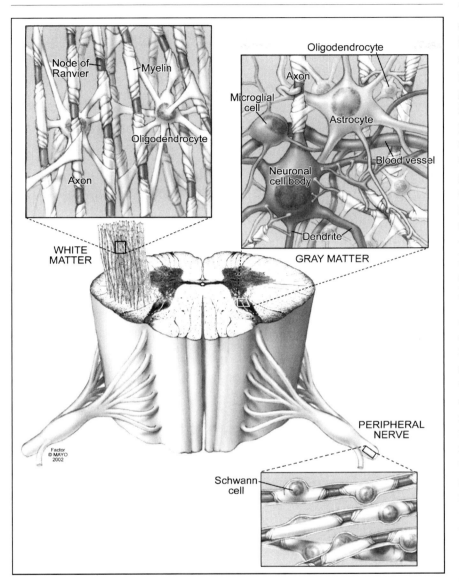

Figure 11 Normal anatomy of the spinal cord. The main components of gray matter consist of neuronal cell bodies and the supporting glial cells including astrocytes, oligodendrocytes, and microglial cells (inset). The white matter is composed of myelinated axons that form ascending and descending tracts (inset). The myelinating cells in the CNS are oligodendrocytes. Schwann cells myelinate axons in the peripheral nervous system (inset). (Reproduced with permission from the Mayo Foundation, Rochester, MN.)

that produce myelin in the peripheral nervous system.[63]

In addition to the properties of myelin, other barriers to regeneration include the glial scar that forms when inhibitory astrocytes and oligodendrocytes migrate into the lesion site.[50] The CNS also lacks the Schwann cells that help guide and stimulate regenerating axons in the peripheral nervous system.[64,65]

CNS neurons have a limited intrinsic capacity to regenerate, determined, in part, by the response of the neuron's cell body. Numerous "regeneration-associated genes" are expressed in response to an axonal injury.[66] A classic study by Richardson and Issa[67] demonstrated that the regenerative capacity of a neuron is greatly influenced by inducible events in the nerve cell. They showed that proximal regeneration of primary sensory neurons into peripheral nerve transplants was 100 times greater when the peripheral nerve axons were also cut. Schreyer and Skene[68] later demonstrated that cutting the peripheral axon leads to upregulation of GAP-43 expression. Induction of GAP-43, a growth cone signaling protein, did not occur following isolated dorsal root lesions.

Experimental Regeneration Strategies

Several events are required to allow axonal regeneration in the CNS.[54,69,70] After the damaged axons sprout, neurotrophic factors are necessary to support their survival; inhibitory molecules, including the myelin and myelin-associated proteins, must be neutralized. The sprouts must cross the zone of injury including the physical and chemical barrier of the glial scar. Once they find their targets, the axons must stop growing and produce a synapse at the right spot. Finally, once they are reconnected, they must be myelinated and morphologically normal to transmit nerve signals. A comprehensive review of regeneration research is beyond the scope of this chapter and only the primary strategies are highlighted here (Figure 13).

Neurotrophic factors have widespread effects including upregulation of regeneration-associated genes and prevention of cell loss and atrophy of neuronal cell bodies after injury.[71,72] Their effectiveness depends on the specific factor administered as well as the timing and site

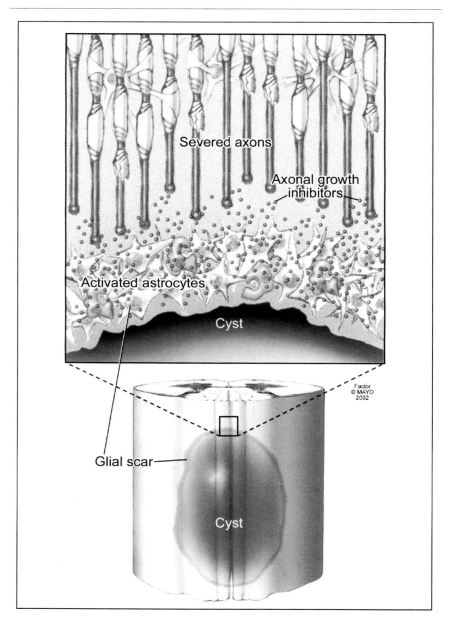

Severed axons

Axonal growth inhibitors

Activated astrocytes

Cyst

Factor
© MAYO
2002

Glial scar

Cyst

Figure 12 Posttraumatic spinal cord cyst. Cavitary defects or cysts result from disruption and loss of neuronal and glial cells. Activated astrocytes proliferate at the edge of the cavitary defect, encapsulating the lesion to form a glial scar (inset). The scar physically blocks the advancement of growth cones and chemically inhibits axonal outgrowth. (Reproduced with permission from the Mayo Foundation, Rochester, MN.)

of application. Gene therapy and tissue engineering techniques are being used to deliver neurotrophic factors in a more sophisticated manner than by simple injection.[73-76]

Strategies to bridge the cavitary defect and overcome the nonpermissive environment have shown promise. Peripheral nerve bridges have been somewhat successful, presumably because they contain Schwann cells to provide guidance channels and produce neurotrophic factors.[77] Fetal CNS tissue transplants have been attemped because fetal cells lack inhibitory myelin-associated molecules and they may provide some intraspinal neurons as relays.[78] Transplants of olfactory ensheathing cells have also shown promise.[79,80] These are specialized CNS glial cells that help support and guide axons from the olfactory mucosa into the olfactory bulbs throughout life. It is postulated that these cells might help axons recognize and grow into their appropriate reentry targets. Tissue engineering strategies involving Schwann cell-seeded guidance channels have been shown to allow some growth of axons through the channel and into the host cord.[81]

In addition to bridging the cavitary defect, some investigators have attempted to removal the glial scar[82] or degrade the inhibitory proteoglycans secreted by the glial cells.[83] The reactive glial cells can also be destroyed by radiation therapy administered during a critical time window after injury.[84]

Attempts at overcoming the inhibitory effects of myelin ignited the recent explosion in spinal cord injury research and is still a cornerstone regeneration strategy.[59-63] Myelin appears to contain numerous inhibitors, and rather than block isolated molecules, it may be more effective to immunologically target the entire myelin sheath.[54,85,86]

Manipulating the guidance of axonal growth cones recently has shown encouraging results. Slit protein,[87] the Rho signaling pathway,[88] and cyclic nucleotides[89] have all been targeted as mediators of axonal growth. Reversal of paralysis will undoubtedly involve multimodality therapy starting with neural protection to prevent secondary injury and followed by a variety of strategies to facilitate regeneration.

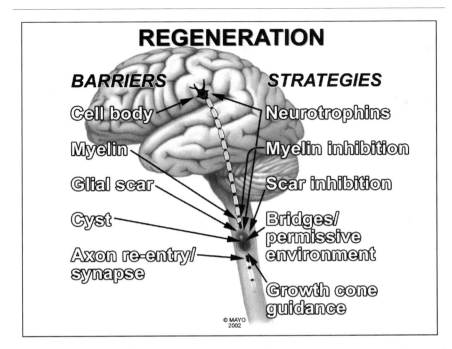

REGENERATION

BARRIERS
Cell body
Myelin
Glial scar
Cyst
Axon re-entry/ synapse

STRATEGIES
Neurotrophins
Myelin inhibition
Scar inhibition
Bridges/ permissive environment
Growth cone guidance

© MAYO 2002

Figure 13 The primary barriers to regeneration in the CNS and current strategies used to overcome them. (Reproduced with permission from the Mayo Foundation, Rochester, MN.)

Current Strategies to Reverse Paralysis

Urgent Surgical Decompression Persistent compression of the cord is a potentially reversible form of secondary injury. Several animal studies have shown a beneficial effect of early decompressive surgery, but there have been no randomized prospective clinical studies to evaluate the effect of surgery in humans.[47,90] Current clinical studies have provided conflicting data, some showing no benefit from early surgery[91-93] and others showing a positive effect.[47,94,95] One area of conflict with these clinical studies is the definition of early surgery. In some studies, early surgery means a decompression in less than 8 hours after injury, whereas in others it means decompression in less than 72 hours.

Considering all the events that occur during the secondary injury cascade, it is likely that the faster the spinal cord can be decompressed, the greater the neurologic benefit. Many surgeons have been reluctant to operate urgently, however, because of a study that showed neurologic deterioration with early surgery.[96] A more recent study, however, showed no increased morbidity or mortality from early surgery.[95] In a recent review of the literature, all pertinent articles were classified based on the quality of the study and the data presented.[97] It was concluded that there are no standards regarding the role and the timing of decompression in acute spinal cord injury. On the basis of prospective, nonrandomized (class 2) studies, early surgery within 24 hours was deemed to be safe. Numerous case series or retrospective (class 3) studies indicate that there are data to support urgent reduction of bilateral locked facets in patients with incomplete tetraplegia. Furthermore, there are limited data to support urgent decompression for

patients with spinal cord injury who are neurologically deteriorating.[47,87]

Pharmacologic Treatment The most widely studied pharmacologic agent for reversing paralysis is methylprednisolone sodium succinate (MPSS). There are compelling animal data[98-102] and several well-designed clinical trials[103,104] that support, to some degree, the use of MPSS to treat spinal cord injury.[105]

The results of the second National Acute Spinal Cord Injury Study (NASCIS II) were reported more than a decade ago and are still the focus of intense scrutiny.[103,105-107] The study concluded that paraplegic patients given MPSS within 8 hours of injury recovered 21% of lost motor function compared with 8% in controls. Paretic patients recovered 75% compared with 59% in controls. Sensory improvement was found to be similar to motor improvement. There was no improvement if MPSS or naloxone was administered more than 8 hours after injury, and naloxone given within 3 hours showed a trend for improvement in motor and sensory recovery. Although most clinicians follow its recommendations, NASCIS II has been widely criticized.[105,106] The overall analysis of the primary outcomes in 487 patients was negative. The only positive effect was seen in a post-hoc analysis of 193 patients who received the treatment within 8 hours. The effect sizes were small, and the functional importance of the changes was questionable. Finally, there is concern regarding the effects of MPSS on wound healing and sepsis.

MPSS is an antioxidant that inhibits lipid peroxidation by its action as a free radical scavenger. It also has potent anti-inflammatory and immunosuppressant effects.[51] The recommended dose of MPSS is 30 mg/kg followed by 5.4 mg/kg/h for 23 hours.[103] That dose is much greater than the dose required to activate glucocorticoid receptors, suggesting that its primary mechanism of action is as an antioxidant.

The third National Acute Spinal Cord Injury Study (NASCIS III) compared the standard 24-hour dose of MPSS with a very potent antioxidant, tirilazad mesylate given within 3 hours of injury.[104] The 48-hour course of MPSS was found to be better than a 24-hour regimen of MPSS or tirilazad mesylate if started 3 to 8 hours, after injury.[104,107] NASCIS III has also been the subject of criticism.[105,106] The study lacked a placebo group, and the overall analysis of the primary outcomes was negative. The effects were limited to post-hoc stratification between 0 to 3 hours and 3 to 8 hours, and there was only modest functional improvement. Concern has also been raised about the risk of increased sepsis and pneumonia with the 48-hour MPSS regimen.

According to a recent spinal focus panel led by Fehlings,[105] use of MPSS should not be a practice standard but rather a guideline. It was concluded that given the devastating impact of spinal cord injury and the evidence of a modest beneficial effect of MPSS, clinicians should consider using this drug despite the well-founded criticisms that have been directed against the NASCIS II and III studies.

There are several other anti-inflammatory and immunosuppressant agents that have been found to be useful in experimental spinal cord injury including naloxone, indocin, cycloheximide, immunosuppressants, and immunofilins.[51] Oddly, some proinflammatory agents may also be beneficial in treating spinal cord injury the most notable of which is monosialotetra-hexosylganglioside GM1 sodium salt (GM1) also known by its trade name, Sygen (Fidia Pharmaceutical Corporation, Washington, DC).

GM1 is a naturally-occurring compound in cell membranes of the CNS that has been found to be neuroprotective and to stimulate axonal growth.[51,108] Interestingly, it antagonizes the beneficial effect of MPSS if it is given shortly after injury.[109] It has been shown to improve recovery rate during the first 3 months after spinal cord injury but not the extent of recovery at 1 year. Geisler and associates[108,110,111] reported the results of a recent multicenter acute spinal cord injury study using GM1. This was a randomized, double-blind, multicenter trial involving 760 patients, comparing two doses of Sygen versus placebo. The primary end point, based on results of a pilot study, was the percentage of patients who experienced marked recovery at 26 weeks. The initial pilot study involved 37 patients and a significant drug effect was found in the proportion of patients able to improve by two Frankel grades (1 of 14 on placebo, 7 of 14 on Sygen). In the multicenter study, marked recovery was defined as "at least a two-grade equivalent improvement in the Modified Benzel Classification from the baseline ASIA impairment scale."[108,111]

The GM1 group did not have a significantly higher proportion of patients with marked recovery at week 26 and so the prospectively chosen primary efficacy analysis was negative. There appeared to be greater beneficial drug effect in the less severely injured patients, most noticeable in the group of patients who did not require surgery. These patients had a contusion but no persistent neural compression. Patients with a suspected central cord injury and those without radiographic evidence of fracture-dislocation showed an early benefit of GM1 but no significant difference at week 26 or at 1 year.

Outcomes
The prognosis for motor recovery after spinal cord injury is based on the severity of the neurologic deficit and the magnitude of recovery during the first week after the injury.[112] Spinal cord injuries is defined as complete when there is no motor or sensory function in the lowest sacral segment, whereas an incomplete injury is characterized by the presence of "sacral sparing."[113] According to ASIA guidelines, spinal cord injuries are classified in decreasing order of severity from A (complete paralysis) to E (normal).[113]

The neurologic level of injury is defined as the most caudal spinal cord segment with normal motor ($\geq 3/5$ muscle strength) and sensory function bilaterally. The motor level is the most caudal spinal cord segment with normal motor function ($\geq 3/5$ muscle strength) bilaterally.[113]

Expected Recovery
Complete Tetraplegia Most patients with complete tetraplegia can expect to eventually regain one motor level.[114,115] There is little chance for functional lower extremity recovery if the injury remains complete for more than 1 month.[115] The initial strength of a muscle is a good predictor of its rate of recovery and the likelihood of achieving antigravity strength. The faster a muscle with 0/5 strength begins to recover, the better its prognosis for recovery. Most upper extremity recovery occurs during the first 6 months, with the greatest rate of change occurring during the first 3 months. Most muscles with some initial power will plateau in their recovery at an earlier time than muscles with no motor

power. Motor recovery can continue into the second year, especially in muscles with initial 0/5 strength. The presence of sensation at the same level increases the chance of recovery of the muscle.

The likelihood that a muscle will recover to at least 3/5 strength 1 year after spinal cord injury is based on the initial examination. If the examination is performed within the first week, then approximately 50% of the muscles with 0/5 strength and almost all of the muscles with 1/5 and 2/5 strength will recover. If the examination is performed 1 month after the spinal cord injury, then recovery to 3/5 strength can be expected in greater than 95% of muscles with 1/5 or 2/5 strength, approximately 25% of the first 0/5 muscles, and 1% of second 0/5 muscles. Furthermore, recovery to 1/5 strength occurs in 50% to 60% of the first 0/5 muscles and less than 10% of second 0/5 muscles.

Sensory Incomplete Tetraplegia The prognosis for motor recovery is more favorable in sensory incomplete tetraplegia if pin sensation is spared than if light touch alone is spared (89% versus 11%). This is presumably because the motor (lateral corticospinal) tracts are close to the pain and temperature (lateral spinothalamic) tracts.[116]

Motor Incomplete Tetraplegia The prognosis for recovery in patients with motor incomplete tetraplegia is markedly better than for patients with complete injuries or those with sensory incomplete tetraplegia.[117] Between 52% and 76% of ASIA C (useless motor) patients recover to ASIA D (useful motor) or E (normal) compared with 20% to 28% of ASIA B (sensory incomplete) patients. Fifty-four percent of muscles that have 0/5 strength at the 1-month examination improve to at

least 1/5 strength and 20% improve to greater than 3/5 strength at 1 year. The majority of functional recovery occurs in the first 6 months and early return of strength is predictive of better functional outcome. Motor recovery occurs concurrently in the upper and lower extremities.

Complete Paraplegia The prognosis for patients with complete paraplegia is based on the neurologic level of injury.[118] When the neurologic level of injury is at T8 or above, no lower extremity motor recovery is expected. When the neurologic level of injury is at T9-11, 15% of patients regain 3/5 strength or greater in hip flexion or knee extension at 1 year. When the neurologic level of injury is at or below T12, 55% of patients recover lower extremity motor function.

Incomplete Paraplegia Patients with incomplete paraplegia have a reasonably good prognosis.[118] Eighty percent of patients regain 3/5 strength or greater in hip flexion and knee extension at 1 year. The greatest motor recovery occurs during the first 3 months, and sensory recovery plateaus 3 months after injury.

Occasionally, patients initially diagnosed with complete lesions convert to incomplete injuries.[119] Ditunno and associates[119] found that 11% of patients with complete loss of motor and sensory function (ASIA A) improve to at least ASIA B (sensory only), 2.9% improve to ASIA C (useless motor), and 2.9% improve to ASIA D (useful motor).

Motor, Functional Independence, Social Integration, and Quality of Life Outcomes
An excellent resource for information on outcomes after spinal cord injury is entitled "The Clinical Practice Guidelines for Health Care Pro-

fessionals." It was prepared by the Consortium for Spinal Cord Medicine and it is available from the Paralyzed Veterans of America.[120]

Summary
Appropriate treatment options for the most common cervical spine injuries and associated spinal cord injury have been described. Thanks to several landmark studies over the past 20 years, the outcomes of patients with spinal cord injury can now be predicted with reasonable accuracy.[121] It is hoped that in the near future, breakthroughs in spinal cord injury research will make current literature on outcomes obsolete.

References
1. McGuire RA, Degnam G, Amundson GM: Evaluation of current extrication orthoses in immbolization of the unstable cervical spine. *Spine* 1990;10:1064-1067.

2. McGuire RA: Physical examination in spinal trauma, in Levine AM, Eismont FJ, Garfin SR, Zigler JE (eds): *Spine Trauma*. Philadelphia, PA, WB Saunders, 1998, pp 16-27.

3. Vaccaro AR, Falatyn SP, Flanders AE, Balderston RA, Northrup BE, Cotler JM: Magnetic resonance evaluation of the intervertebral disc, spinal ligaments, and spinal cord before and after closed traction reduction of cervical spine dislocations. *Spine* 1999;24:1210-1217.

4. Halliday AL, Henderson BR, Hart BL, Benzel EC: The management of unilateral lateral mass/facet fractures of the subaxial cervical spine: The use of magnetic resonance imaging to predict instability. *Spine* 1997;22:2614-2621.

5. Spence KF Jr, Decker S, Sell KW: Bursting atlantal fracture associated with rupture of the transverse ligament. *J Bone Joint Surg Am* 1970;52:543-549.

6. Segal LS, Grimm JO, Stauffer ES: Non-union of fractures of the atlas. *J Bone Joint Surg Am* 1987;69:1423-1434.

7. Levine AM, Edwards CC: Fractures of the atlas. *J Bone Joint Surg Am* 1991;73:680-691.

8. McGuire RA Jr, Harkey HL: Primary treatment of unstable Jefferson's fractures. *J Spinal Disord* 1995;8:233-236.

9. Lee TT, Green BA, Petrin DR: Treatment of stable burst fracture of the atlas (Jefferson fracture) with rigid cervical collar. *Spine* 1998;23:1963-1967.

10. Connolly B, Turner C, DeVine J, Gerlinger T: Jefferson fracture resulting in Collet-Sicard Syndrome. *Spine* 2000;25:395-398.

11. Francis WR, Fielding JW, Hawkins RJ, Pepin J, Hensinger R: Traumatic spondylolisthesis of the axis. *J Bone Joint Surg Br* 1981;63:313-318.

12. Starr JK, Eismont FJ: Atypical hangman's fractures. *Spine* 1993;18:1954-1957.

13. Bucholz RW, Burkhead WZ, Graham W, Petty C: Occult cervical spine injuries in fatal traffic accidents. *J Trauma* 1979;19:768-771.

14. Davis D, Bohlman HH, Walker AE, et al: The pathological findings in fatal craniospinal injuries. *J Neurosurg* 1971;34:603-613.

15. Alker GJ, On YS, Leslie EV, Lehotay J, Panaro YA, Eschner EG: Postmortem radiology of head and neck injuries in fatal traffic accidents. *Radiology* 1975;114:611-617.

16. Montane I, Eismont FJ, Green BA: Traumatic occipitoatlantal dislocation. *Spine* 1991;16:112-116.

17. Eismont FJ, Bohlman HH: Posterior atlanto-occipital dislocation with fractures of the atlas and odontoid process. *J Bone Joint Surg Am* 1978;60:397-399.

18. Bell HS: Paralysis of both arms from injury of the upper portion of the pyramidal decussations: Cruciate paralysis. *J Neurosurg* 1970;33:376-380.

19. Powers B, Miller MD, Kramer RS, Martinez S, Gehweiler JA Jr: Traumatic anterior atlanto-occipital dislocation. *Neurosurgery* 1979;4:12-17.

20. Traynelis VC, Marano GD, Dunker RO, Kaufman HH: Traumatic atlanto-occipital dislocation: Case report. *J Neurosurg* 1986;65:863-870.

21. Werne S: Studies in spontaneous atlas dislocation. *Acta Orthop Scand Suppl* 1957;23:1-150.

22. Anderson PA, Montesano PX: Morphology and treatment of occipital condyle fractures. *Spine* 1988;13:731-736.

23. Anderson LD, D'Alonzo RT: Fractures of the odontoid process of the axis. *J Bone Joint Surg Am* 1974;56:1663-1674.

24. Clark CR, White AA III: Fractures of the dens: A multicenter study. *J Bone Joint Surg Am* 1985;67:1340-1348.

25. Apuzzo MLJ, Heiden JS, Weiss MH, Ackerson TT, Harvey JP, Kurze T: Acute fractures of the odontoid process: An analysis of 45 cases. *J Neurosurg* 1978;48:85-91.

26. Polin RS, Szabo T, Bogaev CA, Replogle RE, Jane JA: Nonoperative management of Types II and III odontoid fractures: The Philidelphia collar versus the halo vest. *Neurosurgery* 1996;38:450-456.

27. Harrop JS, Vaccaro A, Przybylski GJ: Acute respiratory compromise associated with flexed cervical traction after C2 fractures. *Spine* 2001;26:E50-E54.

28. Brooks AL, Jenkins EB: Atlanto-axial arthrodesis by the wedge compression method. *J Bone Joint Surg Am* 1978;60:279-284.

29. Grob D, Jeanneret B, Aebi M, Markwalder TM: Atlanto-axial fusion with transarticular screw fixation. *J Bone Joint Surg Br* 1991;73:972-976.

30. Currier BL, Todd LT, Maus TP, Fisher DR, Yaszemski MJ: Anatomic relationship of the internal carotid artery to the C1 vertebra: A case report of cervical reconstruction for chordoma and pilot study to assess the risk of screw fixation of the atlas. *Spine* 2003;28:E461-467.

31. Jeanneret B, Vernet O, Frei S, Magerl F: Atlantoaxial mobility after screw fixation of the odontoid: A computed tomographic study. *J Spinal Disord* 1991;4:203-211.

32. Chiba K, Fujimura Y, Toyama Y, Fujii E, Nakanishi T, Hirabayashi K: Treatment protocol for fractures of the odontoid process. *J Spinal Disord* 1996;9:267-276.

33. Vieweg U, Meyer B, Schramm J: Differential treatment in acute upper cervical spine injuries: A critical review of a single-institution series. *Surg Neurol* 2000;54:203-210.

34. Allen BL, Ferguson RL, Lehmann TR, O'Brien RP: A mechanistic classification of closed, indirect fractures and dislocations of the lower cervical spine. *Spine* 1982;7:1-27.

35. Koivikko MP, Myllynen P, Karjalainen M, Vornanen M, Santavirta S: Conservative and operative treatment in cervical burst fractures. *Arch Orthop Trauma Surg* 2000;120:448-451.

36. Rushton SA, Vaccaro AR, Levine MJ, Smith M, Balderston RA, Cotler JM: Bivector traction for unstable cervical spine fractures: A description of its application and preliminary results. *J Spinal Disord* 1997;10:436-440.

37. Schneider RC, Kahn EA: Chronic neurological sequelae of acute trauma to the spine and spinal cord: I. The significance of the acute flexion or "teardrop" fracture-dislocation of the cervical spine. *J Bone Joint Surg* 1956;38:985.

38. Fisher CG, Dvorak MR, Leith J, Wing PC: Comparison of outcomes for unstable cervical flexion teardrop fractures managed with halo thoracic vest versus anterior corpectomy and plating. *Spine* 2002;27:160-166.

39. Razack N, Green BA, Levi AD: The management of traumatic cervical bilateral facet fracture-dislocations with unicortical anterior plates. *J Spinal Disord* 2000;13:374-381.

40. Vaccaro AR, Klein GR, Thaller JB, Rushton SA, Cotler JM, Albert TJ: Distraction extension injuries of the cervical spine. *J Spinal Disord* 2001;14:193-200.

41. Eismont FJ, Clifford S, Goldberg M, Green B: Cervical sagittal spinal canal size in spine injury. *Spine* 1984;9:663-666.

42. Eismont FJ, Arena MJ, Green BA: Extrusion of an intervertebral disc associated with traumatic cervical facet subluxation or dislocation of cervical facets: Case report. *J Bone Joint Surg Am* 1991;73:1555-1560.

43. Lu J, Waite P: Advances in spinal cord regeneration. *Spine* 1999;24:926-930.

44. Delamarter R, Coyle J: Acute management of spinal cord injury. *J Am Acad Orthop Surg* 1999;7:166-175.

45. Summa CD, Mirza SK: Epidemiology of traumatic spinal cord injury. *Spine State Art Rev* 1999;13:401-407.

46. Sekhon LH, Fehlings MG: Epidemiology, demographics and pathophysiology of acute spinal cord injury. *Spine* 2001;26(suppl 24):S2-S12.

47. Fehlings MG, Tator CH: An evidence-based review of decompressive surgery in acute spinal cord injury: Rationale, indications, and timing based on experimental and clinical studies. *J Neurosurg* 1999;91(suppl 1):1-11.

48. Slucky AV: Pathomechanisms of spinal cord injury. *Spine State of the Art Reviews* 1999;13:409-417.

49. Beattie MS, Farooqui AA, Bresnahan JC: Review of current evidence for

apoptosis after spinal cord injury. *J Neurotrauma* 2000;17:915-925.

50. Fawcett JW: Spinal cord repair: From experimental models to human application. *Spinal Cord* 1998;36:811-817.

51. Young W: Molecular and cellular mechanisms of spinal cord injury therapies, in Kalb RG, Strittmatter SM (eds): *Neurobiology of Spinal Cord Injury.* Totawa, NJ, Humana Press, 2000, pp 241-276.

52. Hansebout RR, Tanner JA, Romero-Sierra C: Current status of spinal cord cooling in the treatment of acute spinal cord injury. *Spine* 1984;9:508-511.

53. Kuchner EF, Hansebout RR, Pappius HM: Effects of dexamethasone and of local hypothermia on early and late tissue electrolyte changes in experimental spinal cord injury. *J Spinal Disord* 2000;13:391-398.

54. Kwon BK, Tetzlaff W: Spinal cord regeneration: From gene to transplants. *Spine* 2001;26:S13-S22.

55. Ramon Y, Cajal S: *Degeneration and Regeneration of the Nervous System.* London, England, Oxford University Press, Humphrey Milford, 1928.

56. David S, Aguayo DS: Axonal elongation into peripheral nervous system "bridges" after central nervous system injury in adult rats. *Science* 1981;214:931-933.

57. Richardson PM, Issa VM, Aguayo AJ: Regeneration of long spinal axons in the rat. *J Neurocytol* 1984;13:165-182.

58. Richardson PM, McGruinness UM, Aguayo AJ: Axons from CNS neurons regenerate into PNS grafts. *Nature* 1980;284:264-265.

59. Caroni P, Schwab ME: Antibody against myelin-associated inhibitor of neurite growth neutralizes nonpermissive substrate properties of CNS white matter. *Neuron* 1988;1:85-96.

60. Schwab ME, Caroni P: Oligodendrocytes and CNS myelin are nonpermissive substrates for neurite growth and fibroblast spreading in vitro. *J Neurosci* 1988;8:2381-2393.

61. Chen MS, Huber AB, van der Haar ME, et al: Nogo-A is a myelin-associated neurite outgrowth inhibitor and an antigen for monoclonal antibody IN-1. *Nature* 2000;403:434-439.

62. Prinjha R, Moore SE, Vinson M, et al: Inhibitor of neurite outgrowth in humans. *Nature* 2000;403:383-384.

63. GrandPre T, Nakamura F, Vartanian T, Strittmatter SM: Identification of the Nogo inhibitor of axonal regeneration as a Reticulon protein. *Nature* 2000;403:439-444.

64. Oorschott DE, Jones DG: Axonal regeneration in the mammalian central nervous system: A critique of hypotheses. *Adv Anat Embryol Cell Biol* 1990;119:1-121.

65. Li Y, Raisman G: Schwann cells induce sprouting in motor and sensory axons in the adult rat spinal cord. *J Neurosci* 1994;14:4050-4063.

66. Fernandez KJ, Tetzlaff W: Gene expression in axotomized neurons: Identifying the intrinsic determinants of axonal growth, in Ingoglia NA, Murray M (eds): *Axonal Regeneration in the Central Nervous System.* New York, NY, Marcel Dekker, 2001, pp 219-266.

67. Richardson PM, Issa VM: Peripheral injury enhances central regeneration of primary sensory neurons. *Nature* 1984;309:791-793.

68. Schreyer DJ, Skene JH: Injury associated induction of GAP-43 expression displays axon branch specificity in rat dorsal root ganglion neurons. *J Neurobiol* 1993;24:959-970.

69. Fry EJ: Central nervous system regeneration: Mission impossible? *Clin Exp Pharmacol Physiol* 2001;28:253-258.

70. Kwon BK, Borisoff JF, Tetzlaff W: Molecular targets for therapeutic intervention after spinal cord injury. *Molec Interventions* 2002;2:244-258.

71. Kobayashi NR, Fan DP, Giehl KM, Bedard AM, Wiegand SJ, Tetzlaff W: BDNF and NT-4/5 prevent atrophy of rat rubrospinal neurons after cervical oxotomy, stimulate GAP-43 and Talpha1-tubulin mRNA expression, and promote axonal regeneration. *J Neurosci* 1997;17:9583-9595.

72. Messerer C, Kobayashi YN: Abstract: Rubrospinal neurons have undergone massive atrophy, but not death, one year after cervical axotomy in the adult rat. *Soc Neur Abstr* 2000;26:303.

73. Friedman JA, Windebank AJ, Moore MJ, Spinner RJ, Currier BL, Yaszemski MJ: Biodegradable polymer grafts for surgical repair of the injured spinal cord. *Neurosurgery* 2002;51:742-752.

74. Grill R, Murai K, Blesch A, Gage FH, Tuszynski MH: Cellular delivery of neurotrophin-3 promotes corticospinal axonal growth and partial functional recovery after spinal cord injury.

J Neurosci 1997;17:5560-5572.

75. Huber AB, Ehrengruber MU, Schwab ME, Brosamle C: Adenoviral gene transfer to the injured spinal cord of the adult rat. *Eur J Neurosci* 2000;12: 3437-3442.

76. Tresco PA: Tissue engineering strategies for nervous system repair. *Prog Brain Res* 2000;128:349-363.

77. Bunge RP: Expanding roles for the Schwann cell: Ensheathment, myelination, trophism and regeneration. *Curr Opin Neurobiol* 1993;3:805-809.

78. Reier PJ: Neural tissue grafts and repair of hte injured spinal cord. *Neuropathol Appl Neurobiol* 1985;11:81-104.

79. Li H, Filed P, Raisman G: Repair of adult rat corticospinal tract by transplants of olfactory ensheathing cells. *Science* 1997;277:2000-2002.

80. Ramon-Cueto A, Plant G, Avila J, Bung M: Long distance axonal regeneration in the transected adult rat spinal cord is promoted by olfactory ensheathing glia transplants. *J Neurosci* 1998;18:3803-3815.

81. Xu XM, Zhang SX, Li H, Aebischer P, Bunge MB: Regrowth of axons into the distal spinal cord through a Schwann-cell-seeded mini-channel implanted into hemisected adult rat spinal cord. *Eur J Neurosci* 1999;11:1723-1740.

82. Moon LD, Brecknell JE, Franklin RJ, Dunnett SB, Fawcett JW: Robust regeneration of CNS axons through a track depleted of CNS glia. *Exp Neurol* 2000;161:49-66.

83. Muir E, Du JS, Fok-Seang J, et al: Increased axon growth through astrocyte cell lines transfected with urokinase. *Glia* 1998;23:24-34.

84. Kalderon N, Xu S, Koutcher JA, Fuks Z: Fractionated radiation facilitates repair and functional motor recovery after spinal cord transection in rat. *Brain Res* 2001;904:199-207.

85. Dyer JK, Bourque JA, Steeves JD: Regeneration of brainstem-spinal axons after lesion and immunological disruption of myelin in adult rat. *Exp Neurol* 1998;154:12-22.

86. Huang DW, McKerracher L, Braun PE, David S: A therapeutic vaccine approach to stimulate axon regeneration in the adult mammalian spinal cord. *Neuron* 1999;24:639-647.

87. Guthrie S: Axonal guidance: Starting and stopping with slit. *Curr Biol* 1999;9:R432-R435.

88. Lehmann M, Fournier A, Selles-Navarro I, et al: Inactivation of Rho signaling pathway promotes CNS axon regeneration. *J Neurosci* 1999;19:7537-7547.

89. Song HJ, Ming GL, Poo MM: cAMP-induced switching in turning direction of nerve growth cones. *Nature* 1997;388:275-279.

90. Tator CH, Fehlings MG, Thorpe K, Taylor W: Current use and timing of spinal surgery for management of acute spinal surgery for management of acute spinal cord injury in North America: Results of a retrospective multicenter study. *J Neurosurg* 1999;91(suppl 1):12-18.

91. Collins WF: Surgery in the acute treatment of spinal cord injury: A review of the past 40 years. *J Spinal Cord Med* 1995;18:3-8.

92. Vaccaro AR, Daugherty RJ, Sheehan TP, et al: Neurologic outcome of early versus late surgery for cervical spinal cord injury. *Spine* 1997;22:2609-2613.

93. Waters RL, Adkins RH, Yakura JS, Sie I: Effect of surgery on motor recovery following traumatic spinal cord injury. *Spinal Cord* 1996;34:188-192.

94. Chen TY, Dickman CA, Eleraky M, Sonntag VK: The role of decompression for acute incomplete cervical spinal cord injury in cervical spondylosis. *Spine* 1998;23:2398-2403.

95. Mirza SK, Krengel WF III, Chapman JR, et al: Early versus delayed surgery for acute cervical spinal cord injury. *Clin Orthop* 1999;359:104-114.

96. Marshall LF, Knowlton S, Garfin SR, et al: Deterioration following spinal cord injury: A multicenter study. *J Neurosurg* 1987;66:400-404.

97. Fehlings MG, Sekhon HS, Tator CH: The role and timing of decompression in acute spinal cord injury: What do we know? What should we do? *Spine* 2001;26(suppl 24):S101-S110.

98. Chen A, Xu XM, Kleitman N, Bunge MB: Methylprednisolone administration improves axonal regeneration into Schwann cell grafts in transected adult rat thoracic spinal cord. *Exp Neurol* 1996;138:261-276.

99. Hall ED: The neuroprotective pharmacology of methylprednisolone. *J Neurosurg* 1992;76:13-22.

100. Ray SK, Wilford GG, Matzelle DC, Hogan EL, Banik NL: Calpeptin and methylprednisolone inhibit apoptosis in rat spinal cord injury. *Ann N Y Acad Sci* 1999;890:261-269.

101. Xu J, Fan G, Chen S, Wu Y, Xu XM, Hsu CY: Methylprednisolone inhibition of TNF-alpha expression and NF-κB activation after spinal cord injury in rats. *Brain Res Mol Brain Res* 1998;59:135-142.

102. Young W, Flamm ES: Effect of high-dose corticosteroid therapy on blood flow, evoked potentials, and extracellular calcium in experimental spinal injury. *J Neurosurg* 1982;57:667-673.

103. Bracken MB, Shepard MJ, Collins WF, et al: A randomized, controlled trial of methylprednisolone or naloxone in the treatment of acute spinal-cord injury: Results of the second national acute spinal cord injury study. *N Engl J Med* 1990;322:1405-1411.

104. Bracken MB, Shepard MJ, Holford TR, et al: Administration of methylprednisolone for 24 or 48 hours or tirilazad mesylate for 48 hours in the treatment of acute spinal cord injury: Results of the Third National Acute Spinal Cord Injury Randomized Controlled Trial. National Acute Spinal Cord Injury Study. *JAMA* 1997;277:1597-1604.

105. Fehlings MG: Editorial: Recommendations regarding the use of methylprednisolone in acute spinal cord injury: Making sense out of the controversy. *Spine* 2001;26(suppl 24):S56-S57.

106. Hurlbert RJ: The role of steroids in acute spinal cord injury: An evidence-based analysis. *Spine* 2001;26(suppl 24):S39-S46.

107. Bracken MB: Methylprednisolone and acute spinal cord injury: An update of the randomized evidence. *Spine* 2001;26(suppl 24):S47-S54.

108. Geisler FH, Coleman WP, Grieco G, Poonian D, Sygen Study Group: The Sygen multicenter acute spinal cord injury study. *Spine* 2001;26(suppl 24):S87-S98.

109. Constantini S, Young W: The effects of methylprednisolone and the ganglioside GM1 on acute spinal cord injury in rats. *J Neurosurg* 1994;80:97-111.

110. Geisler FH, Coleman WP, Grieco G, Poonian D, Syngen Study Group: Recruitment and early treatment in a multicenter study of acute spinal cord injury. *Spine* 2001;26(suppl 24):S58-S67.

111. Geisler FH, Coleman WP, Grieco G, Poonian D: and Sygen Study Group: Measurements and recovery patterns in a multicenter study of acute spinal cord injury. *Spine* 2001;26(suppl 24):S68-S86.

112. Burns SP, Golding DG, Rolle WA Jr, Graziani V, Ditunno JF Jr: Recovery of ambulation in motor-incomplete tetraplegia. *Arch Phys Med Rehabil* 1997;78:1169-1172.

113. *International Standards for Neurological Classification of Spinal Cord Injury.* Chicago, IL, American Spinal Injury Association, 2002.

114. Kirshblum SC, O'Connor KC: Levels of spinal cord injury and predictors of neurologic recovery, in Kraft GH and Hammon MC (eds): *Physical Medicine and Rehabilitation Clinics of North America: Topics in Spinal Cord Medicine.* Philadelphia, PA, WB Saunders, 2000, pp 1-27.

115. Waters RL, Adkins RH, Yakura JS, Sie I: Motor and sensory recovery following complete tetraplegia. *Arch Phys Med Rehabil* 1993;74:242-247.

116. Crozier KS, Graziani V, Ditunno JF Jr, Herbison GJ: Spinal cord injury: Prognosis for ambulation based on sensory examination in patients who are initially motor complete. *Arch Phys Med Rehabil* 1999;72:119-121.

117. Waters RL, Adkins RH, Yakura JS, Sie I: Motor and sensory recovery following incomplete tetraplegia. *Arch Phys Med Rehabil* 1994;75:306-311.

118. Waters RL, Adkins RH, Yakura JS, Sie I: Motor and sensory recovery following incomplete paraplegia. *Arch Phys Med Rehabil* 1994;75:67-72.

119. Ditunno JF, Cohen MS, Formal C: Functional outcomes, in Stover SI, DeLissa JA, Whiteneck GG (eds): *Spinal Cord Injury: Clinical Outcomes From the Model Systems.* Gaithersburg, MD, Aspen Publishers, 1995, pp 170-184.

120. Consortium for Spinal Cord Medicine: Outcomes following traumatic spinal cord injury: Clinical practice guidelines for health care professionals, Paralyzed Veterans of America, 1999. Available at: http://www.pva.org/NEWPVASITE/publications/cpg_pubs/trauma.htm. Accessed August 29, 2003.

121. Burns AS, Ditunno JF: Establishing prognosis and maximizing functional outcomes after spinal cord injury: A review of current and future directions in rehabilitation management. *Spine* 2001;26(suppl 24):S137-S145.

2

Emergency Evaluation, Imaging, and Classification of Thoracolumbar Injuries

Jeffrey A. Rihn, MD
David T. Anderson, MD
*Rick C. Sasso, MD
*Thomas A. Zdeblick, MD
*Lawrence G. Lenke, MD
*Mitchel B. Harris, MD
*Jens R. Chapman, MD
Alexander R. Vaccaro, MD, PhD

Abstract

Thoracolumbar injuries usually are the result of high-energy trauma and frequently are associated with multisystem concomitant injuries. Whenever a thoracolumbar injury is suspected, a prompt and thorough evaluation should be performed in the emergency department, using the guidelines of the American College of Surgeons and including full primary and secondary surveys as well as resuscitation. Protection of the spine and spinal cord is of paramount importance during the initial evaluation. A careful and complete neurologic examination is warranted as part of the secondary survey. Plain radiography, CT, and MRI studies are useful in diagnosing and classifying thoracolumbar injuries. At many trauma centers, CT has become the standard imaging technology for the initial evaluation of the spine. MRI is particularly accurate in detecting injury to the posterior ligamentous complex of the thoracolumbar spine. Classification and treatment of thoracolumbar injuries are controversial. The comprehensive, reproducible classification system of the Spine Trauma Study Group has prognostic significance and can guide treatment decisions. The Thoracolumbar Injury Classification and Severity scale classifies thoracolumbar injures based on three pivotal characteristics: the morphology of the injury, the integrity of the posterior ligamentous complex, and the patient's neurologic status. A total severity score is used in conjunction with the classification system to determine the treatment.

A thoracolumbar injury usually is the result of high-energy trauma. Multisystem, concomitant injuries are relatively common and often are life-threatening. Prompt and thorough evaluation in the emergency department is therefore imperative. The general surgery trauma team performs a primary survey, including an evaluation of the patient's airway, breathing, and circulation, and begins resuscitation. A thorough secondary survey is then performed, including a careful and complete neurologic examination. The spine must be protected throughout the initial evaluation.

Imaging studies, including plain radiography, CT, and MRI, are essential for diagnosing and classifying a thoracolumbar injury. Many trauma centers have begun using CT, rather than plain radiography, as the initial screening tool for spinal fractures and dislocations. MRI is particularly useful in diagnosing injuries to the soft tissues of the spine, including the intervertebral disk and the posterior ligamentous complex (PLC).

Information from the initial clinical evaluation and imaging studies is important in classifying a thoracolumbar injury. The classification and treatment are controversial, even though a thoracolumbar injury is one of the most common spinal injuries. The Spine Trauma Study Group (STSG) recently developed the comprehensive Thoracolumbar Injury Classification and Severity (TLICS) scale. The TLICS scale is based on the morphology of the injury, the integrity of the PLC, and the patient's neurologic status. A severity score is used in conjunction with the classification system to guide treatment decisions. This classification system has been shown to be valid and reproducible.[1-5]

Evaluation of Injuries

Concomitant injuries are found in 64% of patients with a spinal cord injury and 47% of those with spine trauma.[6,7] These patients require rapid evaluation and resuscitation using the guidelines of the American College of Surgeons.[8] The clinical evaluation begins with assessing the airway, breathing, circulation, disability, and exposure. The airway must be opened, and ventilation and oxygenation must be established. Injuries such as a pneumothorax or a hemothorax must be aggressively treated, and hemodynamic stability must be ensured. Shock in a trauma patient is assumed to be hemorrhagic until proven otherwise. To assess the patient's level of alertness and consciousness, the Glasgow Coma Scale is used to measure eye-opening, verbal, and motor behav-

ioral responses. The secondary survey assesses injuries to the head, chest, abdomen, pelvis, spine, and extremities. It is essential to stabilize the spine during the initial evaluation. The patient should be carefully rolled to evaluate the spinal column. The skin is observed for abrasion or bruising, and the entire spine is palpated for tenderness, step-off, or diastasis between spinous processes. A rectal examination should be performed to evaluate perianal sensation, resting tone, volitional contraction, and bulbocavernosus reflex. The extremities should be examined for injury.

Immediately after initial stabilization, a careful and complete neurologic examination should be performed as part of the secondary survey. The American Spinal Injury Association (ASIA) Impairment Scale can be used to evaluate motor and sensory function; it includes a general impairment scale and functional independence measure.[9,10] The ASIA Impairment Scale's motor score has been shown to be most closely correlated with the potential for functional improvement and rehabilitation performance.[9,11] In general, the neurologic examination in the emergency department should focus on localizing the level of the injury and defining the extent of spinal cord involvement. If the patient is alert, light touch sensation can be assessed by dermatome to locate any

deficits. The contralateral spinothalamic tracts can be evaluated by using pinpricks to elicit pain. If the patient is willing to cooperate, the motor function of the C5 through T1 and L2 through S1 nerve roots can easily be tested to determine the degree of function of the ipsilateral corticospinal tract. Injury to the conus medullaris and cauda equina can be established by testing rectal tone, sacral sensation, and bowel and bladder function. In an unresponsive patient, the neurologic examination should focus on spontaneous movements, motor response to painful stimuli, and the presence or absence of deep tendon reflexes and rectal tone.[10]

Neurogenic and spinal shock are among the spinal cord syndromes that may not be detected during examination of a patient with a spinal cord injury. It is important to distinguish hemorrhagic shock from neurogenic shock because they are treated differently. Hemorrhagic shock is the result of a loss of intravascular volume. Hypotension causes tachycardia, vasoconstriction with cold extremities, and low urine output secondary to simple physiologic response. Hemorrhagic shock is diagnosed and treated simultaneously; the basic treatment principle is to stop the bleeding and restore volume loss. Neurogenic shock refers to the compromise of descending sympathetic outflow, with subsequent loss of vasomotor tone in the heart and peripheral vasculature that occurs with an acute spinal cord injury. Neurogenic shock is more common in cervical and upper thoracic injuries than in thoracolumbar injuries; it leads to hypotension, bradycardia, and venous pooling with warm extremities. Urine output is normal. The patient's heart rate usually is 50 to 70 beats per

Rick C. Sasso, MD or the department with which he is affiliated has received research or institutional support from Medtronic, Stryker, AO Foundation, CeraPedics, and Lilly; has received royalties from Medtronic; holds stock or stock options in Biomet and SpineCore; and is a consultant for or employee of Medtronic. Thomas A. Zdeblick, MD or the department with which he is affiliated has received royalties from Medtronic and is a consultant for or employee of Medtronic and Anulex. Lawrence G. Lenke, MD or the department with which he is affiliated has received research or institutional support from Medtronic and DePuy; has received miscellaneous nonincome support, commercially derived honoraria, or other nonresearch-related funding from Medtronic; has received royalties from Medtronic; and is a consultant for or employee of Medtronic. Mitchel B. Harris, MD or the department with which he is affiliated has received research or institutional support from Synthes, Zimmer, DePuy, and Medtronic; has received miscellaneous nonincome support, commercially-derived honoraria, or other nonresearch-related funding from AO Foundation, and is a consultant for or employee of Globus. Jens R. Chapman, MD or the department with which he is affiliated has received research or institutional support from Synthes, Medtronic, and Johnson & Johnson; has received miscellaneous nonincome support, commercially derived honoraria, or other nonresearch-related funding from Synthes, Medtronic, and Johnson & Johnson; and is a consultant for or employee of Synthes.

minute, and systolic blood pressure is 30 to 50 mm Hg below normal.[12] As a result of the spinal cord injury, the patient may have flaccid paralysis, areflexia, and variable sensory loss. Hypotension is treated with mild fluid resuscitation and the judicious use of vasopressors. Spinal shock, which must be differentiated from neurogenic shock, is the result of a physiologic spinal cord dysfunction after an acute spinal cord injury,[13] causing acute depression of the spinal reflexes caudal to the level of injury. The reflexes gradually return as the physiologic abnormalities are resolved. Although controversial, the belief that resolution of spinal shock is indicated by the return of the bulbocavernosus reflex (usually 24 to 48 hours after the injury) is shared by many authors.[13] Until spinal shock resolves, as indicated by the return of the bulbocavernosus reflex, the presence of a complete neurologic deficit cannot be confirmed. Some neurologic function may return when spinal shock has been resolved, and this development can affect the patient's prognosis.

Treatment: The Role of Steroids

Using glucocorticosteroids to treat acute spinal cord injury is controversial and should be guided by the conclusions of the National Acute Spinal Cord Injury Study (NASCIS). A 1985 NASCIS study[14] found no improvement in the neurologic recovery of patients with acute spinal cord injury after methylprednisolone was administered. A randomized 1990 NASCIS study[15] compared a higher methylprednisolone dosage (30 mg/kg administered intravenously over 15 minutes [followed by a 45-minute rest], then 5.4 mg/kg/h for 23 hours) with naloxone and placebo. Analysis of the

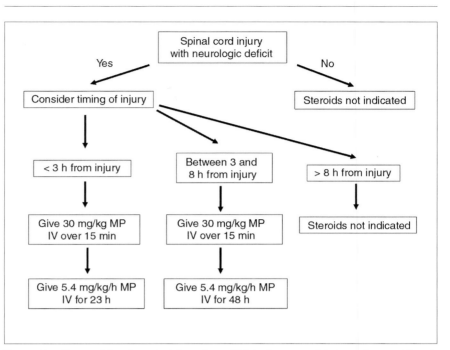

Figure 1 Protocol for the administration of high-dose steroids in patients with spinal cord injury, based on the findings of the NASCIS studies. MP = methylprednisolone, IV = intravenous.

entire study group found no significant difference between the treatments. However, the patients who received methylprednisolone within 8 hours of injury had a significant improvement in neurologic score. Methylprednisolone administered more than 8 hours after the injury was found to cause a significant worsening in the neurologic score. The authors conceded that improvement in the neurologic score is not equivalent to improvement in functional status. Patients with a coexisting life-threatening injury or a spinal cord injury secondary to a gunshot wound were excluded from the study. The first NASCIS study reported an increased rate of infection when steroids were used, but the second NASCIS study did not confirm this finding.

A 1997 NASCIS study[16] found that patients who received a large dose of a steroid 3 to 8 hours after injury had an improved neurologic

outcome when the treatment extended over 48 hours rather than 24 hours. Patients treated for 48 hours had higher rates of severe sepsis and severe pneumonia but did not have higher rates of other complications or mortality. The authors concluded that, if possible, patients with acute spinal cord injury should be treated within 3 hours of injury with a high-dose methylprednisolone regimen (a 30 mg/kg loading dose followed by 5.4 mg/kg/h for 23 hours). Patients treated 3 to 8 hours after spinal cord injury should be maintained on the high-dose steroid regimen for 48 hours. Administration of a high-dose steroid is not indicated for a patient with a life-threatening comorbidity, and a high-dose steroid may be harmful if started more than 8 hours after injury (Figure 1). Several literature reviews concluded that current evidence does not support the use of methylprednisolone to treat an acute

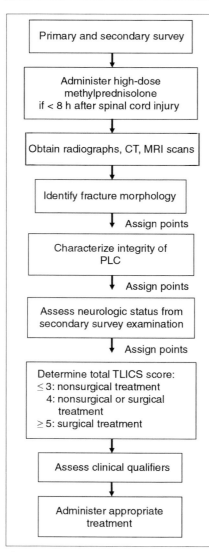

```
Primary and secondary survey
        ↓
Administer high-dose
methylprednisolone
if < 8 h after spinal cord injury
        ↓
Obtain radiographs, CT, MRI scans
        ↓
Identify fracture morphology
        ↓  Assign points
Characterize integrity of
PLC
        ↓  Assign points
Assess neurologic status from
secondary survey examination
        ↓  Assign points
Determine total TLICS score:
≤ 3: nonsurgical treatment
  4: nonsurgical or surgical
     treatment
≥ 5: surgical treatment
        ↓
Assess clinical qualifiers
        ↓
Administer appropriate
treatment
```

Figure 2 Protocol for emergency department evaluation, imaging, and classification of a thoracolumbar injury, based on the TLICS system.

spinal cord injury and suggest that high-dose administration can do more harm than good.[17-19]

Significant research has been conducted on other pharmacologic interventions for acute spinal cord injury, including tirilazad and GM1-ganglioside.[16,20,21] Although some promising clinical results have been reported, these interventions are not routinely used clinically. Additional studies are needed to better understand the risks and benefits of methylprednisolone and other neuroprotective substances.

Imaging Studies

Plain radiography, CT, and MRI are important in the evaluation of thoracolumbar injury. The published selective indications for thoracolumbar radiography appear to be reasonable, although they have not been extensively studied.[22,23] A trauma patient with back pain or tenderness, a neurologic deficit, a distracting injury, altered mental status, and/or a high-energy mechanism of injury requires routine spine radiography; imaging studies are unnecessary if none of these criteria is present.

Standard AP and lateral radiographs have long been the mainstay of initial imaging in trauma patients. Although major fractures or dislocations are readily identifiable from plain radiographs, additional imaging studies usually are required. The presence of neurologic deficit or continued pain also may warrant additional studies.

CT can quickly and accurately characterize most bone injuries. CT is more accurate than plain radiography in revealing the character of a fracture, the extent of bone fragment displacement, and the presence of minor fractures. The standard axial, sagittal, and coronal CT studies are adequate to delineate most injuries. Subtle fractures may not be seen on the coronal and sagittal reconstructions, however. Ongoing investigation is attempting to define the circumstances in which a scout view CT can safely replace AP and lateral radiographs in evaluating the thoracolumbar spine after blunt trauma.[24,25] As CT technology and speed have improved, it has become more widely used for the routine evaluation of blunt thoracolumbar trauma; in many trauma centers, CT has replaced plain radiography as the first imaging study for such patients.

MRI is increasingly used to assess the ligamentous structures and help in surgical planning. MRI allows precise visualization of the spinal cord, ligaments, and soft tissue. As the speed and accessibility of MRI technology improves, it is being used more commonly for routine imaging in patients with spine trauma. STSG members were found to be more likely to use T1-weighted MRI to detect possible injury to the PLC if plain radiographs appeared normal.[26] In a prospective study of established thoracolumbar fractures, Lee and associates[27] assessed the reliability of MRI in detecting PLC injuries. MRI, physical examination, and plain radiographic findings were compared with surgical findings. Fat-suppressed sagittal T2-weighted MRI was found to be far more sensitive, specific, and accurate than palpation or plain radiography in detecting PLC injury. MRI is also useful in classifying thoracolumbar injury and selecting the treatment. Figure 2 presents a protocol for evaluating and classifying thoracolumbar injuries.

Classification of Thoracolumbar Injuries

Information gathered from clinical evaluation and imaging studies is used to classify a thoracolumbar injury. Although considerable research has been devoted to the development of a suitable classification system,[28-35] the shortcomings of the existing systems have limited their clinical use. The Denis system[29] is among the most commonly used. In contrast to the two-column theory first proposed in 1963 by Holdsworth,[30,31] the Denis model is based on a three-column theory of spinal stability (anterior, middle, and posterior columns). The classification of spinal stability and fracture type is based on the mode of failure of the middle column rather than the posterior column. The middle column is the essential contributor to spinal stability; it is composed of the posterior wall of the vertebral body, the posterior anulus fibrosus, and the posterior longitudinal ligament. The most important injury categories in the Denis system are compression fracture, burst fracture, seat belt–type injury, and fracture-dislocation. Each of these categories has three to five subtypes (a total of 16 subtypes).[29]

Magerl and associates[32] introduced the AO classification system for thoracolumbar injuries in 1994. The AO system categorizes a thoracolumbar injury, in order of increasing severity, as a compression fracture (type A), distraction injury (type B), or fracture-dislocation (type C). Each type has three subtypes, each subtype is divided into three subgroups, and each subgroup is further subdivided. The complexity of this classification system limits its use in clinical practice. Studies found the Denis and AO classification systems to have fair to moderate validity and reliability and suggested that their reliability decreases as complexity increases (with inclusion of all subdivisions in the analysis).[36-38]

Oner and associates[37] compared the interobserver and intraobserver reliability of the AO and Denis systems. If only the three major categories were included, the AO classification was found to have fair reliability when used with CT studies and moderate reliability when used with MRI studies. The reliability of the AO system was enhanced

by the use of MRI. Adding subgroups to the evaluation with the AO system decreased the level of interobserver and intraobserver agreement in the AO system.[37] There was greater variance with the Denis system because of the inability to identify categories for certain types of injuries, and information from MRI studies could not easily be incorporated (especially information pertaining to PLC integrity). Using the Denis system, injuries frequently were grouped together based on the pattern of bony involvement, regardless of whether they had a PLC component.

Primary Axes in the TLICS Scale

The goal of the STSG is to improve and standardize the care of spine trauma patients through collaborative research and education.[39] Since its inception in 2002 as an international group of spine trauma experts, the STSG has made considerable progress toward developing a comprehensive classification system for injuries of the thoracolumbar spine. The TLICS scale reflects the consensus of STSG members on the three characteristics of thoracolumbar injury that are essential for clinical decision making: injury morphology, PLC integrity, and neurologic status.[39] These primary axes are believed to be both independently important and complementary. They are divided into a limited number of easily recognizable subgroups to define thoracolumbar injury patterns and are ranked from least significant to most significant.[1]

Injury Morphology

In the TLICS scale, the morphology of a thoracolumbar injury is determined using information from plain radiography, CT, and MRI. The

fracture is described as a compression, translation-rotation, or distraction injury.[1]

The vertebral body fails under an axial load in a compression injury. Less severe injuries affect only the anterior portion of the vertebral body. The posterior vertebral body may be involved in a more severe injury, with retropulsion of bone into the canal (a burst fracture). Based on radiographic, CT, and MRI appearance, the compression injury is further described as axial, flexion, or lateral.

Failure of the spinal column in shear or torsion leads to a rotation or translation injury. This high-energy injury is typically more unstable than a compression injury. Rotation of one vertebra on another can be detected using plain radiography, CT, or MRI. Horizontal rotation of the spinous processes and pedicles can be seen on an AP radiograph or an axial CT scan. Anterior-posterior translation is best seen on a lateral radiograph or a sagittal CT reconstruction. Medial-lateral translation is most often visible on an AP radiograph or a coronal CT reconstruction.

Distraction of the spinal column can occur through the anterior or posterior ligaments, the anterior or posterior bony elements, or both ligamentous and bony elements. A distraction injury results in a circumferential separation of the spinal column and is highly unstable. This type of injury can occur in flexion or extension and can lead to significant angulation across the fracture site. Distraction can be associated with a compression or burst injury to the vertebral body. In a combined ligamentous-bony injury, the classification of the more severely injured component is used to determine the appropriate treatment.

PLC Integrity

The PLC of the spinal column is composed of the bilateral facet capsules, the ligamentum flavum, and the interspinous and supraspinous ligaments. The PLC serves as the posterior tension band of the spinal column, and it significantly contributes to spinal stability.[1] An injured PLC does not heal well in an adult, and therefore surgical stabilization usually is necessary. In a thoracolumbar injury, the PLC is categorized as intact, disrupted, or indeterminate. Disruption of the PLC often appears as splaying of the spinous process and diastasis or subluxation of the facet joints, as seen on AP and lateral plain radiographs or sagittal and axial CT reconstructions.[26] T1-weighted and fat-suppressed T2-weighted sagittal MRI studies have been particularly useful in identifying an injury to the PLC.[26,27]

Neurologic Status

The neurologic status of the patient is important in determining the stability of the spine and the injury prognosis, especially if a neurologic deficit is present. Neurologic status is categorized, in order of increasing injury severity or urgency, as intact or as having a nerve root, cauda equina, incomplete (motor or sensory), or complete (motor and sensory) deficit.[1] In the TLICS grading system, a complete neurologic deficit is that which meets the ASIA grade A criteria, and an incomplete deficit meets the ASIA grade B, C, or D criteria.[1]

TLICS Scoring

In the TLICS scale, a numeric point value is assigned to each subgroup of the three primary axes (injury morphology, PLC integrity, and neurologic status).[1] A higher numeric value is correlated with greater severity or urgency.

The point assignment for morphology is as follows: compression fracture, 1; compression fracture with a burst component, 2; translation or rotation injury, 3; distraction injury, 4. Although combination injuries occur, only the point value of the most severe category is used to calculate the injury severity score. Although a compression fracture with a burst component represents a subset of compression fracture, it has a greater point value because it is a more severe injury. The point value assigned for PLC integrity is as follows: injury with an intact PLC, 0; injury with indeterminate PLC status (seen, for example, as a ligamentous signal change on T2-weighted MRI with no evidence of structural malalignment), 2; injury with a disrupted PLC, 3. A point value is assigned for one of five neurologic status categories: intact neurologic status, 0; simple nerve root deficit, 2; complete neurologic deficit (motor and sensory), 2; incomplete spinal cord deficit (sensory or motor function partially intact below level of injury), 3; cauda equina deficit, 3. Incomplete spinal cord deficit and cauda equina deficit are assigned the highest point value because they represent the most urgent clinical situations.

The TLICS System in Surgical Decision Making

The total TLICS score is the sum of the three component point values. This score has proved to be a useful tool in determining appropriate treatment. A patient whose total severity score is 3 or lower usually can be treated nonsurgically, and a patient whose total score is 5 or higher usually requires surgical treatment. A patient with a total score of 4 is considered to be in a "gray zone" in which surgical and nonsurgical treatment may be equally appropriate. Numerous factors should be considered in deciding on the treatment for a patient with a score of 4, including patient and surgeon preferences and the presence of medical comorbidities or associated injuries (Figure 2).

For a patient requiring surgical treatment, PLC integrity and neurologic status are the most important categories to consider in planning the surgical approach. An anterior approach is recommended if the patient has a neurologic deficit and neural compression from anterior structures (bone or intervertebral disk); the anterior approach can provide adequate decompression of the neural elements. Because the PLC is unable to heal on its own, patients with a disrupted PLC require posterior stabilization. A combined anterior and posterior approach is usually required for a patient with a neurologic deficit and a PLC injury.

The TLICS scale includes guidelines for treatment decision making, in which numerous additional spinal injury and patient characteristics are specified as clinical qualifiers. Among the spinal injury qualifiers are excessive fracture angulation and fracture of associated structures such as the sternum and ribs. The patient qualifiers include systemic conditions such as ankylosing spondylitis, osteoporosis, and obesity as well as age and medical comorbidities. Although the clinical qualifiers are too numerous to be assigned a point value in the treatment algorithm, they must be considered in treatment decision making.[1,40] It is essential that they be used with the total severity score to develop an appropriate treatment plan. Figures 3 and 4 illustrate the

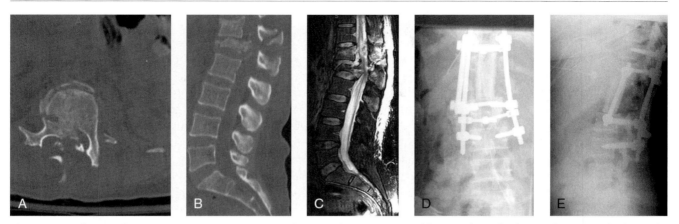

Figure 3 A flexion-distraction injury at T12-L1 was diagnosed in a 19-year-old man after a high-speed motor vehicle crash. **A,** Axial CT scan showing bony involvement of the anterior and posterior spine. **B,** Sagittal CT scan reconstruction showing the burst component of the L1 vertebrae due to flexion and compression, with a fracture through the spinous process of T12 due to distraction. **C,** T2-weighted sagittal MRI study showing disruption of the PLC. This patient had a complete neurologic deficit (ASIA A) with a T12 level. The patient's TLICS total severity score of 9 (4 points for the distraction morphology, 3 points for the disrupted PLC injury, and 2 points for complete neurologic deficit) led to a surgical treatment recommendation. Both anterior and posterior approaches were required because of the neurologic deficit and PLC disruption. **D** and **E,** AP and lateral thoracolumbar radiographs, respectively, showing corpectomies performed anteriorly at T12 and L1, with placement of a humeral allograft strut, anterior instrumentation from T11 to L2, and posterior instrumentation from T10 to L3 with posterior fusion using autograft iliac crest.

application of the TLICS system to two different thoracolumbar injuries.

Validation of the TLICS Scale

The TLICS scale in its current form is the product of extensive reliability and validity studies.[1-5,41] The STSG introduced the Thoracolumbar Injury Severity Score (TLISS) in 2005.[40] The TLISS includes three primary criteria: the mechanism of injury, integrity of the PLC, and neurologic status. Subsequent studies brought into question the use of mechanism of injury as a primary criterion. In a study by Harrop and associates,[2] 48 spine surgeons reviewed 56 thoracolumbar injury patient histories. Intrarater agreement was found to be 59.4% for injury mechanism ($K = 0.429$), 68.4% for PLC integrity ($K = 0.478$), and 91.0% for neurologic status ($K = 0.841$). Interrater agreement was 50.7% for injury mechanism

($K = 0.295$), 59.4% for PLC integrity ($K = 0.336$), and 96.3% for neurologic status ($K = 0.935$). More than 90% of the surgeons agreed with the treatment recommendations specified in the algorithm. Although the TLISS was found to offer acceptable reliability, the authors concluded that the injury mechanism component should be replaced by an injury morphology component.

Vaccaro and associates[3] also evaluated the reliability of the TLISS. Five experienced spine surgeons reviewed 71 thoracolumbar injury patient histories. The interobserver Cohen's kappa scores were injury mechanism, 0.33; PLC integrity, 0.35; and neurologic status, 0.91. The intraobserver Cohen's kappa scores were injury mechanism, 0.57; PLC integrity, 0.48; and neurologic status, 0.93. Surgeons agreed with 96% of the TLISS treatment recommendations. The authors concluded

that the TLISS had excellent construct validity. Its reliability was found to require improvement, although it was comparable with that of other classification systems. The authors believed that either a stricter definition of mechanism of injury should be added to the system or the mechanism of injury component should be altogether changed.

Vaccaro and associates[39] subsequently surveyed 22 experienced spine surgeons from 20 level I trauma centers around the world to determine the thoracolumbar injury characteristics considered essential for developing a treatment plan. The consensus of the surveyed surgeons was that the three most important characteristics of a thoracolumbar injury are injury morphology, PLC integrity, and neurologic status. The STSG used the study by Harrop and associates[2] and the two studies by Vaccaro and associates[3,39] in developing the TLICS scale.

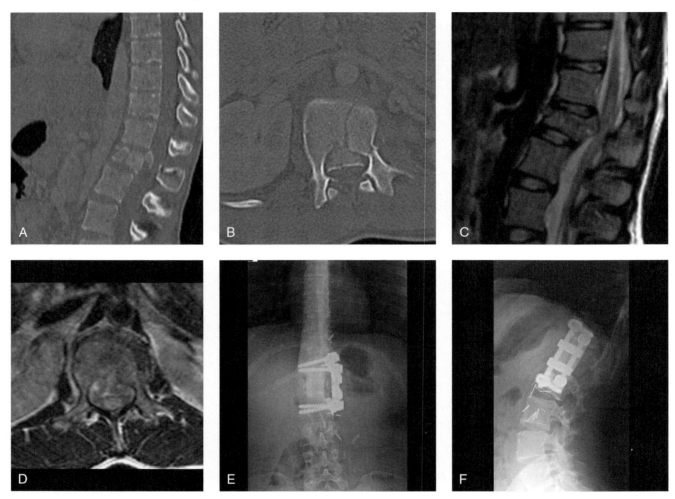

Figure 4 **A** and **B,** Sagittal reconstruction and axial CT images, respectively, showing a burst fracture of the L1 vertebra in a 22-year-old man who fell 20 feet from a ladder. **C** and **D**, Sagittal and axial T2-weighted MRI images, respectively, showing the L1 burst fracture with an intact PLC. The results of the neurologic examination were consistent with cauda equina syndrome. The patient's TLICS total severity score of 5 (2 points for the compression morphology with a burst component, 0 points for the intact PLC, and 3 points for cauda equina syndrome) led to a surgical treatment recommendation. An anterior approach was used because of the neurologic deficit. **E** and **F**, AP and lateral thoracolumbar radiographs, respectively, showing a corpectomy at L1, with placement of a humeral allograft strut and anterior instrumentation from T12 to L2.

In a multicenter study, Raja Rampersaud and associates[4] evaluated agreement between orthopaedic spine surgeons and neurosurgeons using the TLISS to classify thoracolumbar injuries. The TLISS was found to represent a consensus-based algorithm for treating thoracolumbar injuries. Patel and associates[5] recently performed the first prospective validation of the TLISS. Two groups of consecutive patients with acute thoracolumbar injuries were studied at a single institution to evaluate time-dependent changes in interobserver reliability. Interobserver reliability was found to be significantly improved for the second group of patients. This finding suggests that the TLISS classification system can be effectively taught and incorporated into routine clinical practice. Whang and associates[41] compared the reliability and validity of the TLICS scale and the TLISS to characterize the relative importance of injury mechanism and injury morphology for identifying and treating thoracolumbar injury. Thoracolumbar injuries were scored using both systems, and treatment recommendations derived from each system were compared with the actual treatment provided to patients. Interobserver reliability for all scores (injury mechanism or morphology, PLC status, neurologic status, and total severity) as well as recommended treatment were within the range of moderate to substantial reproducibility ($0.45 \leq \kappa \leq 0.74$). Interobserver reliability was higher than that reported in the studies by Harrop and associates[2] and Vaccaro and associates.[3,39] No statistically significant differences were noted between any kappa values for the two systems. Construct validity was excellent for both systems in predicting the actual treatment provided to patients.

Although the TLICS scale has undergone significant validation research, a multicenter prospective study is still lacking to compare the TLICS scale with other systems, such as the AO and Denis systems. In light of the recent results from the study by Whang and associates,[41] debate continues as to whether injury morphology or injury mechanism is a more reliable criterion for classifying thoracolumbar injuries. Studies are underway to clarify such issues.[42]

Summary

Thoracolumbar injury often results from high-energy trauma, with concomitant multisystem involvement. It is essential that a prompt and thorough evaluation be performed in the emergency department whenever thoracolumbar injury is suspected, with protection of the spine throughout the evaluation. When the patient's condition is stable, appropriate imaging, including plain radiography, CT, and MRI, should be obtained. Information from the physical examination and imaging studies is important in classifying a thoracolumbar injury.

The classification and treatment of thoracolumbar injuries are controversial. The TLICS scale is based on three primary axes: morphology

of the injury, PLC integrity, and neurologic status. A severity score used in conjunction with the classification system is useful in guiding treatment decision making and surgical planning. Prospective multicenter studies will in the future provide further information on the validity and reliability of the TLICS scale.

References

1. Vaccaro AR, Lehman RA, Hurlbert RJ, et al: A new classification of thoracolumbar injuries: The importance of injury morphology, the integrity of the posterior ligamentous complex, and neurologic status. *Spine* 2005;30: 2325-2333.

2. Harrop JS, Vaccaro AR, Hurlbert RJ, et al: Intrarater and interrater reliability and validity in the assessment of the mechanism of injury and integrity of the posterior ligamentous complex: A novel injury severity scoring system for thoracolumbar injuries. Invited submission from the Joint Section Meeting on Disorders of the Spine and Peripheral Nerves, March 2005. *J Neurosurg Spine* 2006;4: 118-122.

3. Vaccaro AR, Baron EM, Sanfilippo J, et al: Reliability of a novel classification system for thoracolumbar injuries: The Thoracolumbar Injury Severity Score. *Spine* 2006;31:S62-S69.

4. Raja Rampersaud Y, Fisher C, Wilsey J, et al: Agreement between orthopedic surgeons and neurosurgeons regarding a new algorithm for the treatment of thoracolumbar injuries: A multicenter reliability study. *J Spinal Disord Tech* 2006;19:477-482.

5. Patel AA, Vaccaro AR, Albert TJ, et al: The adoption of a new classification system: Time-dependent variation in interobserver reliability of the thoracolumbar injury severity score classification system. *Spine* 2007;32:E105-E110.

6. Saboe LA, Reid DC, Davis LA, Warren SA, Grace MG: Spine trauma and

associated injuries. *J Trauma* 1991;31: 43-48.

7. Meyer PR Jr, Sullivan DE: Injuries to the spine. *Emerg Med Clin North Am* 1984;2:313-329.

8. American College of Surgeons: *ATLS Advanced Trauma Life Support Program for Doctors*, ed 7. Chicago, IL, American College of Surgeons, 2004.

9. Priebe MM, Waring WP: The interobserver reliability of the revised American Spinal Injury Association standards for neurological classification of spinal injury patients. *Am J Phys Med Rehabil* 1991;70:268-270.

10. Savitsky E, Votey S: Emergency department approach to acute thoracolumbar spine injury. *J Emerg Med* 1997;15:49-60.

11. El Masry WS, Tsubo M, Katoh S, El Miligui YH, Khan A: Validation of the American Spinal Injury Association (ASIA) motor score and the National Acute Spinal Cord Injury Study (NASCIS) motor score. *Spine* 1996;21:614-619.

12. Delamarter RB, Coyle J: Acute management of spinal cord injury. *J Am Acad Orthop Surg* 1999;7:166-175.

13. Ditunno JF, Little JW, Tessler A, Burns AS: Spinal shock revisited: A four-phase model. *Spinal Cord* 2004; 42:383-395.

14. Bracken MB, Shepard MJ, Hellenbrand KG, et al: Methylprednisolone and neurological function 1 year after spinal cord injury: Results of the National Acute Spinal Cord Injury Study. *J Neurosurg* 1985;63:704-713.

15. Bracken MB: Methylprednisolone in the management of acute spinal cord injuries. *Med J Aust* 1990;153:368.

16. Bracken MB, Shepard MJ, Holford TR, et al: Administration of methylprednisolone for 24 or 48 hours or tirilazad mesylate for 48 hours in the treatment of acute spinal cord injury: Results of the Third National Acute Spinal Cord Injury Randomized Controlled Trial. National Acute Spinal Cord Injury Study. *JAMA* 1997; 277:1597-1604.

17. Hurlbert RJ: Methylprednisolone for acute spinal cord injury: An inappropriate standard of care. *J Neurosurg* 2000;93(suppl 1):1-7.

18. Hurlbert RJ: The role of steroids in acute spinal cord injury: An evidence-based analysis. *Spine* 2001;26(suppl 24):S39-S46.

19. Hurlbert RJ: Strategies of medical intervention in the management of acute spinal cord injury. *Spine* 2006; 31:S16-S21.

20. Geisler FH, Dorsey FC, Coleman WP: Recovery of motor function after spinal-cord injury: A randomized, placebo-controlled trial with GM-1 ganglioside. *N Engl J Med* 1991;324: 1829-1838.

21. Geisler FH, Coleman WP, Grieco G, Poonian D: The Sygen multicenter acute spinal cord injury study. *Spine* 2001;26(suppl 24):S87-S98.

22. Terregino CA, Ross SE, Lipinski MF, Foreman J, Hughes R: Selective indications for thoracic and lumbar radiography in blunt trauma. *Ann Emerg Med* 1995;26:126-129.

23. Samuels LE, Kerstein MD: "Routine" radiologic evaluation of the thoracolumbar spine in blunt trauma patients: A reappraisal. *J Trauma* 1993; 34:85-89.

24. Berry GE, Adams S, Harris MB, et al: Are plain radiographs of the spine necessary during evaluation after blunt trauma? Accuracy of screening torso computed tomography in thoracic/lumbar spine fracture diagnosis. *J Trauma* 2005;59:1410-1413.

25. Sroka NL, Combs J, Mood R, Henderson V: Scout anteroposterior and lateral CT scans as a screening test for thoracolumbar spine injury in blunt trauma. *Am Surg* 2007;73:780-785.

26. Lee JY, Vaccaro AR, Schweitzer KM, et al: Assessment of injury to the thoracolumbar posterior ligamentous complex in the setting of normal-appearing plain radiography. *Spine J* 2007;7:422-427.

27. Lee HM, Kim HS, Kim DJ, Suk KS, Park JO, Kim NH: Reliability of magnetic resonance imaging in detecting posterior ligament complex injury in thoracolumbar spinal fractures. *Spine* 2000;25:2079-2084.

28. Kelly RP, Whitesides TE Jr: Treatment of lumbodorsal fracture-dislocations. *Ann Surg* 1968;167: 705-717.

29. Denis F: The three column spine and its significance in the classification of acute thoracolumbar spinal injuries. *Spine* 1983;8:817-831.

30. Holdsworth F: Fractures, dislocations and fracture-dislocations of the spine. *J Bone Joint Surg Br* 1963;45:6-20.

31. Holdsworth F: Fractures, dislocations, and fracture-dislocations of the spine. *J Bone Joint Surg Am* 1970;52: 1534-1551.

32. Magerl F, Aebi M, Gertzbein SD, Harms J, Nazarian S: A comprehensive classification of thoracic and lumbar injuries. *Eur Spine J* 1994;3: 184-201.

33. McAfee PC, Yuan HA, Fredrickson BE, Lubicky JP: The value of computed tomography in thoracolumbar fractures: An analysis of one hundred consecutive cases and a new classification. *J Bone Joint Surg Am* 1983;65:461-473.

34. Ferguson RL, Allen BL Jr: A mechanistic classification of thoracolumbar spine fractures. *Clin Orthop Relat Res* 1984;189:77-88.

35. McCormack T, Karaikovic E, Gaines RW: The load sharing classification of spine fractures. *Spine* 1994;19:1741-1744.

36. Blauth M, Bastian L, Knop C, Lange U, Tusch G: [Inter-observer reliability in the classification of thoracolumbar spinal injuries]. *Orthopade* 1999;28:662-681.

37. Oner FC, Ramos LM, Simmermacher RK, et al: Classification of thoracic and lumbar spine fractures: Problems of reproducibility. A study of 53 patients using CT and MRI. *Eur Spine J* 2002;11:235-245.

38. Wood KB, Khanna G, Vaccaro AR, Arnold PM, Harris MB, Mehbod AA: Assessment of two thoracolumbar fracture classification systems as used by multiple surgeons. *J Bone Joint Surg Am* 2005;87:1423-1429.

39. Vaccaro AR, Lim MR, Hurlbert RJ, et al: Surgical decision making for unstable thoracolumbar spine injuries: Results of a consensus panel review by the Spine Trauma Study Group. *J Spinal Disord Tech* 2006;19:1-10.

40. Vaccaro AR, Zeiller SC, Hulbert RJ, et al: The thoracolumbar injury severity score: A proposed treatment algorithm. *J Spinal Disord Tech* 2005;18: 209-215.

41. Whang PG, Vaccaro AR, Poelstra KA, et al: The influence of fracture mechanism and morphology on the reliability and validity of two novel thoracolumbar injury classification systems. *Spine* 2007;32:791-795.

42. Bono CM, Vaccaro AR, Hurlbert RJ, et al: Validating a newly proposed classification system for thoracolumbar spine trauma: Looking to the future of the thoracolumbar injury classification and severity score. *J Orthop Trauma* 2006;20:567-572.

3

Nonsurgical Treatment of Thoracolumbar Spinal Fractures

*Mitchel B. Harris, MD, FACS
Lewis L. Shi, MD
Alexander R. Vacarro, MD, PhD
*Thomas A. Zdeblick, MD
*Rick C. Sasso, MD

Abstract

The transitional anatomy of the thoracolumbar spine makes it vulnerable to injury from high-energy vehicular crashes and falls. The definitive management of patients with thoracolumbar spinal fractures is dependent on the presence and extent of neurologic injury, the presence and magnitude of acute deformity, and an estimate concerning spinal stability. It is well established that neurologic deficits generally improve without surgery. Nonsurgical treatment leads to decreased pain and improved function. Although there is a dearth of high-quality studies comparing surgical with nonsurgical treatment, the natural course of thoracolumbar fractures usually is benign, and nonsurgical methods should be the standard treatment with few exceptions.

The treatment of thoracolumbar spinal fractures remains controversial. The goal of all spinal fracture management is to maximize functional recovery. This includes optimizing neurologic function, preventing any (further) neurologic injury, restoring spinal stability, and achieving pain-free activity. The key issues in comparing the merits of surgical and nonsurgical treatment are neurology, stability, and complications related to treatment.

Neurology

The natural alignment of the thoracic spine is one of kyphosis with a narrow spinal canal. The rib cage and sternum provide significant additional stability, resisting flexion and lateral stress. The conus medullaris is the termination of the spinal cord, located between T11 and L2; the cauda equina is the collection of nerve roots that continue distally. In the lower lumbar spine, the sagittal alignment becomes lordotic, and the spinal canal is wider. The cauda equina is more resistant to extrinsic pressure than the conus medullaris at the thoracolumbar junction.

Most spinal fractures and dislocations occur at the thoracolumbar junction, which is a transitional zone between a rigid kyphotic thoracic spine and a flexible lordotic lumbar spine. The normal alignment at the junction is neutral. These anatomic features not only predispose this spinal region to injury but also can lead to late sagittal and coronal decompensation if the balance between the anterior and posterior columns is disrupted. The posterior elements and their soft-tissue attachments play an essential role in maintaining stability of the thoracolumbar junction.

Numerous studies have examined the role of imaging as it relates to neurologic injury. Hashimoto

Mitchel B. Harris, MD, FACS or the department with which he is affiliated has received research or institutional support from Synthes and is a consultant for or an employee of Globus and DePuy. Thomas A. Zdeblick, MD or the department with which he is affiliated has received royalties from Medtronic and is a consultant for or an employee of Medtron and Anulex. Rick C. Sasso, MD or the department with which he is affiliated has received research or institutional support from Medtronic, Stryker, AO, Cerapedics, and Lilly; has received royalties from Medtronic; holds stock or stock options in Biomet and SpineCare; and is a consultant for or an employee of Medtronic.

Table 1
Neurologic Improvement of Patients With Thoracolumbar Fractures Undergoing Nonsurgical Treatment (N = 205)

Frankel Grade at Injury (n)	Frankel Grade at Hospital Discharge				
	A	B	C	D	E
A (126)	**102**	12	2	10	0
B (24)	1	**4**	2	15	2
C (25)	1		**4**	16	4
D (27)				**18**	9
E (3)					**3**

Frankel grade: A, complete injury; B, sensory only; C, useless motor; D, useful motor; E, intact

Bold numbers represent patients with no change in grade; the numbers above represent patients whose grade improved, and numbers below represent patients whose grade deteriorated.
Data from Frankel HL, Hancock DO, Hyslop G, et al: The value of postural reduction in the initial management of closed injuries of the spine with paraplegia and tetraplegia. *Paraplegia* 1969;7:179-192.

and associates[1] studied 112 patients with thoracolumbar burst fractures, using CT scans to analyze relationships between spinal canal compromise and neurologic deficits. They concluded that spinal stenosis of 35% or more at the T11-12 level, 45% or more at L1, and 55% or more at L2 and below were significant risk factors for neurologic involvement in burst fractures. These results are consistent with other studies that have shown a poor correlation between canal encroachment measured radiographically and neurologic deficit. In an in vitro study, Panjabi and associates[2] studied dynamic canal encroachment during thoracolumbar burst fractures and found that the dynamic encroachment was 85% more than the static measurement made after trauma. This finding was significant in illustrating to clinicians that radiographs and CT scans often do not adequately describe the situation at the time of trauma. Conversely, in the absence of a neurologic deficit, retropulsed bony fragments can be left alone and do not represent an indication for surgery.

A significant body of literature supports the nonsurgical treatment of thoracolumbar spinal fractures. There is no evidence in the literature demonstrating that surgical decompression improves the neurologic recovery of an incomplete injury any more reliably than nonsurgical management. However, relative indications for surgical management include progressive neurologic deficit, incomplete injury with residual canal compromise in a patient whose improvement has reached a plateau, and patients who present with fracture-dislocations and neurologic injury.

The proponents of surgical treatment often cite animal model studies that advocate immediate decompression. Rivlin and Tator[3,4] and Dolan and associates[5] published a series of studies using a modified aneurysmal clip on rat spines to simulate cord compression. The severity of the injury was related to the time and force of compression. They concluded that compression should be relieved as soon as possible to effect maximal recovery. Delamarter and associates[6] and Carlson and associates[7] provided further support to the importance of early decompression to facilitate neurologic recovery in other animal models.

In humans, nonsurgical treatment leads to neurologic recovery, as has been demonstrated in numerous retrospective studies. In 1969, Frankel and associates[8] described 682 patients with spinal injuries treated with postural reduction; among these, 205 patients had injuries of the thoracolumbar spine. The results of the injuries were presented in Frankel grades: complete injury (A), sensory only (B), motor useless (C), motor useful (D), and intact/full recovery (E). From the time of injury to the time of discharge, the condition of 2 patients (1.0%) deteriorated, 131 (63.9%) remained the same grade, and 72 (35.1%) improved one or more Frankel grades (Table 1).

Davies and associates[9] described the nonsurgical treatment of 34 patients with thoracolumbar injuries with neurologic deficits. Twelve patients (35.3%) had no change in neurologic status, whereas 15 patients (44%) improved one Frankel grade, and 7 (21%) improved two or more grades. No patients deteriorated neurologically (Table 2).

Hartman and associates[10] reported similar results in 32 patients with an average follow-up of 22.3 months. Nine patients who presented with incomplete spinal injuries all improved at least one Frankel grade after nonsurgical treatment. Kinoshita and associates[11] reported similar results.

Studies have consistently demonstrated that there is a definite role for nonsurgical management of thoracolumbar fractures in the presence of a neurologic injury because patients with incomplete spinal cord injury usually improve by one Frankel grade.

Stability

The treatment algorithm for thoracolumbar fractures depends on the ability to accurately assess spinal stability. The clinical definition of spinal instability is the loss of the ability of the spine, under physiologic stress, to maintain its alignment and to prevent increased deformity leading to pain or neurologic deficit.

Neutral Zone Theory

Through in vitro experiments, Panjabi and associates[12,13] developed the neutral zone theory, which emphasizes the nonlinear nature of spinal loading (Figure 1). Loads delivered at the initiation of the load-deformation curve have different effects on displacement of the spine than at later phases. In this theory, the spinal range of motion is separated into two independent motion parameters—the neutral zone and the elastic zone. During loading, both physiologic and traumatic, the ligaments and disk offer resistance to deformation.[13] Within the neutral zone, motion is produced with little internal resistance; that is, the spine is flexible. This represents the ordinary physiologic motion, where there is displacement with minimal force. Within the elastic zone, motion is the result of overcoming internal resistance. Greater force is needed to effect displacement, and at the upper part of the elastic zone curve, tissue injury may occur, leading to later degenerative changes.

With spinal trauma, the neutral zone increases, the elastic zone predominantly decreases, and the spine becomes hypermobile. A modified definition of instability, using the neutral zone theory, includes the capacity of the spine to maintain the size of the neutral zone and to prevent pain, deformity, and neurologic deficit. Rigid fixation, either surgical or through bracing, can restore the neutral zone to normal. This theory has no practical clinical application but does explain the nature of failure of the soft-tissue elements of the spine.

Table 2
Neurologic Improvement of Patients With Thoracolumbar Fractures Undergoing Nonsurgical Treatment (N = 34)

Frankel Grade at Injury (n)	Frankel Grade at Hospital Discharge				
	A	B	C	D	E
A (14)	**11**	1	1	1	
B (5)			1	4	
C (14)			**1**	12	1
D (1)					1
E					

Frankel grade: A, complete injury; B, sensory only; C, useless motor; D, useful motor; E, intact

Bold numbers represent patients with no change in grade; the numbers above represent improvement. Data from Davies WE, Morris JH, Hill V: An analysis of conservative (nonsurgical) management of thoracolumbar fractures and fracture-dislocations with neural damage. *J Bone Joint Surg Am* 1980;62:1324-1328.

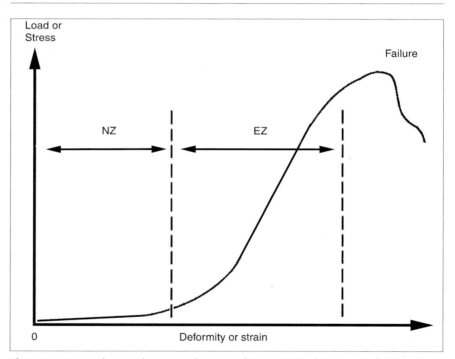

Figure 1 Neutral zone theory. In the neutral zone (NZ), the spine is flexible (such that there is physiologic motion with minimal force). In the elastic zone (EZ), motion is the result of overcoming internal resistance. A greater amount of force is needed to bring about displacement. At the upper part of the EZ curve, as the spine displaces further, tissue injury may occur.

Column Theories and Newer Classifications

Although theoretic constructs make sense in the laboratory, clinicians tend to favor concepts of stability that are applicable to common patient scenarios. Many classification systems have tried to correlate biomechanics or mechanisms of injury with clinical instability. This correlation is understandably difficult, given the heterogeneity of the spine

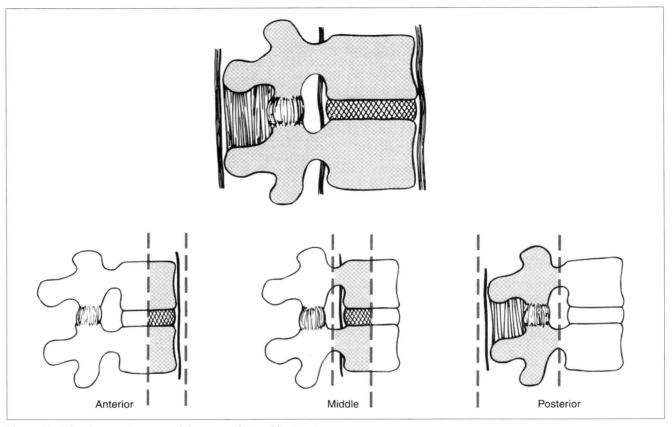

Figure 2   The three-column model, as popularized by Denis.

and the variability of forces applied to it. Most of these classification systems have shortcomings and inconsistencies.

Holdsworth's two-column theory divides the spine into anterior and posterior columns.[14] The anterior column consists of the anterior longitudinal ligament, vertebral body, intervertebral disk, anulus fibrosus, and posterior longitudinal ligament. The posterior column consists of the facet joint complex, ligamentum flavum, and interspinous and supraspinous ligaments. Holdsworth formally introduced his two-column theory in 1962, but in the 1950s he had already recognized the importance of the posterior ligamentous complex (PLC), citing its competence as a crucial determinant

in spinal stability.[15] Modern biomechanical testing of in vitro fracture models confirmed the major contribution of the PLC. James and associates[16] demonstrated that the integrity of the posterior column is far more important in resisting the flexion moment at the T12-L2 motion segment than the middle column.

The three-column theory, which introduced the additional osteoligamentous middle column, was popularized by Denis[17] (Figure 2). He correlated his fracture classification with degrees of instability and provided a basic rationale for treatment. Instability of the first degree, or mechanical instability, occurs when there is a disruption of the anterior and posterior columns, as in a severe compression fracture with distrac-

tion of the posterior elements, or when there is a disruption of the middle and posterior columns, as occurs in a seat-belt–type fracture. These fractures are considered mechanically unstable because they are at risk for either further compression or angulation with increasing kyphotic deformity. External immobilization may not be adequate. Instability of the second degree, or neurologic instability, generally results from a burst fracture or fracture subluxation. There is increased risk for further collapse of the vertebral body with further encroachment of free bone fragments into the spinal canal, leading to the development or worsening of neurologic compromise. In the second degree of instability, the presence of a neurologic injury does not imply that the fracture is biomechanically unstable, although it is a strong indication for surgical intervention. Instability of the third degree, or mechanical and neurologic instability, occurs with severe burst fractures with neurologic injury or with fracture-dislocations involving disruption of all three columns in association with neurologic injury. These fractures are inherently unstable and have a higher likelihood of neurologic deterioration and painful deformity. Fractures with third-degree instability almost always require surgical reduction, decompression, and stabilization.

In 2005, the Spine Trauma Study Group, an international panel of expert spine trauma surgeons, introduced a new classification system called the Thoracolumbar Injury Classification and Severity (TLICS) score to allow a more systematic assessment of fracture morphology in combination with clinical findings of the presence of a neurologic injury.[18-20] Before this initiative, neurologic injury had not been incorporated into a combined classification and scoring system. TLICS assigns points for each of three parameters, involving injury morphology, condition of the PLC, and neurologic status (Table 3). Injury morphology includes compression, burst, translation/rotation, and distraction. The integrity of the PLC is classified as intact, indeterminate, or disrupted. Neurologic status is intact or is a complete or incomplete injury. Nerve root injuries are assigned two points. The TLICS score ranges from 1 to 10 points. The Spine Trauma Study Group recommends that patients whose TLICS is 3 points or lower should be treated nonsurgically, those with scores of 5 points or higher should be treated

surgically, and those with a score of 4 points should be evaluated on a case-by-case basis. This scoring classification has been validated through prospective studies.[21-23]

PLC and the Use of MRI in Spinal Trauma

TLICS places priority on determining the integrity of the PLC to accurately assess spinal stability and guide optimal treatment. The PLC consists of the interspinous ligament, supraspinous ligament, facet capsules, and ligamentum flavum. In a prospective study, Lee and associates[24] showed that fat-suppressed, T2-weighted MRI is accurate in diagnosing posterior ligamentous disruption. Preoperative MRI results of 34 patients with thoracolumbar spinal fractures were compared with the surgical findings of PLC integrity. Positive predictive values were greater than 96% for diagnosing interspinous and supraspinous ligament injuries and 67% for ligamentum flavum injuries. Haba and associates[25] published similar results, using MRI to detect PLC disruption.

In addition to the direct evaluation of the PLC with MRI, indirect methods of assessment can be used. In a panel review published by the Spine Trauma Study Group, most experts believed that radiographic evidence of vertebral body translation was an important factor in determining the integrity of the PLC.[26] Other important clinical and radiographic determinants of PLC incompetence included a palpable interspinous gap, focal kyphosis without vertebral body fracture, and interspinous widening or facet joint diastasis seen on plain radiographs or CT.

Complications

The potential adverse effects of thoracolumbar fracture management

Table 3
Thoracolumbar Injury Classification and Severity Score

Parameter	Points
Mechanism of Injury	
Compression	1
Burst	2
Translation/rotation	3
Distraction	4
Posterior Ligamentous Complex	
Intact	0
Indeterminate	2
Disrupted	3
Neurologic Deficit	
Intact	0
Complete injury	2
Incomplete injury	3
Total	1 to 10

should be taken into account when determining treatment options. These include immediate and long-term complications of the treatment, residual deformity (nonsurgical), neurologic function, pain, and ability to return to work.

In a Scoliosis Research Society–sponsored multicenter prospective study, 1,019 spinal fracture patients were followed for 2 years; the results of surgical and nonsurgical treatment groups were compared.[27] The authors found that neurologic function (improvement) and pain were not statistically different between the surgical and nonsurgical groups; however, 25% of the surgically treated patients had significant complications compared with 3% of the nonsurgical patients. These included both intraoperative and postoperative complications such as a pulmonary embolus, wound infection, and hardware failure.

Weinstein and associates[28,29] evaluated 42 patients (20-year follow-up) with nonsurgically treated thoracolumbar fractures. Eighty-eight percent of the patients returned to work at their preinjury level, and no patients required narcotic medication for low back pain.

The degree of kyphosis did not correlate with pain or function.

In a retrospective study of 24 "unstable" burst fractures, of which 10 were known to have a disrupted PLC, it was shown that treatment with 6 to 8 weeks of recumbency followed by gradual mobilization in a hyperextension brace resulted in a good outcome.[30] Nineteen of 24 patients had minimal or no pain at follow-up, and 18 patients had no work restrictions. The authors concluded that ligamentous injury of the posterior column is not a contraindication to nonsurgical management of thoracolumbar burst fractures.

Shen and Shen[31] evaluated 38 patients with burst fractures with known posterior column involvement. Twenty-nine patients were treated with immediate ambulation and no bracing, and nine patients were treated with a Jewett brace. At 4-year follow-up, 32 of the 38 patients (84%) reported either occasional or no pain. Twenty-nine patients (76%) returned to their previous level of work. Similar to other studies, the authors found no correlation between kyphosis, canal compromise, and clinical outcome.

Rechtine and associates[32] reported on 235 patients with unstable thoracolumbar fractures. The retrospective study compared 117 patients who had surgery with 118 patients who had nonsurgical treatment consisting of 6 weeks on a kinetic bed. There was no statistical difference in the rates of decubitus, pneumonia, deep venous thrombosis, pulmonary embolism, or mortality. The surgical group had an 8% rate of deep wound infections. The nonsurgical group had 24-day longer hospital stays, but the two groups did not have a significant difference in the cost of the hospital stay.

Nonsurgical treatment can yield clinical results similar to surgical treatment but without the inherent risks of surgery.

Search for Evidence-Based Medicine

Although multiple case studies support nonsurgical treatment of thoracolumbar fractures,[9,33-37] there are also case studies that advocate surgical treatment.[38] To date, only two randomized controlled trials have directly compared surgical and nonsurgical treatments.

Wood and associates[39] randomized 47 consecutive neurologically intact patients with burst fractures to either surgical or nonsurgical treatment. Patients with disruption of the PLC were excluded. PLC disruption was defined by plain radiographic or CT evidence of facet fracture-dislocation or flexion-distraction ligamentous disruption. The surgically treated group had anterior or posterior stabilization, without canal decompression. Nonsurgical treatment involved the use of a body cast or a thoracolumbosacral orthosis. After an average follow-up of 44 months, there was no advantage to surgery in fracture alignment, pain, or physical function. There was no statistical difference in the degree of final kyphosis; the surgical group correction changed from 10.1° to 13°, and the nonsurgical group changed from 11.3° to 13.8°. The average visual analog pain scale score at the time of the latest follow-up was 3.3 for the surgical group and 1.9 for the nonsurgical group. Medical Outcomes Study 36-Item Short Form and Oswestry scores favored the nonsurgical group, although the differences were not statistically significant. Differences in return-to-work rates also were not statistically significant—58% in the surgical group and 83% in the nonsurgical group. Complications were more frequent in the surgical group (19) than in the nonsurgical group (2). The average hospital charge was more than four times higher in the surgical group than in the nonsurgical group ($49,063 compared with $11,264). The authors identified several limitations of their study, such as 11% of patients lost to follow-up and a small sample size and thus smaller power; however, they were able to conclude that surgical treatment of stable thoracolumbar burst fractures yields no substantial benefit compared with nonsurgical treatment.

More recently, Siebenga and associates[40] published a European multicenter prospective randomized controlled trial of patients with traumatic thoracolumbar spinal fractures without neurologic deficit; the results were generally in favor of surgical treatment. Thirty-four patients were randomized to receive short-segment posterior stabilization or nonsurgical treatment. These patients were followed for an average of 4.3 years, with a follow-up rate of 94% (32 patients). The length of the hospital stay was similar in both groups. The rates of complications were not significantly different: five complications occurred in the 17 surgically treated patients (broken screws, prominent screws, deep infection, superficial infection, iliac crest donor-site pain), and three complications occurred in the 15 nonsurgically treated patients (scoliosis, conus medullaris syndrome, chronic pain). However, the rest of the variables favored the surgical group. Local and regional kyphotic deformity was significantly improved in patients who had surgery ($P < 0.0001$). Those patients also had higher functional outcome scores (visual analog pain scale, visual analog spine scale, 24-Item Roland-Morris Disability Questionnaire), with *P* values ranging between 0.020 and 0.033. The return-to-work rate was significantly higher in the surgical group (*P* = 0.018), although the Dutch and German welfare systems and insurance policy involvement may have affected this analysis. When compared with the randomized controlled trial of Wood and associates,[39] this study's surgical treatment included more intraoperative reduction of kyphosis with the use of bisegmental pedicle screws as lever arms for reduction. The authors postulated that the surgical patients in the study by Wood and associates[39] may have had more pain because of the more extensive surgical approach needed for multilevel posterior stabilization or postthoracotomy pain after the anterior approach. Other concerns regarding the study by Siebenga and associates[40] are the small sample size, which may affect its generalizability, and the fact that the nonsurgical treatment group used a Jewett brace, which has minimal ability to control lateral and rotational movement. The study also included two cases of missed distraction injuries as confirmed by intraoperative findings; the nonsurgical group may have included patients with missed distraction injuries who would have been inadequately treated with a Jewett brace. These reasons may have directly or indirectly resulted in poorer outcomes for the nonsurgical patients.

In addition to these two randomized controlled trials, several systematic reviews of thoracolumbar fracture treatments have been published in recent years.[41-44] van der Roer and associates[41] evaluated 17 studies from January 1992 to January 2003 and reported that there was not enough evidence to draw any conclusion about whether surgical or nonsurgical treatment is more effective for unstable traumatic thoracolumbar fractures. The Cochrane Library published a review of the prospective trial by Wood and associates.[39,42] Thomas and associates[43] reviewed 141 articles of potential relevance and found that 21 were the most relevant. They concluded that although surgery may result in earlier mobilization and hospital discharge, less initial pain, and faster return to work, there is minimal available evidence to justify the additional risks of surgery. The 2007 review by Dai and associates[44] reached a similar conclusion, with an emphasis that surgical treatment should be considered only if neurologic involvement is significant.

Summary

As a result of ongoing clinical uncertainties, nonsurgical management must be considered the preferred treatment for thoracolumbar fractures, except in patients with progressive kyphosis or a progressive neurologic loss with evidence of canal compromise. The proponents of surgery cite a variety of purported benefits, such as early mobilization, correction and prevention of kyphotic deformity, correction of canal compromise, and protection against potential neurologic injury; however, these arguments are not clearly supported by the literature.

Even though surgery can improve sagittal alignment in the short term, studies have shown that the spine returns to its initial level of deformity over the long term, regardless of nonsurgical treatment or anterior, posterior, or combined surgical approaches.[45] In patients with canal compromise, decompression is unnecessary in the absence of neurologic injury. Spontaneous remodeling of the spinal canal occurs with nonsurgical treatment.[46-48] Mumford and associates[46] showed that in all 41 patients, an average of two thirds of the retropulsed bone was resorbed. As for neurologic injury, new deficits occurring during the course of nonsurgical treatment of a thoracolumbar burst fracture are rare. In nine clinical studies with a total of 274 patients, there was only one case of neurologic deterioration after nonsurgical treatment.[29-31,33-36,46,49]

The natural history of most thoracolumbar fractures is benign. The standard treatment of most thoracolumbar fractures should be nonsurgical. The burden of proof is to demonstrate that surgery, with its attendant morbidity and expense, is superior to nonsurgical care.

References

1. Hashimoto T, Kaneda K, Abumi K: Relationship between traumatic spinal canal stenosis and neurologic deficits in thoracolumbar burst fractures. *Spine* 1988;13:1268-1272.

2. Panjabi MM, Kifune M, Wen L, et al: Dynamic canal encroachment during thoracolumbar burst fractures. *J Spinal Disord* 1995;8:39-48.

3. Rivlin AS, Tator CH: Objective clinical assessment of motor function after experimental spinal cord injury in the rat. *J Neurosurg* 1977;47:577-581.

4. Rivlin AS, Tator CH: Effect of duration of acute spinal cord compression in a new acute cord injury model in the rat. *Surg Neurol* 1978;10:38-43.

5. Dolan EJ, Tator CH, Endrenyi L: The value of decompression for acute experimental spinal cord compression injury. *J Neurosurg* 1980;53:749-755.

6. Delamarter RB, Sherman J, Carr JB: Pathophysiology of spinal cord injury: Recovery after immediate and

delayed decompression. *J Bone Joint Surg Am* 1995;77:1042-1049.

7. Carlson GD, Minato Y, Okada A, et al: Early time-dependent decompression for spinal cord injury: Vascular mechanisms of recovery. *J Neurotrauma* 1997;14:951-962.

8. Frankel HL, Hancock DO, Hyslop G, et al: The value of postural reduction in the initial management of closed injuries of the spine with paraplegia and tetraplegia. *Paraplegia* 1969;7: 179-192.

9. Davies WE, Morris JH, Hill V: An analysis of conservative (nonsurgical) management of thoracolumbar fractures and fracture-dislocations with neural damage. *J Bone Joint Surg Am* 1980;62:1324-1328.

10. Hartman MB, Chrin AM, Rechtine GR: Non-operative treatment of thoracolumbar fractures. *Paraplegia* 1995;33:73-76.

11. Kinoshita H, Nagata Y, Ueda H, Kishi K: Conservative treatment of burst fractures of the thoracolumbar and lumbar spine. *Paraplegia* 1993;31: 58-67.

12. Panjabi MM, Goel VK, Takata K: Physiologic strains in the lumbar spinal ligaments: An in vitro biomechanical study. *Spine* 1982;7:192-203.

13. Panjabi MM, Oxland TR, Lin RM, McGowen TW: Thoracolumbar burst fracture: A biomechanical investigation of its multidirectional flexibility. *Spine* 1994;19:578-585.

14. Holdsworth F: Fractures, dislocations, and fracture-dislocations of the spine. *J Bone Joint Surg Am* 1970;52: 1534-1551.

15. Holdsworth FW, Hardy A: Early treatment of paraplegia from fractures of the thoraco-lumbar spine. *J Bone Joint Surg Br* 1953;35:540-550.

16. James KS, Wenger KH, Schlegel JD, Dunn HK: Biomechanical evaluation of the stability of thoracolumbar burst fractures. *Spine* 1994;19:1731-1740.

17. Denis F: The three column spine and its significance in the classification of acute thoracolumbar spinal injuries. *Spine* 1983;8:817-831.

18. Vaccaro AR, Zeiller SC, Hulbert RJ, et al: The thoracolumbar injury severity score: A proposed treatment algorithm. *J Spinal Disord Tech* 2005;18: 209-215.

19. Vaccaro AR, Lehman RA Jr, Hurlbert RJ, et al: A new classification of thoracolumbar injuries: The importance of injury morphology, the integrity of the posterior ligamentous complex, and neurologic status. *Spine* 2005;30:2325-2333.

20. Lee JY, Vaccaro AR, Lim MR, et al: Thoracolumbar injury classification and severity score: A new paradigm for the treatment of thoracolumbar spine trauma. *J Orthop Sci* 2005;10: 671-675.

21. Patel AA, Vaccaro AR, Albert TJ, et al: The adoption of a new classification system: Time-dependent variation in interobserver reliability of the thoracolumbar injury severity score classification system. *Spine* 2007;32:E105-E110.

22. Whang PG, Vaccaro AR, Poelstra KA, et al: The influence of fracture mechanism and morphology on the reliability and validity of two novel thoracolumbar injury classification systems. *Spine* 2007;32:791-795.

23. Vaccaro AR, Baron EM, Sanfilippo J, et al: Reliability of a novel classification system for thoracolumbar injuries: The thoracolumbar injury severity score. *Spine* 2006;31:S62-S69.

24. Lee HM, Kim HS, Kim DJ, Suk KS, Park JO, Kim NH: Reliability of magnetic resonance imaging in detecting posterior ligament complex injury in thoracolumbar spinal fractures. *Spine* 2000;25:2079-2084.

25. Haba H, Taneichi H, Kotani Y, et al: Diagnostic accuracy of magnetic resonance imaging for detecting posterior ligamentous complex injury associated with thoracic and lumbar fractures. *J Neurosurg* 2003;99(suppl 1): 20-26.

26. Vaccaro AR, Lee JY, Schweitzer KM Jr, et al: Assessment of injury to the posterior ligamentous complex in thoracolumbar spine trauma. *Spine J* 2006;6:524-528.

27. Gertzbein SD: Scoliosis Research Society: Multicenter spine fracture study. *Spine* 1992;17:528-540.

28. Weinstein JN, Collalto P, Lehmann TR: Long-term follow-up of nonoperatively treated thoracolumbar spine fractures. *J Orthop Trauma* 1987; 1:152-159.

29. Weinstein JN, Collalto P, Lehmann TR: Thoracolumbar "burst" fractures treated conservatively: A long-term follow-up. *Spine* 1988;13: 33-38.

30. Chow GH, Nelson BJ, Gebhard JS, Brugman JL, Brown CW, Donaldson DH: Functional outcome of thoracolumbar burst fractures managed with hyperextension casting or bracing and early mobilization. *Spine* 1996;21:2170-2175.

31. Shen WJ, Shen YS: Nonsurgical treatment of three-column thoracolumbar junction burst fractures without neurologic deficit. *Spine* 1999;24: 412-415.

32. Rechtine GR II, Cahill D, Chrin AM: Treatment of thoracolumbar trauma: Comparison of complications of operative versus nonoperative treatment. *J Spinal Disord* 1999;12: 406-409.

33. Cantor JB, Lebwohl NH, Garvey T, Eismont FJ: Nonoperative management of stable thoracolumbar burst fractures with early ambulation and bracing. *Spine* 1993;18:971-976.

34. Tropiano P, Huang RC, Louis CA, Poitout DG, Louis RP: Functional and radiographic outcome of thoracolumbar and lumbar burst fractures managed by closed orthopaedic reduction and casting. *Spine* 2003;28: 2459-2465.

35. Seybold EA, Sweeney CA, Fredrickson BE, Warhold LG, Bernini PM: Functional outcome of low lumbar burst fractures: A multicenter review of operative and nonoperative treatment of L3-L5. *Spine* 1999;24:2154-2161.

36. Kraemer WJ, Schemitsch EH, Lever J, McBroom RJ, McKee MD, Waddell JP: Functional outcome of thoracolumbar burst fractures without neurological deficit. *J Orthop Trauma* 1996;10:541-544.

37. Ohana N, Sheinis D, Rath E, Sasson A, Atar D: Is there a need for lumbar orthosis in mild compression fractures of the thoracolumbar spine? A retrospective study comparing the radiographic results between early ambulation with and without lumbar orthosis. *J Spinal Disord* 2000;13: 305-308.

38. Denis F, Armstrong GW, Searls K, Matta L: Acute thoracolumbar burst fractures in the absence of neurologic deficit: A comparison between operative and nonoperative treatment. *Clin Orthop Relat Res* 1984;189:142-149.

39. Wood K, Buttermann G, Mehbod A, et al: Operative compared with nonoperative treatment of a thoracolumbar burst fracture without neurological deficit: A prospective, randomized study. *J Bone Joint Surg Am* 2003;85: 773-781.

40. Siebenga J, Leferink VJ, Segers MJ, et al: Treatment of traumatic thoracolumbar spine fractures: A multicenter prospective randomized study of operative versus nonsurgical treatment. *Spine* 2006;31:2881-2890.

41. van der Roer N, de Lange ES, Bakker FC, de Vet HC, van Tulder MW: Management of traumatic thoracolumbar fractures: A systematic review of the literature. *Eur Spine J* 2005;14:527-534.

42. Yi L, Jingping B, Gele J, Baoleri X, Taixiang W: Operative versus nonoperative treatment for thoracolumbar burst fractures without neurological deficit. *Cochrane Database Syst Rev* 2006;4:CD005079.

43. Thomas KC, Bailey CS, Dvorak MF, Kwon B, Fisher C: Comparison of operative and nonoperative treatment for thoracolumbar burst fractures in patients without neurological deficit: A systematic review. *J Neurosurg Spine* 2006;4:351-358.

44. Dai LY, Jiang SD, Wang XY, Jiang LS: A review of the management of thoracolumbar burst fractures. *Surg Neurol* 2007;67:221-231.

45. Verlaan JJ, Diekerhof CH, Buskens E, et al: Surgical treatment of traumatic fractures of the thoracic and lumbar spine: A systematic review of the literature on techniques, complications, and outcome. *Spine* 2004;29:803-814.

46. Mumford J, Weinstein JN, Spratt KF, Goel VK: Thoracolumbar burst fractures: The clinical efficacy and outcome of nonoperative management. *Spine* 1993;18:955-970.

47. de Klerk LW, Fontijne WP, Stijnen T, Braakman R, Tanghe HL, van Linge B: Spontaneous remodeling of the spinal canal after conservative management of thoracolumbar burst fractures. *Spine* 1998;23:1057-1060.

48. Sandor L, Barabas D: Spontaneous "regeneration" of the spinal canal in traumatic bone fragments after fractures of the thoraco-lumbar transition and the lumbar spine. *Unfallchirurg* 1994;97:89-91.

49. Reid DC, Hu R, Davis LA, Saboe LA: The nonoperative treatment of burst fractures of the thoracolumbar junction. *J Trauma* 1988;28:1188-1194.

4

Surgical Treatment of Thoracolumbar Fractures

*Thomas A. Zdeblick, MD
*Rick C. Sasso, MD
Alexander R. Vaccaro, MD, PhD
*Jens R. Chapman, MD
*Mitchel B. Harris, MD, FACS

Abstract

Surgical management of a thoracolumbar fracture varies according to many factors. Fracture morphology, neurologic status, and surgeon preference play major roles in deciding on an anterior, a posterior, or a combined approach. The goal is to optimize neural decompression while providing stable internal fixation over the least number of spinal segments. Short-segment constructs through a single-stage approach (anterior or posterior) have become viable options with advances in instrumentation and techniques. Unstable burst fractures can be treated with anterior-only fixation using a strut graft and a modern thoracolumbar plating system or with a posterior-only construct using pedicle screws and possibly hooks. A circumferential construct is considered for extremely unstable injuries.

Unstable fractures of the thoracolumbar spine require internal fixation. Unstable burst fractures generally can be identified by either clinical findings of posterior hematoma, palpable interspinous gap and tenderness, and interspinous widening or by evidence of posterior ligamentous complex failure on appropriate MRI sagittal views or plain radiographs. Stabilization and decompression of these injuries allow early mobilization and the potential for neurologic improvement. Optimal treatment of these injuries remains controversial. Some surgeons prefer to use posterior indirect decompression and instrumentation techniques; others advocate an anterior-only approach to directly decompress the neural elements, followed by internal fixation; and some recommend a combined anterior and posterior approach. Limiting the length of instrumentation is optimal to minimize immobilization of the normal adjacent structures.

Burst Fractures

Burst fractures at the thoracolumbar junction are common and often lead to surgical treatment. Typically, these fractures are caused by a flexion and axial load mechanism that causes failure of the anterior column under compression and the posterior vertebral cortical wall as well. Retropulsion of the "culprit" fragment of the posterior vertebral wall attached to the posterior disk anulus often creates canal compromise and associated neurologic injury. As displacement of the posterior wall occurs, the pedicles often are displaced laterally, with widening of the spine (Figure 1). With continued flexion

★*Thomas A. Zdeblick, MD or the department with which he is affiliated has received royalties from Medtronic and is a consultant for or an employee of Medtronic and Anulex. Rick C. Sasso, MD or the department with which he is affiliated has received research or institutional support from Medtronic, Stryker, AO, Cerapedics, and Lilly; has received royalties from Medtronic; holds stock or stock options in Biomet and SpineCare; and is a consultant for or an employee of Medtronic. Jens R. Chapman, MD or the department with which he is affiliated has received research or institutional support from Synthes, Medtronic, Johnson & Johnson, and Paradigm; has received miscellaneous nonincome support, commercially derived honoraria, or other nonresearch-related funding from Synthes; and is a consultant for or an employee of Synthes. Mitchel B. Harris, MD, FACS or the department with which he is affiliated has received research or institutional support from Synthes, Zimmer, DePuy, and Medtronic; has received miscellaneous nonincome support, commercially derived honoraria, or other nonresearch-related funding from AO Foundation; and is a consultant for or an employee of Globus.*

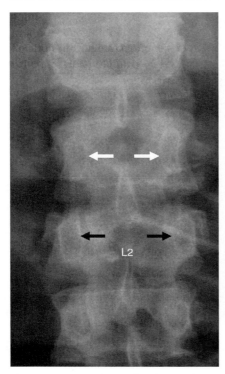

Figure 1 AP radiograph of an L2 burst fracture showing that the pedicles are displaced laterally, widening the spine at L2 (black arrows) compared with the pedicles seen at L1 (white arrows).

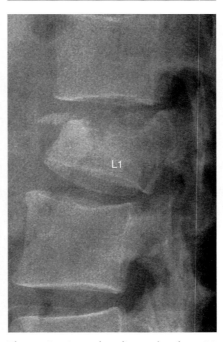

Figure 2 Lateral radiograph of an L1 burst fracture showing compression of the anterior vertebral wall, failure of the superior end plate, and retropulsion of the posterior cortex.

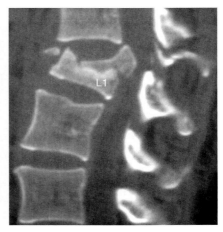

Figure 3 Sagittal reconstruction of CT scan of the L1 burst fracture shown in figure 2, showing retropulsion of the "culprit" fragment of the posterior vertebral wall attached to the posterior disk anulus that creates the canal compromise.

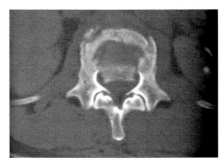

Figure 4 Axial CT scan of the L1 burst fracture shown in figures 2 and 3, showing the retropulsion of the posterior-superior fragment and the degree of canal compromise.

forces, the interspinous ligaments fail posteriorly, leading to subluxation, kyphosis, and instability. Compression of the anterior vertebral wall, failure of the superior or both end plates, and retropulsion of the posterior cortex can be seen on lateral radiographs (Figure 2). The amount of local kyphosis can be determined from the adjacent end plates, and ligamentous injury can be indicated by increased kyphosis and spreading between the spinous process. CT scanning of burst fractures is imperative to help determine the amount of comminution of the vertebral body and the amount of retropulsion and canal compromise (Figures 3 and 4).

The goals of treatment for thoracolumbar burst fractures include re-duction of the deformity, clearance of the spinal canal if there is neurologic deficit, early mobilization of the patient, and long-term stability of the spine. Stable burst fractures can be treated successfully in an orthosis. The surgical treatment of thoracolumbar burst fractures is reserved for unstable burst fractures or those with residual neurologic deficit accompanied by cord or canal compromise. Instability is defined as progressive deformity, pain, or neurologic deficit. A treatment algorithm used at the University of Wisconsin recommends using a thoracolumbosacral orthosis in the setting of thoracolumbar burst fractures without a neurologic deficit and less than 25° of kyphosis. With no neurologic deficit but more than 25° of kyphosis, significant comminution of the vertebral body, or end-plate fractures involving both the superior and inferior end plates, surgical treatment often is recommended; however, substantive literature support is sparse. Surgical treatment can consist of either anterior or posterior internal fixation. If the patient has a neurologic deficit at presentation, anterior corpectomy and anterior plating are indicated. Combined anterior and posterior fixation is reserved for patients with fracture-dislocations or multilevel fractures.

Surgical Treatment
Posterior Treatment

Historically, posterior hook-rod devices were used in the treatment of thoracolumbar burst fractures. These constructs were intended to provide distraction and, through "ligamentotaxis," afford reduction of the deformity. Unfortunately, distraction on the posterior aspect of the spine often resulted in kyphosis. In addition, kyphotic settling and retropulsion usually recurred. Pedicle screw instrumentation provided a more powerful lordosing force to be applied posteriorly; however, with short-segment pedicle screw instrumentation, high percentages of instrumentation failure and progressive kyphosis were seen.[1-3] The goals of posterior treatment of thoracolumbar burst fractures are to reduce the spinal deformity through a combination of lordosis and distraction and maintain this correction throughout the healing period. In general, this requires fixation at least two levels above and two levels below the injured vertebra. Some settling and resulting mild kyphosis usually occur after posterior-only fixation of burst fractures.[4] Posterior fixation is indicated for multilevel fractures or low lumbar burst fractures with neurologic deficit or significant comminution. Posterior pedicle screw instrumentation with vertebral body grafting of the fractured segment has been described. There have been reports of percutaneous posterior pedicle screw fixation without fusion, allowing fracture healing with subsequent fixation removal.[5]

Posterior spinal fixation also is indicated in patients with a thoracolumbar burst fracture and multiple traumas. This "damage control" approach greatly enhances patient survival and treatment by allowing patient transfer, ventilation, and extremity fixation without the need for a more extensive anatomic approach or a cumbersome brace. The focus in these patients is short surgical time, stabilization, and minimal blood loss.

Posterior spinal fixation also is indicated in less common thoracolumbar injuries. Flexion-distraction injuries typically have a tension failure of the posterior vertebral body that may extend through the posterior ligaments or through posterior bony structures. These injuries commonly occur with seat-belt injuries and often are associated with small intestine injuries. In young patients with a completely bony injury, postural reduction and closed treatment may be indicated. More commonly, there is an element of posterior ligamentous damage, and postural reduction, interspinous wire reduction, and fixation of the fracture posteriorly are indicated. Although hook-rod constructs can be used for this, single-level pedicle screw fixation is more frequently advisable.

Translational fracture-dislocation of the spine usually involves some element of facet fracture, sheer or rotational deformity, and neurologic injury. Rarely do these patients escape devastating neurologic injury. Posterior instrumentation is indicated for stabilization following reduction. Typically, these fusions extend two or three levels above and below the dislocation. Multisegment fixation with a combination of screws, hooks, and rods is most common. Anterior and posterior fixation is indicated in patients with incomplete neurologic deficits if bony canal compromise persists after reduction of the dislocation. These anterior bony fragments often are from a burst component in the fracture and are most effectively removed from an anterior approach.

Anterior Treatment

The anterior treatment of thoracolumbar burst fractures has allowed major advances in the recovery of these patients. The most common indication for anterior decompression and stabilization is neurologic injury with a thoracolumbar burst fracture. Fractures at the thoracolumbar junction can cause spinal cord injury, conus medullaris injury, or cauda equina injury. Most fractures below T11 have a mixture of these elements. It is often said that no thoracolumbar injury is ever truly a complete injury because of the recovery potential of the cauda equina components of the injury. Neurologic injury at the thoracolumbar junction can be quite subtle. Often, loss of bladder control may be the only evidence of neurologic damage. Careful physical examination and, occasionally, cystometrograms are indicated to ensure normal neurologic bladder function.

Anterior decompression of burst fractures was first advocated by Dunn[6] and by Kaneda and associates.[7] Their concept was to perform a direct anterior decompression of the spinal canal to remove the bony fragments under direct observation of the dura and spinal cord. The other theoretic advantage is direct reconstruction of the weight-bearing column of the vertebral body, which should prevent settling and recurrence of kyphosis and allow earlier return to function.

Bradford and McBride[8] compared neurologic recovery following posterior and anterior surgical treatment of burst fractures. They found that 64% of patients treated with a posterior approach had neurologic improvement. In those treated with an anterior approach, 88% improved. They concluded that in

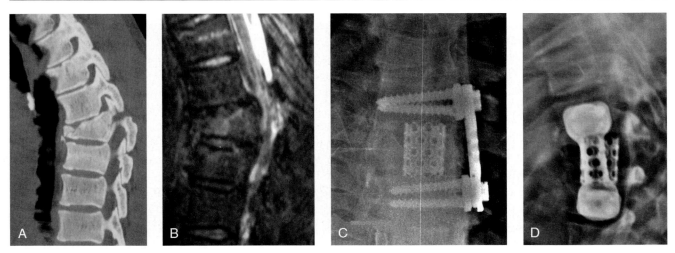

Figure 5 **A,** Lateral radiograph of a T8 fracture. This burst fracture also has a flexion-distraction component with posterior column disruption (AO type B). **B,** Sagittal MRI scan shows compression of the spinal cord caused by retropulsion of the posterior vertebral body and kyphosis across this fracture. The patient had an incomplete spinal cord injury. Postoperative AP radiograph **(C)** and lateral radiograph **(D)** after anterior-only decompression and stabilization. Complete spinal canal clearance was obtained with anatomic reduction of the kyphotic deformity with one approach. The patient had complete resolution of the spinal cord injury.

patients with a neurologic deficit, the anterior approach for decompression yielded a higher percentage of recovery of neurologic function. Gaines and associates[9] developed a load-sharing model to determine which fractures would result in a high incidence of instrumentation failure if treated from a posterior-only approach. They found that fractures with severe comminution of the vertebral body or severe spread of the vertebral body fragments and those patients undergoing significant kyphosis reduction had a much lower hardware failure rate when treated primarily anteriorly than when treated posteriorly. Thus, indications for the anterior treatment of thoracolumbar burst fractures include neurologic deficit, severe vertebral body comminution, kyphosis of more than 30°, and fractured or missing posterior elements. Theoretic disadvantages of the anterior approach include a more difficult exposure, less familiar equipment, and less familiar anatomy.

The advantages, such as direct reconstruction of the weight-bearing column, complete decompression of the spinal canal under direct vision, limiting fusion to only one level above and below the injured vertebra, and no injury of the posterior musculature or prominence of the posterior hardware, outweigh the disadvantages in many patients. Anterior short-segment instrumentation is biomechanically stronger in every loading condition compared with short-segment posterior pedicle screw instrumentation and may be the most reliable method of obtaining optimal decompression and short-segment stabilization.[10] Anterior-only constructs with modern anterior thoracolumbar plates and vertebral body screws have proved successful even for unstable burst fractures with posterior column disruption (AO type B fractures)[11] (Figure 5).

A complete discussion of the surgical approach for the anterior treatment of thoracolumbar burst frac-

tures is beyond the scope of this chapter. In general, for fractures between T3 and T9, right-sided transthoracic approaches are used. For fractures between T10 and T12, a left-sided combined transthoracic and retroperitoneal approach is used. For fractures at L1 or below, a retroperitoneal left-sided approach is indicated. These approaches have become less invasive over the years. Small-incision surgery with thoracoscopic assistance can be used to manage these fractures.

For fractures at the thoracolumbar junction, division of the posterior aspect of the diaphragm usually is indicated. Combined with transpleural and retroperitoneal exposures, this division exposes the T11, T12, and L1 vertebral bodies. The vertebral column must be exposed anteriorly to the midline and posteriorly back to the neural foramen to allow complete definition of the lateral aspect of the vertebral body where fixation devices will be placed. This often helps orient the

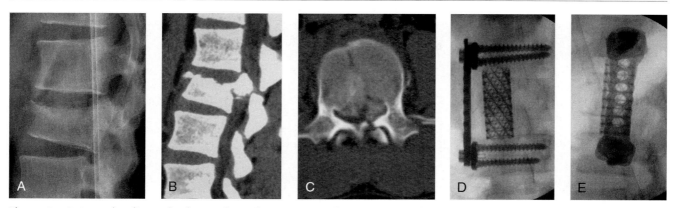

Figure 6 **A,** Lateral radiograph of an L2 burst fracture. Sagittal CT reconstruction **(B)** of the L2 burst fracture and axial CT **(C)** showing the significant retropulsion of the posterior-superior vertebral body and profound spinal canal compromise. The patient had a cauda equina injury with bladder dysfunction. Postoperative AP **(D)** and lateral **(E)** radiographs after anterior-only decompression and stabilization. The cauda equina syndrome was completely resolved, with normalization of bladder function.

surgeon to the spinal canal for decompression. Decompression is performed by removing the fractured vertebral body in its midportion and anterior portions, leaving the retropulsed posterior fragments until later. These fragments are removed with direct visualization of the dura to ensure complete decompression. The decompression must extend across the spinal canal to the contralateral pedicle, which can be palpated. Reconstruction of the vertebral body defect can then be performed with allograft struts (femur or humerus), or titanium structural devices. The placement of lateral fixation devices through vertebral body bolts then maintains the reduction obtained through distraction and lordosis. Lateral devices are either plate- or rod-based but, in general, require bolts placed across the vertebral bodies at the levels above and below the injured vertebra (Figure 6).

In a study of 58 patients treated with anterior decompression and plate fixation, McDonough and associates[12] found that the average kyphosis correction was 13°, with only 2° loss of correction at final follow-up. They reported that of the 46 patients in their study who presented with neurologic deficits, all improved at least one Frankel grade at final follow-up. Eighty-six percent of the patients with neurologic deficit returned to normal function at 2-year follow-up. Anterior-only constructs have demonstrated better restoration and maintenance of sagittal alignment at long-term follow-up compared with posterior-only constructs.[13] In a matched cohort study of unstable thoracolumbar burst fractures with posterior column disruption (AO type B), both techniques resulted in statistically significant initial improvement in sagittal alignment; however, the posterior short-segment group lost this statistical significance at follow-up, whereas the anterior-only group continued to demonstrate statistically significant improvement in sagittal alignment at long-term follow-up compared with preoperative measurements.[13]

Summary

Surgical treatment of thoracic and lumbar fractures is indicated to preserve neurologic integrity, maintain spinal stability, assist in neurologic recovery if deficit is present, and expedite patient rehabilitation. Fracture-dislocations and flexion-distraction injuries usually require posterior spinal instrumentation. Burst fractures can be treated with either anterior or posterior fixation. Patients with neurologic deficit from thoracolumbar burst fractures tend to improve at a greater rate with anterior decompression. Anterior and posterior fixation is reserved for patients with a severe fracture-dislocation with incomplete neurologic deficit, malunion, or severe osteoporosis. For ideal results, the surgeon must plan appropriately, approach the spine without causing complications, perform complete canal decompression when necessary, and pay strict attention to detail in the performance of spinal instrumentation.

References

1. Carl AL, Tromanhauser SG, Roger DJ: Pedicle screw instrumentation for thoracolumbar burst fractures and fracture-dislocations. *Spine* 1992;17:S317-S324.

2. McLain RF, Sparling E, Benson DR: Early failure of short-segment pedicle instrumentation for thoracolumbar fractures. *J Bone Joint Surg Am* 1993; 75:162-167.

3. Sasso RC, Cotler HB, Reuben JD: Posterior fixation of thoracic and lumbar spine fractures using DC plates and pedicle screws. *Spine* 1991; 16:S134-S139.

4. Sasso RC, Cotler HB: Posterior instrumentation and fusion for unstable fractures and fracture dislocations of the thoracic and lumbar spine. *Spine* 1993;18:450-460.

5. Schizas C, Kosmopoulos V: Percutaneous surgical treatment of chance fractures using cannulated pedicle screws: Report of two cases. *J Neurosurg Spine* 2007;7:71-74.

6. Dunn HK: Anterior stabilization of thoracolumbar injuries. *Clin Orthop Relat Res* 1984;189:116-124.

7. Kaneda K, Abumi K, Fujiya M: Burst fractures with neurologic deficits of the thoracolumbar-lumbar spine: Results of anterior decompression and stabilization with anterior instrumentation. *Spine* 1984;9:788-795.

8. Bradford DS, McBride GG: Surgical management of thoracolumbar spine fractures with incomplete neurologic deficits. *Clin Orthop Relat Res* 1987; 218:201-216.

9. Gaines RW Jr, Carson WL, Satterlee CC, Groh GI: Experimental evaluation of seven different spinal fracture internal fixation devices using nonfailure stability testing: The load-sharing and unstable-mechanism concepts. *Spine* 1991;16: 902-909.

10. Shono Y, McAfee PC, Cunningham BW: Experimental study of thoracolumbar burst fractures: A radio-graphic and biomechanical analysis of anterior and posterior instrumentation systems. *Spine* 1994;19: 1711-1722.

11. Sasso RC, Best NM, Reilly TM, McGuire RA: Anterior-only stabilization of three-column thoracolumbar injuries. *J Spinal Disord Tech* 2005;18: S7-S14.

12. McDonough PW, Davis R, Tribus CA, Zdeblick TA: The management of acute thoracolumbar burst fractures with anterior corpectomy and Z-plate fixation. *Spine* 2004;29: 1901-1909.

13. Sasso RC, Renkens K, Hanson D, Reilly T, McGuire RA, Best NM: Unstable thoracolumbar burst fractures: Anterior-only versus short-segment posterior fixation. *J Spinal Disord Tech* 2006;19:242-248.

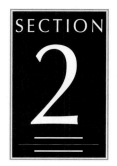

SECTION 2

Pediatric Spinal Deformity

Pediatric Spinal Deformity

This section on pediatric spinal deformity focuses on kyphosis. The four chapters in this section are an excellent review of the subject and include information defining the normal radiographic parameters of kyphosis in the pediatric patient along with a discussion of surgical principles that may help the surgeon avoid complications. Treating pediatric patients with pathologic states that cause kyphosis remains a challenge for the spinal deformity surgeon. This section provides a basic review of the principles necessary to safely and effectively manage these patients.

To provide the basis for understanding the abnormal spine, Betz defines the normal radiographic parameters seen on a lateral standing radiograph. The normal sagittal measurements of kyphosis are reviewed as well as the standard definition of sagittal balance. Spinopelvic balance, which is paramount to understanding spondylolisthesis, is defined by measuring pelvic incidence—a measure of sacral slope and pelvic tilt, both of which are nicely illustrated in this chapter.

Betz also provides a brief synopsis of each of the most common forms of pathologic kyphosis treated by spine surgeons. The author discusses Scheuermann kyphosis (the most common surgically treated deformity), induced kyphosis (such as paralytic and postlaminectomy deformities), kyphosis caused by abnormal biology (such as neurofibromatosis and Marfan syndrome), and kyphosis resulting from congenital spinal malformations.

The second chapter, by Pizzutillo, reviews the available nonsurgical treatment regimens for treating kyphosis. Adolescent postural kyphosis, the kypho-sis most frequently seen by the pediatric orthopaedic surgeon, is reviewed and guidelines are presented regarding treatment of this benign condition. The remainder of the chapter focuses on the nonsurgical treatment of Scheuermann kyphosis, which builds upon Betz's description of this clinical entity. Conservative treatment is indicated in skeletally mature patients with a deformity greater than 60°. The treatment goals are resolution of symptoms, prevention of deformity, and (occasionally) some improvement in sagittal plane measurements. The orthotic treatment options for Scheuermann kyphosis include the Milwaukee brace or a thoracolumbar orthosis. The Milwaukee brace is discussed mainly for historic interest because the popularity of this brace has declined due to the lack of patient compliance. The thoracolumbar orthosis is a reasonable treatment option and should include a sternal pad to extend the spine and control kyphosis. In general, the patient must wear the brace for 16 to 22 hours a day.

Pizzutillo also discusses lumbar Scheuermann kyphosis, a common reason for back pain evaluation referrals, especially in athletic adolescents. The clinical characteristics, radiographic studies, and indications for treatment are discussed for this benign and self-limiting condition.

The chapter by Lowe provides an excellent review of the recommended surgical principles for pediatric kyphosis surgery. We acknowledge Dr. Thomas Lowe's recent death with sincere regret and warmly remember him as both an experienced surgeon and renowned expert and educator in the field of spinal deformity, especially kyphosis. This chapter focuses on large radius and short rigid radius kyphosis. The surgical treatment of both of these types of deformities continues to evolve, especially given the advent of segmental pedicle screw fixation and improved methods of intraoperative neurologic monitoring.[1,2] Most importantly, however, the basic principles detailed in this chapter remain the foundation of effective surgery. Stable zones of instrumentation are defined as well as the needed anchor points above and below the apex of a deformity.

The second part of Lowe's chapter focuses on the surgical treatment of short and angular rigid kyphotic deformities. The principles of neurologic decompression and spinal column shortening are mentioned throughout the chapter and remain a paramount consideration in the safe treatment of these deformities, even as the evolution of posterior-only treatment of these deformities has become much more common. Lowe also discusses the use of traction for these kyphotic deformities, which when applied slowly and under careful clinical monitoring can aid the surgeon in obtaining some preoperative correction of the kyphosis. He also discusses the need for circumferential fusion if the biology of the bone predisposes the patient to pseudarthroses (such as in patients with dystrophic kyphoscoliosis caused by neurofibromatosis).

The Lenke chapter provides an excellent guide and review for preventing and treating surgical complications in the pediatric patient with kyphosis of the thoracic and thoracolumbar spine. This thorough review begins by identifying the causes of surgical complications, such as inadequate planning, poor or inadequate fixation, and implant failures. Perhaps the most important topic is the feared complication of neurologic dysfunction after kyphosis surgery. Lenke discusses the two most common factors involved in this complication: tension applied to the anterior spinal cord and limitation of blood flow to the anterior spinal cord, along with suggestions on how to potentially avoid these two pitfalls.

The second part of the chapter discusses surgical options after failure of a previous surgical procedure for kyphosis.

The potential need for posterior osteotomies (such as pedicle subtraction and Smith-Petersen osteotomies) versus anteroposterior combined procedures is discussed. Lenke also details the occasional need for anterior structural support and its indications, especially at the lumbosacral spine. The use of traction for severe deformities has been shown to be safe and efficacious, especially when improving the preoperative alignment of the spine allows for improved intraoperative correction of the deformity.

This section on pediatric kyphosis serves as an excellent basic reference for treating this challenging condition. Radiographic parameters are defined and nonsurgical and surgical treatments are discussed. Information on avoiding complications and the principles needed to treat complications when they occur will greatly benefit the orthopaedic spine surgeon.

Daniel Hedequist, MD
Assistant Professor of Orthopedics
Department of Orthopedics
Harvard Medical School
Boston, Massachusetts

References

1. Kim YJ, Lenke LG, Bridwell KH, Cho YS, Riew KD: Free hand pedicle screw placement in the thoracic spine: Is it safe? *Spine* (Phila Pa 1976) 2004;29:333-342.

2. Schwartz DM, Auerbach JD, Dormans JP, et al: Neurophysiological detection of impending spinal cord injury during scoliosis surgery. *J Bone Joint Surg Am* 2007;89:2440-2449.

Neither Dr. Hedequist nor any immediate family member has received anything of value from or owns stock in a commercial company or institution related directly or indirectly to the subject of this commentary.

5

Kyphosis of the Thoracic and Thoracolumbar Spine in the Pediatric Patient: Normal Sagittal Parameters and Scope of the Problem

Randal R. Betz, MD

Abstract

As measured by the Cobb angle, normal sagittal kyphosis is 20° to 40°, which encompasses most of the angulated consecutive vertebrae in the thoracic region of the spine. With pathologic kyphosis, however, the segmental analysis of different regions of the thoracic spine plays an important role. Methods of determining sagittal measurements as well as the causes of kyphosis of the thoracic and thoracolumbar spine, including Scheuermann's disease, spinal cord injury, laminectomy, neurofibromatosis, genetic origins, Marfan syndrome, and tuberculosis, are also important in determining treatment.

To assess pediatric patients for abnormal sagittal alignment, physicians must know how normal sagittal measurements are obtained. They must also be aware of the various conditions that are commonly associated with pediatric kyphosis.

Normal Sagittal Measurements

The normal range of kyphosis is described as 20° to 40° as measured by the Cobb angle.[1] When distinguishing pathologic kyphosis from normal kyphosis, the segmental analysis of different regions of the spine is important. Segmental analysis of the spine allows assessment of specific regions. For example, if T10 to L2 is ± 7°, a 20° kyphosis in this region of the spine would be a significant defor-

mity. Similarly, whereas a collective kyphosis of 20° from all the segments in the region from T1 to T5 would be abnormal, the normal collective kyphosis, as described by Bernhardt,[2] would be 12° to 13° across those four segments (Figure 1).

Sagittal balance from C7 to S1 is extremely important in a patient's ability to stand with minimal muscular effort, and a plumb line drawn from the middle of C7 through the posterior vertebral body of S1 should be ± 2 cm. This measurement has significant variability, however, and can be affected by the position of the patient during radiography. Although the correct position for a weight-bearing lateral radiograph has yet to be standardized, variations in positioning (for exam-

ple, arms down, 45° out, or 90° out) can significantly affect this measurement (W Horton, MD, Chicago, IL, unpublished data, 2002).

Spinopelvic balance has been described by Legaye and associates.[3] Pelvic incidence (PI) is an anatomically fixed angle that is specific for each individual (Figure 2). It encompasses the sacral slope (SS) and pelvic tilt (PT), both of which can be altered by the position of the patient, contractures, or surgical intervention (PI = SS + PT). The actual degree of PI varies anatomically and may be a major predisposing factor in developmental spondylolisthesis. Research has shown that there is a progressive increase in PI in progressively severe grades of spondylolisthesis (mean, 72° ± 5°) when compared with normal PI (mean, 52° ± 5°).[4] An increased PI also suggests an increased risk of progression of developmental spondylolisthesis.

Abnormal Sagittal Parameters
Postural Kyphosis

Ascani and associates[5] have described postural kyphosis as a spinal deformity in which there is no vertebral wedging and no end plate irregularities. Because postural ky-

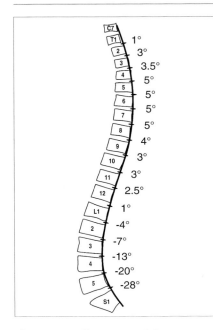

Figure 1 An illustration of the mean segmental sagittal plane angulations of the normal thoracic and lumbar curves using a local coordinate system. (Reproduced with permission from Bernhardt M: Normal spinal anatomy: Normal sagittal plane alignment in Bridwell KH, DeWald RL (eds): *The Textbook of Spinal Surgery*, ed 2. Philadelphia, PA, Lippincott-Raven, 1997, pp185-191.)

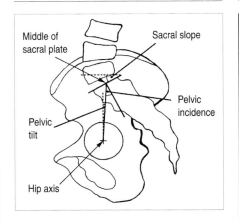

Figure 2 A drawing showing spinal angle: pelvic incidence = sacral slope + pelvic tilt (Reproduced with permission from Mac-Thiong JM, LaBelle H, Charlebois M, Huot MP, De Guise JA: Sagittal plane analysis of the spine and pelvis in adolescent idiopathic scoliosis according to the coronal curve type. *Spine* 2003;28:1404-1409.)

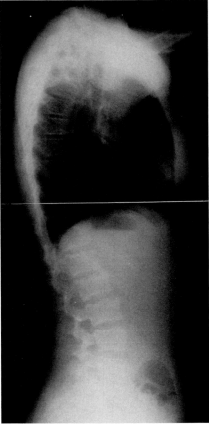

Figure 3 A lateral radiograph of a 13-year-old girl with pain in the lumbar spine region reveals end plate irregularities in L1, L2, L3, and L4 that are consistent with the diagnosis of lumbar Scheuermann's kyphosis.

phosis is nonstructural, complete reduction must be assessed with a hyperextension radiograph. Variants of postural kyphosis that are structural, do not fit the diagnosis for Scheuermann's kyphosis, and do not reduce with hyperextension are referred to as idiopathic kyphosis.[6,7]

Scheuermann's Kyphosis

The abnormal sagittal parameters for Scheuermann's kyphosis are determined from the thoracic, thoracolumbar, and lumbar regions of the spine. For a diagnosis of thoracic Scheuermann's kyphosis, the thoracic sagittal Cobb angle must to be greater than 40°, with wedging of greater than 5° of more than three consecutive vertebrae; the deformity must also be associated with end plate irregularities.[1] The apex of the deformity in patients with thoracic Scheuermann's kyphosis is generally between T7 and T9. Prevalence ranges from 0.4 to 8%,[8] and 20% to 30% of patients also have scoliosis.[5] Additionally, there is an increased incidence of spondylolysis in patients with thoracic Scheuermann's kyphosis.[9]

If the residual kyphosis in these patients remains less than 50° to 60°, there is usually little if any discomfort in adult life.[10] Murray and associates[11] reviewed 61 patients who were observed into adulthood and confirmed that the clinical and functional natural history of thoracic Scheuermann's kyphosis tends to be benign. Nonetheless, cosmesis and patient comfort with the appearance of the deformity should also be assessed when considering treatment, and these parameters cannot be easily or adequately quantified on the basis of questionnaires.[12,13] Thoracic Scheuermann's kyphosis greater than 100° can be associated with reduced pulmonary function.[11]

A 20° kyphosis in the area of T10 to L2 may be indicative of thoracolumbar Scheuermann's kyphosis (normal range, ± 7°).[2] The apex of a thoracolumbar Scheuermann's kyphosis is generally between T10 to T12 and may be associated with considerable pain and significant cosmetic deformity.[4]

Patients with lumbar Scheuermann's kyphosis typically have little deformity and primarily report pain.[14] The diagnosis is usually made when radiographs show irregular end plates, Schmorl's nodes (end plate-disk herniations), and decreased disk height[15] (Figure 3).

Paralytic Kyphosis

Most patients with a spinal cord injury also have a paralytic kyphosis. This abnormal kyphosis is usually noted in the lumbar or thoracolumbar region. In the lumbar region, where lordosis is normally 57° ± 9°, it averages only 8° in patients with spinal cord injury. In the thoracolumbar region (T10 to L2), where lordosis normally measures 5° ± 10°, it averages 19° ± 8° in patients with spinal cord injury (Table 1) (RR Betz, MD; MJ Mulcahey, MS; E Lebby, M; D'Andrea, MD; MD Antonacci, MD; Las Vegas, NV, unpublished data, 2002).

Treatment of paralytic kyphosis is typically done alone or in conjunction with spinal instrumentation for the correction of scoliosis (Figure 4, *A* and *B*). Standard practice calls for the use of a unit rod, which has a fixed kyphosis and lordosis (Figure 4, *C* through *E*). Although this type of

Table 1
Cobb Angle Sagittal Profiles

	Normal Spine, mean ± SD	Spinal Cord Injury, mean ± SD
Thoracic kyphosis	38.5 ± 8.1°	+40.2 ± 9°
Thoracolumbar region	5 ± 10°	+19.1 ± 8°
Lumbar lordosis	-56.6 ± 9.1	-8 ± 12°

(RR Betz, MD; MJ Mulcahey, MS; E Lebby, MD; D'Andrea, MD; MD Antonacci, MD; Las Vegas, NV, unpublished data, September 2002)

spinal instrumentation with a fixed lordosis may be appropriate for treating patients with neuromuscular scoliosis who are ambulatory, in patients with a spinal cord injury and scoliosis who are primarily sedentary, it can have adverse effects because thoracolumbar and lumbar kyphosis is required to enable a patient to sit properly in a chair (RR Betz, MD; MJ Mulcahey, MD; Sydney, Australia, unpublished data, 2000).

Postlaminectomy Kyphosis

The prevalence of kyphosis following laminectomy is 30% to 80%.[16-19] Various risk factors have been reported, including irradiation,[20-22] paralysis,[23] age younger than 15 years, and the location of the laminectomy.[19] The prevalence of postlaminectomy kyphosis is 100% in patients who underwent cervical laminectomy, 36% of those who underwent thoracic laminectomy, and only rarely in those who underwent lumbar laminectomy.[19] Prevention of postlaminectomy kyphosis should be addressed at the time of the laminectomy by using prophylactic fusion and instrumentation.[24-27] If this cannot be done at that time, use of a cervicothoracolumbosacral brace is recommended, and fusion and instrumentation should be done as soon as possible. Bracing alone has not been shown to be effective in long-term studies.[28,29]

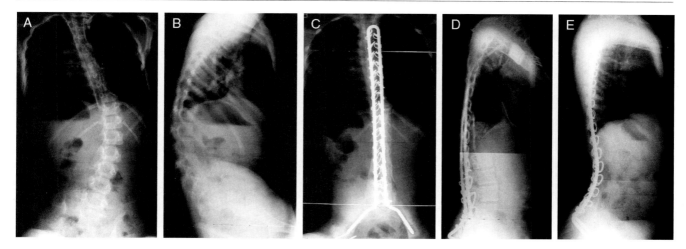

Figure 4 A and **B,** Radiographs of a 12-year-old boy with a paralytic scoliosis and associated paralytic kyphosis that typically develops in patients with scoliosis. **C** and **D,** The patient underwent a posterior spinal fusion with a unit rod fixing a standard amount of lumbar lordosis and thoracic kyphosis. Note that the sitting position in D is dramatically different from the patient's preoperative sitting posture as seen in B. **E,** Radiograph showing the sagittal profile of instrumentation used in an attempt to simulate the preoperative sitting position with decreased lumbar lordosis and some kyphosis across the thoracolumbar region.

Table 2
Dysmorphic Features of Neurofibromatosis

Feature	%
Rib penciling	62
Vertebral rotation	51
Posterior vertebral scalloping	31
Vertebral wedging	36
Spindling of transverse processes	31
Anterior wedging	31
Widened interpedicular distances	29
Enlarged intervertebral foraminae	25
Lateral vertebral scalloping	13

(Reproduced with permission from Durrani AA, Crawford AH, Choudhary SN, Saifuddin A, Morley TR: Modulation of spinal deformities in patients with neurofibromatosis type 1. *Spine* 2000;25:69-75.)

Kyphosis Associated With Neurofibromatosis

Kyphosis resulting from neurofibromatosis (NF-1) is almost always associated with scoliosis and is therefore referred to as kyphoscoliosis. This deformity is diagnosed by identifying scoliosis with a kyphosis greater than 50° on a weight-bearing lateral radiograph. Additionally, kyphosis resulting from NF-1 is usually associated with dysmorphic features.[30] The dysmorphic features of patients with NF-1 have been described elsewhere in the literature[31] and are listed in Table 2.

Curtis and associates[32] suggest that in patients with NF-1, kyphosis contributes more to the production of paraplegia than scoliosis. This view is supported Breig's[33] biomechanical studies, showing that flexion of the spine causes elongation of the spinal canal and deformation of the spinal cord. Pathologically increased spine flexion, as occurs with a kyphotic deformity, leads to excessive axial tension of the spinal cord

parenchyma and may result in neurologic impairment. Miller[34] found that among 20 patients with paraplegia associated with NF-1, severe angulation of the spine was responsible for the paraplegia in more than 50%. Lonstein and associates[35] reviewed 45 patients with spinal cord compression caused by spinal curvature and found NF-1 to be second only to congenital kyphosis as the cause of the compression.

Rotatory dislocation of the spine is a mechanical deformity caused by the sudden presence of a kyphotic zone between two areas of scoliosis, each of them often in lordosis and rotating in opposite directions. Duval-Beaupère and Dubousset[17] described three patients (one with neurofibromatosis, one with chondrodystrophy, and one with congenital vertebral anomalies). They reported that although the deformity may occur anywhere in the spine, it is generally located in the upper thoracic or thoracolumbar region. They also reported that sudden kyphosis is usually angular, with a scissoring effect at the apex of the deformity often occurring in association with considerable collapse of the spine. Because the apex of the deformity is abrupt and because the spinal cord twists inside the spine, neurologic complications are common. Therefore, a complete spinal MRI or a complete high-volume CT myelogram should be performed before surgical treatment of patients with kyphosis associated with NF-1. If spinal cord impingement is detected, a corpectomy may be indicated, followed by anterior and posterior fusions. Anteriorly, an anterior disk excision with tibial or fibular strut bone graft followed by posterior arthrodesis and instrumentation should be extended one to two levels past

both end vertebrae. The patient should be surgically reexamined posteriorly 6 months postoperatively and the fusion mass augmented at that time.

Congenital Kyphosis

McMaster and Singh[36] described the natural history of congenital kyphosis and kyphoscoliosis and reported that congenital scoliosis, kyphoscoliosis, and kyphosis are part of a gradually blending spectrum of spinal deformities caused by developmental anomalies that produce a localized imbalance in the longitudinal growth of the spine. The type of deformity that develops depends on whether the impaired growth occurs unilaterally, producing a pure scoliosis, or occurs anteriorly or anterolaterally to the transverse axis of vertebral rotation in the sagittal plane, producing kyphosis or kyphoscoliosis. In a study of 584 consecutive patients with closed congenital spine deformities, McMaster and Singh[36] found that 472 patients had pure congenital scoliosis, 76 had kyphoscoliosis, and 36 had a pure kyphosis. Of the 36 patients with pure kyphosis, the cause was failure of formation in one half of patients, and failure of segmentation in the other half.

Three types of failure of formation can be identified: (1) partial failure of formation with a well-aligned canal, (2) partial failure of formation with a dislocated canal, and (3) total failure of formation of the vertebral bodies. Pure anterior and symmetric failure is rare and results in an angular kyphosis. The differential growth potential results in a kyphosis and spinal cord tethering that may progress 5° to 7° per year. In partial failure of formation, the offset is clear, and the neurologic risk for the spinal cord is greater.

Neurologic injury can occur suddenly (for example, as the result of a minor trauma). If the offset is clear on the sagittal radiograph, it can also frequently be seen in the coronal plane and almost always has a bayonet-type appearance. If instability is present, minor trauma to a normal spinal cord can lead to a nonreversible, acute paraplegia, in contrast to those instances in which the spinal cord is progressively stretched. Total failure of formation of the vertebral bodies results in the agenesis of one, two, or three or more vertebral bodies, usually with agenesis of the posterior arches as occurs in myelodysplasia.[37] This occurs more frequently in the lumbar spine and almost always in patients with a congenital paraplegia.

Kyphosis Associated With Marfan Syndrome

Patients with Marfan syndrome usually are classified as belonging to one of two groups—those having Marfan syndrome and those having the Marfan habitus (marfanoid). This variability can make prognosis and genetic counseling difficult and inconclusive.[38-40] Marfan syndrome often is misdiagnosed as homocystinuria, Ehlers-Danlos syndrome, congenital contractural arachnodactyly, and many other conditions because of the wide expression of the gene.[41-46] The prevalence of Marfan syndrome has been estimated to be 1 in 10,000 persons in the United States.[47] Approximately 10% of patients with Marfan syndrome have thoracic and thoracolumbar kyphosis,[48,49] which usually manifests late in infancy or early in childhood and is most apparent when the child is sitting. Exercises to improve muscle tone often result in improvement, but kyphosis associated with Marfan syndrome can persist and progress during

adolescence.[48] Sponseller and associates[50] reported that 41% of the patients studied had kyphosis greater than 50°. Taneja and Manning[49] found a 45% incidence of marked kyphosis among patients with Marfan syndrome and an 11% incidence among patients with Marfan habitus.

The reversal of the normal sagittal alignment of the spine is unique to patients with Marfan syndrome. Thoracic lordosis with lumbar kyphosis occurs in some of these patients. Thoracic lordosis, especially in combination with pectus excavatum, can cause respiratory difficulty because of the narrowed anteroposterior (sternovertebral) diameter of the chest.

Posttubercular Kyphosis

Kyphosis caused by tuberculosis has been discussed extensively in the literature, and its natural history has recently been described by Rajasekaran,[51] who identified signs that may predict when instability would be present and deformity would develop. He reported that when a patient has more than two of the following signs—dislocation of facets, posterior retropulsion of the diseased fragments, lateral translation of the vertebrae in the AP view, or toppling of the superior vertebrae—it provided a reliable predictor that the kyphosis would increase to more than 30° of deformity and the final deformity to more than 60°.

Summary

Many conditions other than those discussed can cause kyphosis,[52] but a discussion of causes is beyond the scope of this chapter. Kyphosis can result from a variety of pathologic conditions, each with a unique aspect. The cause of kyphosis must be clearly understood before treatment is considered.

References

1. Bradford DS: Juvenile kyphosis. *Clin Orthop* 1977;128:45-55.

2. Bernhardt M: Normal spinal anatomy: Normal sagittal plane alignment, in Bridwell KH, DeWald RL, Hammerberg KW, et al (eds): *The Textbook of Spinal Surgery*, ed 2. Philadelphia, PA, Lippincott-Raven Publishers, 1997, pp 185-191.

3. Legaye J, Duval-Beaupere G, Hecquet J, Marty C: Pelvic incidence: A fundamental pelvic parameter for three-dimensional regulation of spinal sagittal curves. *Eur Spine J* 1998;7:99-103.

4. Mac-Thiong JM, LaBelle H, Charlebois M, Huot MP, De Guise JA: Sagittal plane analysis of the spine and pelvis in adolescent idiopathic scoliosis according to the coronal curve type. *Spine* 2003;28:1404-1409.

5. Ascani E, La Rosa G, Ascani C: Scheuermann kyphosis, in Weinstein SL (ed): *The Pediatric Spine: Principles and Practice*, ed 2. Philadelphia, PA, Lippincott Williams & Wilkins, 2001, pp 413-431.

6. De Mauroy JC, Gonon G, Stagnara P: *Courbures Saggitales, Types, Morphologiques: Essai de Classification: Criteres Cliniques et Radiologiques Dans le Cyphoses Regulieres.* Reunion du Groupe d'Etude de la Scoliose, Aix en Provence, France, 1988, vol 1, p 11.

7. De Mauroy JC, Stagnara P: *Cyphose Idiopatique: Entite Pathologique. Reunion du Groupe d'Edute de la Scoliose*, Aix en Provence, France, 1978, vol 1, p 24.

8. Lowe TG, Kasten MD: An analysis of sagittal curves and balance after Cotrel-Dubousset instrumentation for kyphosis secondary to Scheuermann's disease: A review of 32 patients. *Spine* 1994;19:1680-1685.

9. Ogilvie JW, Sherman J: Spondylolysis in Scheuermann's disease. *Spine* 1987;12:251-253.

10. Lowe TG: Scheuermann disease. *J Bone Joint Surg Am* 1990;72:940-945.

11. Murray PM, Weinstein SL, Spratt KF: The natural history and long-term follow-up of Scheuermann kyphosis. *J Bone Joint Surg Am* 1993;75:236-248.

12. McCallum MJ: Letter: Scheuermann's disease: The result of emotional stress? *Med J Aust* 1984;140:184.

13. Southwick SM, White AA: The use of psychological tests in the evaluation of low-back pain. *J Bone Joint Surg Am* 1983;65:560-565.

14. Greene TL, Hensinger RN, Hunter LY: Back pain and vertebral changes simulating Scheuermann's disease. *J Pediatr Orthop* 1985;5:1-7.

15. Blumenthal SL, Roach J, Herring JA: Lumbar Scheuermann's: A clinical series and classification. *Spine* 1987;12:929-932.

16. Boersma G (ed): *Verkrommingen van de Wervelkolom na Laminectomieën bij Kinderen: Een Klinisch Onderzoek en een Literatuurstudie Over Normale en Mechanisch Verstoorde Wervelgroei.* Amsterdam, Netherlands, Born, 1969.

17. Duval-Beaupere G, Dubousset J: Progressive rotational dislocation of the spine: Mechanical process common to evolutive kyphoscoliosis complicated by neurologic disorders: Apropos of 16 cases. *Rev Chir Orthop Reparatrice Appar Mot* 1972;58:323-334.

18. Haft H, Ransohoff J, Carter S: Spinal cord tumors in children. *Pediatrics* 1959;23:1152-1159.

19. Yasuoka S, Peterson HA, MacCarty CS: Incidence of spinal column deformity after multilevel laminectomy in children and adults. *J Neurosurg* 1982;57:441-445.

20. Arkin AM, Simon N: Radiation scoliosis: An experimental study. *J Bone Joint Surg Am* 1950;32:396-401.

21. Arkin A, Simon N, Siffert R: Asymmetrical suppression of vertebral epiphyseal growth with ionizing radiation. *Proc Soc Exp Biol Med* 1948;69:171-173.

22. Donaldson WF, Wissinger HA: Abstract: Axial skeletal changes following tumor dose radiation therapy. *J Bone Joint Surg Am* 1967;49:1469-1470.

23. Brown HP, Bonnett CC: Abstract: Spine deformity subsequent to spinal cord injury. *J Bone Joint Surg Am* 1973;55:441.

24. Hopf C, Heine J: Operative therapy in metastases and primary tumors of the spine. *Neurosurg Rev* 1990;13:205-210.

25. Natelson SE: The injudicious laminectomy. *Spine* 1986;11:966-969.

26. Perra JH: Iatrogenic spinal deformities, in Weinstein SL (ed): *The Pediatric Spine: Principles and Practice,* ed 2. Philadelphia, PA, Lippincott Williams & Wilkins, 2001, pp 491-504.

27. Winter RB: Postlaminectomy kyphosis, in Lovell WW, Winter RB (eds): *Pediatric Orthopaedics.* Philadelphia, PA, JB Lippincott, 1978, vol 2, pp 645-646.

28. Sim FH, Svien HJ, Bickel WH, Janes JM: Swan-neck deformity following extensive cervical laminectomy: A review of twenty-one cases. *J Bone Joint Surg Am* 1974;56:564-580.

29. Steinbok P, Boyd M, Cochrane D: Cervical spinal deformity following craniotomy and upper cervical laminectomy for posterior fossa tumors in children. *Childs Nerv Sys* 1989;5:25-28.

30. Crawford AH: Neurofibromatosis, in Weinstein SL (ed): *The Pediatric Spine: Principles and Practice,* ed 2. Philadelphia, PA, Lippincott Williams & Wilkins, 2001, pp 471-490.

31. Durrani AA, Crawford AH, Choudhary SN, Saifuddin A, Morley TR: Modulation of spinal deformities in patients with neurofibromatosis type 1. *Spine* 2000;25:69-75.

32. Curtis BH, Fisher RL, Butterfield WL, Saunders FP: Neurofibromatosis with paraplegia: Report of 8 cases. *J Bone Joint Surg Am* 1969;51:843-861.

33. Breig A: *Biomechanics of the Central Nervous System: Some Basic and Normal Pathological Phenomena Concerning Spine, Disc, and Cord.* Stockholm, Sweden, Almquist and Wiskel, 1960.

34. Miller A: NF-1 with reference to skeletal changes, compression myelitis, and malignant degeneration. *Arch Surg* 1936;32:109.

35. Lonstein JE, Winter RB, Moe JH, Bradford DS, Chou SN, Pinto WC: Neurologic deficits secondary to spinal deformity: A review of the literature and report of 43 cases. *Spine* 1980;5:331-355.

36. McMaster MJ, Singh H: Natural history of congenital kyphosis and kyphoscoliosis: A study of one hundred and twelve patients. *J Bone Joint Surg Am* 1999;81:1367-1383.

37. Bradford DS, Hensinger RN: *The Pediatric Spine.* Stuttgart, Germany, Thieme Verlag, 1985.

38. Health supervision for children with Marfan syndrome: American Academy of Pediatrics Committee on Genetics. *Pediatrics* 1996;98:978-982.

39. Pyeritz RE: The Marfan phenotype: Pleiotropy and variability as clues to genetic heterogeneity, in Akeson WH, Bornstein P, Glimcher MJ (eds): *Symposium on Heritable Disorders of Connective Tissue.* St Louis, MO, CV Mosby, 1983, pp 114-121.

40. Pyeritz RE, Murphy EA, McKusick VA: Clinical variability in the Marfan syndrome(s). *Birth Defects Orig Artic Ser* 1979;15:155-178.

41. Beals RK, Hecht F: Congenital contractual arachnodactyly: A heritable disorder of connective tissue. *J Bone Joint Surg Am* 1971;53:987-993.

42. Birkenstock WE, Louw JH, Maze A, Sladen RN: Combined Ehlers-Danlos and Marfan syndromes, with a case report. *S Afr Med J* 1973;47:2097-2102.

43. Brenton DP, Dow CJ, James JIP, Hay RL, Wynne-Davies R: Homocystinuria and Marfan's syndrome: A comparison. *J Bone Joint Surg Br* 1972;54:277-298.

44. Jaffer J, Beighton P: Syndrome identification case report 98: Arachnodactyly, joint laxity, and spondylolisthesis. *J Clin Dysmorphol* 1983;1:14-18.

45. Lowry RB, Guichon VC: Congenital contractural arachnodactyly: A syndrome simulating Marfan's syndrome. *Can Med Assoc J* 1972;107:531-532.

46. Wilner HI, Finby N: Skeletal manifestations in the Marfan syndrome. *JAMA* 1964;187:490-495.

47. Francke U, Furthmayr H: Marfan's syndrome and other disorders of fibrillin. *N Engl J Med* 1994;330:1384-1385.

48. Goldberg MJ: Marfan and the marfanoid habitus, in Goldberg MJ (ed): *The Dysmorphic Child: An Orthopaedic Perspective.* New York, NY, Raven Press, 1987, pp 83-108.

49. Taneja DK, Manning CW: Scoliosis in Marfan syndrome and arachnodactyly, in Zorab PA (ed): *Scoliosis.* London, England, Academic Press, 1977, pp 261-281.

50. Sponseller PD, Hobbs W, Riley LH III, Pyeritz RE: The thoracolumbar spine in Marfan syndrome. *J Bone Joint Surg Am* 1995;77:867-876.

51. Rajasekaran S: The natural history of post-tubercular kyphosis in children: Radiological signs which predict late increase in deformity. *J Bone Joint Surg Br* 2001;83:954-962.

52. Winter RB, Hall JE: Kyphosis in childhood and adolescence. *Spine* 1978;3:285-308.

6

Nonsurgical Treatment of Kyphosis

Peter D. Pizzutillo, MD

Abstract

An increase in thoracic kyphosis in children and adolescents is usually the result of postural kyphosis or Scheuermann's kyphosis. Although no structural deformity of the spine is observed in postural kyphosis, wedging of vertebral bodies and disk space narrowing are noted radiographically in patients with Scheuermann's kyphosis. Effective interventions for adolescents with postural kyphosis include exercises to relieve lower extremity contractures and strengthen abdominal musculature coupled with practiced normal posture in stance and in sitting. Skeletally immature patients with Scheuermann's kyphosis benefit from a similar exercise program but also require the use of a spinal orthosis. Bracing of the spine in patients with Scheuermann's kyphosis results in permanent correction of vertebral deformity, unlike bracing in patients with idiopathic scoliosis. The evaluation of children and adolescents with increased thoracic kyphosis is an important aspect of the decision process used to determine appropriate interventions.

The term kyphosis is derived from the Greek work kyphos, meaning humpbacked, and refers to the posterior rounding of the spine when viewed from the side. Conversely, lordosis refers to the anterior curving of the spine in the sagittal plane. In the past 2 decades, there have been extensive efforts to better understand and define the sagittal alignment of the human spine.[1-5] Although this work may have been initiated to improve surgical techniques for correction of spinal deformity, the observations have had broader applications for understanding the normal human spine and its development at various stages of growth and development. The normal mature pattern of sagittal alignment of the spine is established by 6 years of age. The average cervical lordosis, measured from C2 to C7, is 15°; thoracic kyphosis, measured from T5 to T12 ranges between 20° and 40°; and lumbar lordosis, measured from L1 to L5, ranges between 20° and 55°.

A host of clinical problems may result in increased or decreased kyphosis. Although congenital, neuromuscular, infectious, iatrogenic, and neoplastic etiologies exist, the most common causes of increased kyphosis are postural kyphosis and Scheuermann's kyphosis. Decreased kyphosis or flattening of the thoracic spine is observed in patients with bone dysplasia, myopathy, myelodysplasia, idiopathic scoliosis, congenital scoliosis, and as a secondary deformity in association with severe spondylolisthesis and lumbar Scheuermann's disease. Decreased kyphosis may create significant cosmetic concerns because of the flat appearance of the back; of even greater importance is the development of restrictive pulmonary disorder that has implications for impaired health and decreased longevity.

Postural Kyphosis

Increased kyphosis in the preadolescent and adolescent patient often causes parental anxiety because of the child's development of back pain or the possibility of permanent spinal deformity. Patients with postural kyphosis are readily identified because of their ability to voluntarily correct their deformity. They are asymptomatic, unconcerned about the appearance of their back, and may be tall for their peer group. Early breast development is also a common reason for adolescent girls to stand with a round-back posture. The older adolescent female, with ponderous breasts and increased thoracic kyphosis, may experience significant upper back pain that will require intervention. Strengthening exercises for the upper back and abdominal muscles, the use of a supportive figure-of-8 brace, or breast reduction may be indicated for relief of pain.

Physical examination of the erect patient shows forward posturing of the shoulders, gentle posterior rounding of the thoracic spine, increased lumbar lordosis, and mild protuberance of the abdomen. The increased thoracic kyphosis and lumbar lordosis are flexible. No focal areas of back deformity, tenderness, or spasm are found. Physical examination also reveals contracture of the pectoral and hamstring muscle groups and weakness of the abdominal muscles.

Radiographic evaluation of the spine is not necessary in postural kyphosis unless there is concern that structural changes may be present. The AP radiograph taken with the patient in an erect position is normal. Standing lateral radiographs of the thoracic and lumbar spine may show increased dorsal kyphosis, but no vertebral body wedging, end plate irregularity, disk space narrowing, or Schmorl's nodes will be observed. In clinical practice, there is great variation in the quality of standing lateral radiographs of the spine. Radiologic techniques may result in overexposure or underexposure with resultant difficulty in seeing clear anatomic landmarks for measurement of curve magnitude. The interobserver error in measurement of lateral radiographs of the spine is 11°.[6] In addition, unorthodox positioning of the upper extremities as well as the tendency to lean forward or backward will alter the true spinal curve measurements. The current positioning technique requires the patient to stand erect with hips and knees in extension and with the arms resting comfort-

ably at shoulder height on a crossbar positioned directly in front of the patient. Positioning for more reliable and reproducible evaluation of lateral radiographs of the spine is currently under investigation.

The motivated patient is able to correct the postural kyphosis by practicing more normal posture and by performing exercises to stretch contracted pectoral and hamstring muscles and strengthen abdominal muscles. The use of figure-of-8 straps or spinal orthoses is not indicated in this patient population. An exercise program, which eliminates contracture and weakness, will facilitate the patient's efforts to stand in a more normal posture. There is no evidence that persistence of postural kyphosis will result in the development of fixed spinal deformity or an increased risk for back pain.

Scheuermann's Kyphosis

Scheuermann's kyphosis refers to the condition characterized by increased posterior rounding of the thoracic spine in association with structural deformity of the vertebral elements. Multiple theories on the etiology of Scheuermann's kyphosis have suggested osteonecrosis of the vertebral ring apophyses, intrinsic weakness of the cartilaginous end plate, osteochondrosis, transient osteoporosis, malabsorption, infection, and endocrine disorders as contributing factors; none have been established as the primary cause. Histologic evaluations of vertebrae from patients with Scheuermann's kyphosis have not confirmed the presence of osteoporosis or osteonecrosis; however, altered endochondral ossification in the vertebral end plates and growth cartilage has been found, which results in abnormal longitudinal growth of the end plate.[7] These biologic alter-

ations may then be worsened by mechanical factors that increase compressive forces on the anterior portion of the vertebral body. Although familial incidence of this condition has been recognized, recent studies suggest that Scheuermann's kyphosis is inherited by a major gene allele model in which all male carriers of the mutant gene and one half of the female carriers will manifest the kyphosis.[8] The study group showed a higher frequency of scoliosis with 0.08 per 1,000 compared with 0.02 per 1,000 for the general population.

Scheuermann's kyphosis occurs more often in males and typically develops between 10 and 14 years of age. Preadolescent and adolescent patients seek evaluation for increased rounding of the thoracic spine and infrequently report back pain. When pain is present, it is usually localized at the interscapular area. Parental concerns primarily involve cosmetic deformity, progressive spinal deformity, and the possible development of back pain in the asymptomatic patient.

The natural history of patients with Scheuermann's kyphosis has been reported by several investigators. Progression of deformity has been documented by Travaglini and Conte[9] who noted increased structural spinal changes in 40 of 50 untreated patients who had been followed for 25 years. Pain developed more frequently in those patients with thoracolumbar kyphosis; however, no significant functional problems were noted. Lowe[10] reported that, with deformity less than 75°, no long-term disability or significant pain problems should be expected. Murray and associates'[11] review indicated that low back pain occurs in patients with Scheuermann's kyphosis but patients do not experience a major effect on life activities. No correlations were found for pain that interfered with activities of daily living, numbness of lower extremities, use of medication for back pain, level of recreational activity, fatigue, self-esteem, social limitations, occupation, sick leave usage, psychologic disorders, or cardiopulmonary insufficiency when comparing patients with Scheuermann's kyphosis with a control group. Spondylolisthesis was not observed in their study population.

Physical examination of the standing patient shows findings similar to those seen in postural kyphosis except for the inability to voluntarily correct the deformity. Young patients, who are referred for evaluation after school screening for scoliosis, may show a mild thoracic scoliosis but may also exhibit a previously undetected increase in thoracic kyphosis. In the erect position, increased thoracic kyphosis with sloping shoulders and forward posturing of the head and neck and increased lumbar lordosis will be seen. The Adam's forward flexion test is used to critically observe the patient from behind to detect truncal asymmetry associated with scoliosis. Although forward flexion of the back is typically restricted in these patients, examination from the side is important because increases in thoracic kyphosis will be exaggerated and easier to identify (Figure 1). Patients with Scheuermann's kyphosis will show abrupt posterior angulation of a segment of the thoracic spine compared with the harmonious curvature of the normal flexed spine. A frequently observed pattern of deformity in forward flexion is that of a sharply angulated, short segment kyphosis of the midthoracic spine with flattening of the upper thoracic spine and loss of reversal of

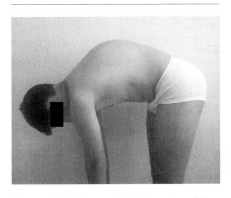

Figure 1 In forward flexion, dorsal kyphosis is accentuated and more easily detected.

the lumbar spine. A less common pattern of deformity is the sharply angulated kyphosis that is centered at the low thoracic or thoracolumbar junction and is associated with marked hypokyphosis of the upper thoracic spine. The latter pattern is usually evident on observation of the erect patient and results in greater cosmetic deformity.

The patient with Scheuermann's kyphosis is not able to voluntarily correct the sagittal deformity of the spine. When the patient is examined prone or supine, it is difficult to passively correct the increased kyphosis by direct pressure, whereas the increased lumbar lordosis may be reversible. Increased lordosis of the cervical spine is cosmetically objectionable and may become fixed. Contracture of the pectoral and hamstring muscle groups is common, as is weakness of the abdominal and upper paraspinal muscle groups. Neurologic evaluation is normal.

Standing AP radiographs of the spine will show scoliosis of the thoracic or thoracolumbar spine. Scoliosis associated with Scheuermann's kyphosis is characterized by a thoracic curve that is not progressive and rarely exceeds a 25° Cobb angle.

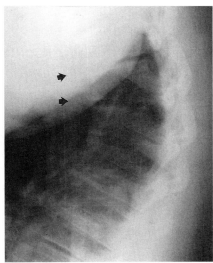

Figure 2 A lateral radiograph shows wedging of vertebrae with end plate irregularities and Schmorl's nodes (*arrows*).

This radiographic view also provides an estimate of skeletal maturity by inspection of the Risser sign.

A standing lateral radiograph of the spine will show thoracic kyphosis greater than 40° with anterior wedging of three or more vertebral bodies, end plate irregularities, disk space narrowing, and Schmorl's nodes (Figure 2). There is also a concomitant increase in cervical lordosis and lumbar lordosis. Attention to the increased lordosis of the cervical spine associated with Scheuermann's kyphosis has not been emphasized in medical literature. Loder[2] studied the sagittal profile of the cervical and lumbar spine in children with Scheuermann's kyphosis to determine whether significant correlations existed. He found that the flexible cervical and lumbar areas are linked by a rigid intermediate thoracic segment. As the residual sagittal difference (for example, thoracic kyphosis/lumbar lordosis) became more kyphotic, the cervical lordosis became more lordotic. Significant fixed deformity of the cervical spine may be an important limiting factor in the surgical correction of the thoracic kyphosis.

When the initial clinical and radiographic evaluation is consistent with a diagnosis of Scheuermann's kyphosis in a skeletally immature patient, brace treatment may be considered. The use of a cross-table stress lateral radiographic view of the spine, which passively extends the kyphos, provides helpful information to determine the appropriateness of bracing for a given patient. The stress radiograph is obtained by placing the patient supine with a bolster positioned at or below the apex of the kyphosis. The patient should be resting comfortably with hips and knees flexed to control the lumbar spine. The weight of the freely hanging head and upper back provide the force needed to passively extend the thoracic spine. After a 5-minute period, a cross-table lateral radiograph is obtained in the stress position. It is important to measure the stress lateral radiograph at the same vertebral landmarks as the previously obtained standing lateral radiograph.

If the kyphosis is flexible and reduces to less than 40° on the stress radiograph, brace treatment may be initiated. If the kyphosis remains more than 40°, there is a decreased likelihood of success with the use of bracing. In the patient with rigid kyphosis that exceeds 50°, surgical intervention may be more appropriate.

In an immature patient with rigid kyphosis that does not reduce to less than 40° on the stress lateral radiograph, serial casting may result in reduction of kyphosis to normal parameters that would then allow application of a brace. An underarm cast is applied with the patient supine on a Risser table with hips and knees in flexed position to reduce

the lumbar lordosis; the cast is molded well over the pectorals anteriorly. By using a muslin strap that is positioned under the apex of the kyphosis, a posterior mold is created to provide strong anterior forces directed at passive correction of the kyphosis. The patient will require cast changes every 2 weeks until the thoracic kyphosis is reduced to less than 40°. At that time, the patient may be transitioned from cast to brace treatment.

Brace treatment for patients with Scheuermann's kyphosis includes a regular program of physical therapy to complement the effects of bracing. Stretching of pectoral muscles, lumbosacral fascia, and hamstring muscles is uniformly indicated. Supine hyperextension maneuvers over a bolster or exercise ball aid in stretching the thoracic spine and are helpful in achieving passive correction. Strengthening of thoracic paraspinal muscles and abdominal muscles is important for maintenance of good postural alignment.

Orthotic treatment of Scheuermann's kyphosis is indicated in the skeletally immature patient with progressive kyphosis, unacceptable cosmesis, or kyphosis greater than 60° that is flexible. The goals of orthotic treatment include the prevention of increasing deformity, the reduction of compressive forces on the anterior aspect of the vertebral bodies to foster restoration of vertebral height, the reduction of hyperlordosis of the lumbar spine, and the restoration of normal sagittal alignment of the spine. Orthotic treatment of patients with idiopathic scoliosis can prevent curve progression but does not offer the likelihood of curve correction. Orthotic treatment of patients with Scheuermann's kyphosis not only prevents curve progression but may result in

significant curve correction.

The Milwaukee brace is the most commonly used brace for the treatment of Scheuermann's disease. It is indicated when the apex of the kyphosis is at or above T8 and for the overweight patient or the female patient with large breasts. The pelvic girdle serves as the base for the superstructure and decreases the lumbar lordosis. Posterior pads are positioned at or just below the apex of the kyphosis but should not be placed above the apex where they would apply forces that block correction or increase deformity. The Milwaukee brace neck ring and occipital pads are rarely used.

The underarm orthosis or thoracolumbosacral orthosis (TLSO) is indicated in the trim patient when the apex of the kyphosis is at or below T9. The anterior upper portion of the TLSO is molded tightly to the sternal area or is augmented with shoulder outrigger extensions. As the patient's kyphosis becomes more flexible, the shoulder outriggers may be adjusted or anterior chest pads may be added to the TLSO to obtain more correction in the brace. The upper border of the posterior aspect of the TLSO is trimmed at the level of the apex of the kyphosis and the lower portion of the TLSO is molded to decrease lumbar lordosis (Figure 3).

Treatment protocols for brace treatment of Scheuermann's kyphosis are similar for all of the spinal orthoses and all include a concomitant exercise regimen. Wear time varies from 16 to 22 hours per day. Earlier treatment programs recommended continued bracing until vertebral ring apophyses were fused; more recent studies suggest that weaning from brace usage may proceed rapidly when Risser 4 capping of the iliac crest is observed.[12]

Sachs and associates[12] reported on 120 patients with an established diagnosis of Scheuermann's kyphosis who were treated with the Milwaukee brace and reevaluated at least 5 years after completion of treatment. Ten patients showed no change in kyphosis when final radiographic studies were compared with initial studies. Seventy-six patients had improvement in the kyphosis and 24 patients had more kyphosis than found in their initial studies. Ten patients did not fully comply with the recommended brace treatment and were included in the failure group of 44 patients; ie, 37% of the 120 in the study sample group. One third of patients with initial kyphosis of 75° or greater subsequently underwent surgical treatment. The authors noted a 41% correction of the prebrace kyphosis with 69% maintenance of correction when evaluated 5 years after completion of brace wear.

Gutowski and Renshaw[13] reported the results of 41 patients with Scheuermann's kyphosis who were treated with either a Milwaukee or Boston brace. The authors noted significant difficulty in determining actual hours of brace usage and documented a progressive degradation in curve improvement with 30% correction recorded at evaluation 2 years after completion of brace wear.

Ponte and associates[14,15] reported the results of using antigravity and localizer-type casts in 1,043 patients with Scheuermann's kyphosis. Patients with mean initial curves of 57° were treated in casts from 8 to 16 months with 40% improvement. Subsequent treatment included night wear of a Milwaukee brace and physical therapy until maturity. At 3-year follow-up, an average 62% mean wedge improvement was observed, thus suggesting that pro-

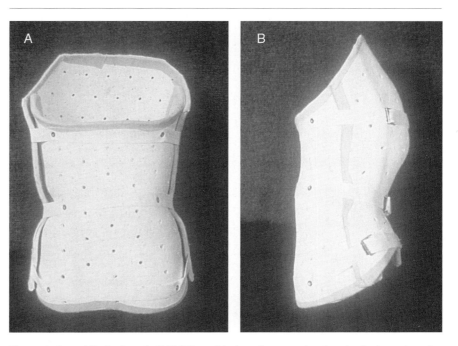

Figure 3 A and **B**, A clamshell TLSO molded to decrease lumbar lordosis and to decrease dorsal kyphosis.

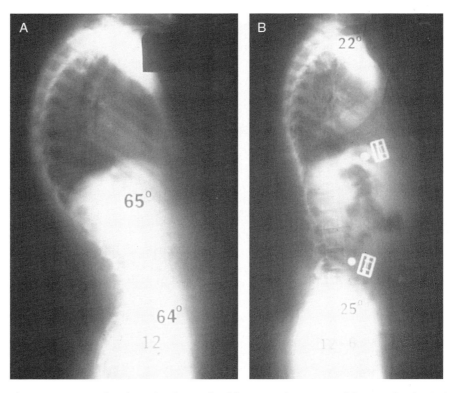

Figure 4 A, A standing lateral radiograph of the spine shows 65° of thoracic kyphosis. **B,** A standing lateral radiograph of the spine in a TLSO show reduction of dorsal kyphosis and lumbar lordosis.

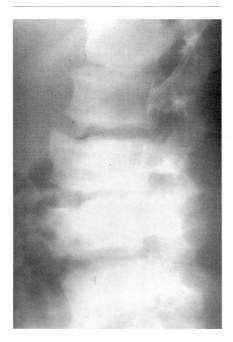

Figure 5 Lateral radiograph of the thoracolumbar spine shows anterosuperior segmental defects of the vertebral body with significant enlargement of involved vertebral bodies.

longed use of the Milwaukee brace lessens the loss of correction.

The nonsurgical treatment of Scheuermann's kyphosis is effective if brace treatment is pursued in the skeletally immature patient with flexible kyphosis less than 74° (Figure 4). The best results have been achieved with full-time use of the Milwaukee brace program. With more rigid kyphosis (more than 75°) surgical intervention becomes more appropriate.

Lumbar Scheuermann's Disease

Adolescent patients with lumbar Scheuermann's disease typically have insidious onset of severe low back pain that is unrelated to activity.[16] Progressive increase in severity of pain precludes involvement in athletic activities and may even interfere with activities of daily living.

Radiation of pain to the buttocks or lower extremities, night pain that awakens the patient, and episodes of sphincter dysfunction are not present in this population. These patients are in good health and have no prior experience of similar back pain. In general, although significant deformity may be obvious on physical examination, neither the patients nor their family members will initially report cosmetic concerns.

Physical examination reveals significant flattening of the lumbar lordosis with a thoracolumbar kyphosis. In more advanced stages of this disorder, the patient may exhibit kyphosis of the lumbar spine and compensatory thoracic lordosis. Although true muscle spasm is not usually present, the rigidity of the flat lumbar region may suggest spasm. Spinal movement is painful and markedly limited in flexion, extension, and rotation. No scoliosis is noted, and the neurologic evaluation is normal. No tenderness is noted with palpation of the sacroiliac joints or the sciatic notch. Severe contracture of the hamstrings is present with no evidence of knee flexion contractures.

Standing AP radiographs of the spine usually will not show scoliosis. If a mild curvature is noted, there is usually no rotational change. Standing lateral radiographs of the spine show marked distortions from normal sagittal alignment. The lumbar spine is minimally lordotic to kyphotic with a concomitant kyphotic deformity at the thoracolumbar junction. Scalloped, lucent defects are noted at the anterosuperior corner of involved vertebral bodies (Figure 5). Schmorl's nodes are not typical but end plate irregularities may be seen. The involved vertebrae are significantly larger in the AP dimension when compared with more

normal vertebral bodies.

Orthotic treatment is indicated for the relief of pain and to halt progressive deformity of the spine. The TLSO used for patients with lumbar Scheuermann's disease is molded or padded in a manner to encourage more normal lumbar lordosis compared with the TLSO used in patients with Scheuermann's kyphosis. In the author's experience, low back pain quickly subsides with brace treatment. The patient is instructed to wear the brace between 16 and 22 hours per day for a period of 18 months in conjunction with an exercise program of abdominal strengthening and hamstring stretching exercises.

Brace treatment quickly relieves pain and stimulates bone formation in the lucent defects of the anterosuperior corner of vertebral bodies but has been ineffective in improving the sagittal alignment of the spine.

Lumbar Scheuermann's disease is not hereditary but is believed to be caused by anterior herniation of disk material under the anterior longitudinal ligament.[17] Longitudinal studies of patients with lumbar Scheuermann's kyphosis are not available but concern exists for future disk degeneration in this population.

Summary

Increased roundback deformity of the upper back or kyphosis may be postural or structural in nature. Patients with postural kyphosis will respond to an exercise program, whereas those with Scheuermann's kyphosis will demonstrate improved spinal alignment and relief of pain after a combined program of exercises and bracing.

References

1. Bernhardt M: Spinal anatomy: Normal sagittal plane alignment, in Bridwell KH,

DeWald RL (eds): *The Textbook of Spinal Surgery*, ed 2. Philadelphia, PA, Lippincott-Raven, 1997, pp 185-191.

2. Loder RT: The sagittal profile of the cervical and lumbosacral spine in Scheuermann thoracic kyphosis. *J Spinal Disord* 2001;14:226-231.

3. Propst-Poctor L, Bleck EE: Radiographic determination of lordosis and kyphosis in normal and scoliotic children. *J Pediatr Orthop* 1983;3:344-346.

4. Stagnara P, De Mauroy JC, Dran G, et al: Reciprocal angulation of vertebral bodies in the sagittal plane: Approach to references for the evaluation of kyphosis and lordosis. *Spine* 1982;7:335-342.

5. Voutsinas SA, MacEwen GD: Sagittal profiles of the spine. *Clin Orthop* 1986;210:235-242.

6. Stotts AK, Smith JT, Santora SD, Roach JW, D'Astous JL: Measurement of spinal kyphosis: Implications for the management of Scheuermann's kyphosis. *Spine* 2002;27:2143-2146.

7. Ippolito E, Ponseti IV: Juvenile kyphosis: Histologic and histochemical studies. *J Bone Joint Surg Am* 1981;63:175-182.

8. Axenovich TI, Zaidman AM, Zorkoltseva IV, Kalashnikova EV, Borodin PM: Segregation analysis of Scheuermann disease in ninety families from Siberia. *Am J Med Genet* 2001;100:275-279.

9. Travaglini F, Conte M: Untreated kyphosis: 25 years later, in *Kyphosis*. Bologna, Italy, Italian Scoliosis Research Group, 1984, pp 21-27.

10. Lowe TG: Scheuermann's disease. *Orthop Clin North Am* 1999;30:475-487.

11. Murray PM, Weinstein SL, Spratt KF: The natural history and long-term follow-up of Scheuermann kyphosis. *J Bone Joint Surg Am* 1993;75:236-248.

12. Sachs B, Bradford DS, Winter R, Lonstein J, Moe J, Willson S: Scheuermann kyphosis: Follow-up of Milwaukee brace treatment. *J Bone Joint Surg Am* 1987;69:50-57.

13. Gutowski WT, Renshaw TS: Orthotic results in adolescent kyphosis. *Spine* 1988;13:485-489.

14. Ponte A, Gebbia F, Eliseo F: Nonoperative treatment of adolescent hyperkyphosis. *Annual Meeting Proceedings*. Milwaukee, WI, Scoliosis Research Society, 1984.

15. Ponte A, Vero B: Siccardi Gl, et al: Ipercifosi Dell' adolescenza: Il trattamento incruento. *Prog Pat Vert* 1988;12:85.

16. Edgren W, Vaino S: Osteochondrosis juvenilis lumbalis. *Acta Chir Scand Suppl* 1957;227:1.

17. Blumenthal SL, Roach J, Herring JA: Lumbar Scheuermann's: A clinical series and classification. *Spine* 1987;12:929-932.

Kyphosis of the Thoracic and Thoracolumbar Spine in the Pediatric Patient: Surgical Treatment

Thomas G. Lowe, MD

Abstract

Kyphosis of the thoracic or thoracolumbar spine is a common deformity in pediatric and adolescent populations. When it progresses to the point at which nonsurgical treatment is no longer an option, surgery is indicated. Surgical options available for the treatment of different types of pediatric kyphosis of the thoracic and thoracolumbar spine include posterior instrumentation and fusion, posterior instrumentation and fusion combined with anterior fusion, and anterior instrumentation and fusion.

Two basic patterns of kyphosis are found in pediatric patients: nonfixed and fixed. Nonfixed kyphosis, the most common pattern, is a rounded, flexible deformity commonly associated with postural kyphosis and Scheuermann's disease. Nonfixed kyphosis is rarely associated with neurologic compromise. Progression of the deformity and/or significant pain in adults may occur when kyphosis is greater than 80° in the thoracic spine or greater than 50° in the thoracolumbar spine. Kyphosis of lesser degree rarely results in progressive deformity or significant pain.

Fixed kyphosis is an angular, rigid deformity that is often associated with congenital kyphosis, neurofibromatosis, postlaminectomy kyphosis, and infectious diseases of the spine. This curve pattern has a high incidence of neurologic compromise if a high degree of deformity develops and is untreated.[1,2] Progression of fixed kyphosis into adulthood is an unpredictable but frequent sequelae.

Differences in pediatric kyphotic deformities are based on the location of the apex of the deformity. Kyphosis, which occurs in the thoracic spine, is inherently stable because of the rib cage, and pulmonary complications are rare unless kyphosis exceeds 100°.[3-5] Pediatric patients who seek surgical treatment for thoracic kyphosis usually do so because of pain, progression of the deformity, or poor cosmesis.[3,4] Thoracolumbar kyphosis has a much higher incidence of progression because of the lack of support provided by surrounding musculature. When the deformity exceeds 50° to 55°,

sagittal imbalance and pain are common, and the deformity is readily apparent.

Clinical Evaluation

Preoperative clinical evaluation should include a history of the onset and progression of the deformity, degree of severity, and location of associated pain. The flexibility, severity, and location of the deformity and any associated coronal deformity should be carefully assessed. When any cutaneous lesions, foot deformities, or muscle contractures are present, a complete neurologic examination should be done to determine the etiology of the deformity and the urgency of treatment.

Diagnostic Studies

Routine preoperative radiographic studies should include standing PA and lateral 36-inch radiographs as well as a supine hyperextension bolster lateral at the level of the apex of the deformity. A preoperative MRI should be obtained for patients with atypical or rapidly progressive kyphosis, any neurologic signs and symptoms, or congenital kyphosis or neurofibromatosis. A three-dimensional CT with coronal and sagittal reconstruction

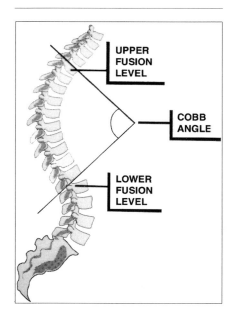

UPPER
FUSION
LEVEL

COBB
ANGLE

LOWER
FUSION
LEVEL

Figure 1 The degree of kyphosis is determined by measuring the intersecting lines of the most tilted vertebrae above and below the apex of the deformity. Levels of fusion should include the upper Cobb vertebra and the first lordotic vertebra and the first lordotic vertebra below the lower Cobb vertebra. (Reproduced with permission from Lowe TG: Scheuermann's disease, in Bridwell K, DeWald R (eds): *The Textbook of Spinal Surgery*. Philadelphia, PA, Lippincott-Raven, 1997, pp 1173-1198.)

should be obtained for patients with congenital deformities for preoperative planning.

Large Radius Kyphosis
Surgical Indications and Options
Surgical indications for large radius, flexible kyphosis include thoracic kyphosis greater than 80° or thoracolumbar kyphosis greater than 50° and progression of the deformity despite brace treatment, thoracic back pain interfering with activities of daily living, or cosmetic deformity that the surgeon, patient, and patient's family believe to be significant.[4] Unusual indications include pulmonary or neurologic compro-

mise, both of which would be unusual in kyphosis less than 100°.

Surgical options for large radius kyphosis include posterior instrumentation and fusion alone, posterior instrumentation and fusion combined with anterior fusion, and occasionally anterior instrumentation and fusion alone.

Posterior Instrumentation and Fusion Posterior instrumentation and fusion is useful in the skeletally immature individual with a flexible deformity. Because of remaining anterior vertebral body growth, continued anterior growth will frequently occur, creating a stable anterior column for load sharing. Posterior instrumentation and fusion should also be considered for skeletally mature individuals in whom the deformity corrects to less than 50° on the hyperextension bolster lateral radiograph. Levels of posterior instrumentation, shown in Figure 1, should include the upper and lower Cobb levels and the first lordotic level distally to minimize the risk of junctional kyphosis.[6] If there is a significant associated thoracolumbar coronal deformity, a lower level of instrumentation may be required.

The basic posterior instrumentation construct should include a minimum of eight anchors above and below the apex of the kyphosis. Pedicle screws below the apex provide better fixation than hooks. Above the apex, either two double-level, pedicle-transverse process claws with hooks (Figure 2) or five or six pedicle screws on each side (Figure 3) provide the best fixation. Smooth 5.5- to 6.0-mm rods are first contoured to the anticipated corrected kyphosis based on the hyperextension lateral radiograph. The rods are then inserted into the hooks or screws above the apex of the ky-

phosis and cantilevered into the distal implants below the apex; compression is applied toward the apex of the kyphosis. Transverse connectors are applied to the proximal and distal ends of the construct. Iliac and local bone graft are packed into each of the facetectomy sites and along the transverse processes. For additional correction, two to three periapical Smith-Petersen osteotomies are often helpful.

Posterior Instrumentation and Fusion Combined With Anterior Fusion Posterior instrumentation and fusion combined with anterior fusion is recommended for adolescent patients with less flexible kyphotic deformities (> 50° on the hyperextension lateral radiograph).[3,4,7] Combined procedures are normally done at the same sitting. An anterior release and fusion is usually done first to achieve increased flexibility of the deformity. Levels for anterior release and fusion should include all "fixed" levels above and below the apex of the kyphosis based on the hyperextension lateral radiographs (usually six to eight segments) and distally across the thoracolumbar junction to the distal level of the planned posterior instrumented fusion. This would generally include the distal Cobb level and the first lordotic level. Single-lung ventilation is mandatory to achieve adequate exposure whether a thorascopic or open approach is selected. For an open procedure, a standard right-sided thoracotomy or thoracoabdominal approach is usually used, depending on whether exposure below L1 is needed. During the exposure, segmental vessels can easily be preserved and retracted with vessel loops while the diskectomies are being performed.[4] Morcellized rib graft alone is normally used above T10, whereas structural cages or grafts should be

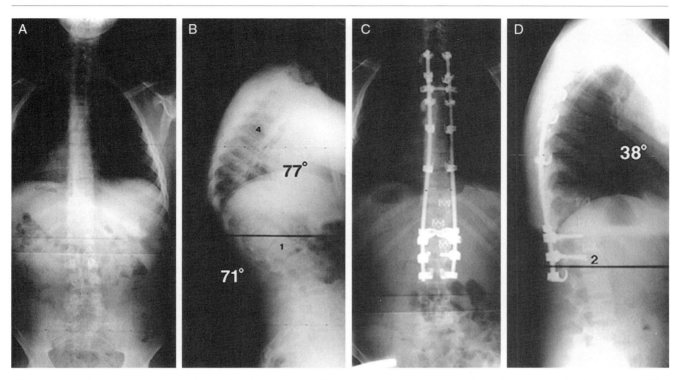

Figure 2 A and **B,** Preoperative radiographs of a 16-year-old patient with a progressive low thoracic 77° kyphosis caused by Scheuermann's disease. **C** and **D,** Postoperative radiographs at 2-year follow-up. Double two-level pediculotransverse process claws with hooks for fixation above the apex and an additional pedicle hook just below the apex of the deformity were used. Pedicle screws and infralaminar hooks were used distally.

added from T10 distally where the disk spaces are larger to provide load sharing. After the insertion of a chest tube and wound closure, the patient is positioned for the posterior procedure.

Anterior Instrumentation and Fusion In pediatric patients with flexible kyphosis, the deformity can be corrected with anterior instrumentation and fusion[4] (Figure 4). This technique allows for saving several fusion levels proximally and distally. In addition to complete diskectomy, structural grafts or cages must be inserted at each level for arthrodesis and instrumentation. Next, bicortical vertebral body screws are inserted transversely at each level, followed by insertion of a single 6.5- to 7.0-mm rod that is contoured to the corrected sagittal profile of the kyphotic deformity.

Surgical Outcomes
Surgical outcomes for correction of this type of kyphosis in the pediatric population have been very good, with long-term correction returning the spinal curvature to within normal range and maintaining good sagittal and coronal balance. In general, clinical outcomes have been good, with patients reporting significant improvements in back pain and cosmesis.[4,6,8,9]

Short Radius Kyphosis
Surgical Indications and Options
Several special considerations must be taken into account in the treatment of short radius, rigid kyphosis in pediatric patients. Kyphosis created by congenital spine deformity is related to developmental vertebral anomalies that impair longitudinal

growth anteriorly or anterolaterally. These curves have been classified as caused by anterior failure of vertebral body formation (type I), anterior failure of vertebral body segmentation (type II), and a combination of failure of formation and segmentation (type III).[1,2,10] All three types may cause potentially serious deformities; even type I congenital spinal deformity can lead to cord compression and paraplegia. As a result, brace treatment is ineffective, and surgery is frequently necessary. No single surgical procedure is effective for all types and magnitudes of congenital spinal deformity. The method of treatment depends on the age of the patient, size of the deformity, type of anomaly, and presence or absence of spinal cord compression. Before surgical treatment is undertaken, possible cardiopulmonary, urinary, and neurologic

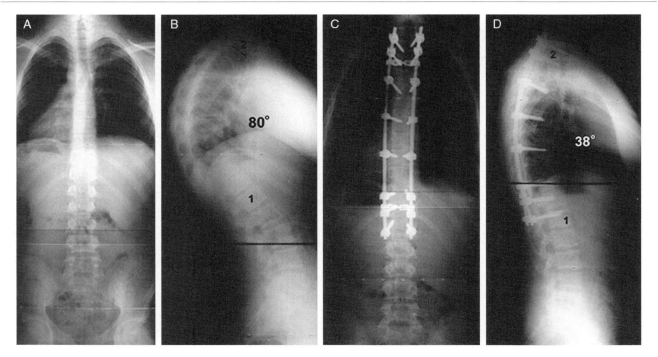

Figure 3 A and **B,** Preoperative radiographs of a 17-year-old boy with a painful 80° thoracic kyphosis caused by Scheuermann's disease. **C** and **D,** Postoperative radiographs following a combined anterior-posterior spinal fusion using a pedicle screw construct extending from T2 to L1. Note that pedicle screws are used distally and proximally in two levels and then every other level in between.

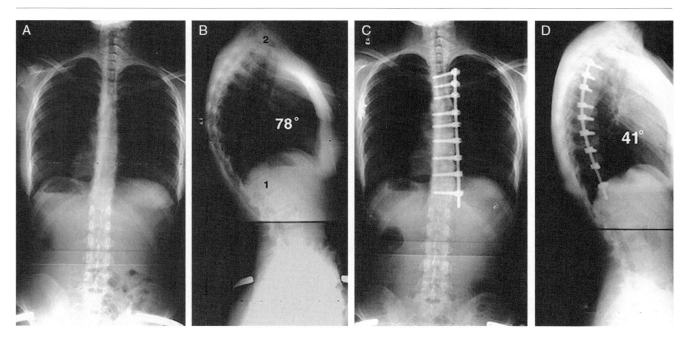

Figure 4 A and **B,** Preoperative radiographs of a 16-year-old girl with a progressive flexible 78° kyphotic deformity caused by Scheuermann's disease. Postoperative PA (**C**) and lateral (**D**) radiographs 2 years after an anterior instrumented fusion. Structural interbody support was placed at each instrumented level, followed by a single anterior rod and vertebral screws. One level was saved distally by this technique.

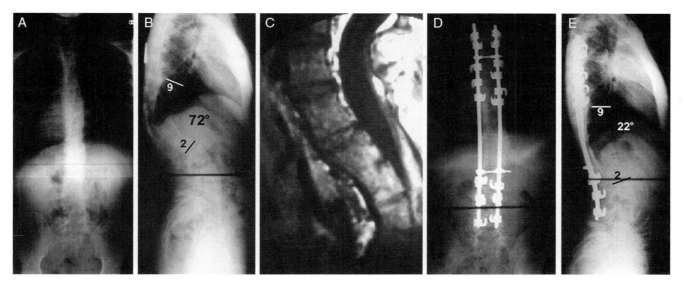

Figure 5 A and **B,** Preoperative radiographs of a 15-year-old boy with a progressive thoracolumbar kyphosis caused by a congenital anterior bar. Congenital kyphosis extends from T9 to L2. Preoperative kyphosis was 72°. **C,** MRI scan of the thoracolumbar spine shows the anterior bar with formation of a portion of the disks posteriorly. **D** and **E,** Postoperative radiographs 4 years after three osteotomies of the bar and posterior instrumentation and fusion. Postoperative kyphosis was 22°.

anomalies must be assessed because such anomalies may affect the timing and approach to treatment.

Posterior In Situ Fusion With or Without Instrumentation In pediatric patients with a congenital spinal deformity that meets treatment criteria, a posterior in situ fusion with or without instrumentation is usually all that is necessary to treat both type I and II deformities.[1,10] A posterior epiphysiodesis is created that allows for continued anterior growth through the remaining anterior growth plates and some degree of correction. Posterior instrumentation may decrease the incidence of pseudarthrosis and provide some additional correction.

Combined Anterior and Posterior Fusion With Instrumentation In pediatric patients with a congenital spinal deformity greater than 60° to 70° and for whom correction of the deformity is appropriate, a combined anterior and posterior fusion with instrumentation is indicated.[1,10] For type I deformities, the anterior procedure should consist of a release of

ligamentous structures and any remaining disk followed by grafting with morcellized autogenous graft and strut grafting to fill in large gaps. For type II deformities, the anterior procedure should consist of one or more osteotomies of the unsegmented bar followed by packing of the defects with morcellized autograft. After the anterior procedure is completed, a posterior instrumented fusion of the entire deformity is performed.

Combined Anterior and Posterior Instrumented Fusion In pediatric patients with a congenital spinal deformity ranging from 60° to 80°, a combined anterior and posterior instrumented fusion of the entire deformity is usually the treatment of choice.[1] Excessive correction should be avoided because of the high risk of neurologic complications. In type I deformities, the anterior procedure consists of an anterior soft-tissue release and diskectomy followed by strut grafting. In type II deformities, single or multiple osteotomies of the anterior bar

followed by grafting of the defects should be done to facilitate correction (Figure 5).

Combined Anterior-Posterior In Situ Fusion With Strut Grafting or Spine Shortening In pediatric patients with a congenital spinal deformity greater than 80°, either a combined anterior-posterior in situ fusion with strut grafting or a spine shortening procedure can limit the risk of neurologic complications (Figure 6). If a spine shortening procedure is selected, a single-stage posterior vertebrectomy is the best option for treating type I deformities. Following the hemivertebrectomy, a posterior fusion with instrumentation should be done to maximize correction of the spine. For type II deformities, a pedicle subtraction osteotomy offers the best solution.[11] Before the osteotomy, pedicle screws should be inserted above and below the proposed osteotomy site. After completion of one side of the osteotomy, temporary fixation should always be inserted to avoid displacement and possible spinal cord injury once the opposite side

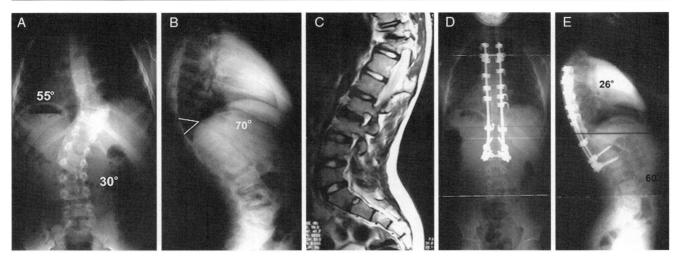

Figure 6 **A** and **B,** Preoperative radiographs of an 11-year-old boy with a progressive thoracic kyphoscoliosis (55°) caused by a posterolateral hemivertebra. Lumbar scoliosis was 30°. Thoracic kyphosis was 70°. **C,** MRI of the hemivertebra reveals no spinal cord impingement. **D** and **E,** Postoperative radiographs 2 years after excision of the hemivertebra and correction of the thoracic hyperkyphosis, which were done through a posterior approach. Thoracic kyphosis was 26°.

of the osteotomy is completed. After controlled correction of the osteotomy, bilateral pedicle screw fixation is obtained. Although excellent correction can be obtained with either of these procedures, they require the expertise of experienced surgeons to avoid neurologic complications.

Other Surgical Options When there is major spinal cord compression, either formal anterior cord decompression or a spine shortening procedure combined with correction of the kyphosis should be done along with a posterior fusion with instrumentation (Figure 7). Mild spinal cord compression without motor loss can usually be treated effectively with a standard combined anterior-posterior instrumented fusion. This procedure achieves only a

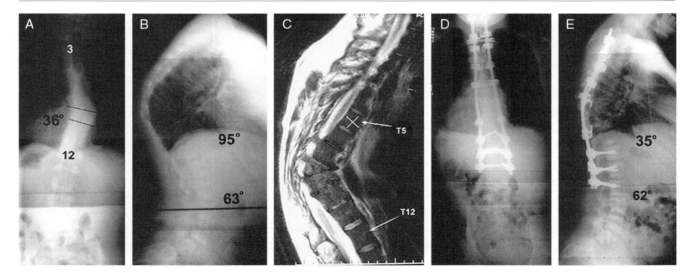

Figure 7 **A** and **B,** Radiographs of a 17-year-old boy with a progressive thoracic kyphosis caused by two hemivertebrae (T8-T9) and the subsequent acute onset of paraparesis. The patient was also undergoing routine renal dialysis because of chronic renal failure. Scoliosis extends from T3 to T12 and measures 32°. Thoracic kyphosis is 95° and lumbar lordosis is 62°. **C,** Sagittal MRI of the spine shows severe stenosis at the apex of the deformity. **D** and **E,** Postoperative radiographs 2 years after complete excision of T8 and partial excision of T9, which was done through a posterior approach. A long construct was required because of osteopenia related to dialysis. 35° is the corrected thoracic kyphosis.

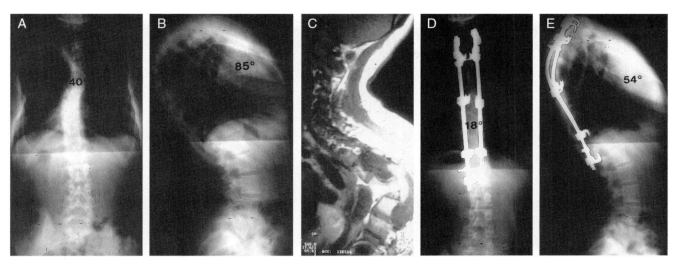

Figure 8 A and **B,** Preoperative radiographs of a 12-year-old girl with a fixed 85° thoracic kyphosis and an associated 40° thoracic scoliosis caused by neurofibromatosis. She reported mild weakness in both lower extremities, hyperreflexia, and bilateral ankle clonus. Thoracic scoliosis is 40°. Thoracic kyphosis is 85°. **C,** MRI shows the sharp angular deformity as well as compression of the spinal cord. **D** and **E,** Postoperative radiographs 3 years after a combined anterior cord decompression and strut grafting followed by posterior instrumentation and fusion. The patient's myelopathic findings resolved postoperatively.

modest amount of correction of the kyphosis, but it is often enough to resolve the paresis.

The role of skeletal traction for fixed deformities remains controversial because of an increased risk of neurologic complications.[1] It may, however, be useful in the treatment of flexible, high-magnitude deformities. A pretraction MRI and frequent, careful neuromonitoring are essential.

Patients with dystrophic kyphoscoliosis caused by neurofibromatosis usually require a combined anterior-posterior fusion.[12-14] These patients have an increased risk of spinal cord compression if a high-magnitude deformity develops. These deformities are usually fixed and difficult to correct. The surgical goal in kyphosis associated with neurofibromatosis is to achieve permanent stabilization of the spine and avoid neurologic injury. Surgical treatment should consist of a combined anterior-posterior in situ fusion. When a high-magnitude residual deformity is present, either a vascularized rib pedicle graft and/or

fibular strut grafts should be considered[15] (Figure 8). Dystrophic thinning of posterior elements and dural ectasia make posterior instrumentation more difficult, resulting in a high rate of pseudarthrosis. Any loss of correction or implant failure warrants reexploration and reinforcement of the fusion mass.[12,14,16]

With aggressive surgical treatment of malignant spinal tumors with laminectomy, chemotherapy, and radiation, many children survive and develop postlaminectomy kyphosis.[17-19] The treatment of postlaminectomy kyphosis poses some special problems. Obviously, prevention of the deformity is the best treatment. In pediatric patients, the younger the patient and the higher the level of the laminectomy, the greater the likelihood of postlaminectomy kyphosis to occur.[17,18] A posterolateral fusion should always accompany a multilevel decompression, especially if facetectomies are a required part of the decompression. Bracing after decompression is ineffective in preventing or treating the deformity.

A combined anterior-posterior fusion of the entire deformity is required because of the poor posterior fusion bed related to missing posterior elements.[17,19] Although posterior instrumentation is often difficult because of missing posterior elements and osteopenia, pedicle screws can usually be used and provide excellent fixation when combined with double-rod systems; postoperative bracing is usually not needed (Figure 9).

Summary

The treatment of large radius kyphosis in pediatric patients is primarily nonsurgical. Surgery should be reserved for patients with kyphosis of 80° or more and painful or progressive deformities. Congenital kyphosis requires early diagnosis and treatment using posterior fusion to prevent worsening of the deformity. Short radius, fixed deformities that have progressed significantly before initial evaluation require combined anterior-posterior fusion. Patients who have developed neurologic complications require a formal anterior decompres-

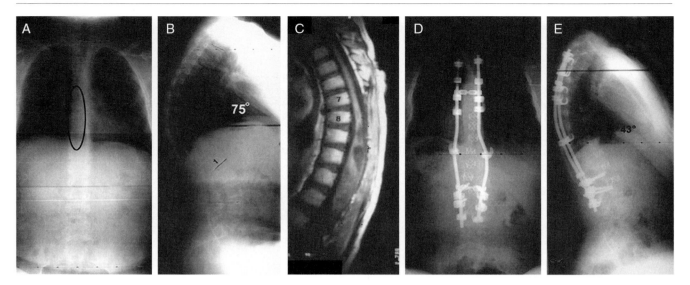

Figure 9 A and **B,** Radiographs of a 12-year-old boy 1 year after he underwent a multilevel laminectomy; a progressive thoracic kyphosis developed within a few months of the surgery. The black line in **A** identifies the extent of the multilevel laminectomy. **B,** thoracic kyphosis that developed after the laminectomy was 75°; the levels of kyphosis are identified by the lines and spaces. **C,** MRI scan demonstrates the presence of a spinal cord tumor (astrocytoma). **D** and **E,** Postoperative radiographs following a combined anterior-posterior fusion. Note that anterior cages were used for structural support for the length of the laminectomy defect.

sion and strut grafting as well as an instrumented posterior fusion. Patients with kyphosis caused by neurofibromatosis or postlaminectomy always require combined anterior-posterior fusion because of a high risk of pseudarthrosis.

References

1. Lonstein JE: Congenital spine deformities: Scoliosis, kyphosis, and lordosis. *Orthop Clin North Am* 1999;30:387-405.

2. McMaster MJ, Singh H: Natural history of congenital kyphosis and kyphoscoliosis: A study of one hundred and twelve patients. *J Bone Joint Surg Am* 1999;81:1367-1383.

3. Lowe TG: Scheuermann disease. *J Bone Joint Surg Am* 1990;72:940-945.

4. Lowe TG: Scheuermann's disease. *Orthop Clin North Am* 1999;30:475-487.

5. Murray PM, Weinstein SL, Spratt KF: The natural history and long-term follow-up of Scheuermann kyphosis. *J Bone Joint Surg Am* 1993;75:236-248

6. Lowe TG, Kasten MD: An analysis of sagittal curves and balance after Cotrel-Dubousset instrumentation for kyphosis secondary to Scheuermann's disease: A review of 32 patients. *Spine* 1994;19:1680-1685.

7. Bradford DS, Ahmed KB, Moe JH, Winter RB, Lonstein JE: The surgical management of patients with Scheuermann's disease: A review of twenty-four cases managed by combined anterior and posterior spine fusion. *J Bone Joint Surg Am* 1980;62:705-712.

8. Bradford DS, Moe JH, Montalvo FJ, Winter RB: Scheuermann's kyphosis: Results of surgical treatment by posterior spine arthrodesis in twenty-two patients. *J Bone Joint Surg Am* 1975;57:439-448.

9. Bradford DS, Ahmed KB, Moe JH, Winter RB, Lonstein JE: The surgical management of patients with Scheuermann's disease: A review of twenty-four cases managed by combined anterior and posterior spine fusion. *J Bone Joint Surg Am* 1980;62:705-712.

10. McMaster MJ, Singh H: The surgical management of congenital kyphosis and kyphoscoliosis. *Spine* 2001;26:2146-2155.

11. Thiranont N, Netrawichien P: Transpedicular decancellation closed wedge vertebral osteotomy for treatment of fixed flexion deformity of spine in ankylosing spondylitis. *Spine* 1993;18:2517-2522.

12. Crawford AH: Neurofibromatosis, in Weinstein SL (ed): *The Pediatric Spine: Principles and Practice*, ed 2. Philadelphia, PA, Lippincott Williams & Wilkins, 2001, pp 471-490.

13. Fienman NL: Pediatric neurofibromatosis: Review. *Compr Ther* 1981;7:66-72.

14. Kim HW, Weinstein SL: Spine update: The management of scoliosis in neurofibromatosis. *Spine* 1997;22:2770-2776.

15. Bradford DS, Daher YH: Vascularised rib grafts for stabilisation of kyphosis. *J Bone Joint Surg Br* 1986;68:357-361.

16. Hsu LC, Lee PC, Leong JC: Dystrophic spinal deformities in neurofibromatosis: Treatment by anterior and posterior fusion. *J Bone Joint Surg Br* 1984;66:495-499.

17. Lonstein JE: Post-laminectomy kyphosis. *Clin Orthop* 1977;128:93-100.

18. Munechica Y: Influence of laminectomy on the stability of the spine. *J Jpn Orthop Assoc* 1973;47:111-126.

19. Peterson HA: Spinal deformity secondary to tumor, irradiation and laminectomy, in Bradford DS, Hensinger RN (eds): *The Pediatric Spine*. New York, NY, Thieme, 1985, pp 273-285.

8

Kyphosis of the Thoracic and Thoracolumbar Spine in the Pediatric Patient: Prevention and Treatment of Surgical Complications

Lawrence G. Lenke, MD

Abstract

The successful outcome of surgical treatment of pediatric kyphosis depends on careful preoperative identification of the etiology of the problem as well as identification of any associated medical conditions or syndromes that may render surgical reconstruction more challenging. Many perioperative surgical factors can lead to an unsuccessful surgical outcome, including inadequate preoperative patient or kyphosis assessment; inappropriate selection of proximal and/or distal instrumentation and fusion levels; inadequate spinal fixation applied at the ends of the posterior construct where tension forces are greatest; inadequate performance of a meticulous posterior spinal fusion; absence and/or an inadequate performance of an anterior spinal fusion when required either before or after the posterior procedure; overcorrection of the kyphotic deformity based on the ability of the spine above and below to compensate for the correction; a higher risk of neurologic complications with correction of kyphotic deformities; and inadequate postoperative support with an orthosis. Revision surgery for failed pediatric kyphosis surgeries requires careful reexamination of all these factors to correct any shortcomings. In addition, adjunctive procedures such as spinal osteotomies, perioperative traction, and/or anterior fusion techniques may be required to optimize spinal alignment, balance, and ultimate successful fusion. When following these guidelines, pediatric spinal kyphosis disorders can be successfully treated and complications avoided.

It is generally more difficult and dangerous to surgically treat kyphosis pathology than scoliosis pathology.[1] Because the management of complications related to the surgical treatment of pediatric kyphosis can be particularly challenging, it is important to stress preventive measures to avoid complications in the first place. When postoperative problems arise, however, the reasons why the kyphosis reconstruction failed must be identified and a treatment plan developed to correct and overcome the complications.

This chapter discusses the etiology of failed pediatric kyphosis reconstructive surgery along with spe-cific treatment plans to surgically manage these difficult complications. Preventive measures are also discussed that can help avoid the complications of failed surgery.

Etiology

Before treating complications arising from failed pediatric kyphosis surgery, it is extremely important to accurately determine what caused the initial reconstruction to fail.[2,3] Various causes include but are not limited to the following: inadequate preoperative patient or deformity assessment; fusion done at inappropriate proximal and/or distal levels; the application of inadequate fixation, especially at the ends of the posterior construct; inadequate abundant posterior spinal fusion; inadequate anterior spinal fusion; overcorrection of kyphosis as determined by the ability of the spine above and below to compensate for the correction; neurologic complications; and any combination of the above. The type of kyphosis and the particular patient characteristics must also be determined. For example, the surgical treatment of kypho-

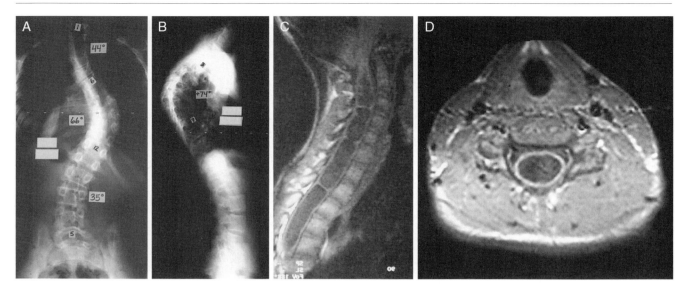

Figure 1 A and **B**, Radiographs of a 15-year-old boy with a 44° proximal thoracic and 66° main thoracic double-thoracic curve pattern. Although the coronal plane is idiopathic in presentation, the sagittal plane demonstrates 74° of kyphosis in the mid-thoracic region. Because of the presence of thoracic hyperkyphosis, which is atypical for adolescent idiopathic scoliosis, the patient underwent total spine MRI examination. **C** and **D**, Total spine MRI scans show a large cervical-thoracic syrinx extending from C2 down to T10 as well as an Arnold-Chiari malformation. This condition required neurosurgical intervention before anterior and posterior spinal fusion.

sis will fail for different reasons in a 3-year-old patient who weighs 30 lb and has a congenital dislocation of the proximal thoracic spine and an adult patient who weighs 275 lb and has a Scheuermann's kyphosis. In addition to identifying the type of kyphosis being treated (for example, congenital, Scheuermann's, post-laminectomy, posttraumatic, or my-elokyphosis), it must also be determined whether sagittal plane malalignment is associated with any coronal plane malalignment (scoliosis). Although rare, an otherwise idiopathic scoliosis apparent on a coronal plane radiograph can be associated with a thoracic hyperky-phosis malalignment.[4] Therefore, a preoperative total spine MRI should be obtained to exclude any associated spinal canal anomalies (Figure 1). Because medical problems such as heart disease, lung disease, and connective tissue disorders can complicate the surgical treatment of

pediatric kyphosis, a thorough medical history must be obtained and a careful physical examination performed when revision surgery is being planned.

Problems with the surgical treatment of pediatric kyphosis most often arise as the result of inappropriate selection of proximal and/or distal fusion levels, which often occurs in combination with inadequate fixation.[3,5] Much has been written regarding the selection of appropriate proximal and distal fusion levels in the treatment of coronal plane abnormalities such as scoliosis; however, much less has been written regarding the selection of appropriate proximal and distal fusion levels in the treatment of kyphosis. One published method recommends including the first lordotic disk in the upper to midlumbar spine as the distal fusion level.[5] This will usually be a safe distal fusion level in the majority of patients.

However, in some patients, a neutral disk above the first lordotic disk is present, and the vertebra between these disks can occasionally be the distal fusion level. The concept of the "stable" vertebra on the sagittal radiographs can be used to denote the safe distal fusion level and draw the posterior sacral vertical line, a vertical line drawn from the posterior edge of the S1 body, proximally until it intersects (or bisects) one of the lumbar vertebra (Figure 2). Similarly, the center sacral vertical line is drawn on the coronal plane radiograph to determine the "stable" vertebra in the coronal plane. As is true in the coronal plane, occasionally the vertebra immediately above the true "stable" vertebra can be the distal fusion level in the sagittal plane. As long as the posterior sacral vertical line intersects some part of this more proximal vertebra, this vertebra is a safe distal fusion level, particularly when the disk above it is lordotic or neutral. If the disk above it is in any degree of kyphosis, the safe fusion level normally will have to be extended one level more distal.

For choosing the proximal level of instrumentation and fusion, symmetry is normally defined above the apex of a deformity to make symmetric moment arms both above and below the apex. For example, if a kyphosis has an apex of T10, and the posterior sacral vertical line selected L3 as the stable vertebra (five levels below the apex T10), then T4 would be selected as the proximal starting point, which is five levels above the apex. Occasionally, one more proximal level can be added for additional fixation, if required.

With posterior fixation, the strength and security of the fixation increases as sublaminar wires, various supralaminar and infralaminar hooks, and then pedicle screws are used for fixation.[6-11] The three-column support of multisegmented pedicle screw constructs provides extremely secure purchase and construct stability for primary and revision kyphosis reconstructions. The number of pedicle screw implants required to optimally stabilize a kyphosis reconstruction, especially in a revision reconstruction, is unknown. But because of the difficulty in healing of kyphosis surgeries as a result of the tension-band forces of posteriorly applied implants, more fixation points are used.[7,12] This is particularly appropriate in a revision reconstruction for which previous posterior implants have failed to secure a strong posterior fusion mass for long-term stability. Also, failed hook purchase in the low thoracic and upper- and midlumbar spine can be revised with appropriate distal screw fixation (Figure 3).

Another distinct advantage of using transpedicular fixation for proxi-

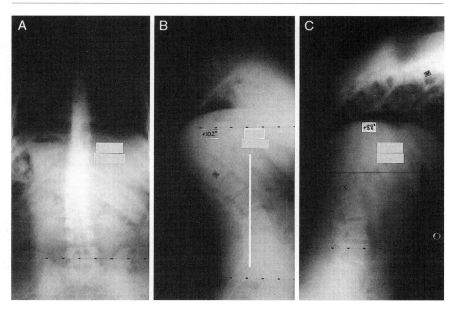

Figure 2 A through **C**, Radiographs of a 17-year-old boy with a large Scheuermann's kyphosis. The posterior sacral vertical line as drawn from the back edge of the sacrum most closely bisects the L3 vertebral body, which is known as the "stable" sagittal vertebra. This was the lowest instrumented vertebra for anterior and posterior spinal reconstruction.

mal and distal kyphosis implants is the lack of any iatrogenic ligamentous injury when the implants are properly placed. Generally, with any type of sublaminar wire or hook fixation, implants placed supra-adjacent to the proximal fusion level and infra-adjacent to the inferior instrumented level will disrupt ligamentous tissue. To avoid junctional problems, it is important to maintain the posterior ligamentous tension band. If radical posterior tension-band disruption occurs, as it can when the bilateral supralaminar hooks used as proximal implants are placed following complete removal of the interspinous ligaments and ligamentum flavum at the supra-adjacent level, then proximal junctional kyphosis will ensue (Figure 4). Regardless of the type of implant used, injury to the supra-adjacent and infra-adjacent soft tissue and ligamentous structures must also be avoided when per-

forming any type of primary or revision reconstruction for kyphosis.

Overcorrection of the kyphotic deformity can also cause surgery to fail.[5] If overcorrection occurs, a problem is usually evident more proximally at the cervicothoracic junction than distally at the lumbosacral junction. Thus, for severe kyphotic deformities, such as those associated with Scheuermann's disease, it is advisable to plan for correction of approximately 50%. Attempting to correct these deformities to within the 25° to 30° range may result in overcorrection for those patients with deformities within the 80° to 100° range. Regardless of the amount of correction, a thorough posterior fusion with autogenous bone graft is mandatory to create a thick posterior fusion mass that will prevent loss of correction, which can occur over time as a result of constant posterior tension forces. Additionally,

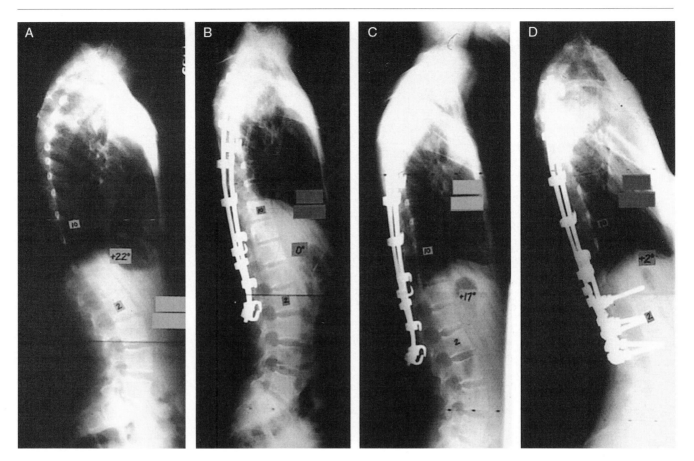

Figure 3 A, Preoperative radiograph of a female patient with adolescent idiopathic scoliosis and a 22° T10-L2 thoracolumbar kyphosis. **B**, The patient underwent posterior instrumentation and fusion down to L2 with a segmental hook construct. **C**, Four weeks postoperatively, the patient reported increased pain and a palpable mass in the lower part of her incision. A lateral radiograph demonstrated hook pull-off distally. **D**, The patient had a revision posterior instrumentation with extension to L3 with transpedicular screws with good sagittal realignment.

posterior implants should be left in place long term, even when a solid posterior fusion mass is present. A fusion mass with a residual large kyphosis can still bend and/or break over time, in which case revision surgery involving an anterior fusion mass (intradiskal and/or strut) will be required to prevent further bending (Figure 5).

Some of the more common complications associated with pediatric kyphosis surgery are neurologic. It is well known that the primary and revision surgical treatment of conditions such as congenital kyphosis have an extremely high rate of neu-

rologic complications. Two factors account for this high rate: tension applied to the anterior portion of the spinal cord[13,14] and limitation of the anterior spinal cord blood supply[15-17] resulting from straightening of the kyphosis. Although it is difficult to distinguish these two etiologies clinically, spinal cord monitoring during pediatric kyphosis surgery can help identify problems occurring as a result of concomitant hypotension. With combined somatosensory-evoked potential and neurogenic motor-evoked potential monitoring, hypotension-induced spinal cord monitoring signal losses can be

abruptly reversed by the delivery of hypertensive agents. This intervention occasionally requires administering a dopamine drip intraoperatively and immediately postoperatively to maintain blood pressures at a level that will maintain adequate spinal cord blood flow.

Because it is so important to maximize spinal cord blood flow during kyphosis reconstruction, harvesting of segmental vessels anteriorly should be avoided. The placement of instrumentation anteriorly should also be avoided because it often requires segmental vessel ligation. Inducing hypotension during the posterior

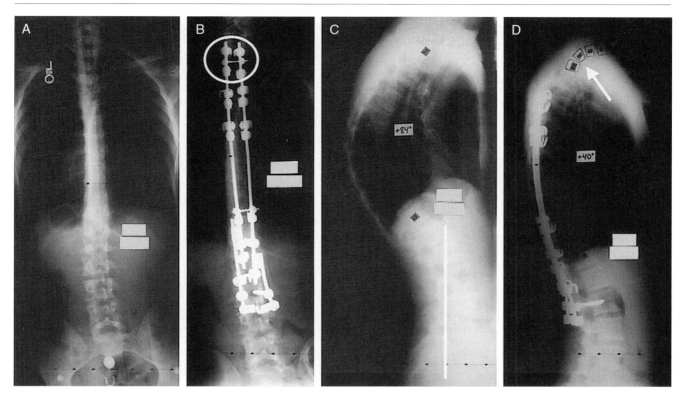

Figure 4 A, Preoperative radiograph of a male patient with a Scheuermann's kyphosis. **B**, The patient underwent anterior and posterior spinal fusion with posterior instrumentation from T2 to L3. His proximal construct consisted of bilateral pedicle-supralaminar claw hooks. **C**, These bilateral supralaminar hooks are detrimental for cervical thoracic junctional stability because of the iatrogenic ligamentous disruption required to place the hooks. **D**, The patient subsequently developed a cervicothoracic junctional kyphosis.

correction of kyphosis is not recommended. A mean arterial blood pressure of 70 to 80 mm Hg can maintain optimal spinal cord perfusion. Because diminution of spinal cord data with hypotension is more often seen initially with neurogenic motor-evoked potential than somatosensory-evoked potential monitoring, multimodality spinal cord monitoring should be used when surgically treating patients with kyphosis.[15,18-21] The intraoperative wake-up test can definitively confirm appropriate lower extremity neurologic function; however, results of this test provide data for only one moment in time, and waiting for results may delay the correction of a hypotension-induced

neurologic dysfunction. In addition, the problem may not be appropriately identified if correction of deformity has not yet been performed.

The etiology of failed pediatric kyphosis surgery may be multifactorial, with several of the previously discussed factors resulting in an unsuccessful reconstruction that requires revision. Thus, before revision takes place, all previous surgical procedures must be carefully reviewed and the factors that contributed to the ultimate failure definitively identified (Figures 6 through 8). Only then can corrective surgery be planned that will ultimately result in a solid spinal fusion and a well-balanced spine.

Surgical Treatment
The basic options available for pediatric patients in whom previous kyphosis surgery has failed include revision posterior spinal fusion with instrumentation; anterior spinal fusion either as a primary or revision procedure; spinal osteotomies to improve segmental, regional, and global spinal kyphotic malalignment; and potentially adjunctive procedures, such as halo traction, to assist in overall realignment.

If the previous fusion and existing instrumentation needs to be extended proximally and/or distally, the entire spinal region can be exposed to confirm that adequate fusion exists in those regions as well.

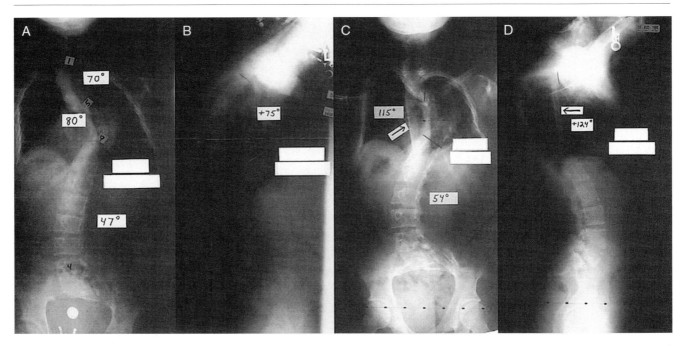

Figure 5 A, Preoperative radiographs of a 17-year-old boy with a congenital kyphoscoliosis with an 80° coronal and 75° sagittal plane deformity and a solid posterior fusion. A progressive deformity occurred as a result of chronic bending of the fusion mass caused by severe residual kyphosis. **B**, Radiographs of the same patient at 5-year follow-up. The patient underwent an anterior allograft fibular structural fusion from a concave thoracotomy approach. This vertically placed fibular graft supports the spine from bending, providing an "I" beam type of support for the 115° coronal and 124° sagittal plane deformity.

Although an existing rod can be added to extend the patient's proximal and/or distal fusion and instrumentation in simple reconstructions, in complex reconstructions (ie, in patients who have undergone multiple previous surgeries), the entire "fusion" mass should be explored to make sure that it is solid rather than simply noting pseudarthrotic areas that will require revision posteriorly and/or anteriorly. Previous fixation points, such as hooks or screws, can be reused, although it is recommended that old implants be exchanged for new implants to ensure that the connection between the longitudinal member and the implants is as strong and secure as possible. If the previous wire or hook fixation was inadequate, then placing pedicle screws is usually possible in these regions, even

with altered anatomy. Fluoroscopy or image-guided techniques (eg, computerized stealth systems) can be helpful, if required. In these situations, more rather than less fixation will be indicated to fully immobilize the spine and provide the best chance of obtaining a solid fusion.

Posterior osteotomies may help realign the kyphotic spine into a more neutral or even lordotic position. Osteotomies may also improve segmental and regional lordosis and sagittal balance. Three types of osteotomies can be used: the Smith-Petersen osteotomy (SPO), the pedicle subtraction osteotomy (PSO), and the anterior-posterior osteotomy (APO).

The SPO is a posterior column osteotomy that opens the anterior column (disk), hinges on the middle column, and closes the posterior column the amount that is removed posteri-

orly. This is done in a V-shaped fashion in the infralaminar spaces posteriorly between the spinous processes and lamina. Five to 10 mm of posterior element bone and ligament is usually removed to allow posterior closure, which is best accomplished with multisegmented screw fixation. If the anterior column is fused, SPO may not work. Additionally, once done, the anterior defects created by closing the posterior column must be examined and may require secondary intradiskal grafting to optimize the fusion rate. SPO can be very helpful in the treatment of thoracic and thoracolumbar pathologies in which a modest amount of correction can be obtained over multiple segments to nicely contour the spine into a better alignment.

The PSO is a more extensive three-column osteotomy that re-

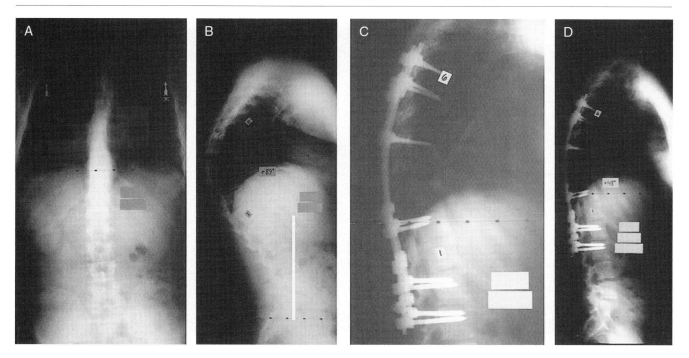

Figure 6 Preoperative PA (**A**) and lateral (**B**) radiographs of an 18-year-old man with a presumed Scheuermann's kyphosis. **C** and **D**, The patient underwent anterior and posterior spinal fusion. A diagnosis of connective tissue disorder was made later. His posterior instrumentation initially ended at L1, which was far proximal to his stable vertebra at L3. He experienced early screw pull-out and 1 week postoperatively underwent surgery for extension down to L3. However, because of the connective tissue disorder in his neutral thoracolumbar alignment, his deformity below the instrumentation progressed with a rounded kyphosis extending to L5.

sects the posterior column, the pedicles (middle column), and the lateral portion of the vertebral body, while hinging on the anterior aspect of the body. Approximately 30° to 40° of kyphosis correction can often be obtained at one level. The PSO is quite stable because, when done correctly, a bone-on-bone position of all three columns of the spine is produced once the posterior column is closed. It is preferable to perform this osteotomy in the midlumbar and upper-lumbar spine (below the spinal cord) because of the amount of dural retraction and tension created when this osteotomy is closed. A PSO in the midlumbar spine can be combined with multiple SPOs in the thoracolumbar junction and thoracic spine for marked deformity correction of stiff global ky-

photic deformities (Figure 6).

The APO is rarely used because it is only indicated to treat fixed kyphosis in the thoracic spine and thoracolumbar junction for which the PSO may not be as appropriate. For example, an APO is potentially indicated to correct congenital kyphosis over multiple segments in the thoracic spine. Regardless of the posterior approach used, secure segmental instrumentation and the abundant application of autogenous bone graft from either the iliac crest or ribs (as in a thoracoplasty procedure) are mandatory for the long-term success of primary and/or revision posterior kyphosis surgery.

Appropriate anterior spinal fusion can also help achieve long-term fusion in patients undergoing posterior kyphosis surgery. If the anterior

spine has not been approached during the initial operation, then performing anterior spinal fusion either before or after the posterior procedure may be indicated, especially over any pseudarthrotic area where the posterior fusion bed may not be adequate for obtaining a secure fusion. In the thoracic spine, this usually entails the application of morcellized autogenous bone after a thorough diskectomy. However, in the lower thoracic and throughout the lumbar and lumbosacral spine, intradiskal structural support should be provided using allograft bone or vertical mesh cages that help support the loads applied to the anterior and middle columns through the disk spaces. Applying strut graft as an "I" beam support is indicated for large severe kyphoses in which intradiskal

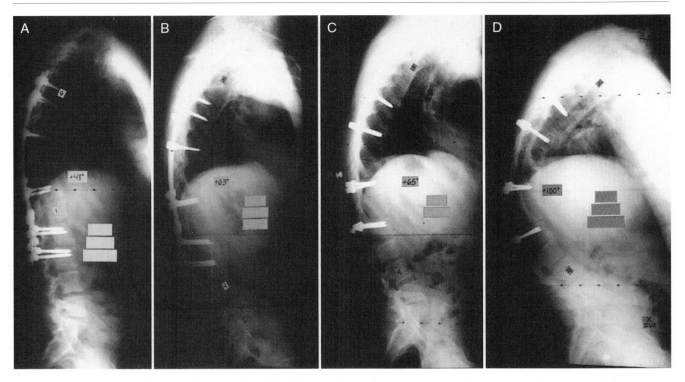

Figure 7 Same patient as shown in Figure 6. **A** and **B,** When exploring the patient's posterior wound, a deep wound infection was noted with multiple organisms cultured out. Thus, the rods were removed, several critical screws kept and he was placed on long-term intravenous antibiotics. **C** and **D,** Although the patient's wound infection healed, he developed a stiff progressive global thoracic and lumbar kyphosis all the way to his sacrum measuring 100°.

grafting alone may not provide enough support to prevent postoperative fusion mass bending or breakage because of the large kyphotic angulation and long moment arm involved in the spinal malalignment. Applying allograft or autograft fibula is the preferred method of treatment of these types of deformities in pediatric patients with vertebral bodies large enough to accept these grafts. Rarely, a vascularized rib or autogenous fibula graft will be required for high-risk patients undergoing revision kyphosis surgery.[22-24]

Perioperative or intraoperative halo traction can be used to help realign the kyphotic spine. When used perioperatively, halo traction can gradually and safely stretch the spinal column and cord, with the patient awake and able to respond to any type of excessive stretching to the neural axis. Although halo traction has been used selectively to treat very severe deformities, it can be especially helpful in patients who have undergone surgical revision because previous anterior surgery and vessel harvest or ligation or anterior or posterior scar formation with previous laminectomies can put them at increased risk for neurologic complications. Additionally, the halo device can be used to optimize intraoperative positioning for deformity correction. Preoperative halo traction can be used for patients with kyphosis greater than 100°, especially those who will undergo revision and those who are smaller or in ill health to maximize their respiratory status perioperatively. In addition, patients with a concomitant scoliosis deformity greater than 90° to 100° would also be candidates for simultaneous coronal and sagittal plane correction. Thus far, no major complications resulting from the use of perioperative halo gravity traction have been reported, and traction has not been stopped because of any type of cranial nerve or upper or lower extremity neurologic complication (A Rinella, MD, LG Lenke, MD, St Louis, MO, unpublished data, 2003).

Summary

Although prevention is often the best way to avoid the need for revision surgery, surgical treatment of pediatric kyphosis is a significant undertaking. Thorough preoperative evaluation is required to identify not only the nature of the defor-

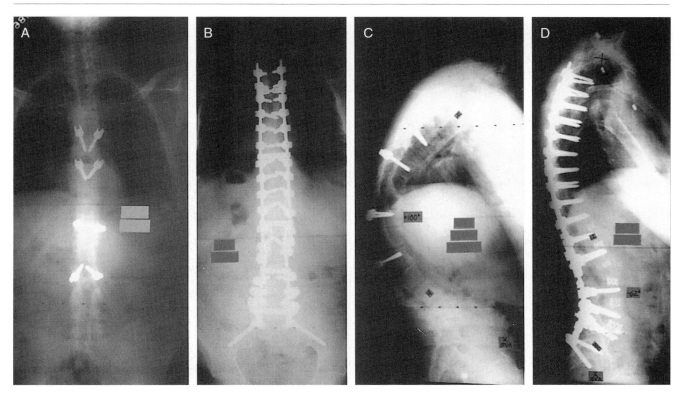

Figure 8 Same patient as shown in Figure 6. **A** through **D,** The patient's spinal reconstruction was extensive because of the complicated nature of his pathology. He underwent a first-stage posterior instrumentation and fusion with bilateral transpedicular screws at every level from T3 to the sacrum except L3, where a PSO was done. Pseudarthrosis was noted at every level of his previous fusion attempt. Thus, multilevel SPOs were done to contour his lower thoracic and thoracolumbar junction and to achieve a more appropriate amount of sagittal alignment. An anterior spinal fusion was subsequently done from T10 to the sacrum using structural cages, autogenous, and allograft bone. Postoperative radiographs show excellent sagittal realignment with normal sagittal contours throughout.

mity but also the patient's overall health and any existing conditions/syndromes. Selection of the best approach (posterior alone or circumferential), appropriate fusion levels, placement of secure segmental spinal instrumentation, the judicious use of both anterior (if needed) and posterior spinal fusion techniques with autogenous bone are necessary for success. Revision for failed surgery requires careful reexamination of all of these factors and compensation for any shortcomings. In addition, adjunctive procedures such as spinal osteotomies, perioperative traction, and anterior fusion techniques may be required to optimize spinal alignment, balance, and ultimately successful fusion. When following these guidelines, kyphosis in pediatric patients can be successfully treated and complications avoided.

References

1. Bridwell KH, Lenke LG, Baldus C, Blanke K: Major intraoperative neurologic deficits in pediatric and adult spinal deformity patients: Incidence and etiology at one institution. *Spine* 1998;23:324-331.

2. Johnston CE II, Schoenecker PL: Letter: Cervical kyphosis in patients who have Larsen syndrome. *J Bone Joint Surg Am* 1997;79:1590-1591.

3. Wiggins GC, Rauzzino MJ, Bartkowski HM, Nockels RP, Shaffrey CI: Management of complex pediatric and adolescent spinal deformity. *J Neurosurg* 2001;95(suppl 1):17-24.

4. Betz RR, Harms J, Clements DH III, et al: Comparison of anterior and posterior instrumentation for correction of adolescent thoracic idiopathic scoliosis. *Spine* 1999;24:225-239.

5. Wenger DR, Frick SL: Scheuermann kyphosis. *Spine* 1999;24:2630-2639.

6. Abumi K, Shono Y, Taneichi H, Ito M, Kaneda K: Correction of cervical kyphosis using pedicle screw fixation systems. *Spine* 1999;24:2389-2396.

7. Belmont PJ Jr, Polly DW Jr, Cunningham BW, Klemme WR: The effects of hook pattern and kyphotic angulation on mechanical strength and apical rod strain in a long-segment posterior construct using a synthetic model. *Spine* 2001;26:627-635.

8. Brown CA, Lenke LG, Bridwell KH, Greideman WM, Hasan SA, Blanke K: Complications of pediatric thoracolumbar and lumbar pedicle screws. *Spine* 1998;23:1566-1571.

9. Lenke LG, Padberg AM, Russo MH, Bridwell KH, Gelb DE: Triggered electromyographic threshold for accuracy of pedicle screw placement: An animal model and clinical correlation. *Spine* 1995;20:1585-1591.

10. Lewis SJ, Lenke LG, Raynor B, Long J, Bridwell KH, Padberg A: Triggered electromyographic threshold for accuracy of thoracic pedicle screw placement in a porcine model. *Spine* 2001;26:2485-2490.

11. Papagelopoulos PJ, Klassen RA, Peterson HA, Dekutoski MB: Surgical treatment of Scheuermann's disease with segmental compression instrumentation. *Clin Orthop* 2001;386:139-149.

12. Oda I, Cunningham BW, Buckley RA, et al: Does spinal kyphotic deformity influence the biomechanical characteristics of the adjacent motion segments? An in vivo animal model. *Spine* 1999;24:2139-2146.

13. Birnbaum K, Siebert CH, Hinkelmann J, Prescher A, Niethard FU: Correction of kyphotic deformity before and after transection of the anterior longitudinal ligament: A cadaver study. *Arch Orthop Trauma Surg* 2001;121:142-147.

14. Bridwell KH, Kuklo TR, Lewis SJ, Sweet FA, Lenke LG, Baldus C: String test measurement to assess the effect of spinal deformity correction on spinal canal length. *Spine* 2001;26:2013-2019.

15. Kai Y, Owen JH, Lenke LG, Bridwell KH, Oakley DM, Sugioka Y: Use of sciatic neurogenic motor evoked potentials versus spinal potentials to predict early-onset neurologic deficits when intervention is still possible during overdistraction. *Spine* 1993;18:1134-1139.

16. Pelosi L, Jardine A, Webb JK: Neurological complications of anterior spinal surgery for kyphosis with normal somatosensory evoked potentials (SEPs). *J Neurol Neurosurg Psychiatry* 1999;66:662-664.

17. Tribus CB: Transient paraparesis: A complication of the surgical management of Scheuermann's kyphosis secondary to thoracic stenosis. *Spine* 2001;26: 1086-1089.

18. Komanetsky RM, Padberg AM, Lenke LG, et al: Neurogenic motor evoked potentials: A prospective comparison of stimulation methods in spinal deformity surgery. *J Spinal Disord* 1998;11:21-28.

19. Padberg AM, Russo MH, Lenke LG, Bridwell KH, Komanetsky RM: Validity and reliability of spinal cord monitoring in neuromuscular spinal deformity surgery. *J Spinal Disord* 1996;9:150-158.

20. Wilson-Holden TJ, Padberg AM, Parkinson JD, Bridwell KH, Lenke LG, Bassett GS: A prospective comparison of neurogenic mixed evoked potential stimulation methods: Utility of epidural elicitation during posterior spinal surgery. *Spine* 2000;25:2364-2371.

21. Wilson-Holden TJ, Padberg AM, Lenke LG, Larson BJ, Bridwell KH, Bassett GS: Efficacy of intraoperative monitoring for pediatric patients with spinal cord pathology undergoing spinal deformity surgery. *Spine* 1999;24:1685-1692.

22. Govender S, Kumar KP, Med PC: Long-term follow-up assessment of vascularized rib pedicle graft for tuberculosis kyphosis. *J Pediatr Orthop* 2001;21:281-284.

23. Harwant S: Factors influencing the outcome of arthrodesis for congenital kyphosis and kyphoscoliosis. *Med J Malaysia* 2001;56:18-24.

24. Zeller RD, Dubousset J: Progressive rotational dislocation in kyphoscoliotic deformities: Presentation and treatment. *Spine* 2000;25:1092-1097.

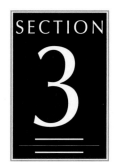

SECTION 3

Adolescent Idiopathic Scoliosis

Adolescent Idiopathic Scoliosis

The three chapters in this section provide a thorough discussion of adolescent idiopathic scoliosis (AIS). In the first chapter, Parent and associates provide information to convey a basic understanding of this disorder. In the two subsequent chapters, Lenke and Newton discuss the areas of their expertise, the classification and surgical approaches to AIS, respectively. The information within each chapter provides an excellent springboard for comprehending subsequent developments in the field.

In the first chapter, Parent and associates begin with a discussion of the influences that may play a role in the development of AIS—genetics, hormonal factors, tissue abnormalities, neuromuscular pathology, and biomechanics. Although the exact etiology of this disorder is unknown, it is believed to be multifactorial, with genetic influences the most documented of the aforementioned factors. New research continues to validate the genetic basis for AIS;[1,2] however, the variable clinical expression and lack of consistent identifiable inheritance patterns reinforces the complexity of this disease.

Parent and associates provide an excellent description of the structural deformity in AIS, which consists of a three-dimensional rotational change that is most commonly characterized with two orthogonal plain radiographs showing a thoracic, coronal plane, convex, right-sided curve with hypokyphosis. The rotational deformity results in morphometric changes in the ribs and components of the vertebrae, which are most discernible at the apex of the curve. At this location, the rib prominence is greatest, the concave pedicles have the smallest diameter, and the vertebral bodies are the most wedged and rotated. An understanding of these three-dimensional anatomic changes is crucial in safely instrumenting the spine.

Parent and associates also highlight the influence of thresholds in calculating the prevalence of AIS. When a low threshold is used (for example, a curve magnitude greater than 10°), the prevalence of AIS is between 2% and 3% and occurs equally in males and females. However, curves greater than 30° are approximately 10 times less common and are overrepresented in females compared with males by an 8:1 ratio. The authors also undertake the difficult task of discussing the natural history of AIS. Curves that appear similar may progress differently. This is the central issue in treating AIS. Understanding the factors that influence curve progression is imperative. Gender, the initial curve pattern, and the curve magnitude in relationship to skeletal maturity influence curve progression. Monitoring and screening for the stage of skeletal maturity is time and resource intensive.

Parent and associates also discuss bracing, which is the sole nonsurgical treatment of AIS. Bracing for adolescent scoliosis remains controversial. It is generally believed that increasing the time the brace is worn will increase the success rate in preventing curve progression. Although the Boston brace remains the gold standard for the nonsurgical treatment of AIS, the Charleston nighttime brace has proven valuable in patients with single lumbar and thoracolumbar curves.

Lenke led the development of an AIS classification system designed to characterize curves in both the sagittal and coronal planes while denoting the flexibility of the spine to establish surgical treatment. His chapter reviews this classification system. Although some physicians disagree regarding the use of this system in making surgical decisions, the Lenke classification system has substantially improved communication about AIS. This improvement is seen at many levels: literature reviews, clinical discussions among peers, and in the instruction of residents and fellows. Perhaps the most important contribution of this classification system has been its recognition that optimal surgical treatment of AIS requires a more thorough evaluation of the curve than indicated by previous classification systems. In the future, computerized databases that can be used to collect and organize a large amount of data from radiographs and clinical measurements may provide information for a more thorough evaluation and assistance in surgical planning.[3,4]

The chapter by Newton discusses the thoracoscopic approach to the spine in scoliosis management. This surgical approach has similar merit to other minimally invasive endoscopic procedures in that less dissection is required and visualization is improved. The proposed decreased morbidity coupled with the surge in popularity of anterior spine surgery during the 1990s helped advance this technique.

The indications for anterior endoscopic instrumentation are reserved for patients with Lenke type 1 AIS with nonstructural proximal thoracic and lumbar curves. Although the technique has been perfected by a select number of surgeons, the benefits are diminished when compared with more recent posterior instrumentation techniques. These posterior techniques use more pedicle screws and involve more aggressive posterior releases.[5] These changes largely negate the previously touted benefits of anterior instrumentation, namely improved correction through fewer instrumented levels. Proponents of the newer posterior techniques also provide good argument against the need for anterior release in large, rigid curves because equivalent corrections can be achieved with all-posterior pedicle screw constructs as with combined anterior-posterior approaches.[6] This viewpoint has been nicely summarized by Arlet.[7]

These three chapters provide a wonderful base of knowledge for those who devote or plan to devote their practice to the management of AIS. These chapters highlight many of the changes that have occurred over the past decade and introduce upcoming advances in the treatment of AIS.

Jeffrey S. Shilt, MD
Medical Director of Pediatric
    Orthopaedics
St. Alphonsus Regional Medical Center
Boise, Idaho

References

1. Raggio CL, Giampietro PF, Dobrin S, et al: A novel locus for adolescent idiopathic scoliosis on chromosome 12p. *J Orthop Res* 2009;27(10):1366-1372.

2. Kouwenhoven JW, Castelein RM: The pathogenesis of adolescent idiopathic scoliosis: review of the literature. *Spine* (Phila Pa 1976) 2008;33(26):2898-2908.

3. Arlet V, Shilt J, Bersusky E, et al: Experience with an online prospective database on adolescent idiopathic scoliosis: Development and implementation. *Eur Spine J* 2008;17(11): 1497-1506.

4. Sangole AP, Aubin CE, Labelle H, et al: Three-dimensional classification of thoracic scoliotic curves. *Spine (Phila Pa 1976)* 2009;34(1):91-99.

5   Cuartas E, Rasouli A, O'Brien M, Shufflebarger HL: Use of all-pedicle-screw constructs in the treatment of adolescent idiopathic scoliosis. *J Am Acad Orthop Surg* 2009;17(9):550-561.

6. Li M, Ni J, Fang X, et al: Comparison of selective anterior versus posterior screw instrumentation in Lenke5C adolescent idiopathic scoliosis. *Spine* (Phila Pa 1976) 2009;34(11): 1162-1166.

7. Arlet V: Comment regarding "Is anterior release effective to increase flexibility in idiopathic thoracic scoliosis? Assessment by traction films" (A. Hempfing et al). *Eur Spine J* 2007;16(4):521-522.

Dr. Shilt or an immediate family member is a member of a speakers' bureau or has made paid presentations on behalf of Medtronic and is a consultant for or is an employee of Ellipse Technologies.

9

Adolescent Idiopathic Scoliosis: Etiology, Anatomy, Natural History, and Bracing

Stefan Parent, MD, PhD
Peter O. Newton, MD
Dennis R. Wenger, MD

Abstract

Adolescent idiopathic scoliosis is a three-dimensional deformity of the spine. Despite active efforts by different research teams, the etiology of scoliosis remains unclear. Treatment of scoliosis requires a solid understanding of the natural history of the disorder as well as sound clinical judgment. The evaluation, monitoring, and institution of conservative treatment such as bracing can present a challenge to the orthopaedic surgeon. Clinical monitoring is the only intervention necessary in most patients. A detailed review of the patient's history as well as a careful physical examination can help establish the diagnosis and the risk for progression. Skeletal maturity, gender, growth velocity, curve location, and magnitude are factors that can help assess the likelihood of progression. Bracing is the only nonsurgical measure proven to have any effect on halting the progression of scoliosis. Other forms of conservative treatment have not been shown to significantly modify the natural history of idiopathic scoliosis. Bracing results are directly related to compliance with brace treatment; therefore, optimal results cannot be achieved without the patient's cooperation and family support.

The etiology of idiopathic scoliosis remains unknown, but recent developments in the fields of genetics and molecular biology may ultimately provide insights into the etiology and pathophysiology of scoliosis. Several etiologic theories exist and include genetic factors, hormonal factors, growth abnormalities, biomechanical and neuromuscular theories, as well as different tissue disorders of bone, muscle, and fibrous tissue.

Etiology
Genetic Factors

Several studies suggest there is a genetic component in the development of idiopathic scoliosis. Population studies have shown an increased incidence in families of patients with idiopathic scoliosis compared with the general population.[1-7] In one study, daughters of women with idiopathic scoliosis had a 27% prevalence of scoliotic curves greater than 15°.[8] Another study on familial prevalence showed an 11% prevalence for first-degree relatives, and a 2.4% and 1.4% prevalence for second- and third-degree relatives, respectively.[2] A meta-analysis of 68 sets of twins with scoliotic curves (37 sets of monozygotic and 31 sets of dizygotic twins) showed a prevalence of scoliosis in 73% of monozygous twins compared with 36% in dizygous twins.[9] Curve severity has also been evaluated, and monozygotic twins had greater correlation than in dizygotic twins.

Despite the accumulating evidence for a genetic etiology, the exact inheritance pattern, genes, and gene product causing scoliosis remain unknown. The most likely inheritance pattern is multifactorial.[2] Genomic screening and statistical linkage analysis are research methods used to help identify the genetic features of scoliosis.[10]

Hormonal Factors

An observation that pinealectomized chickens develop scoliosis has led to the hypothesis that melatonin (secreted by the pineal gland) deficiency may lead to scoliosis.[11,12] Levels of melatonin were then evaluated in a group of 30 patients with idiopathic scoliosis. Patients showing curve progression of more than 10° in 1 year showed a decrease of 35% of nighttime melatonin secretion compared with the patients without progression and normal controls.[13] However, in another study, Bagnall and associates[14] could not demonstrate a statistically significant difference in melatonin secretion in a group of patients with idiopathic scoliosis.

Rapid progression of scoliotic curves has been reported in patients taking growth hormone, but scoliosis is a problem in less than 1% of patients taking growth hormone.[15] Growth hormone seems to be related to melatonin activity because it has a diurnal secretion pattern, but unlike melatonin, the concentrations of growth hormone are higher during the daytime. The pineal gland could be responsible for growth control by melatonin's modulation on growth hormone activity.[14] Injection of growth hormone in pinealectomized chickens also seems to produce greater scoliotic curves.[14] An attractive theory relating to melatonin is that a deficiency in the receptor, not the ligand, is responsible for curve development. If changes in the receptor for melatonin render the hormone inactive, this could explain the variations in melatonin levels observed in different studies. Melatonin receptors have been identified in different tissues including bones and muscle. However, the exact relationship between melatonin and scoliosis development, if one exists, remains to be elucidated.

Tissue Abnormalities

The observed associations between scoliosis and disorders such as Marfan syndrome and osteogenesis imperfecta have led to research efforts evaluating the role of connective tissue in the pathogenesis of scoliosis. Collagen fibers and elastin fibers are important components of the spine that provide stability and support. A histomorphometric study of intervertebral disks has shown changes associated with the distribution of collagen fibers in patients with scoliosis, but these changes were not constant.[16]

Several investigators have proposed that scoliosis could be secondary to a functional deficit of muscular components.[17-21] Several studies have demonstrated structural changes in muscle fibers, with asymmetric changes found on the concavity and convexity of scoliotic curves.[22-25] However, these convexity/concavity modifications could easily be secondary changes associated with the alterations in muscle length or loading that follow scoliosis development.

Similarities between platelet contractile elements and skeletal muscle fibers have led researchers to study the cellular structure of thrombocytes. Because platelets are not located primarily in the spine, the changes observed in their contractile elements could represent a primary systemic process as opposed to secondary changes caused by scoliosis.[7] Elevated levels of intracellular calcium and phosphorus have been observed in patients with scoliosis.[25] Other investigators have identified abnormal calmodulin levels in patients with scoliosis.[26,27] These observations support the hypothesis of a general cellular membrane anomaly (possibly present in both platelets and muscle fibers) as a cause for idiopathic scoliosis, but this theory remains to be proven.

Neuromuscular Theories

Neuromuscular theories are based on the observations that patients with neuromuscular disease often develop scoliosis. The hypothesis is that a subclinical dysfunction of the central nervous system could result in scoliosis. Syringomyelia is associated with an increase in scoliosis incidence, possibly secondary to direct pressure on the sensory or motor tracts of the spinal cord.[28,29] Irritation of the brain stem may result from Chiari malformation or enlargement of the fourth ventricle and result in scoliosis. Cerebral asymmetry[30] and postural equilibrium dysfunction[31] have been observed in patients with scoliosis. These changes in equilibrium have been shown to be proportional to curve severity but returned to normal at maturity.[32,33] Abnormalities in the vestibulo-ocular system have also been identified in patients with scoliosis.[34,35]

Spinal Growth/Biomechanical Theories

Mechanical influences on spinal growth are thought to play an important role in curve progression because scoliosis occurs mainly during the rapid growth period of adolescence. The biomechanical theories can be divided between the causative (etiologic) theories and the secondary, self-sustaining curve progression model occurring after an initial event. Several authors have proposed an etiologic theory for the development of scoliosis based on the modification of the sagittal profile.[36-42] According to this model, patients with idiopathic scoliosis develop progressive hypokyphosis, followed by lordosis of the thoracic spine, causing the spine to "buckle" under the physiologic load applied on the spine. Smith and associates[43] later described a transverse plane deformity and a bone drift phenomenon toward the concavity of the curve. More recently, Porter[44] proposed that the length of the spinal canal was shorter than the anterior length of the vertebral body, thus creating an effect similar to a posterior tether causing spinal "buckling" and finally the typical three-dimensional deformity of idiopathic scoliosis. However, the cause for this theorized "mismatch" of anterior and posterior spinal column growth has not been determined. It may relate to differences in the rates of endochondral and intramembranous growth of the vertebral elements.[27]

Once the scoliotic deformity has been established, most agree that some component of curve progression is regulated by the Hueter-Volkmann principle,[45,46] which states that growth is retarded by increased compression and accelerated when compressive loads are reduced. Stokes and associates[47,48] have proposed a mechanical modulation theory of vertebral growth based on the Hueter-Volkmann principle, and they believe that once asymmetric loading occurs, a "vicious circle" ensues, with progressive vertebral wedging promoting further asymmetric loading and further vertebral deformity. Perdriolle and associates[49] have proposed that a small thoracic curve could create asymmetric loading causing curve progression once the curve reaches a certain level.

Spinal Anatomy

The vertebral column constitutes the central structure of the human body. Along with the thoracic cage, it serves as a scaffold attaching the upper and lower extremities while supporting the head. It surrounds and protects the spinal cord and transfers the weight of the trunk to the lower extremities through the pelvis. Because of the erect posture adopted by humans during evolution, the vertebral column is composed of physiologic curvatures allowing prolonged standing. Cervical lordosis, thoracic kyphosis, and lumbar lordosis constitute the normal sagittal contour. In the frontal plane, the vertebral column is normally straight.

Idiopathic scoliosis is a three-dimensional deformity affecting the orientation and position of the spinal elements in space (Figure 1). The regional and global changes are characterized by a deviation in the frontal plane, a modification of the sagittal profile, as well as alterations in the shape of the rib cage. The most characteristic feature of scoliosis is the coronal plane curvature of the spine, the most common being a right-sided convex deviation of the thoracic spine. Although originally thought to be associated with kyphosis, in most instances the apical region of thoracic scoliosis is in fact hypokyphotic. The "apparent kyphosis" results from the convex side rib prominence that results from axial rotation of the vertebra in the transverse plane. Maximal at the apex, vertebral rotation alters the shape and orientation of the ribs, creating the rib prominence that makes the trunk appear kyphotic.

A morphometric analysis of anatomic specimens with scoliosis has demonstrated deformation of the vertebrae. This altered shape consists of progressive vertebral wedging with the transitional vertebra demonstrating minimal or no wedging and maximum wedging located at the apex of a typical scoliotic curve. In addition, pedicle width was modified significantly on the concave side of the sco-

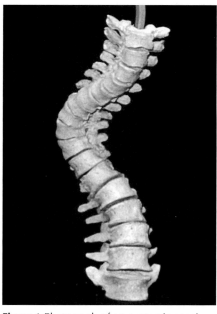

Figure 1 Photograph of an anatomic specimen with right thoracic scoliosis, demonstrating a marked change in shape of the spinal column (anterior view).

liotic curve with progressive thinning of the pedicle toward the apex of the curve.[50,51] Because of the scoliosis, the spinal cord tends to lie closer to this smaller concave apical pedicle[52] (Figure 2).

Prevalence and Natural History of Idiopathic Scoliosis

The prevalence of idiopathic scoliosis varies greatly based on the minimal curvature selected as the lower limit for diagnosis. The reported prevalence for scoliotic curves greater than 10° ranges from 0.5% to 3%.[53-58] For curves greater than 30°, the prevalence decreases to 1.5 to 3 per 1,000.[58,59] Thus, small to moderate curves are common and severe curves that require treatment are rare. Idiopathic scoliosis is most common during adolescence. The ratio of boys to girls affected is equal for minor curves, yet dominated by girls as the curve magnitude increases, reaching a ratio of 1:8 for those requiring treatment.[60]

Risk factors for scoliosis progression

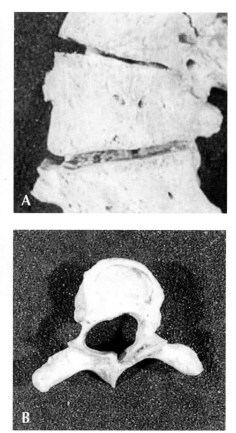

Figure 2 A, Anterior view photograph of an anatomic specimen demonstrating the vertebral wedging that results from long-standing scoliotic deformity. The Hueter-Volkmann principles result in alterations in growth, resulting in these shape changes. **B,** Superior view photograph of an anatomic specimen with scoliotic deformity, demonstrating asymmetry of the pedicles.[51]

that have been identified include gender, remaining skeletal growth, curve location, and curve magnitude, with scoliosis progression being the most rapid during peak skeletal growth. Peak growth velocity of adolescence averages 6 to 8 cm of overall height gain per year. Bone age and menarcheal status help determine the growth spurt in females, with the onset of menses generally following the most rapid stage of skeletal growth by approximately 12 months. When the Risser sign is grade 1 or less, the risk for progression is increased to 60% to 70%. However, if

Table 1
Risk of Scoliosis Progression and Relation to Curve Magnitude and Patient Skeletal Maturity

	Curves That Progressed (%)	
	5° to 19° Curves	20° to 29° Curves
Risser sign		
Grade 0 or 1	22	68
Grade 2, 3, or 4	2	23

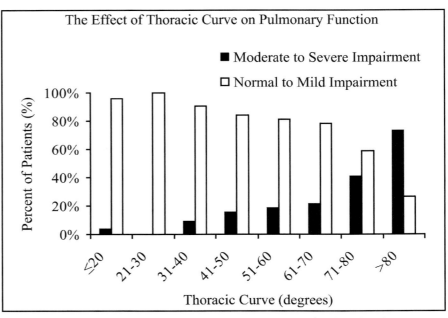

Figure 3 Graphic representation of the relationship between predicted forced vital capacity (% predicted) and thoracic Cobb angle.

the Risser sign is grade 3, the risk is reduced to less than 10%.[61,62] Unfortunately, many of the readily identified markers of maturity (for example, menarcheal status and Risser sign) are variable and appear just after the adolescent growth spurt. Therefore, it is impossible to tell whether a patient who is premenarcheal and has a Risser sign of grade 0 is approaching, in the midst of, or past the most rapid growth stage and thus at risk for scoliosis progression. Closure of the triradiate cartilage of the acetabulum has been identified as a radiographic sign, which more closely approximates the time of peak growth velocity.[63]

Curve pattern has also been identified as an important variable for predicting the probability of progression. Curves with an apex above T12 are more likely to progress than isolated lumbar curves.[61] Curve magnitude at the initial diagnosis appears to be a factor predicting progression.[62,64] Larger curves are more likely to continue to increase in magnitude with growth (Table 1).

Pulmonary function becomes limited as thoracic scoliosis becomes more severe (> 60° to 70°).[65,66] Forced vital capacity and forced expiratory volume in 1 second decrease linearly, with an approximate 20% reduction in predicted values with 100° curves.[66] The associated deformity of the chest cavity causes restrictive lung disease. Thoracic lordosis also decreases lung volume and increases the deleterious effects of scoliosis on pulmonary function[67] (Figure 3).

Estimates regarding the frequency of back pain and associated disability in adults with scoliosis vary, but most studies have shown slightly higher rates of back pain compared with control groups.[66-69] Although the risk of curve progression is highest during the rapid phases of growth, not all curves stabilize after growth. In long-term studies, many patients experience progression after skeletal maturity.[70,71] Curves less than 30° tend not to progress, with the most marked progression occurring in curves that are between 50° and 75° at the completion of growth (progression continuing at a rate of nearly 1° per year). Lumbar curves are more likely to progress if they are greater than 30° at skeletal maturity. This risk of progression in adults after skeletal maturity has led to many of the treatment recommendations regarding surgical management of scoliosis.

Nonsurgical Treatment and Bracing
The treatment approach for any condition should be based on both long-term

and short-term outcomes. Treatment decisions often are made with incomplete data, particularly with regard to the longer-term results. The three general options for treatment are observation, use of an orthotic device, or some form of surgical stabilization (Figure 4). Although other forms of treatment have been proposed (such as electrical muscle stimulation, exercise, postural training, spinal manipulation, and nutritional supplementation), it seems that only bracing and surgical fusion have scientific evidence of affecting the outcome compared with observation alone. Even the efficacy of brace treatment, which has been extensively evaluated, remains in question.

Early Detection/School Screening Programs
The objective of school screening for scoliosis is to detect scoliosis early enough to allow brace treatment instead of a later time when surgical correction is the only option. To be effective, screening programs must have early treatment

methods available for the specific disorder, and the condition must be frequent enough to justify the cost of screening. Although screening programs for scoliosis are widespread in North America, some authors have suggested that school screening is not justified based on variable sensitivity and specificity of the screening examination and the efficacy of bracing.[72-74]

School screening is routinely performed in children in the fifth and sixth grades (age 10 to 12 years). The Adams forward-bend test and the scoliometer are used in combination to evaluate the maximal angle of trunk rotation[75] (Figure 5). It has been shown that an angle of trunk rotation greater than 7° detects nearly all curves over 30°, but also refers a large number of patients (2 to 3 per 100 children screened)[74,75] for radiographs in children only presenting with spinal asymmetry (Cobb angle < 10°) or mild scoliosis (Cobb angle < 25°) not needing treatment. Despite the high number of referrals and the high costs associated with school screening, these programs have increased the awareness of scoliosis among primary care physician and the general population.

Observational Monitoring

Most patients with adolescent idiopathic scoliosis only require observational monitoring, which may create anxiety in the patient and family who are concerned about living with scoliosis. However, the natural history of most minor curves is benign. Patients with growth remaining are at risk for progression, and thus those skeletally immature patients with curves between 11° and 25° warrant periodic evaluation. Radiographs (standing PA view) are recommended every 4 to 12 months depending on the rate of growth at the time. During peak adolescent growth (6 to 10 cm per year), monitoring every 4 to 6 months may be appropriate, especially if the scoliosis is approaching a magnitude to consider brace treatment.

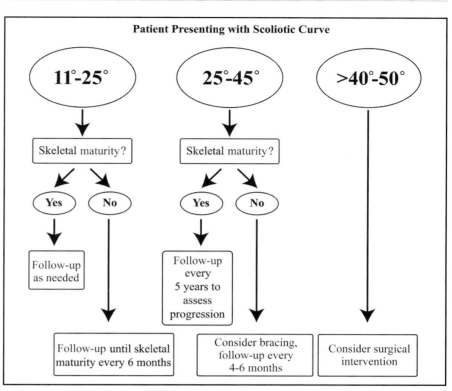

Figure 4 Treatment algorithm for adolescent idiopathic scoliosis based on curve magnitude and skeletal maturity at presentation.

Once skeletal maturity is reached, the rate of scoliosis progression, when it occurs, is much slower (approximately 1° per year) than during adolescent growth. As such, the requirements for monitoring are much less. Curves less than 25° in adults are at low risk for progression and do not require routine follow-up. Above this 25° limit, follow-up every 5 to 10 years will allow detection of a slow progression should it occur.

Brace Treatment

The use of a thoracolumbosacral orthosis is the only nonsurgical method of controlling scoliosis progression that has had any evidence of success. Current recommendations are to use a scoliosis brace to prevent progression of moderate curves only during growth. The exact upper and lower limits of curve magnitude that are appropriate for brace usage are debatable; however, the Scoliosis Research Society

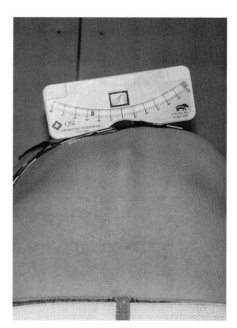

Figure 5 Photograph of a patient during Adams forward bending test, with scoliometer demonstrating right thoracic prominence and angle of trunk rotation.

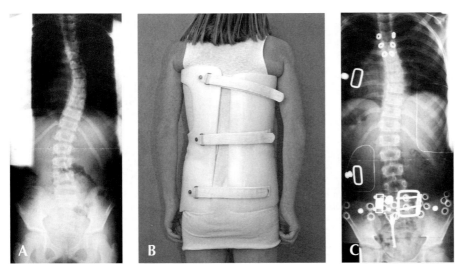

Figure 6 A, PA radiograph of patient before bracing with a Boston brace. **B,** Photograph of a patient wearing a Boston brace. **C,** PA radiograph of patient in a Boston brace shows good correction of the main thoracic curve.

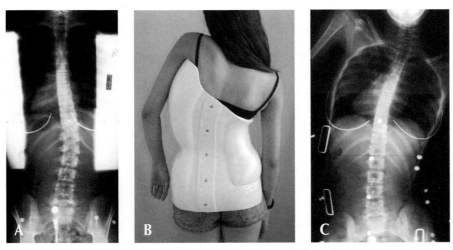

Figure 7 A, PA radiograph of patient before bracing with a Charleston brace. **B,** Photograph of a patient in Charleston nighttime bending brace. **C,** PA radiograph of patient in a Charleston brace shows good correction of the main lumbar curve.

has stated the following guidelines: a curve that has documented progression to greater than 25° or a patient presenting with a curve initially greater than 30° should be treated with bracing if the patients is still growing (Risser grade 0, 1, or 2). It is clear that brace efficacy is impacted by curve size, and those curves greater than 45° to 50° will likely benefit little from bracing.

The goal of brace treatment is to limit further curve progression, ideally keeping the scoliosis from reaching surgical indications. Although curve severity is reduced after appropriate brace fitting, this correction primarily occurs only when the brace is worn. In most patients, lasting correction of the deformity does not remain when use of the brace is discontinued. Thus, if a patient presents with a clinical deformity and scoliosis that suggests a need for surgical treatment, the same situation is likely to remain even if a brace is worn during the period of remaining growth. Currently, methods for nonsurgical reversal of a scoliotic curvature do not exist. This is often a difficult and frustrating circumstance for the patient and family because the best outcome of brace treatment is only prevention of further progression.

Brace correction is thought to occur by constant molding of the trunk and spine during growth. Full-time bracing was therefore originally suggested and remains the method of choice at several centers.[76,77] However, full-time brace wear is difficult. As such, brace-wearing schedules have been modified, reducing the time in the brace to 15 to 16 hours per day.[78,79] A dose-dependent relationship between the time per day in the brace and success in preventing curve progression was found in a meta-analysis of the literature[80] and suggests that the more time the patient spends in the brace, the less likely the curve is to progress.

Although brace treatment was deemed successful for many years, only recently have controlled treatment trials been completed.[81,82] The Scoliosis Research Society sponsored a study that compared the results of observation, bracing, and electrical stimulation in 286 patients in a prospective controlled trial.[81] Curve progression at the end of treatment was limited to less than 5° in 74% of patients treated with a brace compared with 34% in the group without treatment and 33% in the group that received electrical stimulation. Although the methodology of this study was criticized,[55] many centers continue to advise brace treatment in adolescent idiopathic scoliosis patients presenting with substantial growth remaining.

The effect of brace design on outcome is difficult to compare because most studies do not use the same inclusion criteria, and indications for brace use depends on the type and localization of the curve. In two recent studies, the underarm brace design worn full time was found to be more effective both at preventing progression and preventing further surgery than the Charleston nighttime brace design.[82,83] However, for single lumbar and thoracolumbar curves, the results of using the Charleston nighttime brace equaled those of the Boston brace.[82] (Figures 6 and 7)

The decision to include bracing in the treatment algorithm is debatable; however, if bracing is to have any chance of success, a coordinated effort must be made among the treating physician, the patient, and family as well as an orthotist with a strong interest in scoliosis treatment. Careful fitting and continued adjustment of the brace optimize curve correction while intermittent radiographs (every 4 to 6 months) are used to monitor for progression. Optimal curve correction cannot be achieved without the patient's cooperation in conforming to the brace-wearing schedule.

Summary

The cause of scoliosis remains a subject of active research. Many etiologic theories exist with different levels of evidence to support them. Adolescent idiopathic scoliosis carries a strong genetic component. Both the parents and the patient with scoliosis should be advised about the increased risk to siblings and offspring of developing scoliosis.

Treatment of scoliosis requires a solid understanding of the natural history of the disorder as well as sound clinical judgment. Adolescent idiopathic scoliosis treatment is based on curve magnitude at presentation, skeletal maturity, risk factors for progression, and clinical deformity (Figure 4). Clinical monitoring is the only intervention necessary in most patients. Brace treatment remains the standard of care in several countries for curves between 25° and 45° when significant growth remains. However, the sci-entific basis for brace use in scoliosis is limited. Surgical treatment is advocated in skeletally immature patients when the curve reaches 40° to 50°. The small margin between bracing and surgical indications represents a challenge to the treating physician, the patient, and the family.

References

1. De George FV, Fisher RL: Idiopathic scoliosis: genetic and environmental aspects. *J Med Genet* 1967;4:251-257.

2. Risenborough EJ, Wynne-Davies R: A genetic survey of idiopathic scoliosis in Boston, Massachusetts. *J Bone Joint Surg Am* 1973;55:974-982.

3. Robin GC, Cohen T: Familial scoliosis: A clinical report. *J Bone Joint Surg Br* 1975;57:146-148.

4. Wynne-Davies R: Familial (idiopathic) scoliosis: A family survey. *J Bone Joint Surg Br* 1968;50:24-30.

5. Wynne-Davies R: Genetic aspects of idiopathic scoliosis. *Dev Med Child Neurol* 1973;15:809-811.

6. Hadley MN: Spine update: Genetics of familial idiopathic scoliosis. *Spine* 2000;25:2416-2418.

7. Miller NH: Cause and natural history of adolescent idiopathic scoliosis. *Orthop Clin North Am* 1999;30:343-352.

8. Harrington PR: The etiology of idiopathic scoliosis. *Clin Orthop* 1977;126:17-25.

9. Kesling KL, Reinker KA: Scoliosis in twins: A meta-analysis of the literature and report of six cases. *Spine* 1997;22:2009-2014.

10. Justice CM, Miller NH, Marosy B, Zhang J, Wilson AF: Familial idiopathic scoliosis: Evidence of an X-linked susceptibility locus. *Spine* 2003;28:589-594.

11. Machida M, Dubousset J, Imamura Y, Iwaya T, Yamada T, Kimura J: An experimental study in chickens for the pathogenesis of idiopathic scoliosis. *Spine* 1993;18:1609-1615.

12. Machida M, Dubousset J, Imamura Y, Iwaya T, Yamada T, Kimura J: Role of melatonin deficiency in the development of scoliosis in pinealectomised chickens. *J Bone Joint Surg Br* 1995;77:134-138.

13. Machida M, Dubousset J, Imamura Y, Miyashita Y, Yamada T, Kimura J: Melatonin: A possible role in pathogenesis of adolescent idiopathic scoliosis. *Spine* 1996;21:1147-1152.

14. Bagnall KM, Raso VJ, Hill DL, et al: Melatonin levels in idiopathic scoliosis: Diurnal and nocturnal serum melatonin levels in girls with adolescent idiopathic scoliosis. *Spine* 1996;21:1974-1978.

15. Allen DB: Safety of human growth hormone therapy: Current topics. *J Pediatr* 1996;128:S8-13.

16. Roberts S, Menage J, Eisenstein SM: The cartilage end-plate and intervertebral disc in scolio-sis: Calcification and other sequelae. *J Orthop Res* 1993;11:747-757.

17. Fidler MW, Jowett RL: Muscle imbalance in the aetiology of scoliosis. *J Bone Joint Surg Br* 1976;58:200-201.

18. Langenskiold A, Michelsson J: Experimental progressive scoliosis in the rabbit. *J Bone Joint Surg Br* 1961;43:116.

19. Spencer GS, Zorab PA: Spinal muscle in scoliosis: Comparison of normal and scoliotic rabbits. *J Neurol Sci* 1976;30:405-410.

20. Spencer GS, Eccles MJ: Spinal muscle in scoliosis: Part 2. The proportion and size of type 1 and type 2 skeletal muscle fibres measured using a computer-controlled microscope. *J Neurol Sci* 1976;30:143-154.

21. Spencer GS, Zorab PA: Spinal muscle in scoliosis: Part 1. Histology and histochemistry. *J Neurol Sci* 1976;30:137-142.

22. Bylund P, Jansson E, Dahlberg E, Eriksson E: Muscle fiber types in thoracic erector spinae muscles: Fiber types in idiopathic and other forms of scoliosis. *Clin Orthop* 1987;214:222-228.

23. Yarom R, Robin GC, Gorodetsky R: X-ray fluorescence analysis of muscles in scoliosis. *Spine* 1978;3:142-145.

24. Yarom R, Robin GC: Studies on spinal and peripheral muscles from patients with scoliosis. *Spine* 1979;4:12-21.

25. Yarom R, Blatt J, Gorodetsky R, Robin GC: Microanalysis and x-ray fluorescence spectrometry of platelets in diseases with elevated muscle calcium. *Eur J Clin Invest* 1980;10:143-147.

26. Cheung WY: Calmodulin. *Sci Am* 1982;246:62-70.

27. Kindsfater K, Lowe T, Lawellin D, Weinstein D, Akmakjian J: Levels of platelet calmodulin for the prediction of progression and severity of adolescent idiopathic scoliosis. *J Bone Joint Surg Am* 1994;76:1186-1192.

28. Zadeh HG, Sakka SA, Powell MP, Mehta MH: Absent superficial abdominal reflexes in children with scoliosis: An early indicator of syringomyelia. *J Bone Joint Surg Br* 1995;77:762-767.

29. Samuelsson L, Lindell D: Scoliosis as the first sign of a cystic spinal cord lesion. *Eur Spine J* 1995;4:284-290.

30. Goldberg CJ, Dowling FE, Fogarty EE, Moore DP: Adolescent idiopathic scoliosis and cerebral asymmetry: An examination of a nonspinal perceptual system. *Spine* 1995;20:1685-1691.

31. Yamada K, Yamamoto H, Nakagawa Y, Tezuka A, Tamura T, Kawata S: Etiology of idiopathic scoliosis. *Clin Orthop* 1984;184:50-57.

32. Sahlstrand T, Lidstrom J: Equilibrium factors as predictors of the prognosis in adolescent idiopathic scoliosis. *Clin Orthop* 1980;152:232-236.

33. Lidstrom J, Friberg S, Lindstrom L, Sahlstrand T: Postural control in siblings to scoliosis patients and scoliosis patients. *Spine* 1988;13:1070-1074.

34. Sahlstrand T, Petruson B: A study of labyrinthine function in patients with adoles-

cent idiopathic scoliosis: I. An electro-nystag-mographic study. *Acta Orthop Scand* 1979;50: 759-769.

35. Sahlstrand T, Petruson B, Ortengren R: Vestibulospinal reflex activity in patients with adolescent idiopathic scoliosis: Postural effects during caloric labyrinthine stimulation recorded by stabilometry. *Acta Orthop Scand* 1979;50:275-281.

36. Somerville EW: Rotational lordosis: The development of the single curve. *J Bone Joint Surg Br* 1952;34:421-427.

37. Deacon P, Berkin CR, Dickson RA: Combined idiopathic kyphosis and scoliosis: An analysis of the lateral spinal curvatures associated with Scheuermann's disease. *J Bone Joint Surg Br* 1985;67:189-192.

38. Dickson RA: The etiology and pathogenesis of idiopathic scoliosis. *Acta Orthop Belg* 1992;58(suppl 1):21-25.

39. Roaf R: The basic anatomy of scoliosis. *J Bone Joint Surg Br* 1966;48:786-792.

40. Cruickshank JL, Koike M, Dickson RA: Curve patterns in idiopathic scoliosis: A clinical and radiographic study. *J Bone Joint Surg Br* 1989;71:259-263.

41. Murray DW, Bulstrode CJ: The development of adolescent idiopathic scoliosis. *Eur Spine J* 1996;5:251-257.

42. Willner S, Johnson B: Thoracic kyphosis and lumbar lordosis during the growth period in children. *Acta Paediatr Scand* 1983;72:873-878.

43. Smith RM, Pool RD, Butt WP, Dickson RA: The transverse plane deformity of structural scoliosis. *Spine* 1991;16:1126-1129.

44. Porter RW: Idiopathic scoliosis: The relation between the vertebral canal and the vertebral bodies. *Spine* 2000;25:1360-1366.

45. Hueter C: Anatomische Studien an den Extramitaetengelenken Neugeborener en Erwachsener. *Virkows Archiv Path Anat Physiol* 1862;25:572-599.

46. Volkmann R: Verletzungen end Krankenheiten des Bewegungsorgane, in von Pitha B (ed): *Handbuch der allgemeine und speciellen Chirurgie Bd II Teil II.* Stuttgart, Germany, Ferdinanc Enke, 1882.

47. Stokes IA, Aronsson DD, Spence H, Iatridis JC: Mechanical modulation of intervertebral disc thickness in growing rat tails. *J Spinal Disord* 1998;11:261-265.

48. Stokes IA, Spence H, Aronsson DD, Kilmer N: Mechanical modulation of vertebral body growth: Implications for scoliosis progression. *Spine* 1996;21:1162-1167.

49. Perdriolle R, Becchetti S, Vidal J, Lopez P Mechanical process and growth cartilages: Essential factors in the progression of scoliosis. *Spine* 1993;18:343-349.

50. Parent S, Labelle H, Skalli W, Latimer B, De Guise J: Morphometric analysis of anatomic scoliotic specimens. *Spine* 2002;27:2305-2311.

51. Parent S, Labelle H, Skalli W, De Guise J: Thoracic pedicle morphometry in vertebrae from scoliotic spines. *Spine* 2004;29:239-248.

52. Liljenqvist UR, Allkemper T, Hackenberg L, Link TM, Steinbeck J, Halm HF: Analysis of vertebral morphology in idiopathic scoliosis with use of magnetic resonance imaging and multiplanar reconstruction. *J Bone Joint Surg Am* 2002;84:359-368.

53. Kane WJ, Moe JH: A scoliosis-prevalence survey in Minnesota. *Clin Orthop* 1970;69: 216-218.

54. Stirling AJ, Howel D, Millner PA, Sadiq S, Sharples D, Dickson RA: Late-onset idiopathic scoliosis in children six to fourteen years old: A cross-sectional prevalence study. *J Bone Joint Surg Am* 1996;78:1330-1336.

55. Dickson RA, Weinstein SL: Bracing (and screening): Yes or no? *J Bone Joint Surg Br* 1999;81:193-198.

56. Rogala EJ, Drummond DS, Gurr J: Scoliosis: Incidence and natural history. A prospective epidemiological study. *J Bone Joint Surg Am* 1978;60:173-176.

57. Morais T, Bernier M, Turcotte F: Age- and sex-specific prevalence of scoliosis and the value of school screening programs. *Am J Public Health* 1985;75:1377-1380.

58. Montgomery F, Willner S: The natural history of idiopathic scoliosis: Incidence of treatment in 15 cohorts of children born between 1963 and 1977. *Spine* 1997;22:772-774.

59. Kane WJ: Scoliosis prevalence: A call for a statement of terms. *Clin Orthop* 1977;126: 43-46.

60. Bunnell WP: The natural history of idiopathic scoliosis before skeletal maturity. *Spine* 1986;11:773-776.

61. Peterson LE, Nachemson AL: Prediction of progression of the curve in girls who have adolescent idiopathic scoliosis of moderate severity: Logistic regression analysis based on data from The Brace Study of the Scoliosis Research Society. *J Bone Joint Surg Am* 1995;77:823-827.

62. Lonstein JE, Carlson JM: The prediction of curve progression in untreated idiopathic scoliosis during growth. *J Bone Joint Surg Am* 1984;66:1061-1071.

63. Sanders JO, Little DG, Richards BS: Prediction of the crankshaft phenomenon by peak height velocity. *Spine* 1997;22:1352-1356.

64. Karol LA, Johnston CE, Browne RH, Madison M: Progression of the curve in boys who have idiopathic scoliosis. *J Bone Joint Surg Am* 1993;75:1804-1810.

65. Pehrsson K, Bake B, Larsson S, Nachemson A: Lung function in adult idiopathic scoliosis: A 20 year follow up. *Thorax* 1991;46:474-478.

66. Weinstein SL, Zavala DC, Ponseti IV: Idiopathic scoliosis: Long-term follow-up and prognosis in untreated patients. *J Bone Joint Surg Am* 1981;63:702-712.

67. Winter RB, Lovell WW, Moe JH: Excessive thoracic lordosis and loss of pulmonary function in patients with idiopathic scoliosis. *J Bone Joint Surg Am* 1975;57:972-977.

68. Mayo NE, Goldberg MS, Poitras B, Scott S, Hanley J: The Ste-Justine Adolescent Idiopathic Scoliosis Cohort Study: Part III. Back pain. *Spine* 1994;19:1573-1581.

69. Dickson JH, Erwin WD, Rossi D: Harrington instrumentation and arthrodesis for idiopathic scoliosis: A twenty-one-year follow-up. *J Bone Joint Surg Am* 1990;72:678-683.

70. Weinstein SL: Idiopathic scoliosis: Natural history. *Spine* 1986;11:780-783.

71. Weinstein SL, Ponseti IV: Curve progression in idiopathic scoliosis. *J Bone Joint Surg Am* 1983;65:447-455.

72. Pruijs JE: van der MR, Hageman MA, Keessen W, van Wieringen JC. The benefits of school screening for scoliosis in the central part of The Netherlands. *Eur Spine J* 1996;5:374-379.

73. Goldberg CJ, Dowling FE, Fogarty EE, Moore DP: School scoliosis screening and the United States Preventive Services Task Force: An examination of long-term results. *Spine* 1995;20:1368-1374.

74. Grossman TW, Mazur JM, Cummings RJ: An evaluation of the Adams forward bend test and the scoliometer in a scoliosis school screening setting. *J Pediatr Orthop* 1995;15:535-538.

75. Bunnell WP: Outcome of spinal screening. *Spine* 1993;18:1572-1580.

76. Price CT, Scott DS, Reed FE Jr, Riddick MF: Nighttime bracing for adolescent idiopathic scoliosis with the Charleston bending brace: Preliminary report. *Spine* 1990;15:1294-1299.

77. Blount WP, Schmidt A: The Milwaukee brace in the treatment of scoliosis. *J Bone Joint Surg Am* 1957;39:693.

78. Allington NJ, Bowen JR: Adolescent idiopathic scoliosis: treatment with the Wilmington brace: A comparison of full-time and part-time use. *J Bone Joint Surg Am* 1996;78:1056-1062.

79. Green NE: Part-time bracing of adolescent idiopathic scoliosis. *J Bone Joint Surg Am* 1986;68:738-742.

80. Rowe DE, Bernstein SM, Riddick MF, Adler F, Emans JB, Gardner-Bonneau D: A meta-analysis of the efficacy of non-operative treatments for idiopathic scoliosis. *J Bone Joint Surg Am* 1997;79:664-674.

81. Nachemson AL, Peterson LE: Effectiveness of treatment with a brace in girls who have adolescent idiopathic scoliosis: A prospective, controlled study based on data from the Brace Study of the Scoliosis Research Society. *J Bone Joint Surg Am* 1995;77:815-822.

82. Howard A, Wright JG, Hedden D: A comparative study of TLSO, Charleston, and Milwaukee braces for idiopathic scoliosis. *Spine* 1998;23:2404-2411.

83. Katz DE, Richards BS, Browne RH, Herring JA: A comparison between the Boston brace and the Charleston bending brace in adolescent idiopathic scoliosis. *Spine* 1997;22:1302-1312.

10

Lenke Classification System of Adolescent Idiopathic Scoliosis: Treatment Recommendations

Lawrence G. Lenke, MD

Abstract

The Lenke and associates classification system of adolescent idiopathic scoliosis (AIS) was developed to provide a comprehensive and reliable means to categorize all surgical AIS curves. This classification system requires analysis of the upright coronal and sagittal radiographs along with the supine side bending radiographic views. The triad classification system consists of a curve type (1-6), a lumbar spine modifier (A, B, C), and a sagittal thoracic modifier (-, N, +). All three regions of the radiographic coronal and sagittal planes, the proximal thoracic, main thoracic, and thoracolumbar/lumbar are designated as either the major curve (largest Cobb measurement) or minor curves with the minor curves separated into structural and nonstructural types. The recommendations are that the major and structural minor curves are included in the instrumentation and fusion and the nonstructural minor curves are excluded. Overall, the classification system is treatment directed; however, there are other aspects of the radiographic and clinical deformity that may suggest deviation from the recommendations of the classification system. The ultimate goal of this classification system is to allow organization of similar curve patterns to provide comparisons of various treatment methods to provide optimal treatment for each AIS surgical patient.

Although the King-Moe system has been the gold standard for classification of adolescent idiopathic scoliosis (AIS) since its publication in 1983,[1] several authors have found that the system has several shortcomings when used to evaluate the surgical treatment of various types of scoliosis curves with modern segmental spinal instrumentation.[2,3] Thus, a new classification system was developed that requires use of the upright coronal and sagittal radiographs, along with the supine side bending views for complete curve classification.

The development of this new triad, modular classification system for the surgical treatment of AIS was based on six goals:[4] the classification system would be comprehensive for all curve types; two-dimensional, with increased emphasis placed on the sagittal plane; treatment-based to recommend surgery on the major and structural minor regions of the spine but not on the nonstructural minor regions; able to recommend selective fusions of the spine when appropriate; able to have specific objective criteria to help separate curve types which would then optimize both interobserver and intraobserver reliability; and easily understood and usable for surgeons and their trainees on a routine basis.

Using the Lenke Classification System

The classification system begins with the evaluation of the upright coronal, sagittal, and right and left side bending radiographs. On the upright coronal radiograph, the three spinal column regions that may develop surgical curves are evaluated: the proximal thoracic (PT), main thoracic (MT), and thoracolumbar/lumbar (TL/L) regions. The major curve is the curve with the largest Cobb measurement, and that will always be included in the fusion of surgical AIS. The minor curves are the two other regions, and one of the main decisions in scoliosis surgery is whether or not to include these minor curves in the fusion along with the major curve. To help in this decision, minor curve structural criteria were established to help guide the surgeon and also create a classification scheme template. In the coronal plane, inflexibility on side bending radiographs where the residual minor curve is greater than or equal to 25° in each of the three regions will render that region a structural minor curve. In addition, hyperkyphosis greater than or equal to 20° in the PT region (T2-T5) or TL junction (T10-L2) renders the associated region of the spine a structural minor curve as well. Thus, a schematic can be created for six different curve types that are defined in this new

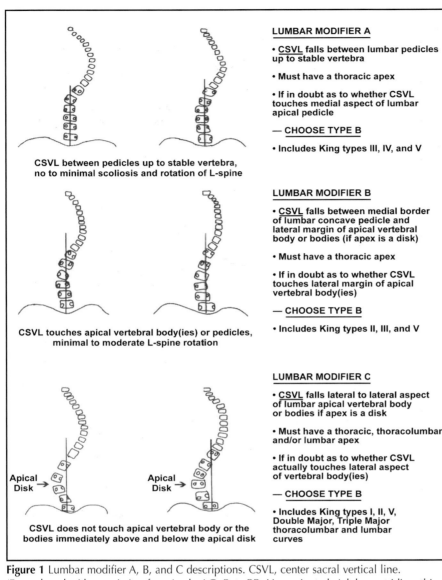

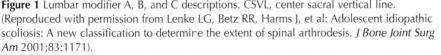

Figure 1 Lumbar modifier A, B, and C descriptions. CSVL, center sacral vertical line. (Reproduced with permission from Lenke LG, Betz RR, Harms J, et al: Adolescent idiopathic scoliosis: A new classification to determine the extent of spinal arthrodesis. *J Bone Joint Surg Am* 2001;83:1171).

LUMBAR MODIFIER A

- <u>CSVL</u> falls between lumbar pedicles up to stable vertebra

- Must have a thoracic apex

- If in doubt as to whether CSVL touches medial aspect of lumbar apical pedicle

— CHOOSE TYPE B

- Includes King types III, IV, and V

LUMBAR MODIFIER B

- <u>CSVL</u> falls between medial border of lumbar concave pedicle and lateral margin of apical vertebral body or bodies (if apex is a disk)

- Must have a thoracic apex

- If in doubt as to whether CSVL touches lateral margin of apical vertebral body(ies)

— CHOOSE TYPE B

- Includes King types II, III, and V

LUMBAR MODIFIER C

- <u>CSVL</u> falls lateral to lateral aspect of lumbar apical vertebral body or bodies if apex is a disk

- Must have a thoracic, thoracolumbar and/or lumbar apex

- If in doubt as to whether CSVL actually touches lateral aspect of vertebral body(ies)

— CHOOSE TYPE B

- Includes King types I, II, V, Double Major, Triple Major thoracolumbar and lumbar curves

center sacral vertical line, thus documenting complete deviation of the apex of the lumbar curve off the midline. Finally, a sagittal thoracic modifier is added based on the T5-T12 sagittal Cobb measurement. When the T5-T12 Cobb measurement is less than +10°, a "-" modifier signifying thoracic hypokyphosis or lordosis is assigned. When the T5-T12 Cobb measurement is between +10° and +40°, a normal or "N" sagittal thoracic modifier is assigned. When the T5-T12 Cobb measurement is more than +40° a "+" or hyperkyphotic sagittal modifier is assigned.

Thus, this triad classification system of AIS combines the three components of curve type (1-6), lumbar spine modifier (A, B, C), plus the sagittal thoracic modifier (-, N, or +) to create the full classification system (eg, 1BN). There are 42 different curve classifications possible with this system. Thus it is very important to use the modularity of this system to help determine the appropriate classification. One must determine the curve type, then add the lumbar spine and sagittal thoracic modifiers to the curve type rather than trying to memorize all 42 different configurations. On premeasured radiographs, this classification system has been evaluated by the developers of the system, as well as an independent group of Scoliosis Research Society surgeons, and also an independent group of surgeons from a different country.[2,6] These studies have all found this system to be more reliable than the King-Moe system in its interobserver and intraobserver reliability.

Specific Treatment Recommendations

One of the general guidelines from this classification system is that the major structural curve as well as the structural minor curves should be fused, but not the nonstructural minor curves. In addition, for type 1, MT curves, the MT region should be fused exclusively either

system based on whether each of the regions, the PT, MT, or TL/L, is a structural curve (major or minor) or a minor nonstructural curve. The six curve types are type 1, main thoracic (MT); type 2, double thoracic (DT); type 3, double major (DM); type 4, triple major (TM); type 5, thoracolumbar/lumbar (TL/L); and type 6, thoracolumbar/lumbar—main thoracic (TL/L-MT).

Next, two modifiers are added to the curve type—a lumbar spine modifier and a sagittal thoracic modifier. The lumbar spine modifier is based on the position of the center sacral vertical line to the apex of the lumbar curve preoperatively[5] (Figure 1). For lumbar modifier A, the center sacral vertical line falls between the pedicles of the lumbar spine up to the stable vertebra. For lumbar modifier B, the center sacral vertical line touches the apex of the lumbar curve (pedicles). For lumbar modifier C, the apex (pedicles) of the lumbar curve falls completely off the

posteriorly or anteriorly. For type 2, DT curves, both the PT and MT regions should be fused posteriorly. For type 3, DM curves, both the MT and TL/L regions should be fused posteriorly. For type 4, TM major curves, all three regions, the PT, MT, and TL/L should be fused posteriorly. For type 5, TL/L curves, the TL/L region should be fused either anteriorly or posteriorly. Finally, for type 6, TL/L—MT curves, the MT and TL/L regions should be fused posteriorly. Obviously, there are certain circumstances where a circumferential approach will be considered for either the MT or TL/L regions for very large curve magnitudes, increased stiffness on side bending, increased kyphosis, or skeletal immaturity with those patients at risk for crankshaft phenomenon. The general rules of fusing the major and structural minor curves will still need to be followed as described.

Type 1: MT Curves

In type 1, MT curves, the general rule is to fuse the MT region only either via a posterior or anterior route.[7] These curve patterns can either have a lumbar modifier A, B, or C, with the 1C pattern representing a true selective fusion of the MT region. The sagittal modifier can be -, N, or +, which may affect whether the curve is approached posteriorly or anteriorly.[7]

Type 1, MT curves are primarily treated posteriorly. The posterior approach for these curves is universal, with all type 1 curves being amenable to posterior instrumentation and fusion.[8] Recently, pedicle screw anchors have been used as the spinal implants of choice for AIS surgeries.[9] In addition to the strong corrective forces applied by these posterior screw constructs, the ability to truly derotate the apical vertebrae is being achieved with multilevel segmental pedicle screw constructs through direct apical vertebral derotation maneuvers[10] (Figure 2).

However, an anterior approach could

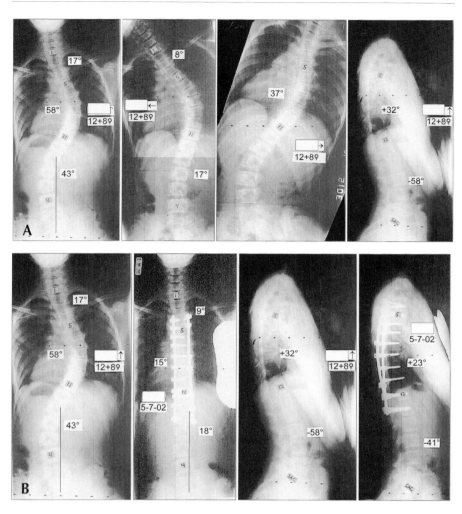

Figure 2 Radiographs of a 12-year-old girl with a 17° PT, 58° MT, 43° lumbar AIS curve. **A,** The left side bender shows the PT curve decreases to 8°, and the lumbar curve to 17°. The right side bender shows the MT curve decreases to 37°. T5-T12 kyphosis is +32°, thus the sagittal modifier is "N." The center sacral vertical line falls just off the apical lumbar pedicles, thus the lumbar modifier is a C. The PT and lumbar curves are nonstructural, and the Lenke curve classification is 1CN. **B,** The patient underwent a segmental pedicle screw instrumentation and fusion from T4 to L1 for correction of the MT curve to 15° and excellent overall coronal and sagittal balance.

be considered for a type 1 curve in those patients who have a lordotic sagittal thoracic alignment with a minus sagittal modifier; those with a true C lumbar modifier position where selective anterior thoracic fusion may optimize spontaneous lumbar curve positioning; those patients who are skeletally immature and are at risk for crankshaft phenomenon with posterior-only fusion without the use of apical pedicle screws (which may

prevent crankshaft phenomenon by the posterior route); when one to three distal fusion levels can be saved with an anterior approach by stopping at the thoracic lower end vertebra; and for those patients who can be treated with an endoscopic anterior approach to minimize morbidity during the surgical instrumentation and fusion. An anterior approach for main thoracic curves can be performed with an open, mini-open, or pure endoscopic approach, and pulmonary function should be evaluated because of the anticipated postoperative decline[11,12,] similar to that seen with a posterior thoracoplasty.[13] The instrumentation choices include a single screw/single rod, single screw/dual rod, or dual screw/dual rod construct. An anterior release and fusion combined with a posterior instrumentation and fusion of a type 1 main thoracic curve can also be done. Indications for this would be for those MT curves with very large curve magnitudes (> 90°-100° upright, with increased stiffness on side bending with a > 60°-70° residual Cobb measurement), severe lordosis or hyperkyphosis in the sagittal plane, and in those patients who are very skeletally immature and thus at high risk for crankshaft phenomenon. Currently, this circumferential approach is being used less frequently because of the powerful corrective and holding forces of multilevel segmental pedicle screw constructs, which are commonly used on these patients.

Type 2: DT Curves

Type 2, DT curve patterns require posterior instrumentation and fusion of the PT and MT regions.[14] Occasionally, a preliminary anterior release and fusion will be required for a very large and/or stiff main thoracic curve, similar to the criteria listed for type 1 MT curves. Most commonly, posterior instrumentation and fusion will extend from T2, or occasionally T3, down to the most proximal lumbar vertebra intersected by the center sacral vertical line, whether the lumbar spine modifier is A, B, or C.[15] It is very important to optimize clinical and radiographic shoulder alignment when treating the type 2, DT curve patterns, for it is not uncommon that the left shoulder will be elevated with maximal correction of the right MT curve.[16] This is especially true when the left shoulder is clinically elevated preoperatively, or even when the shoulders are level preoperatively.[17] The PT region must be corrected with poste-

rior convex compression forces and concave distraction forces on the appropriate sides of the curve. Usually the convex compression force is applied first to reverse kyphosis in that region.

Type 3: DM Curves

The type 3, DM curve pattern requires posterior instrumentation and fusion of the MT and TL/L regions. The most common DM curve pattern will have a lumbar C modifier position with the lumbar curve completely deviated from the midline. Varying degrees of thoracolumbar kyphosis can be seen in the junction between the thoracic and lumbar curves, and a significant amount of thoracolumbar kyphosis, 20° or more between T10 and L2, will automatically designate both curves as structural when surgically planning to treat one of them as the major curve. These DM curve patterns usually require posterior instrumentation and fusion down to either L3 or L4[9,15] (Figure 3). Occasionally a 3C curve can undergo a selective thoracic fusion if the spine can be maintained in good balance and there is a lack of junctional kyphosis between the two curves preoperatively.[18,19] In this circumstance, it is extremely important to evaluate the clinical examination of the patient very carefully to make sure that the thoracic region is still the more prominent clinical part of the deformity and will allow a successful selective thoracic fusion procedure to be performed. Also, occasionally a circumferential approach will be required for either the thoracic or lumbar portions of a double major curve pattern in those curves that are very large in curve magnitude, and/or have marked sagittal plane malalignment as described above.

Type 4: TM Curves

Type 4, TM curves are somewhat rare curve patterns that require all three structural regions of the spine (PT, MT, and TL/L) to be instrumented and fused posteriorly. Commonly, these are 4C pat-

terns with complete apical deviation off of the midline of the lumbar curve. Fusion levels normally need to extend from T2 or T3 proximal to L3 or L4 distal. Occasionally, a preliminary anterior release and fusion of the MT or TL/L regions may be required when one of those regions is disproportionately much larger and stiffer than the other region.

Type 5: TL/L Curves

In this curve pattern, the major curve is in the TL/L region, and the minor PT and MT curves above are nonstructural. Thus, the isolated TL/L curve can be treated anteriorly or posteriorly. Traditionally, most of these curves have been treated anteriorly either using single or dual rod anterior instrumentation systems.[20,21,22] In this manner, these curves are fused from the upper end vertebra to the lower end vertebra. Usually this will be one level shorter distally than what posterior instrumentation would require. It is important to maintain adequate sagittal alignment during these anterior procedures with the use of structural interbody grafts or cages, appropriate rod contouring, and/or the use of dual rod instrumentation constructs to maintain sagittal alignment over time during healing.[21] With the use of transpedicular screw fixation, these curve patterns can also be treated posteriorly, occasionally to the lower end vertebra of the TL/L curve, or one level caudal to that.

Type 6: TL/L-MT Curves

The type 6 curve pattern has the major curve in the TL/L region, with the MT region being the structural minor curve above. These curves will require posterior instrumentation and fusion of both the MT and TL/L regions. Normally the instrumentation and fusion will extend down to L3 or L4. Occasionally, an isolated selective TL/L fusion may be performed, leaving the MT region unfused when specific clinical and radiograph criteria are met that will allow the selective TL/L fusion.

Curve Prevalence

A multicenter study was performed to evaluate 606 surgical AIS cases to determine the prevalence of various curve types, lumbar and sagittal modifiers, and overall curve classification.[23] With respect to the curve types, type 1 MT curves were found in 51% of all cases; type 2 DT in 20%; type 3 DM in 11%; type 4 TM in 3%; type 5 TL/L in 12%; type 6 TL/L-MT curves, in 3%. For the lumbar spine modifiers, the lumbar modifier A position was found in 41%, lumbar spine modifier B in 37% , and lumbar spine modifier C in 32%. Finally, with respect to sagittal thoracic spine modifier, the "-" or hypokyphotic modifier was found in 14%, the "N" or normal sagittal thoracic modifier was found in 75%, and the "+" or hyperkyphotic sagittal thoracic modifier was found in 11%. Although there are 42 different configurations of all curve classifications, the top five most commonly seen curves accounted for almost 60% of all curves treated surgically. The most common classifications include: 1AN (19%), 1BN (11%), 2AN (10%), 5CN (10%), and 1CN (8%).

To help judge whether the classification system truly makes treatment recommendations, a retrospective review of 606 surgical curves (treated before the classification system was developed) was performed to investigate whether the treatment recommendations by this new system were actually used.[23] In this manner, it was investigated whether the instrumentation and fusion included the major and structural minor curves, and excluded the nonstructural minor curves during surgical treatment. The study found that for approximately 90% of cases, the treatment guidelines were followed as recommended by the classification system. Looking at individual curve types, the results ranged from a low of 75% to a high of 95% as far as following

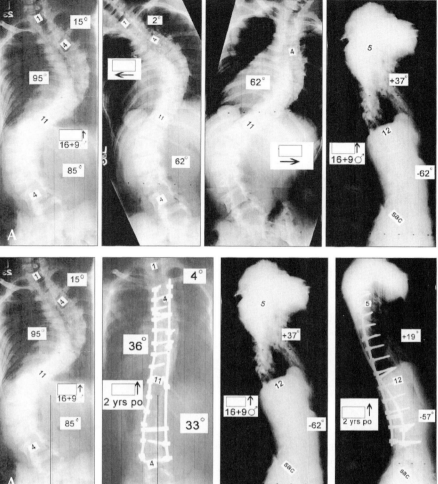

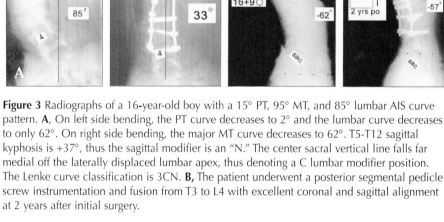

Figure 3 Radiographs of a 16-year-old boy with a 15° PT, 95° MT, and 85° lumbar AIS curve pattern. **A**, On left side bending, the PT curve decreases to 2° and the lumbar curve decreases to only 62°. On right side bending, the major MT curve decreases to 62°. T5-T12 sagittal kyphosis is +37°, thus the sagittal modifier is an "N." The center sacral vertical line falls far medial off the laterally displaced lumbar apex, thus denoting a C lumbar modifier position. The Lenke curve classification is 3CN. **B**, The patient underwent a posterior segmental pedicle screw instrumentation and fusion from T3 to L4 with excellent coronal and sagittal alignment at 2 years after initial surgery.

the treatment guidelines. Obviously, no radiographic classification system will ever be 100% predictive of treatment. Other important issues such as the clinical examination, the level of skeletal maturity of the patient, surgeon bias, and the overall radiographic structural criteria ratios between the MT and TL/L regions will often provide significant input to the surgical treatments rendered.[24]

Summary

The Lenke classification system of AIS is a comprehensive, two-dimensional, and reliable system. It is not completely treatment directed because of variations that will occur in the radiographic and clinical examination of the patient that will suggest deviation from the recommendations of the system. The ultimate goal of this classification system is to allow organization of similar patterns of surgical curves to allow comparison of various treatment methods. This will then provide surgeons with the information needed to select the optimal treatment of each particular curve pattern when discussing treatment options with AIS surgical patients and their families.

References

1. King HA, Moe J, Bradford DS, Winter RB: The selection of fusion levels in thoracic idiopathic scoliosis. *J Bone Joint Surg Am* 1983;65:1302-1313.

2. Lenke LG, Betz RR, Bridwell KH, et al: Intraobserver and interobserver reliability of the classification of thoracic adolescent idiopathic scoliosis. *J Bone Joint Surg Am* 1998;80:1097-1106.

3. Cummings RJ, Loveless EA, Campbell J, Samelson S, Mazur JM: Interobserver reliability and intraobserver reproducibility of the system of King et al for the classification of adolescent idiopathic scoliosis. *J Bone Joint Surg Am* 1998;80:1107-1111.

4. Lenke LG, Betz RR, Harms J, et al: Adolescent idiopathic scoliosis: A new classification to determine extent of spinal arthrodesis. *J Bone Joint Surg Am* 2001;83:1169-1181.

5. Lenke LG, Betz RR, Bridwell KH, Harms J, Clements DH, Love TG: Spontaneous lumbar curve coronal correction after selective anterior or posterior thoracic fusion in adolescent idiopathic scoliosis. *Spine* 1999;24:1663-1671.

6. Ogon M, Giesinger K, Behensky H, et al: Interobserver and intraobserver reliability of Lenke's new scoliosis classification system. *Spine* 2002;27:858-862.

7. Betz RR, Harms J, Clements DH III, et al: Comparison of anterior and posterior instrumentation for correction of adolescent thoracic idiopathic scoliosis. *Spine* 1999;24:225-239.

8. Lenke LG, Bridwell KH, Blanke K, Baldus C, Weston J: Radiographic results of arthrodesis with Cotrel-Dubousset instrumentation for the treatment of adolescent idiopathic scoliosis: A five to ten-year follow-up study. *J Bone Joint Surg Am* 1998;80:807-814.

9. Hamill CL, Lenke LG, Bridwell KH, Chapman MP, Blanke K, Baldus C: The use of pedicle screws to improve correction in the lumbar spine of patients with idiopathic scoliosis: Is it warranted? *Spine* 1996;21:1241-1249.

10. Rinella AS, Kim JA, Lenke LG: Posterior spinal instrumentation techniques for spinal deformity, in Bradford DS (ed): *Masters Series in Orthopaedic Surgery*. Philadelphia, PA, Lippincott Williams and Wilkins, 2004, pp 231-246.

11. Vedantam R, Lenke LG, Bridwell KH, Haas J, Linville DA: A prospective evaluation of pulmonary function in patients with adolescent idiopathic scoliotics relative to the surgical approach used for spinal arthrodesis. *Spine* 2000;25:82-90.

12. Graham EJ, Lenke LG, Lowe TG, et al: Prospective pulmonary function evaluation following open thoracotomy for anterior spinal fusion in adolescent idiopathic scoliosis. *Spine* 2000;25:2319-2325.

13. Lenke LG, Bridwell KH, Blanke K, Baldus C: Analysis of pulmonary function and chest cage dimension changes after thoracoplasty in idiopathic scoliosis. *Spine* 1995;20:1343-1350.

14. Lenke LG, Bridwell KH, O'Brien MF, Baldus C, Blanke K: Recognition and treatment of the proximal thoracic curve in adolescent idiopathic scoliosis treated with Cotrel-Dubousset instrumentation. *Spine* 1994;19:1589-1597.

15. Lenke LG, Bridwell KH, Baldus C, Blanke K, Schoenecker PL: Ability of Cotrel-Dubousset instrumentation to preserve distal lumbar motion segments in adolescent idiopathic scoliosis. *J Spinal Disord* 1993;6:339-350.

16. Kuklo T, Lenke LG, Won DS, et al: Spontaneous proximal thoracic curve correction following isolated fusion of the main thoracic curve in adolescent idiopathic scoliosis. *Spine* 2001;26:1966-1975.

17. Kuklo TR, Lenke LG, Graham EJ, et al: Correlation of radiographic, clinical, and patient assessment of shoulder balance following fusion versus nonfusion of the proximal thoracic curve in adolescent idiopathic scoliosis. *Spine* 2002;27:2013-2020.

18. Lenke LG, Bridwell KH, Baldus C, Blanke K: Preventing decompensation in King Type II curves treated with Cotrel-Dubousset instrumentation: Strict guidelines for selective thoracic fusion. *Spine* 1992;17(suppl 8):S274-S281.

19. Edwards CC II, Lenke LG, Peelle M, Sides B, Rinella AS, Bridwell KH: Time dependent response of the unfused lumbar curve after selective thoracic fusion: A 2-16 year radiographic and clinical follow-up. *Spine* 2004;29:536-546.

20. Lenke LG, Rhee J: Adolescent scoliosis: Anterior surgical techniques for adolescent idiopathic scoliosis. *Curr Opin Orthop* 2001;12:199-205.

21. Sweet FA, Lenke LG, Bridwell KH, Blanke KM: Maintaining lumbar lordosis with anterior single solid-rod instrumentation in thoracolumbar and lumbar adolescent idiopathic scoliosis. *Spine* 1999;24:1655-1662.

22. Sweet F, Lenke LG, Bridwell KH, Blanke KM, Whorton J: Prospective radiographic and clinical outcomes and complications of single solid rod instrumented anterior spinal fusion in adolescent idiopathic scoliosis. *Spine* 2001;26:1956-1965.

23. Lenke LG, Betz RR, Clements D, et al: Curve prevalence of a new classification of operative adolescent idiopathic scoliosis: Does classification correlate with treatment? *Spine* 2002;27:604-611.

24. Lenke LG, Betz RR, Haher T, et al: Multisurgeon assessment of surgical decision-making in adolescent idiopathic scoliosis: Curve classification, operative approach, and fusion levels. *Spine* 2001;26:2347-2353.

11

The Use of Video-Assisted Thoracoscopic Surgery in the Treatment of Adolescent Idiopathic Scoliosis

Peter O. Newton, MD

Abstract

The video-assisted thoracoscopic approach has become a useful adjunct in the treatment of scoliosis. This minimally invasive anterior approach allows access to the thoracic spine, providing a means of achieving disk excision and anterior body fusion. The advantage of this technique is the limited chest wall dissection required to reach the anterior thoracic spine. More recently, techniques have been developed to allow anterior instrumentation for an entirely endoscopic method of performing scoliosis correction. This approach is appropriate for curves less than 70° when only the thoracic curve is structural. The outcomes of this approach are promising and suggest reduced morbidity compared with open anterior approaches.

The video-assisted thoracoscopic approach has been used for a variety of diagnoses in the chest cavity,[1-3] and more recently, it has been used for spinal deformity treatment.[4-6] The thoracoscopic approach is a minimally invasive method of accessing the anterior spine through the chest cavity. It has its appeal in the limited chest wall dissection required to reach the anterior spine. In the surgical treatment of scoliosis, the anterior approach to the thoracic spine is commonly indicated. Anterior thoracic scoliosis procedures are often well suited for the thoracoscopic approach because the chest cavity is typically spacious and it is relatively easy to manipulate the endoscope and instruments within.

The thoracoscopic approach uses three to five small incisions through which instruments can be placed to visualize and perform anterior spinal surgery.

Visualization using the latest video technology can be quite spectacular; however, loss of this visualization (because of poor camera position, bleeding, and lung tissue) can make it impossible to safely perform surgery. Thoracoscopic anterior spinal release and fusion for the treatment of scoliosis continues to gain acceptance and popularity within the orthopaedic community. In addition, thoracoscopic anterior instrumentation techniques, which now allow for an entirely endoscopic correction of scoliosis, have been developed and may be appropriate for select patients.

Thoracoscopic Anterior Release and Fusion

The indications for anterior release and fusion in patients with scoliosis generally relate to the treatment of large or rigid curves,[6,7] which require increased flexi-

bility to obtain maximal correction during posterior instrumentation and fusion. The upper limits of curve magnitude as well as flexibility may be debated. However, it is clear that removal of the disk anteriorly increases curve flexibility,[8-11] providing both greater coronal and sagittal plane correction with posterior implant systems. The degree to which flexibility can be increased is dependent on the completeness of removal of both the anulus fibrosus and internal disk material. In the most severe cases of scoliosis, resection of the rib head and/or costovertebral joint may be required to optimize mobility. An additional indication for anterior disk excision and fusion is in the prevention of crankshaft growth, which has been reported to occur following an isolated posterior instrumentation and fusion procedure in skeletally immature patients.[12] In general, patients being treated posteriorly before their peak growth are at risk for crankshaft development.[13] The triradiate cartilage closure may be a reasonable marker to determine which patients such an anterior procedure would benefit. Thus, patients being treated posteriorly with open triradiate cartilage who are Risser 0 are considered for an anterior release and fusion with the primary goal of limiting later anterior growth.[14,15] An additional indication for anterior release and fusion may exist in those patients at greater risk for pseudarthrosis. Examples include patients with the diagnosis of neurofibromatosis, Marfan syndrome, or prior irradiation. Anterior fusion generally provides a large cancellous bony surface for fusion once the disk has been adequately removed, increasing the likelihood of solid arthrodesis. The thoracoscopic approach is applicable for release and fusion between the T4-T12 vertebral levels and may be extended both proximally to T2 and distally to L1 as additional experience is gained.[16] As with any open procedure, the goal is to obtain complete release with thorough disk excision to allow grafting and ultimately solid interbody arthrodesis.

Contraindications to the Thoracoscopic Approach

The thoracoscopic approach requires an adequate working space within the chest cavity to manipulate both the endoscope and working instruments. This generally requires selective ventilation of the lungs, with collapse of the lung in the chest cavity to be operated. As such, the pulmonary status of the patient must allow single lung ventilation. In addition, any past medical history that would suggest intrathoracic pleural adhesions should be considered a relative contraindication. Pleural adhesions between the lung and chest wall limit the ability of the lung to adequately collapse. If minor, these adhesions can be divided, although a nearly complete pleural symphysis between the chest and lung can make this an extremely challenging proposition. This scenario is most often encountered in patients with a prior thoracotomy or significant pulmonary infection. In addition, the requirement for an adequate working space dictates that curves in which the spine has become closely approximated to the rib cage may also be relatively contraindicated. A working distance of 2 to 3 cm should be considered the minimum when reviewing the preoperative radio-

graphs. Achieving single lung ventilation in young children as well as having an adequate space to work within the chest is a challenge. Children who weigh less than 30 kg have been safely treated with this method;[17] however, the relative benefit of the minimally invasive approach seems to be reduced in very small patients.

If visualization is inadequate at any point during the endoscopic procedure, conversion to an open approach must be considered. It is certainly unwise to proceed with an operation when visualization is compromised. Visualization is most often limited by excessive bleeding or inconsistent lung deflation.

Surgical Technique for Thoracoscopic Disk Excision

Thoracoscopic removal of multiple thoracic disks for the purpose of increasing flexibility of the spine, as mentioned, requires single lung ventilation. The patient is placed in the lateral decubitus position with plans to approach the chest via the convex side of the curve. In the typical right thoracic scoliosis pattern, the right lung is deflated with either a double lumen endotracheal tube or a mainstem bronchial blocker on the right side. There are occasions in which the prone position may be used rather than the lateral decubitus position. In the prone position it is possible to reach the spine endoscopically without complete deflation of the lung. With the lungs hypoventilated, a posterior working space is created that, when combined with a retractor, allows access to the spine. This situation has been found to be less satisfactory than the lateral approach, which allows for more anterior portals and greater access to the concave side of the spine.

In either position, typically three to four portals are used for both visualization and working instruments. Skin incisions (1.5 cm in length) are used to place rigid tubular ports between the ribs along the anterior axillary line. A 10-mm endo-

scope, both with straight-ahead and angled optics, is used for visualization. A 45° angulation of the endoscope provides the best opportunity to see deep within the disk space during disk removal and is recommended over the 30° angulated endoscope. Care should be taken in placing the portals, particularly when placing them distally to avoid penetration below the diaphragm. Upon entering the chest cavity with the endoscope, a fan retractor is often required to provide initial additional displacement and protection of the lung. After establishing the levels of release by counting from the proximal ribs, a longitudinal opening of the pleura is performed using an ultrasonic dissecting device. Segmental vessels may be isolated and preserved or more commonly coagulated with the ultrasonic device. This provides excellent hemostasis and allows circumferential exposure of the spine. The azygos vein, esophagus, and aorta are reflected anteriorly off the spine, and a space between the anterior longitudinal ligament and these structures is maintained by packing sponges within the interval (Figure 1).

Following exposure of the spine, disk excision is initiated after incising the anulus of the disk with an ultrasonic scalpel. Diskectomy is performed using a combination of rongeurs and curets, first removing the most anterior and concave aspects of the anulus. Clear identification of the direction and path of diskectomy is required to avoid removing excessive bone, which will result in additional bleeding and difficulties in visualization. Additional disk material is then removed centrally and on the convex lateral side of the spine. Disk mobility can be confirmed with the use of an end plate shaver. By carefully peeling the end plate cartilage off the vertebral body, in most pediatric patients the disk can be excised with very little bleeding from the vertebral body itself (Figure 2). In patients with osteopenia or when the disk excision inadvertently involves portions of

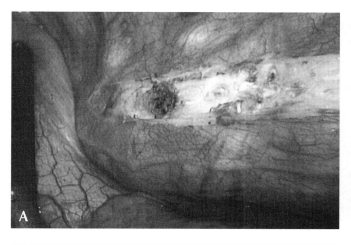

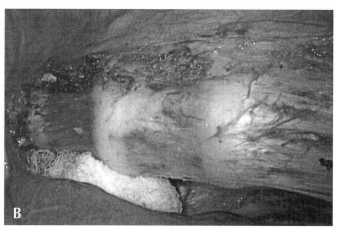

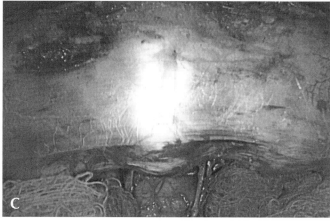

Figure 1 A, Endoscopic view of the midthoracic spine demonstrating a longitudinal incision of the pleura just anterior to the rib heads. The segmental vessels have been divided using the ultrasonic device. **B,** After stripping the pleura from the anterior aspect of the spine, a sponge has been packed in this interval, protecting the azygos vein, aorta, and esophagus. **C,** A close-up view of the concave side of the spine demonstrates that the segmental vessels have been pushed off of the concave lateral aspect of the spine. The view is directly anterior with the margins of the anterior longitudinal ligament easily seen.

the vertebral body, bleeding can make visualization more problematic. The deep aspects of the disk should only be taken under direct visualization, maintaining the integrity of the posterior longitudinal ligament to protect the neural elements. Bone grafting of the disk space can be performed with either autograft or allograft bone, based on the surgeon's preference and requirements of the individual patient. The endoscope and working instruments are moved within the various portals to gain access to each disk space with the rongeur or other working instrument directed inline with the disk space. Following diskectomy and grafting, it is recommended that the pleura be closed with a running suture using the Endo-Stitch (US Surgical, Norwalk, CT) device. The running closure reapproxi-

mates the pleura, minimizing intrathoracic scar and chest tube drainage, while maintaining the graft within the intervertebral spaces.

Results Following Thoracoscopic Release and Fusion

The thoracoscopic method of removing disk and performing anterior interbody fusion is comparable to that of open approaches.[4] There is, however, a substantial learning curve associated with this procedure.[16] The procedure typically requires the skills of both an endoscopic surgeon as well as a spinal surgeon. As with any endoscopic approach, the limitation in direct visualization can be challenging but generally mastered. There have been several studies published in the literature that demonstrate comparable

degrees of disk excision in both clinical series and animal models.[8-11] The safety of the thoracoscopic approach has been evaluated in clinical series with relatively few perioperative complications and rates similar to those for open procedures.[16] The potential complications include excessive bleeding, injury to the lung parenchyma, spinal cord injury, chylothorax, nonunion, and postoperative pulmonary complications typical for anterior thoracic surgery. The surgical time for many of these procedures has been longer than in the open series; however, with experience surgical time has been consistently reduced. In one study, the length of the procedure is comparable to that of an open thoracotomy, with a surgical time of 2 to 2.5 hours.[17] In most series, patients with neuromuscular con-

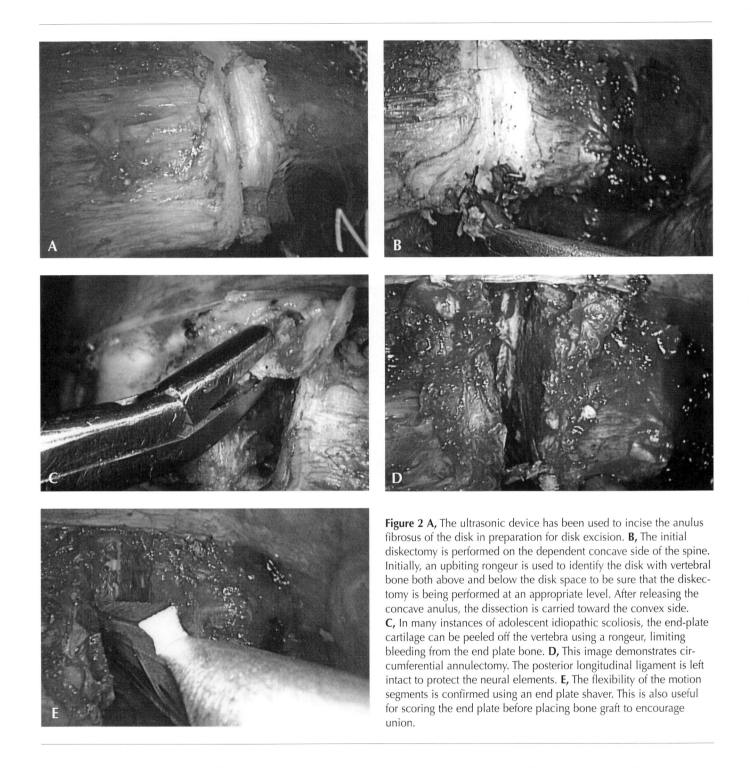

Figure 2 A, The ultrasonic device has been used to incise the anulus fibrosus of the disk in preparation for disk excision. **B,** The initial diskectomy is performed on the dependent concave side of the spine. Initially, an upbiting rongeur is used to identify the disk with vertebral bone both above and below the disk space to be sure that the diskectomy is being performed at an appropriate level. After releasing the concave anulus, the dissection is carried toward the convex side. **C,** In many instances of adolescent idiopathic scoliosis, the end-plate cartilage can be peeled off the vertebra using a rongeur, limiting bleeding from the end plate bone. **D,** This image demonstrates circumferential annulectomy. The posterior longitudinal ligament is left intact to protect the neural elements. **E,** The flexibility of the motion segments is confirmed using an end plate shaver. This is also useful for scoring the end plate before placing bone graft to encourage union.

ditions provide the greatest challenges because of curve magnitude, small patient size, preoperative pulmonary compromise, and osteopenia associated with increased blood loss. However, in patients with idiopathic scoliosis, many of these issues are less problematic and outcomes have been similar to open series but without the chest wall dissection required of an open thoracotomy. Anterior fusion rates have been measured and assessed critically, demonstrating that in most of the disk spaces treated with either autograft or allograft some degree of fusion exists.[18] Clinical failures associated with a thoracoscopic anterior release/fusion followed by posterior instrumentation and fusion have been exceedingly rare.

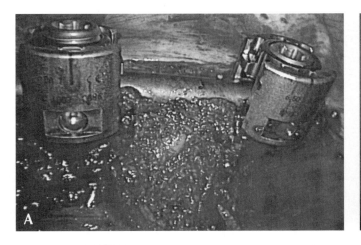
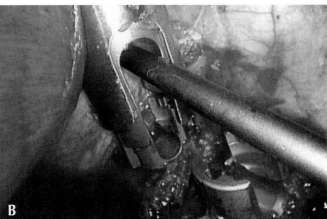
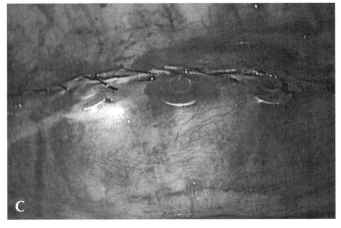

Figure 3 A, This photograph demonstrates the rod having been placed in the proximal two screws of a scoliosis construct. The disk space has been fully packed with autogenous iliac crest bone, which has been placed through a bone mill. Prior to tightening the screw on the left, interbody compression will be performed. **B,** Distally, the rod requires cantilevering to engage the lower screws. An approximating device is used to achieve this aspect of the correction. **C,** This photograph demonstrates the closure of the pleura following multilevel scoliosis instrumentation performed endoscopically.

Indications for Thoracoscopic Anterior Scoliosis Correction

Anterior scoliosis correction has been popularized over the past 10 years with the use of single-rod thoracic constructs placed generally through a thoracotomy approach.[19] These techniques have been adapted for thoracoscopic placement as well. Single structural thoracic scoliosis is generally amenable to a selective fusion of the thoracic curve.[20-22] This may be accomplished by either anterior or posterior methods. The anterior approach has the advantage of typically fewer levels of instrumentation. However, the open anterior approach has had the disadvantages of the morbidity associated with an extensive thoracotomy. As such, the thoracoscopic minimally invasive approach has been developed to limit the morbidi-

ty associated with this approach. The specific curve patterns that are appropriate for such instrumentation include the Lenke 1A, 1B, and 1C curve patterns in which there is reduced or normal kyphosis (see chapter 51). The anterior approach tends to be kyphogenic, and the use of this approach in patients with increased thoracic kyphosis should be avoided. In addition, the approach is believed to be contraindicated in obese patients, who will overstress a single rod anterior construct. The upper limit in weight is roughly 60 to 70 kg. In addition, the approach is contraindicated in very small patients in whom the vertebral bodies have limited ability to maintain the purchase of a vertebral body screw. Curves less than 70° with greater than 50% flexibility are amenable to the thora-

coscopic approach. Larger curves have been instrumented; however, the challenges associated with such curves seem to favor a posterior approach.

Surgical Technique for Anterior Thoracoscopic Scoliosis Correction

The patient is positioned and prepared for surgery just as for a thoracoscopic release and rigidly stabilized in the direct lateral position. The image intensifier is critical for identifying the orientation of each vertebra in the coronal plane within the levels to be instrumented. In this way, the trajectory of each screw can be anticipated before making skin incisions for screw placement. Generally, three portals are required along the posterior axillary line for screw insertion. This is supple-

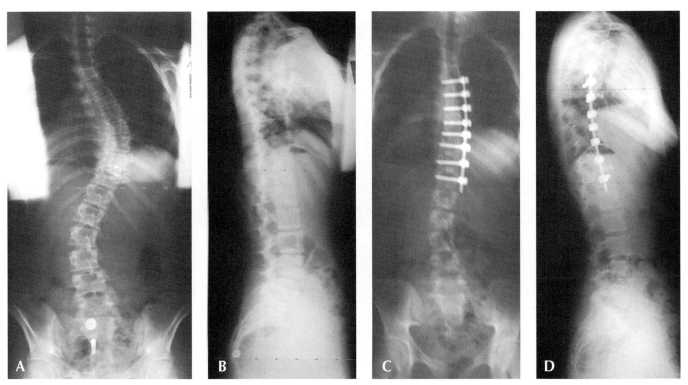

Figure 4 Preoperative standing PA (**A**) and lateral (**B**) radiographs demonstrate the typical right thoracic adolescent idiopathic scoliosis, which is appropriate for thoracoscopic anterior instrumentation. Postoperative PA (**C**) and lateral (**D**) radiographs demonstrate the correction achieved with a thoracoscopic instrumentation system. This was accomplished using five portals. The iliac crest was harvested for graft material, and the patient wore a brace for 3 months postoperatively.

mented by two anterior axillary line portals, which are used during disk excision and for placement of the endoscope. The levels to be instrumented generally include those of the measured Cobb angle. The procedure is initiated by thoracoscopic exposure of the spine and disk excision as described previously. The disk spaces are packed with an oxidized cellulose hemostat to reduce bleeding from the vertebral end plates. Next, screw insertion is initiated proximally. A 15-mm Thoracoport (US Surgical) is placed between the ribs through the proximal skin incision. The starting point for the screw is in the mid to superior aspect of the vertebral body just anterior to the rib head articulation with the vertebral body. An awl is used to initiate the hole, followed by a tap. The screw path is tapped through the far cortex, and using a ball-

tipped calibrated probe the exact length of the screw is determined. Typically, 6.5-mm diameter screws are used. Moving the portal one rib space distally, the adjacent screw is placed in similar fashion, with care being taken to appropriately align each screw to make later rod insertion as straightforward as possible. Each of the screws should be placed with bicortical purchase; however, excessive screw penetration should be avoided, given the location of the aorta on the left side of the vertebral bodies. Following screw placement, each of the disk spaces should be grafted with autogenous bone, from either the iliac crest or rib. At more distal levels, the interspace may require structural support, in which case an interbody device or cortical allograft is used. Deformity correction is accomplished by cantilevering a rod into posi-

tion, beginning by engaging the proximal screws first. Segmental compression is performed at each of the levels with an endoscopic compressing device. This combination of rod cantilevering facilitated with an approximating device and segmental vertebral body compression provide coronal plane correction of the scoliosis, sagittal restoration of kyphosis, and axial plane derotation of the spine. Following rod insertion, the pleura may be closed with a running suture (Figure 3).

Outcomes of Thoracoscopic Anterior Scoliosis Correction

The thoracoscopic method of anterior scoliosis correction remains relatively new, but follow-up data are limited. In 1998, Picetti and associates[23] first reported on the clinical use of a thoracoscopic anterior scoliosis system. The worldwide experience since then has been increasing.[24,25] In the author's initial experience, curve correction has averaged 60%, with operating time averaging 5.5 hours.[24] The number of vertebra instrumented in such constructs has ranged from six to nine levels, with the uppermost instrumented vertebra being T4 and the distal most level being L1. The author continues to brace thoracoscopically instrumented patients for 3 months postoperatively; with this protocol, one instance of rod failure has occurred in the first 30 idiopathic cases performed (follow-up of 2 years or longer). Comparative studies of anterior and posterior approaches have suggested similar degrees of deformity correction when curve patterns were matched.[24] Complication rates, however, have been greater in nearly all surgeons' initial experience with the technique. This approach remains technically demanding and requires thorough disk excision and grafting to obtain early solid union (Figure 4).

The functional benefits associated with the thoracoscopic approach have begun to be quantified. Shoulder girdle strength and range of motion return to normal within 3 to 6 months following surgery. This is a more rapid return than noted in open anterior procedures. In addition, the reduction in pulmonary function following thoracoscopic instrumentation is less than that associated with open anterior instrumentation (Figure 5). All of these data suggest that there are benefits to the thoracoscopic approach that may be realized once the surgeon is able to master the technique.

Summary

The role of thoracoscopy in the treatment of pediatric spinal deformity is evolving, and surgeon experience with the technique continues to grow. Early reports of this approach suggested its safety and efficacy. Refinements in the technique and instrumentation used for

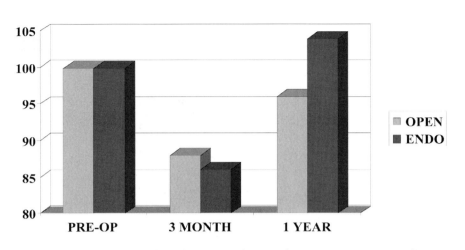

Figure 5 This graph represents the reduction in pulmonary function, as a percentage of preoperative value (y-axis), associated with open and thoracoscopic (endoscopic) anterior scoliosis correction. At 1 year, the thoracoscopic group has returned to greater than baseline forced vital capacity, whereas the open anterior instrumentation patients have not completely recovered to baseline. The difference in the return of function between these two groups is statistically significant. Pre-op = preoperative; endo = endoscopic.

this surgery will also continue to evolve. There is room for cautious optimism with regard to the continued development of this field. The approach requires the careful selection of patients and a surgeon with the appropriate temperament and judgment to negotiate the challenges of the early learning curve. It is likely that continued advances with this technique will reduce the learning curve and allow this technique to have greater indications in the future.

References

1. Dickman CA, Karahalios DG: Thoracoscopic spinal surgery. *Clin Neurosurg* 1996;43:392-422.

2. Mack MJ, Regan JJ, Bobechko WP, et al: Application of thoracoscopy for diseases of the spine. *Ann Thorac Surg* 1993;56:736-738.

3. Dickman CA, Rosenthal D, Karahalios DG, et al: Thoracic vertebrectomy and reconstruction using a microsurgical thoracoscopic approach. *Neurosurgery* 1996;38:279-293.

4. Newton PO, Wenger DR, Mubarak SJ, et al: Anterior release and fusion in pediatric spinal deformity: A comparison of early outcome and cost of thoracoscopic and open thoracotomy approaches. *Spine* 1997;22:1398-1406.

5. Crawford AH, Wall EJ, Wolf R: Video-assisted thoracoscopy. *Orthop Clin North Am* 1999;30:367-385.

6. Waisman M, Saute M: Thoracoscopic spine release before posterior instrumentation in scoliosis. *Clin Orthop* 1997:130-136.

7. Kokoska ER, Gabriel KR, Silen ML: Minimally invasive anterior spinal exposure and release in children with scoliosis. *J Soc Laparoendosc Surg* 1998;2:255-258.

8. Wall EJ, Bylski-Austrow DI, Shelton FS, et al: Endoscopic discectomy increases thoracic spine flexibility as effectively as open discectomy: A mechanical study in a porcine model. *Spine* 1998;23:9-15.

9. Newton PO, Cardelia JM, Farnsworth CL, et al: A biomechanical comparison of open and thoracoscopic anterior spinal release in a goat model. *Spine* 1998;23:530-535.

10. Huntington CF, Murrell WD, Betz RR, et al: Comparison of thoracoscopic and open thoracic discectomy in a live ovine model for anterior spinal fusion. *Spine* 1998;23:1699-1702.

11. Connolly PJ, Ordway NR, Sacks T, et al: Video-assisted thoracic diskectomy and anterior release: A biomechanical analysis of an endoscopic technique. *Orthopedics* 1999;22:923-926.

12. Dubousset J, Herring JA, Shufflebarger H: The crankshaft phenomenon. *J Pediatr Orthop* 1989;9:541-550.

13. Sanders JO, Little DG, Richards BS: Prediction of the crankshaft phenomenon by peak height velocity. *Spine* 1997;22:1352-1356.

14. Gonzalez Barrios I, Fuentes Caparros S, Avila Jurado MM: Anterior thoracoscopic epiphysiodesis in the treatment of a crankshaft phenomenon. *Eur Spine J* 1995;4:343-346.

15. Lapinksy AS, Richards BS: Preventing the crankshaft phenomenon by combining anterior fusion with posterior instrumentation. Does it work? *Spine* 1995;20:1392-1398.

16. Newton PO, Shea KG, Granlund KF: Defining the pediatric spinal thoracoscopy learning curve: sixty-five consecutive cases. *Spine* 2000;25:1028-1035.

17. Early SD, Newton PO, White KK, et al: The feasibility of anterior thoracoscopic spine surgery in children under 30 kilograms. *Spine* 2002;27:2368-2373.

18. Newton PO, Faro F, Gaynor TP, et al: Anterior fusion after thoracoscopic disc excision: Analysis of 112 consecutive deformity cases. *71st Annual Meeting Proceedings*. Rosemont, IL, American Academy of Orthopaedic Surgeons, 2004, p 541.

19. Betz RR, Harms J, Clements DH, et al: Comparison of anterior and posterior instrumentation for correction of adolescent thoracic idiopathic scoliosis. *Spine* 1999;24:225-239.

20. Newton PO, Faro FD, Lenke LG, et al: Factors involved in the decision to perform a selective versus nonselective fusion of Lenke 1B and 1C (King-Moe II) curves in adolescent idiopathic scoliosis. *Spine* 2003;28:S217-S223.

21. Lenke LG, Betz RR, Clements D, et al: Curve prevalence of a new classification of operative adolescent idiopathic scoliosis: does classification correlate with treatment? *Spine* 2002;27:604-611.

22. Lenke LG, Betz RR, Bridwell KH, et al: Spontaneous lumbar curve coronal correction after selective anterior or posterior thoracic fusion in adolescent idiopathic scoliosis. *Spine* 1999;24:1663-1671.

23. Picetti G III, Blackman RG, O'Neal K, et al: Anterior endoscopic correction and fusion of scoliosis. *Orthopedics* 1998;21:1285-1287.

24. Newton PO, Marks M, Faro F, et al: Use of video-assisted thoracoscopic surgery to reduce perioperative morbidity in scoliosis surgery. *Spine* 2003;28:S249-S254.

25. Sucato DJ: Thoracoscopic anterior instrumentation and fusion for idiopathic scoliosis. *J Am Acad Orthop Surg* 2003;11:221-227.

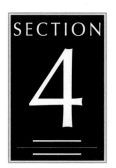

SECTION

4

Adult Spinal Deformity

Adult Spinal Deformity

This section includes three chapters that discuss complex adult spinal deformities, specifically those deformities that cause significant coronal and sagittal imbalance. Complex adult spinal deformity as a diagnostic category unfortunately includes a high proportion of previously operated spines. It has been shown in recent years that the restoration or maintenance of sagittal balance is one of the most important factors affecting patient function and outcome after spinal surgery. Bridwell's chapter discusses the causes of sagittal imbalance and its assessment in regard to surgical planning. The chapter authored by Burton details the importance and versatility of the Smith-Petersen osteotomy technique as originally described, and adds pearls gained from current experience in treating patients with the technique at the author's institution. Boachie-Adjei's expertise in vertebral column resection and the use of eggshell osteotomies is delineated in the last of these three important chapters.

Bridwell's chapter begins with a description of a classification system of sagittal imbalance, which is applied in assessing an affected patient. The most common causes of sagittal imbalance are described: the postoperative development of the condition after surgery for idiopathic scoliosis, degenerative loss of lumbar lordosis, posttraumatic kyphosis, and ankylosing spondylitis. An understanding of the causes of sagittal imbalance is critical in surgical planning and in preventing complications during surgical spine procedures that could lead to the development of sagittal imbalance. Information is presented on how surgeons can influence the so-called natural

history of a patient's deformity. The importance of intraoperative patient positioning with the hips extended to maintain lordosis, avoiding distraction in the lumbar spine, and being cognizant of the effect of fusion on adjacent levels are noted. Important assessment parameters, including measurements of the pelvic incidence, sacral slope, pelvic tilt, relative thoracic kyphosis and lumbar lordosis, as well as the C7 plumb line are reviewed. Orthopaedic surgeons are only beginning to understand the importance of individual patient factors that influence the ability to achieve sagittal balance. The chapter concludes with an overview of the Smith-Petersen osteotomy, pedicle subtraction osteotomy, and expectations when extending fusion levels. A review of this information will help the surgeon better understand the advantages and limitations of each of these options when assessing a patient for sagittal correction. An algorithm to aid in surgical planning is included for determining whether the Smith-Petersen osteotomy or pedicle subtraction osteotomy is best suited for a specific patient. It is also necessary to consider if a prior circumferential fusion has been performed, if there is coexisting spinal stenosis or pseudoarthrosis, and if comorbidities are present (including osteoporosis).

The Burton chapter on Smith-Petersen osteotomies describes the use of this osteotomy in classic cases—for patients with ankylosing spondylitis—and in its more recent application as a salvage surgical procedure for patients with noninflammatory arthritic spinal deformity. An illustration from Smith-Petersen's classic 1945 article is included and speaks volumes. This chapter

includes technical details and pearls, and highlights the significant differences in treating patients with ankylosing spondylitis and those with noninflammatory arthritic spinal deformities. The complexity of positioning the patient with ankylosing spondylitis, the adherence of the dura mater to the lamina that is usually present, and the osteoclasis that can allow more dramatic correction in these patients (as well as the caveat that the anterior opening is contraindicated in a patient with a calcified aorta) are discussed. The published outcomes in both types of patients are nicely summarized in this chapter. Reported outcomes for patients with ankylosing spondylitis include results from older studies in which surgeries were performed with less advanced instrumentation and anesthetic techniques. These studies report on numerous complications, including death, neurologic injury, infection, loss of correction, and implant failures. Similar complications can occur in patients undergoing salvage deformity surgery, although more recent studies report fewer deaths and permanent neurologic deficits. These better outcomes may be due in part to improved techniques of fixation and anesthesia rather than differences in the patient populations.

In the last chapter in this section, Boachie-Adjei reviews eggshell osteotomies, pedicle subtraction osteotomies, and vertebral column resection. These procedures should be considered for patients who have severe truncal imbalance, including those with combined deformities. The pedicle subtraction osteotomy can be considered for patients with flatback deformity, moderate amounts of lumbar kyphosis, and less severe coronal deformity. The classic correction technique of resecting a wedge of vertebral body and bilateral pedicles in a closing wedge is described. The author notes that the surgeon can choose whether to resect through the pedicles or to preserve the medial wall of the pedicle to protect the neural elements until just before the final correction. Additional correction can be achieved if an adjacent open disk space is resected. These techniques can be augmented with an anteriorly placed cage filled with bone graft, which permits greater angular correction. The posterior vertebral column resection is Boachie-Adjei's preferred technique for treating thoracic and thoracolumbar hyperkyphosis. This technique involves skeletonizing the apex of the kyphosis prior to its resection, including dissecting the pleura and segmental and great vessels free from the spine. Thoracic nerve roots can be sacrificed; however, lumbar roots must be preserved. The spinal column must be stabilized with temporary rods during the resection and shortened adequately during correction to minimize the risk of neurologic injury. Final correction is achieved over a structural strut, usually a cage filled with bone graft, and manipulation of the rods either by in situ bending of the provisional rods or by cantilever correction with rods controlling proximal and distal portions of the spine. Curve corrections averaging 50% can be achieved in both the coronal and sagittal planes. Despite the risk of significant complications, including neurologic injury, instrumentation failure, pseudarthrosis, adjacent segment disease, and significant blood loss, patient satisfaction rates are reported at 70% to 85%, which underscores the severe baseline disability that such patients experience from the effects of the spinal deformity prior to surgery.

Although these surgeries are involved and the potential complications are quite serious, modern techniques of surgery, instrumentation, anesthesia, and critical care have made major reconstruction of severe and complex spinal deformities feasible when performed by experienced surgeons. The chapters in this section provide descriptions of powerful techniques to correct adult spinal deformities and detail indications for these procedures along with their risks and complications. Careful patient selection, preoperative planning, meticulous surgical technique, and postoperative care are all important for achieving the desired outcomes in this challenging patient population.

Serena S. Hu, MD
Professor and Vice Chair
Chief, Spine Surgery
Department of Orthopaedic Surgery
University of California, San Francisco
San Francisco, California

Dr. Hu or an immediate family member serves as a board member, owner, officer, or committee member for American Orthopaedic Association and Socliosis Research Society; has received royalties from Pioneer; is a member of a speakers' bureau or has made paid presentations on behalf of Synthes and DePuy; serves as a paid consultant for or is an employee of Pioneer; and has received research or institutional support from DePuy and Medtronic Sofamor Danek.

12

Causes of Sagittal Spinal Imbalance and Assessment of the Extent of Needed Correction

Keith H. Bridwell, MD

Abstract

Most patients with spinal sagittal imbalance have a fusion mass that is either kyphotic or hypolordotic, with segments above or below the fusion that have subsequently degenerated. The four most common presentations include a patient who had a long fusion for adolescent idiopathic scoliosis with subsequent degeneration distally; a patient with degenerative sagittal imbalance in whom fusions have initially been performed in the distal lumbar spine in a somewhat hypolordotic or kyphotic position with subsequent degeneration of segments above the fusion; a patient with posttraumatic kyphosis; and a patient with ankylosing spondylitis.

The surgical solutions usually involve a combination of osteotomies through the fusion mass and extension of the fusion to include degenerated segments. Most of the correction is accomplished by the osteotomies with additional correction achieved by adding the degenerated segments to the fusion in patients with idiopathic scoliosis, degenerative sagittal imbalance, or posttraumatic kyphosis. For patients with ankylosing spondylitis, the correction is achieved entirely with osteotomies.

The usual goal is to normalize the regional segmental spinal alignment as much as possible and to achieve global balance. Global balance is confirmed when the C7 plumb falls over the lumbosacral disk on a standing long cassette lateral radiograph taken with the patient standing with knees fully extended in a natural, comfortable position. Most patients should have at least 10° to 20° more lumbar lordosis than thoracic kyphosis. Usually a Smith-Petersen osteotomy will achieve 10° of correction and a pedicle subtraction osteotomy will produce 30° to 35° of lordization of the spine.

Many factors contribute to fixed sagittal imbalance. A hypolordotic or hyperkyphotic fusion mass with subsequent disk degeneration above or below the fusion is common. Subsequent disk degeneration leads to loss of anterior column height and increased kyphosis. In most patients, both aging and iatrogenic factors contribute to fixed sagittal imbalance.

Sagittal Imbalance

Sagittal balance is most frequently defined by the position of the C7 plumb on a standing lateral radiograph. When a C7 plumb is dropped, neutral balance is suggested if the plumb falls through the lumbosacral disk. If the C7 plumb falls behind the lumbosacral disk, sagittal balance is defined as negative, whereas if it falls in front of the lumbosacral disk it is positive. The most commonly used specific reference point for the C7 plumb is the posterior aspect of the L5-S1 disk. Most investigators consider normal sagittal balance as the C7 plumb falling through the lumbosacral disk or 2 cm in front or behind it. It is known that the C7 plumb and the center of gravity are not identical. In most circumstances the center of gravity falls in front of the C7 plumb and slightly behind the hip joints (P Roussouly, MD, Lyon, France, personal communication, 2004).

There is a range of sagittal imbalance (Figure 1). Booth and associates[1] refer to a type I imbalance as a segmental kyphosis, with global balance in which the C7 plumb (on a long cassette standing radiograph) falls over the lumbosacral disk. Patients with this type of imbalance frequently have to hyperextend segments above or below the kyphosis to maintain balance. It is believed that this compensatory mechanism predisposes the patient to accelerated disk degeneration. In a type II sagittal imbalance,

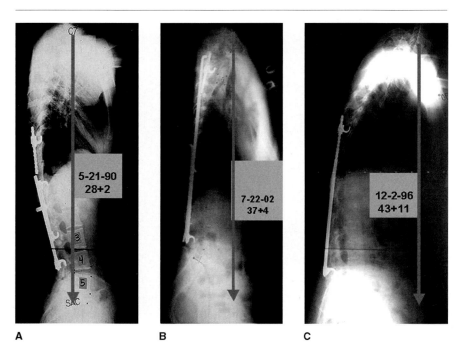

A　　　　　　　　**B**　　　　　　　　**C**

Figure 1　In a type I deformity (**A**), the patient is able to maintain balance (the C7 plumb falls over the lumbosacral disk) by substantially hyperextending segments below a hypolordotic fusion mass as shown on this long cassette sagittal radiograph. In a mild to moderate type II deformity (**B**), the patient is not able to hyperextend the segments below the fusion because of moderate to severe degeneration of those segments; the C7 plumb falls a few centimeters anterior to the lumbosacral disk. In a patient with major sagittal imbalance (**C**), the spinal fusion is sufficiently kyphotic and the segments above and below have degenerated to the extent that the C7 plumb falls more than 10 cm in front of the lumbosacral disk.

the C7 plumb is so far anterior to the lumbosacral disk that the patient is not able to compensate to maintain global balance. In this situation, there is usually substantial disk degeneration above or below an area of prior fusion or pathology that makes it impossible for the patient to hyperextend segments enough to maintain balance. Sagittal imbalance is the most poorly tolerated and debilitating form of adult spinal deformity. Sagittal imbalance is more poorly tolerated than coronal imbalance or large coronal deformities that are not associated with sagittal imbalance.[2]

Idiopathic Scoliosis

Idiopathic scoliosis usually results in a long hypolordotic fusion mass. In the past, this condition was associated with the use of Harrington distraction instrumentation (which reduces lumbar lordosis) that had been placed to L3, L4, or L5. If this hypolordotic fusion mass is combined with subsequent disk degeneration of segments below, then sagittal imbalance ensues. This condition also can occur with more modern segmental implants if the final result is that the patient loses lordosis within the fusion mass. Full-blown sagittal imbalance syndrome most commonly occurs in the fourth decade of life in a patient who had undergone fusion as a teenager.

The goal of surgical treatment of a sagittal imbalance that occurs after fusion for scoliosis is to normalize the patient's sagittal plane within the fusion mass and extend the fusion down to the sacrum. A potential complication of this surgical strategy is that the sacral fixation points often loosen, pull out, or fail. If sacral fixation is lost, the patient will develop a pseudarthrosis at L5-S1. Most commonly this pseudarthrosis will have some degree of kyphosis and further contribute to the patient's sagittal imbalance. Because of the possibility of pseudarthrosis, structural grafting at L5-S1 and protection of the sacral screws with iliac screws to reduce the likelihood of failure of the sacral screw implants is recommended.[3]

Degenerative Sagittal Imbalance

Patients with degenerative sagittal imbalance are usually older than patients with idiopathic scoliosis. Most patients with degenerative sagittal imbalance have undergone fusions of the distal one, two, or three segments of the lumbar spine. Often these distal segments have been fused in a somewhat hypolordotic position. Disk degeneration leads to loss of anterior column height; therefore, most degenerative lumbar fusions tend to solidify in a position of hypolordosis. As the patient ages, segments above the fusion degenerate. When these proximal segments degenerate, kyphosis is exaggerated and the patient is no longer able to maintain sagittal balance. Some component of spinal extensor muscle denervation as well as ligamentous disruption and decompression that extends above the prior fusion mass also may be involved.[4]

Posttraumatic Kyphosis

Posttraumatic kyphosis may occur in patients who have received either surgical or nonsurgical treatment. It is more common to see full-blown sagittal imbalance syndrome in a patient who has been treated surgically. Possible presentation scenarios include patients who had prior anterior surgery, prior posterior surgery, or prior decompressions with or without pseudarthrosis. The longer the length of the prior fusion and the greater the degree of kyphosis with the prior fusion, the more likely there is to be a complication. Subsequently, segments degenerate above or below the kyphosis. These additional degenerative segments further contribute to sagittal imbalance as is the case in patients with degenerative sagittal imbalance and idiopathic scoliosis. Patients with posttraumatic kyphosis most commonly present with a type I imbalance, although this condition may progress to a type II imbalance. A change in the patient's neurologic status will affect decisions concerning surgical treatment.[5]

Ankylosing Spondylitis

The natural history of a patient with ankylosing spondylitis is characterized by a progressive fusion of spinal segments, atrophy of spinal extensor muscles, and progressive kyphosis. This condition may occur with a coexistent spondylodiskitis, which refers to a three-column fracture that often is initially unrecognized and presents in a manner similar to a neuropathic spine. Ankylosing spondylitis is usually characterized by a rounded kyphosis that occurs from the sacrum upward into the cervical spine and occiput. Some patients with ankylosing spondylitis present with more of a cervicothoracic kyphosis, subsequent to a fracture in the upper thoracic or lower cervical spine. Another presentation is characterized by reasonable cervical alignment and a long rounded kyphosis that affects the lumbar and thoracic spine and creates fixed sagittal imbalance. The amount of sagittal imbalance may be very dramatic.[6-23]

How Surgeons Can Impact the Natural History

When performing a spinal fusion it has been recommended that the patient be positioned on a four- or six-poster frame with the hips relatively extended to maintain lordosis. Using instrumentation that does not distract the posterior column also prevents complications. The risk of sagittal imbalance increases to some extent as the fusion is increased in length; however, performing a fusion that is too short may predispose the patient to junctional kyphosis.

For a patient with degenerative sagittal imbalance, it is beneficial to attempt to perform distal lumbar fusion with the patient in a position of normal segmental lordosis. There are many strategies to potentially normalize the segmental sagittal plane when performing a lumbar fusion.[24] Circumferential fusion seems to accelerate disk degeneration at levels above the fusion. Pedicle screw implants may violate the facet capsule of the segment above the fusion. Anterior threaded cage constructs have a tendency to settle and to lose some of the lordosis that was initially achieved. There are no precise remedies for the preservation and enhancement of distal lumbar lordosis in a patient with a degenerative spine.

For a patient with a fracture, the use of distraction instrumentation is now largely obsolete. Distraction instrumentation, with or without three-point fixation, may create an initial ligamentotaxis effect that is radiographically desirable. Unfortunately, the usual long-term outcome involves settling of the reduction and ultimate healing with segmental kyphosis. Other strategies such as anterior-only treatment or posterior pedicle screw constructs have evolved to accomplish ultimate physiologic segmental lordosis.

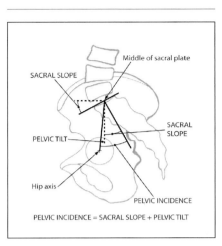

Figure 2 Sagittal pelvic parameters are assessed from the standing lateral radiograph. The hip axis is located midway between the center of the femoral heads. The pelvic incidence is defined as the angle between the perpendicular of the sacral plate and the line joining the middle of the sacral plate and the hip axis. The sacral slope represents the angle between the sacral plate and the horizontal line. The pelvic tilt is measured from the angle between the vertical line and the line joining the middle of the sacral plate and the hip axis and is positive when the hip axis lies in front of the vertical line through the middle of the sacral plate. (Reproduced with permission from Mac-Thiong J, Berthonnaud E, Dimar JR II, Betz RR, Labelle H: Sagittal alignment of the spine and pelvis during growth. *Spine* 2004;29:1642-1647.)

Assessment of Correction
Pelvic Incidence

Duval-Beaupère and associates[25] defined the term pelvic incidence and the term has been further popularized by Labelle and associates.[26] Pelvic incidence measures a combination of pelvic tilt and sacral slope (Figure 2). The higher the pelvic incidence the more lumbar lordosis a patient needs to maintain balance. A higher pelvic incidence is associated with a more horizontal sacrum; the hip joints are situated more anterior to the L5-S1 disk. The measurement of pelvic incidence is made by drawing a line between the midpoint of the L5-S1 disk connecting the midpoint of the femoral heads. The intersection between this line and a line that is perpendicular to the L5-S1 end plate determines the pelvic incidence.[27]

Thoracic Kyphosis Relative to Lumbar Lordosis

There is a wide variation in the normal range of the measurements of thoracic kyphosis and lumbar lordosis.[28] The middle of the bell-shaped curve is 30° to 35° of thoracic kyphosis measured from T5 to T12 and 55° to 60° of lumbar lordosis measured from T12 to the sacrum. Lumbar lordosis usually begins at T12-L1. Between two thirds and three fourths of lumbar lordosis is located in the distal two disks. However, there is substantial individual variation. If a patient has only 10° of thoracic lordosis, then less lumbar lordosis is required to maintain balance. One guideline is that the measurement of lumbar lordosis from T12 to S1 should exceed the measurement of thoracic kyphosis from T5 to T12 by at least 10° to 20°.[12,29]

The C7 Plumb

The C7 plumb will be affected by the patient's positioning. When a long cassette lateral radiograph is taken, the patient is usually asked to extend the shoulders and arms out in front of the trunk to allow the spine to be seen on the radiograph. This positioning may have a tendency to posteriorly displace the C7 plumb. The effect of arm position on the C7 plumb was studied and it was concluded that a position in which the shoulders are flexed approximately 30° and the fists are placed in the supraclavicular fossa was the most desirable position to allow for visualization of the anatomic landmarks (W Horton, MD, Atlanta, GA, personal communication, 2004). The upper thoracic spine is the area most difficult to see on radiographs because of the overlap with the shoulder girdle.

Patients with sagittal imbalance will frequently stand with their feet further apart and their knees flexed to better position their head over their feet. This posture will adversely affect the C7 plumb assessment. Therefore, it is preferable to ask the patient to stand with knees fully extended and feet no more than shoulder width apart. Also, there are limitations to the assessment of a C7 static plumb. As the patient ambulates, the hip extensors tend to fatigue; therefore, after walking a certain distance a patient's posture will clinically be more pitched forward than it was at stance.[30-32]

The C7 plumb is the best assessment for sagittal balance, but it is not perfect because it does not always directly correlate with the center of gravity, which is the element that is actually being assessed. A patient's center of gravity should always fall either through the hip joints or somewhat behind it. Usually the center of gravity is in front of the C7 plumb.

Expectations With Smith-Petersen Osteotomies

The extent of correction achieved with a Smith-Petersen osteotomy depends on the characteristics of the anterior column of the spine and the amount of bone that is resected posteriorly.[18,33-38] In patients with ankylosing spondylitis, corrections up to 50° have been achieved with this osteotomy. However, for patients who do not have ankylosing spondylitis the amount of correction that is achieved per level is approximately 10°.[30] Therefore, three Smith-Petersen osteotomies usually achieve the same

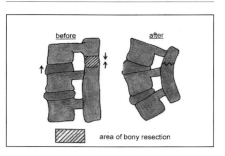

Figure 3 A Smith-Petersen osteotomy shortens the posterior column that is resected. The middle column is shortened and the anterior column is lengthened through the disk space, which must be mobile. Usually approximately 10° of correction is achieved through each segment of a Smith-Petersen osteotomy.

amount of correction as one pedicle subtraction procedure. To close a Smith-Petersen osteotomy it is necessary to have a mobile anterior column. In the presence of an anterior fusion, it will not be possible to close a Smith-Petersen osteotomy without releasing the spine anteriorly. If there is an open visible disk space, then it usually is possible to close a Smith-Petersen osteotomy without an anterior operation (Figure 3).

A Smith-Petersen osteotomy shortens the posterior column and lengthens the anterior column. Therefore, if these osteotomies are done symmetrically at the apex of a residual scoliosis with residual rotation, there is potential to decompensate the patient's spine in the coronal plane.[1] With residual rotation the posterior column is on the concave side of the spine and the anterior column is on the convexity. Shortening the posterior column and lengthening the anterior column has a tendency to shorten the concavity, lengthen the convexity, and pitch the patient's spinal alignment to the concavity (Figure 4). When performing multiple Smith-Petersen osteotomies through seg-

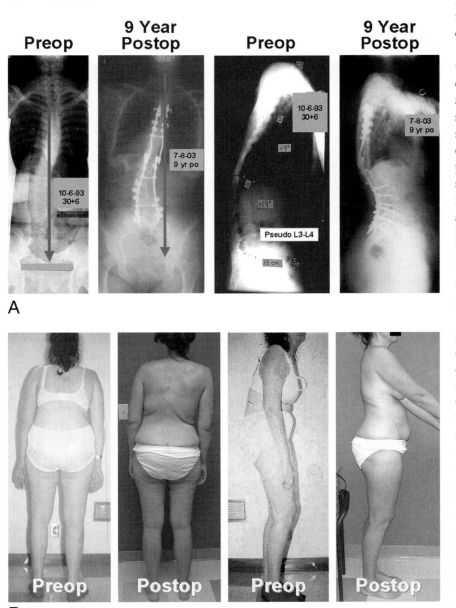

Figure 4   A, Composite long cassette radiographs of a patient who presented with good coronal balance, very positive sagittal balance, and pseudarthrosis of the lumbar spine are shown. The patient was treated with circumferential surgery in the lumbar spine and multiple Smith-Petersen osteotomies that were done symmetrically at several segments through areas of residual rotation. This treatment shortened the posterior column and lengthened the anterior column. Postoperative results at 9 years were satisfactory. Sagittal balance was excellent; however, in the coronal plane the patient decompensated to the right side. **B,** Clinical photographs of the same patient showing the correction of the sagittal deformity with somewhat worsened balance in the coronal plane. In the preoperative photographs the patient was asked to keep her knees extended, but otherwise to stand as erect as possible. In the postoperative photographs the patient was asked to stand naturally.

ments with residual rotation, care must be taken to avoid increasing coronal deformity.

Smith-Petersen osteotomies can be used to treat mild or moderate type II deformities if care is taken not to create a coronal imbalance. Figure 5 shows a patient who had severe spinal stenosis of distal segments and degeneration of two segments below the prior fusion mass. Rebalancing in the sagittal plane was achieved by extending the fusion down to the sacrum and pelvis and by performing Smith-Petersen osteotomies at the two distal levels of the prior fusion (L2-L3 and L3-L4). The Smith-Petersen osteotomy is discussed in greater detail in chapter 13.

Expectations With Pedicle Subtraction Osteotomies

A pedicle subtraction procedure may achieve up to 50° to 60° of correction, depending on the size of the wedge that is resected and whether the disk above is also resected. However, a more typical correction is approximately 35°.[39-41] Pedicle subtraction procedures can be performed through the apex of a deformity in the presence of substantial rotation. If the procedure is performed symmetrically on both sides, there does not appear to be a tendency to pitch the patient's spinal alignment to the concavity as can occur in Smith-Petersen osteotomies. A pedicle subtraction procedure shortens the posterior column and hinges on the anterior column in contrast to the Smith-Petersen procedure, which lengthens the anterior column (Figure 6). One pedicle subtraction procedure accomplishes approximately as much correction as three Smith-Petersen osteotomies. A pedicle subtraction procedure is usually associated with more blood loss than three Smith-Petersen osteotomies.[30] It is

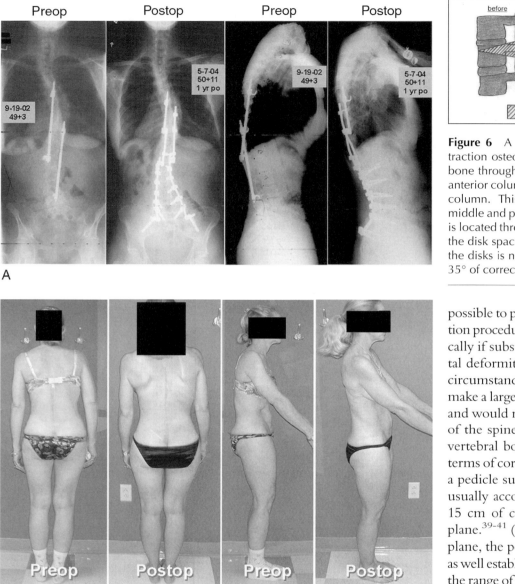

A

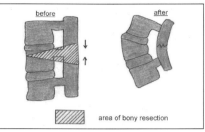

Figure 6 A three-column pedicle subtraction osteotomy involves resection of bone through the posterior, middle, and anterior columns, hinging on the anterior column. This procedure shortens the middle and posterior columns. The hinge is located through the vertebral body, not the disk space, therefore, the mobility of the disks is not germane. Approximately 35° of correction is usually achieved.

B

Figure 5 **A,** Composite preoperative and 1-year postoperative long cassette radiographs of a patient with a prior Harrington fusion and instrumentation to L4. The patient presented with a kyphotic fusion mass, marked degeneration of the two segments below the fusion, and marked spinal stenosis of those segments. Her sagittal imbalance was moderate. Treatment involved appropriate decompressions at the lower two segments and subsequent correction of the sagittal deformity with two Smith-Petersen osteotomies in the mid lumbar spine. Some lordization of the segments at L4-L5 and L5-S1 was accomplished with intraoperative table positioning. **B,** Clinical photographs of the same patient showing substantial improvement in the deformity. In the preoperative photographs she was asked to keep her knees extended, but to stand as erect as possible. In the postoperatively photographs the patient was asked to stand naturally.

possible to perform a pedicle subtraction procedure somewhat asymmetrically if substantial coronal and sagittal deformities both exist. In such a circumstance, the surgeon would make a larger wedge on the convexity and would reach around to the front of the spine and resect more of the vertebral body on the convexity. In terms of correction of the C7 plumb, a pedicle subtraction procedure will usually accomplish between 12 and 15 cm of correction in the sagittal plane.[39-41] (Figure 7). In the coronal plane, the potential correction is not as well established but appears to be in the range of 5 to 7 cm.[21,22,42,43] An algorithm summarizing strategy for deciding when to perform Smith-Petersen osteotomies versus pedicle subtraction procedures for various types of sagittal imbalance is shown in Figure 8. The pedicle subtraction osteotomy is also discussed in chapter 14.

Expectations With Adding Levels to an Existing Fusion

In patients with fixed sagittal imbalance, degenerated segments that develop either above or below a prior

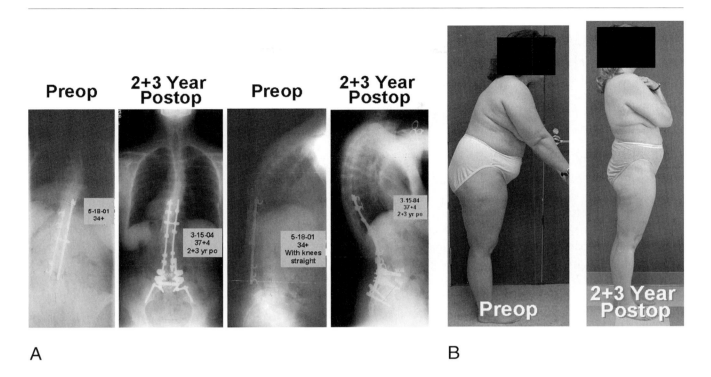

A   **B**

Figure 7   **A,** Composite preoperative and postoperative (2 years and 3 months) long cassette radiographs of a patient who presented with a kyphotic fusion mass after prior surgery (many years before) for idiopathic scoliosis and marked degeneration of the segments below. The C7 plumb was greater than 10 cm in front of the lumbosacral disk. Surgical treatment included pedicle subtraction osteotomy, structurally grafting the degenerated segments below, and performing instrumented fusion to the sacrum and pelvis. Most of the correction was accomplished with the pedicle subtraction procedure, although some correction was achieved with the structural grafting of segments below. **B,** Clinical photographs of the same patient. In the preoperative photograph the patient was asked to keep her knees extended, but to stand as erect as possible. In the postoperative photograph she was asked to stand naturally.

fusion are logically included in the revision surgical construct. It may be possible to achieve additional lordosis of the spine when adding those segments. Most commonly, if distal segments (for example, L4-L5 and L5-S1) are being added, those segments first will be structurally grafted anteriorly and then fixed posteriorly. The anterior structural grafting will open up the disk spaces and create a ligamentotaxis effect that both reduces subluxations and also provides additional lordosis. Also, in segments with severe degeneration, placing the patient in a prone position under anesthesia may open up disk spaces and provide more lordosis than was apparent when the patient was standing.

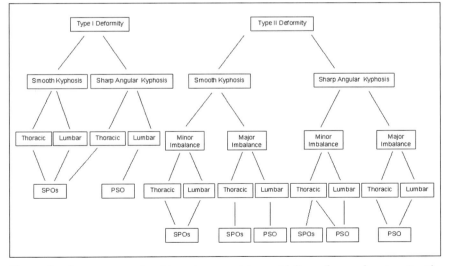

Figure 8   A treatment algorithm that provides guidelines for performing Smith-Petersen versus pedicle subtraction osteotomies based on the characteristics of the sagittal deformity and its anatomic location. SPO = Smith-Petersen osteotomy; PSO = pedicle subtraction osteotomy.

The amount of additional lordosis that can be achieved by adding segments above and below the prior fusion is quite variable. The additional amount of lordosis that can be achieved by adding segments is on average 5° per level.

Summary

There are multiple causes of sagittal spinal imbalance. Historically, distraction instrumentation (specifically, the posterior Harrington implant) was the principal cause of this condition. The most common causes of sagittal imbalance are degeneration at L3-L4, L4-L5, or L5-S1 distal to a fusion for idiopathic scoliosis; multiple fusions performed in the middle to distal lumbar spine with each level being fused in a somewhat hypolordotic position and subsequent degeneration of the segments above; posttraumatic kyphosis; and ankylosing spondylitis. When performing an instrumented fusion in the lumbar spine to treat a fracture it is important to always place the fused segment(s) in lordosis. When treating degenerative fusions, the fusing of a segment in a kyphotic position should be avoided. Although a one-level fusion in a slightly kyphotic position may be tolerated, the subsequent addition of more segments may make it impossible for the patient to compensate by hyperextending unfused segments and will contribute to sagittal imbalance syndrome.

For a patient with sagittal imbalance the most common radiographic measure used to characterize the imbalance is the C7 plumb relative to the posterior aspect of the L5-S1 disk. Because the C7 plumb does not always correlate with the center of gravity, studies are underway to investigate this parameter.

In most circumstances the patient should have 10° to 30° more lumbar lordosis than thoracic kyphosis to have ideal balance. Usually a Smith-Petersen osteotomy will accomplish approximately 10° of spinal lordosis. A pedicle subtraction procedure will accomplish approximately 30° of additional lordosis. Usually 30° to 35° of correction will displace the C7 plumb posteriorly between 12 and 15 cm in a patient with type II major sagittal imbalance. Many investigators believe that the more distal the osteotomy, more correction will be achieved in the C7 plumb. Some investigators find it useful to cut wedges from photocopies of the long cassette radiograph in an effort to assess the extent of correction in overall sagittal balance that will be achieved by performing various osteotomies at various locations. The reproducibility and reliability of such practices has not been documented in the peer-reviewed literature.

For the treatment of sagittal imbalance within a solid spinal fusion from T3 to the sacrum, osteotomies will achieve correction. This situation, however, is somewhat unusual. More commonly, the patient also has either multiple pseudarthroses or very degenerated segments that need to be added to the fusion. Correction may also be achieved by adding pseudarthrotic or degenerated segments to the prior fusion.

References

1. Booth KC, Bridwell KH, Lenke LG, Baldus CR, Blanke KM: Complications and predictive factors for the successful treatment of flatback deformity (fixed sagittal imbalance). *Spine* 1999;24:1712-1720.

2. Glassman SD, Berven S, Bridwell K, Horton W, Dimar JR: Correlation of radiographic parameters and clinical symptoms in adult scoliosis. *Spine* 2005;30:682-688.

3. Kuklo TR, Bridwell KH, Lewis SJ, et al: Minimum two-year analysis of sacropelvic fixation and L5/S1 fusion utilizing S1 and iliac screws. *Spine* 2001;26:1976-1983.

4. Farcy JP, Schwab FJ: Management of flatback and related kyphotic decompensation syndromes. *Spine* 1997;22:2452-2457.

5. Gertzbein SD, Harris MB: Wedge osteotomy for the correction of post-traumatic kyphosis: A new technique and a report of three cases. *Spine* 1992;17:374-379.

6. Bradford DS, Schumacker WL, Lonstein JE, Winter RB: Ankylosing spondylitis: Experience and surgical management of 21 patients. *Spine* 1987;12:590-592.

7. Camargo FP, Cordeiro EN, Napoli MM: Corrective osteotomy of the spine in ankylosing spondylitis: Experience with 66 cases. *Clin Orthop* 1986;208:157-167.

8. Chen IH, Chien JT, Yu TC: Transpedicular wedge osteotomy for correction of thoracolumbar kyphosis in ankylosing spondylitis: Experience with 78 patients. *Spine* 2001;26:E354-E360.

9. Emneus H: Wedge osteotomy of spine in ankylosing spondylitis. *Acta Orthop Scand* 1968;39:321-326.

10. Goel MK: Vertebral osteotomy for correction of fixed flexion deformity of the spine. *J Bone Joint Surg Am* 1968;50:287-294.

11. Halm H, Metz-Stavenhagen P, Zielke K: Results of surgical correction of kyphotic deformities of the spine in ankylosing spondylitis on the basis of the modified arthritis impact measurement scales. *Spine* 1995;20:1612-1619.

12. Hehne HJ, Zielke K, Bohm H: Polysegmental lumbar osteotomies and transpedicled fixation for correction of long-curved kyphotic deformities in ankylosing spondylitis: Report on 177 cases. *Clin Orthop* 1990;258:49-55.

13. Herbert JJ: Vertebral osteotomy for kyphosis, especially in Marie-Strumpell arthritis. *J Bone Joint Surg Am* 1959;41:291-302.

14. Jaffray D, Becker V, Eisenstein S: Closing wedge osteotomy with transpedicular fixation in ankylosing spondylitis. *Clin Orthop* 1992;279:122-126.

15. LaChapelle EH: Osteotomy of the lumbar spine for correction of kyphosis in a case of ankylosing spondylarthritis. *J Bone Joint Surg* 1946;28:851-858.

16. Law WA: Lumbar spinal osteotomy. *J Bone Joint Surg Br* 1959;41:270-278.

17. McMaster MJ: A technique for lumbar spinal osteotomy in ankylosing spondylitis. *J Bone Joint Surg Br* 1985;67:204-210.

18. Nash CL, Moe JH: A study of vertebral rotation. *J Bone Joint Surg Am* 1969;51:223-229.

19. Simmons EH: Kyphotic deformity of the spine in ankylosing spondylitis. *Clin Orthop* 1977;128:65-77.

20. Styblo K, Bossers GT, Slot GH: Osteotomy for kyphosis in ankylosing spondylitis. *Acta Orthop Scand* 1985;56:294-297.

21. Thiranont N, Netrawinchien P: Transpedicular decancellation closed wedge vertebral osteotomy for treatment of fixed flexion deformity of the spine in ankylosing spondylitis. *Spine* 1993;18:2517-2522.

22. Thomasen E: Vertebral osteotomy for correction of kyphosis in ankylosing spondylitis. *Clin Orthop* 1985;194:142-152.

23. van Royen BJ, Slot GH: Closing-wedge posterior osteotomy for ankylosing spondylitis: Partial corporectomy and transpedicular fixation in 22 cases. *J Bone Joint Surg Br* 1995;77:117-121.

24. Bridwell KH: Lumbosacral junction and sacrum stabilization, in Kim D, Vaccaro A, Fessler R (eds): *Surgical Techniques in Spinal Instrumentation.* New York, NY, Thieme, 2005.

25. Duval-Beaupère G, Schimdt C, Cosson P: A barycentremetric study of the sagittal shape of spine and pelvis: The conditions required for an economic standing position. *Ann Biomed Eng* 1992;20:451-462.

26. Mac-Thiong J, Berthonnaud E, Dimar II Jr, Betz RR, Labelle H: Sagittal alignment of the spine and pelvis during growth. *Spine* 2004;29:1642-1647.

27. Legaye J, Duval-Beaupère G, Hecquet J, Marty C: Pelvic incidence: A fundamental pelvic parameter for three-dimensional regulation of spinal sagittal curves. *Eur Spine J* 1998;7:99-103.

28. Wambolt A, Spencer DL: A segmental analysis of the distribution of lumbar lordosis in the normal spine. *Orthop Trans* 1987;11:92-93.

29. Bernhardt M, Bridwell KH: Segmental analysis of the sagittal plane alignment of the normal thoracic and lumbar spines and thoracolumbar junction. *Spine* 1989;14:717-721.

30. Cho K, Bridwell KH, Lenke LG, Berra A, Baldus C: Comparison of Smith-Petersen osteotomy versus pedicle subtraction osteotomy for the correction of fixed sagittal imbalance. *Spine* 2005;30:2030-2037.

31. Engsberg JR, Bridwell KH, Reitenbach AK, et al: Preoperative gait comparisons between adults undergoing long spinal deformity fusion surgery (thoracic to L4, L5, or sacrum) and controls. *Spine* 2001;26:2020-2028.

32. Engsberg JR, Bridwell KH, Wagner JM, Uhrich ML, Blanke K, Lenke LG: Gait changes as the result of deformity reconstruction surgery in a group of adults with lumbar scoliosis. *Spine* 2003;28:1836-1843.

33. Berven SH, Deviren V, Smith JA, Hu SH, Bradford DS: Management of fixed sagittal plane deformity: Outcome of combined anterior and posterior surgery. *Spine* 2003;28:1710-1715.

34. Floman Y, Penny JN, Micheli LJ, Riseborough EJ, Hall JE: Osteotomy of the fusion mass in scoliosis. *J Bone Joint Surg Am* 1982;64:1307-1316.

35. Kostuik JP, Maurais GR, Richardson WJ, Okajima Y: Combined single stage anterior and posterior osteotomy for correction of iatrogenic lumbar kyphosis. *Spine* 1988;13:257-266.

36. LaGrone MO, Bradford DS, Moe JH, Lonstein JE, Winter RB, Ogilvie JW: Treatment of symptomatic flatback after spinal fusion. *J Bone Joint Surg Am* 1988;70:569-580.

37. Shufflebarger HL, Clark CE: Thoracolumbar osteotomy for postsurgical sagittal imbalance. *Spine* 1992;17:S287-S290.

38. Smith-Petersen MN, Larson CB, Aufranc OE: Osteotomy of the spine for correction of flexion deformity in rheumatoid arthritis. *J Bone Joint Surg* 1945;27:1-11.

39. Bridwell KH, Lewis S, Edwards C, et al: Complications and outcomes of pedicle subtraction osteotomies for fixed sagittal imbalance. *Spine* 2003;28:2093-2101.

40. Bridwell KH, Lewis SJ, Lenke LG, Baldus C, Blanke K: Pedicle subtraction osteotomy for the treatment of fixed sagittal imbalance. *J Bone Joint Surg Am* 2003;85-A:454-463.

41. Bridwell KH, Lewis SJ, Rinella A, Lenke LG, Baldus C, Blanke K: Pedicle subtraction osteotomy for the treatment of fixed sagittal imbalance: Surgical technique. *J Bone Joint Surg Am* 2004;86-A:44-50.

42. Danisa OA, Turner D, Richardson WJ: Surgical correction of lumbar kyphotic deformity: posterior reduction "eggshell" osteotomy. *J Neurosurg Spine* 2000;92:50-56.

43. Lehmer SM, Keppler L, Biscup RS, Enker P, Miller SD, Steffee AD: Posterior transvertebral osteotomy for adult thoracolumbar kyphosis. *Spine* 1994;19:2060-2067.

Smith-Petersen Osteotomy of the Spine

Douglas C. Burton, MD

Abstract

The Smith-Petersen osteotomy has been a mainstay in the treatment of sagittal deformity since it was first described in 1945. The primary indication for an osteotomy is fixed sagittal deformity. When an osteotomy is performed in a patient with ankylosing spondylitis, it can be combined with an anterior column osteoclasis to achieve a correction of up to 40° to 50°. When performed for other indications, the osteotomy can result in approximately 10° of correction per level treated.

Osteotomy of the spine was first reported in 1945 by Smith-Petersen and associates[1] as a treatment for sagittal imbalance caused by ankylosing spondylitis. They reported on six patients who were treated with a posterior opening wedge osteotomy that now bears Smith-Petersen's name. All patients were immobilized in a plaster cast for 1 year.

A year later, La Chapelle[2] reported on a similar osteotomy, which was done in two stages with a second anterior operation performed to divide the ossified anterior longitudinal ligament using direct vision. Several other early studies were published on the Smith-Petersen osteotomy used in the treatment of ankylosing spondylitis.[3-8] Adams[9] reported on a modification of the technique, which involved performing the surgery on a patient who was placed in a lateral rather than a prone position.

In 1955, Meiss[10] was the first physician to use this technique to treat a condition other than ankylosing spondylitis. He performed a two-stage biplanar correction on a patient with severe kyphoscoliosis who had been previously treated with fusion. Meiss' article was the first to highlight the two different methods of using this technique, depending on the diagnosis. Because of the brittle nature of the anterior column in patients with ankylosing spondylitis, an anterior osteoclasis can be performed from a posterior approach. Other diagnoses do not allow this approach; therefore, to obtain corrections greater than 10° to 15° per level, multiple level osteotomies must be performed with or without anterior release.

Indications

The indication for an osteotomy of the spine is spinal imbalance in the sagittal and/or coronal plane that does not correct on bending radiographs. The options for osteotomy are numerous and include the Smith-Petersen osteotomy and posterior osteotomy techniques such as the pedicle centered osteotomy, also called the eggshell osteotomy.[11,12] This procedure can be combined with anterior diskectomy or osteotomy. The choice of technique depends on the amount of correction desired and the etiology of the deformity. More information on eggshell osteotomies can be found in chapter 14.

The Smith-Petersen osteotomy was developed to treat sagittal deformity caused by ankylosing spondylitis. Because of the brittle nature of the ossified anterior longitudinal ligament and disk, an anterior osteoclasis (fracture) was performed through the anterior column. This aspect of the technique allowed large corrections to be achieved. Smith-Petersen's original description of the technique used elevation of the head and feet to affect the anterior column osteoclasis.[1] La Chapelle[2] used a second stage anterior approach to osteotomize the bamboo spine. In both approaches, the correction is obtained through an anterior opening wedge osteotomy. The fulcrum of the osteotomy is the posterior longitudinal ligament and the amount of angular

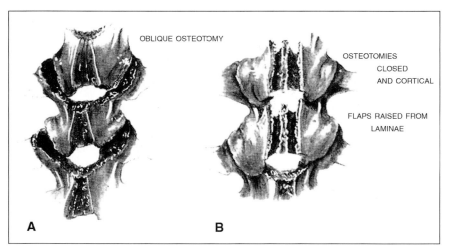

Figure 1 Drawing of the Smith-Petersen osteotomy before (**A**) and after (**B**) closure. (Reproduced with permission from Smith-Petersen MN, Larson CB, and Aufranc OE: Osteotomy of the spine for correction of flexion deformity in rheumatoid arthritis. *J Bone Joint Surg Am* 1945;27:1-11.)

correction is limited by the amount of anterior opening. A calcified aorta is a contraindication to this procedure because of the potential for aortic rupture.[13]

If the patient does not have ankylosing spondylitis, osteoclasis cannot be performed and the amount of correction that can be obtained is considerably limited. Without anterior osteoclasis, each millimeter of posterior bone resection yields 1° of angular correction for a maximal correction of 10° to 15°.[14] These results also are reliant on the presence of relatively "fat" anterior disks (at least 5 mm in height without bridging osteophytes).[14] If the disks are narrowed, an anterior release may be necessary to obtain the desired correction.

Technique

At the author's institution, spinal monitoring including transcranial motor-evoked potentials, somatosensory-evoked potentials, and continuous electromyograms are used for all osteotomy procedures. A central venous line, arterial line, Foley catheter, and nasogastric tube are placed. The patient is carefully positioned prone on a Relton-Hall frame (Imperial Surgical Co, Toronto, Canada). If there is any question concerning neck stability, such as in patients with ankylosing spondylitis, the head is placed in Mayfield tongs. A flexed bed is not routinely used for positioning, but may be helpful in certain situations.

The choice of osteotomy level depends on the apex of the deformity. The normal apex of the lumbar lordosis is L3-4 and this level is usually chosen. It is preferable to stay below the level of the conus medullaris if possible.

After the patient is positioned, the spine is exposed and the spinal fixation is placed. This technique allows a temporary stabilizing rod to be used if the spine becomes unstable before the osteotomy is completed, permits rapid closure of the osteotomy, and usually diminishes the epidural bleeding that occurs.

It is important to identify the pedicles above and below the osteotomy site; this is usually done by dissecting out the transverse processes. The resection is wedge- or chevron-shaped, with the point distal (Figure 1). If posterior elements are intact, such as in ankylosing spondylitis, the initial resection is performed on the spinous process at the level to be resected. Portions of the spinous processes above and below also are removed. It is important to keep both limbs of the wedge symmetrical, unless some coronal plane correction is desired. In this situation, one side of the wedge is widened with respect to the other. The area to be resected can be outlined with an oscillating saw from the apex of the wedge out laterally to the notch. The bone between the cut lines is then thinned with an osteotome. This technique preserves as much local bone as possible for the arthrodesis.

The canal is entered in the midline and a dural elevator is used to free any dural adhesions if present. In patients with ankylosing spondylitis, the dura may strongly adhere to the ossified ligamentum flavum. Incidental durotomies are repaired before closure of the osteotomy. The osteotomy is carried laterally out to the intervertebral notch using small Kerrison rongeurs. Epidural bleeding is controlled with thrombin-soaked absorbable gelatin and cottonoid. Special care is taken to undercut the osteotomy to avoid any neural compression associated with closing the osteotomy. If there is any indication of dural compression during osteotomy closure, the osteotomy should be enlarged centrally.

If the osteotomy is performed at a level with significant rotational deformity, the osteotomy should be opened to a greater degree on the side of the convexity.[15] This technique will minimize coronal plane

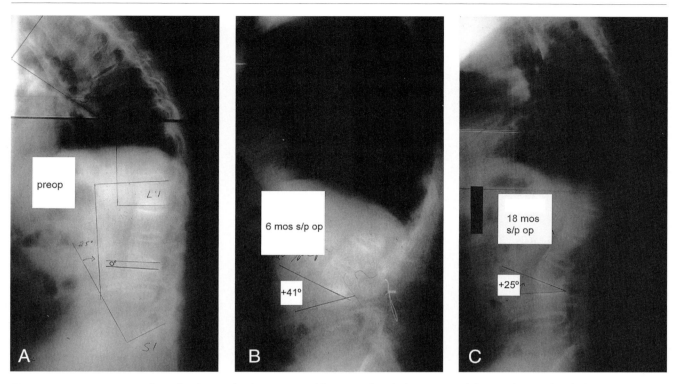

Figure 2 **A**, Preoperative lateral radiograph of a 36-year-old man with ankylosing spondylitis and sagittal imbalance. **B**, Immediate postoperative radiograph after a Smith-Petersen osteotomy and spinous process wiring showing a 41° correction. Patient was immobilized in a cast for 6 months. **C**, Postoperative radiograph taken 18 months after surgery. The patient has lost 16° of correction, but is satisfied with the result.

decompensation when the osteotomy is closed.

After the osteotomy is completed, it is closed. Closure may occur passively as a result of lordosis induced by the surgical frame, or prebent rods can be added to the previously placed bone anchors and a combination of maneuvers of cantilever correction and compression should achieve the necessary reduction. If osteoclasis is planned, manual pressure on the fusion mass or elevation of the feet may aid in fracturing the anterior column. Osteoclasis should be accomplished in a slow and controlled manner. After the correction is completed and the rods are set, it is imperative to obtain intraoperative radiographs to verify appropriate sagittal and coronal balance. At the author's institution, coronal balance is assessed using

36-inch posteroanterior radiographs that are double exposed proximally and distally with a sterile, wrapped, lead apron protecting the nonexposed portion of the cassette. A lateral 17- × 14-inch radiograph is used to document the sagittal correction. At this stage of the procedure, the surgeon must confirm that adequate correction has been obtained. Failure to achieve appropriate sagittal alignment will result in an unsatisfactory outcome for the patient (Figure 2).

Treatment Results: Ankylosing Spondylitis

In 1945, Smith-Petersen and associates[1] initially reported on six patients. All patients had good outcomes with only one complication (a retained iliac sponge). In 1958, Sotelo-Ortiz[6] reported on two patients who had an

osteotomy for ankylosing spondylitis. Both had good outcomes; however, temporary anterior thigh paresthesia was reported. In 1958, McMaster[5] added information on five additional patients who all had good results and no complications after osteotomy. Although these early reports did not document the amount of correction obtained from the osteotomy procedure, all patients were reportedly satisfied with the outcomes.

In 1959, Law[4] published his results in treating 80 patients with extension osteotomy. The average correction achieved was between 25° to 45°. Complications included eight perioperative deaths, two from gastrointestinal causes and six from neurologic injuries. Recurrence of deformity occurred in three patients. Law's study is the largest series documented in the early literature and is the most cited study providing data on rates of death and neurologic injury.

Goel[7] studied 15 patients treated with a Smith-Petersen osteotomy in 1968. He reported an average correction of 37° along with seven complications, including two pressure sores, two cases of ileus, two root irritations, and one recurrence of deformity. Emnéus[8] reported on five patients in 1968, finding an average correction of 24° and two complications (one dural laceration and one pseudarthrosis). In 1986, Camargo and associates[16] reported on 66 patients who had been treated with lumbar osteotomy for ankylosing spondylitis and had a 2- to 30-year follow-up after surgery. Corrections ranged from 22° to 55°. Complications included one ileus, one aortic rupture, and two patients with neurologic deficits who recovered spontaneously.

In 1977, Simmons[17] published a study on results using a variation of the original Smith-Petersen osteotomy technique. He retained the technical methods of the osteotomy as they were originally described, but performed the surgery with the patient in the lateral position using local anesthetic. Simmons achieved an average correction of 47° with no reported complications. The nasogastric tube was routinely left in place for 2 to 3 days postoperatively to avoid gastrointestinal complications. Spinous process wiring and external casting for immobilization was used.

By the 1970s, surgeons had begun adding Harrington instrumentation to the procedure for additional internal fixation. In 1985, McMaster[18] described the use of modified Harrington compression instrumentation to aid in both the correction maneuver as well as the postoperative immobilization. He

treated 14 patients and obtained an average correction of 38°, which was maintained at 33° at final follow-up. Complications included three dural tears and two instances of ileus. Bradford and associates[19] also used Harrington instrumentation with the Smith-Petersen osteotomy and reported on eight patients treated with posterior osteotomy alone and compression instrumentation. Four complications occurred in these eight patients including two partial neurologic injuries that resolved and two hook cutouts.

The development of pedicle screw systems in the 1980s led to the use of these systems for internal fixation after the osteotomy. In 1990, Hehne and associates[20] reported on 177 patients treated with polysegmental osteotomies and pedicle screw fixation. They reported an average correction of 10° per osteotomy. Complications included 4 deaths, 4 permanent root injuries, 19 resolved neurologic deficits, 4 implant failures, and 6 deep wound infections.

van Royen and associates[21] subsequently reported on the same surgery in 21 patients; an average correction of 25° was achieved. Complications included nine implant failures and seven deep wound infections. The use of polysegmental osteotomies for deformity correction in ankylosing spondylitis is no longer recommended.

All of these studies highlight the variety of complications that can result from this procedure. Complications are common even for an experienced surgeon.

Treatment Results: Deformity Salvage

The increased use of surgical treatment for patients with scoliosis that followed the advent of Harrington

instrumentation also led to complex revision surgeries (Figure 3). The term flatback syndrome, arising from the loss of iatrogenic lumbar lordosis, was popularized by LaGrone and associates in 1988.[22] The use of distraction instrumentation in the lumbar spine was identified as the most common etiology of this disorder. LaGrone and associates performed 66 osteotomies on 55 patients, with 19 concomitant anterior procedures to treat flatback syndrome. There were 33 complications, but no deaths nor patients with permanent neurologic deficits. The anterior sagittal displacement improved from 8.2 cm preoperatively to an average of 0.1 cm after surgery and to 4.2 cm at final follow-up. Twenty-six patients with an average displacement of 5.4 cm believed that they were still leaning forward after surgery. These results are contrasted with 24 patients with an average displacement of 1.3 cm who did not believe that they were leaning forward after the procedure. These data support the observation that in patients who undergo revision surgery for sagittal imbalance, satisfaction with the surgery is dependent on the restoration of adequate lordosis.

Floman and associates[23] reported on 154 osteotomies in 55 patients who required revision surgery because of imbalance following previous spinal fusion. Nine patients had additional anterior surgery. There were 32 complications, including one death and nine neurologic deficits (eight of which resolved). Spinal imbalance was improved to within 2 cm on average; only five patients continued to report back pain.

More recently, Voos and associates[24] reported on 27 patients with rigid deformity treated with multiple osteotomies. The average sagittal

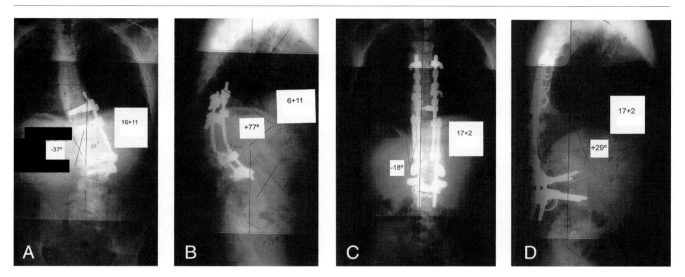

Figure 3 PA **(A)** and lateral **(B)** 36-inch radiographs of a 16-year-old boy with congenital scoliosis. The patient had two previous anterior surgeries and one anterior and posterior surgery. He had a presumed pseudarthrosis and broken anterior implants with thoracolumbar junctional kyphosis of 77°. Postoperative PA **(C)** and lateral **(D)** radiographs after staged reconstruction. The initial stage of reconstruction consisted of anchor placement and three Smith-Petersen osteotomies through the fusion mass. The second stage of the procedure consisted of anterior implant removal, osteotomy, pseudarthrosis takedown, and sequential posterior implant placement and deformity correction. Note the correction of both the kyphosis as well as the coronal imbalance.

balance was corrected 6.5 cm. Nine complications occurred in eight patients: three pseudoarthroses, five implant failures, and one transient neurologic deficit. There were no deaths or permanent neurologic deficits.

Summary

Smith-Petersen's admonition that "the operative procedure must not be belittled–there are many points in the technique that we have found difficult," remains as true today as it was in 1945.[1] The complication rate associated with this procedure is high when performed in patients with ankylosing spondylitis or for iatrogenic spinal imbalance in patients who have had multiple surgeries. The keys to a successful outcome lie in careful assessment of the deformity and the amount of correction desired, understanding of the etiology of the deformity and comorbidities, meticulous surgical technique, and prompt attention to postoperative complications when they occur.

References

1. Smith-Petersen MN, Larson CB, Aufranc OE: Osteotomy of the spine for correction of flexion deformity in rheumatoid arthritis. *J Bone Joint Surg Am* 1945;27:1-11.

2. La Chapelle EH: Osteotomy of the lumbar spine for correction of kyphosis in a case of ankylosing spondylarthritis. *J Bone Joint Surg Am* 1946;28:851-858.

3. Herbert JJ: Vertebral osteotomy. *J Bone Joint Surg Am* 1948;30:680-689.

4. Law WA: Lumbar spinal osteotomy. *J Bone Joint Surg Br* 1959;41:270-278.

5. McMaster PE: Osteotomy of the spine for correction of fixed flexion deformity. *AMA Arch Surg* 1958;76:603-610.

6. Sotelo-Ortiz F: Results of osteotomy of the spine according to the type of curvature. *Surg Gynecol Obstet* 1958;107:47-54.

7. Goel MK: Vertebral osteotomy for correction of fixed flexion deformity of the spine. *J Bone Joint Surg Am* 1968;50:287-294.

8. Emnéus H: Wedge osteotomy of spine in ankylosing spondylitis. *Acta Orthop Scand* 1968;39:321-326.

9. Adams JC: Technique, dangers and safeguards in osteotomy of the spine. *J Bone Joint Surg Br* 1952;34:226-232.

10. Meiss WC: Spinal osteotomy following fusion for paralytic scoliosis. *J Bone Joint Surg Am* 1955;37:73-77.

11. Thomasen E: Vertebral osteotomy for correction of kyphosis in ankylosing spondylitis. *Clin Orthop* 1985;194:142-152.

12. Heinig CF: The eggshell procedure, in Luque E (ed): *Segmental Spinal Instrumentation.* Thorofare, NJ, Slack Inc, 1985.

13. Lichtblau PO, Wilson PD: Possible mechanism of aortic rupture in orthopaedic correction of rheumatoid spondylitis. *J Bone Joint Surg Am* 1956;38:123-127.

14. Bridwell KH: Osteotomies for fixed deformities in the thoracic and lumbar spine, in Bridwell KH, Dewald RL (eds): *The Textbook of Spinal Surgery*, ed 2. Philadelphia, PA, Lippincott-Raven Publishers, 1997, pp 821-835.

15. Bridwell KH, Lenke LG, Lewis SJ: Treatment of spinal stenosis and fixed sagittal imbalance. *Clin Orthop* 2001;384:35-44.

16. Camargo FP, Cordeiro EN, Napoli MMM: Corrective osteotomy of the spine in ankylosing spondylitis. *Clin Orthop* 1986;208:157-166.

17. Simmons EH: Kyphotic deformity of the spine in ankylosing spondylitis. *Clin Orthop* 1977;128:65-77.

18. McMaster MJ: A technique for lumbar spinal osteotomy in ankylosing spondylitis. *J Bone Joint Surg Br* 1985;67:204-210.

19. Bradford DS, Schumacher WL, Lonstein JE, Winter RB: Ankylosing spondylitis: Experience in surgical management of 21 patients. *Spine* 1987;12:238-243.

20. Hehne HJ, Zielke K, Bohm H: Polysegmental lumbar osteotomies and transpedicled fixation for correction of long-curved kyphotic deformities in ankylosing spondylitis. *Clin Orthop* 1990;258:49-55.

21. van Royen BJ, de Kleuver M, Slot GH: Polysegmental lumbar posterior wedge osteotomies for correction of kyphosis in ankylosing spondylitis. *Eur Spine J* 1998;7:104-110.

22. LaGrone MO, Bradford DS, Moe JH, Lonstein JE, Winter RB, Ogilvie JW: Treatment of symptomatic flatback after spinal fusion. *J Bone Joint Surg Am* 1988;70:569-579.

23. Floman Y, Penny N, Micheli LJ, Riseborough EJ, Hall JE: Osteotomy of the fusion mass in scoliosis. *J Bone Joint Surg Am* 1982;64:1307-1316.

24. Voos K, Boachie-Adjei O, Rawlins B: Multiple vertebral osteotomies n the treatment of rigid adult spine deformities. *Spine* 2001;26:526-533.

Role and Technique of Eggshell Osteotomies and Vertebral Column Resections in the Treatment of Fixed Sagittal Imbalance

Oheneba Boachie-Adjei, MD

Abstract

Fixed sagittal imbalance of the spine leads to a disabling posture with compensatory hip and knee flexion. The most common causes of fixed sagittal imbalance include degenerative lumbar disease, complications from the use of distraction instrumentation in the lower lumbar spine, ankylosing spondylitis, and posttraumatic kyphosis. Surgical procedures to correct sagittal deformities include the posterior Smith-Petersen osteotomy, pedicle subtraction osteotomy, and posterior vertebral column resection. For complex multiplanar deformities, combined anterior and posterior vertebral column resection may be needed to provide vertebral column shortening and balanced correction in the coronal and sagittal planes. Current reports of these procedures stress the importance of patient selection, radiographic evaluation, and meticulous surgical technique. Complications include excessive blood loss, incomplete correction, wound infection, and pseudarthrosis. Most patients who are treated with these procedures report a high level of satisfaction with the outcome.

The patient with a fixed, decompensated spinal deformity is easy to recognize and is challenging to treat. The potential risks and benefits of surgery must be carefully considered along with the patient's expectations before undertaking this significant reconstruction procedure. For deformities that exist predominantly in the sagittal plane, posterior procedures such as decancellation, also known as the eggshell posterior pedicle subtraction osteotomy, and posterior vertebral column resection with posterior segmental instrumentation can achieve balanced correction in the sagittal plane and improve function[1-4] (Boachie-Adjei and associates, Quebec City, Canada, unpublished data, 2003). Severe rigid multiplane deformities are best treated by circumferential osteotomy with vertebral column shortening.[3,5] Patients with fixed sagittal deformities are often disabled and may have deformity secondary to conditions such as ankylosing spondylitis or from complications of previous spinal surgery. The most common cause of iatrogenic flatback is distraction instrumentation used in the lower lumbar spine during spinal deformity surgery, which causes a loss of lumbar lordosis.[6,7] Other, less common causes of sagittal deformities are posttraumatic, neuromuscular, congenital, or degenerative disorders.

Because patients with fixed sagittal imbalance are unable to stand with hips and knees extended, compensation for this limitation is attempted by using a crouched knee and hip flexion posture. They often report decreased ability to ambulate, severe back pain, and fatigue. The gait in patients with fixed sagittal imbalance shows significant abnormalities in all gait parameters, implying that the patients exert an increased effort during locomotion that results in easy fatigability and joint degeneration.[8]

Historical Background

In 1973, Doherty[6] first reported postfusion decompensation in patients with thoracolumbar scoliosis who were treated with Harrington rod instrumentation (Figure 1). Bilateral innominate osteotomy was used to improve upright posture.

The transpedicular approach for biopsy and drainage of a vertebral

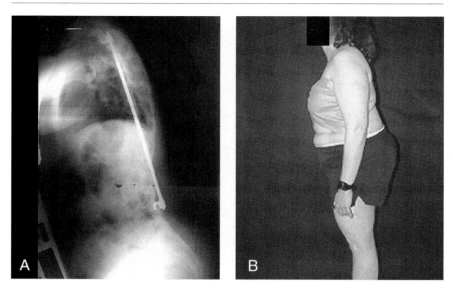

Figure 1 **A,** Standing lateral radiograph of a 44-year-old woman treated with Harrington instrumentation 20 years previously. **B,** The patient has a typical flatback deformity with sagittal imbalance and loss of lumbar lordosis.

body was initially described by Michelle and Krueger[9] in 1949. Hening and Chewning[3] popularized the term "eggshell decancellation," which has now been modified to include a posterior shortening osteotomy such as pedicle subtraction. In 1985, Thomasen[10] reported the results of corrective osteotomy by removal of a posterior wedge vertebra, the spinous process, neuroarch of the second lumbar vertebra, and removal of the cancellous portion of the posterior part of the vertebral body of L2. This technique provided overall vertebral column shortening posteriorly with a fulcrum at the anterior aspect of the vertebral body and produced an average correction of 30° to 50° at a single level in patients with ankylosing spondylitis who had not undergone previous procedures.

Indications and Preoperative Planning

A pedicle subtraction osteotomy, or posterior vertebral column resection, is performed to enable the patient to assume a more erect posture (thereby restoring horizontal gaze), relieving compression on the abdominal contents, and improving diaphragmatic breathing and appearance. Before undertaking this procedure, detailed radiographic evaluation is mandatory. Evaluation of the spinal canal can be obtained using MRI or myelography with a CT scan used with sagittal reconstruction. The desired amount of correction should be estimated on full-length, standing, lateral spinal radiographs. For patients with loss of lumbar lordosis or with lumbar kyphosis, the osteotomy level is best placed at the mid lumbar spine (L2 or L3) to allow adequate proximal and distal fixation points. Pelvic fixation may be needed to provide the strong distal foundation necessary to support the long lever arm created by previous long fusions. Approximately 30° to 50° of correction can be achieved per osteotomy; a 6- to 13.5-cm correction of the sagittal vertical axis is also anticipated. The osteotomy can be performed in rotated scoliotic segments, preferably at the apex, which can be corrected if a trapezoidal shape is

given to the osteotomy. Ideally, the osteotomy is performed in an area of previous fusion. If the osteotomy is performed through a motion segment, neither the bone stock nor stability after the procedure will be ideal and the outcome of the fusion may be compromised.

Surgical Technique
Pedicle Subtraction Osteotomy

To perform the pedicle subtraction osteotomy, the patient is prone and provision is made for extension at the osteotomy site (Figure 2). The author recommends that three levels of rigid transpedicular fixation both above and below the level of the osteotomy be placed before any destabilization of the spine is begun. The entire neural arch of the selected level and a portion of the cephalad and caudal neural arches are also resected. To avoid central canal stenosis with closure of the osteotomy, it is safer to perform an extended central laminectomy. The dura and the nerve roots above and below the pedicle that is to be resected are freed. Transverse processes and the muscle attachments to the transverse processes are detached from the vertebra.

Two approaches to resection are possible. One approach involves decancellation of the vertebral body directly or through the pedicles, excising the entire pedicle, and performing the decancellation at the bases of the pedicle. Alternatively, the second approach preserves the medial pedicle wall for provisional protection of the neural elements. Copious bleeding should be anticipated; this bleeding can be controlled either with bipolar electrocautery or with the application of absorbable gelatin and thrombin. During the decancellation it is important to prevent inadvertent col-

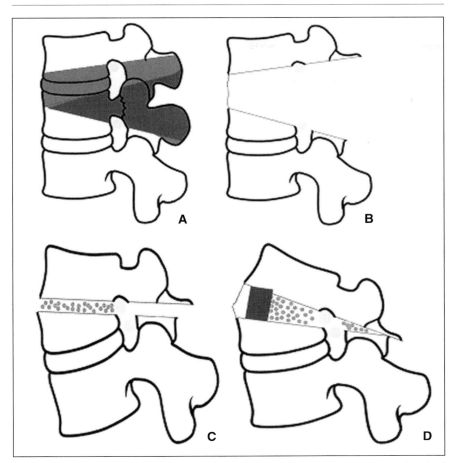

Figure 2   Schematic representation of a pedicle subtraction osteotomy. **A,** Surgical planning of the wedge resection. Note that bone and disk are resected. **B,** Resected area of the posterior arch and vertebral body. **C,** Correction following bony apposition of bone graft. **D,** Global correction with added anterior strut graft.

ing the decancellation is placed on the posterior lateral elements and the rods are secured in the corrected position.

In some instances, the osteotomy may not hinge on the anterior column and can open through the disk spaces above and below, or the bone interposition in the anterior column may be insufficient. In such cases, a cage filled with autograft can be positioned anteriorly, and a posterior lumbar interbody fusion can be added to the procedure or the anterior column can be reconstructed later through an anterior approach. Anterior surgery or posterior lumbar interbody fusion at adjacent segments may be used if there is compromised bone stock, concomitant pseudarthrosis, or extension to the sacrum. For long fusions and for extension to the sacrum, fusion of the two lowest intervertebral disks and pelvic fixation should be considered. Intraoperative monitoring with somatosensory-evoked potentials, motor-evoked potentials, or wake-up tests should be performed to assess neurologic function.

Posterior Vertebral Column Resection

The author prefers posterior vertebral column resection to treat patients with thoracic or thoracolumbar hyperkyphosis (Figure 3). The patient is placed prone on a four-poster frame. No provision for spinal extension is made. The apical vertebra is identified and wide exposure is performed proximally, distally, and laterally along the surrounding ribs. Transverse processes and 2 to 3 cm of the proximal part of the periapical ribs are excised and the parietal pleura are pushed away from the anterior vertebral body. The segmental vessels are identified and ligated, thus freeing the aorta,

lapse by placing temporary fixation rods opposite the resection site. Next, the remaining medial pedicle cortex (if preserved) and the posterior vertebral cortex are resected. An adequate amount of posterior vertebral cortical bone is resected with Woodson elevators or reverse-angle curets.

At this stage of the procedure, the choice can be made to resect the proximal intervertebral disk and proceed with an eggshell osteotomy, which causes a type of compression fracture of the vertebral body, or to resect the lateral vertebral wall with a rongeur or an osteotome to create a wedge osteotomy. When perform-

ing the wedge osteotomy, the soft tissues should be dissected from the lateral wall either with a curet or with cautery. Care should be taken to avoid the segmental vessels, mainly those below the pedicle.

Correction is achieved as gradual extension of the operating table results in closing of the osteotomy site. This process brings the remaining superior and inferior posterior arches together. The neurologic elements are viewed directly during closure. The enlarged foramen that was created by the pedicle resection now contains two nerve roots. The foramen can be probed with a ball tip probe. Bone graft removed dur-

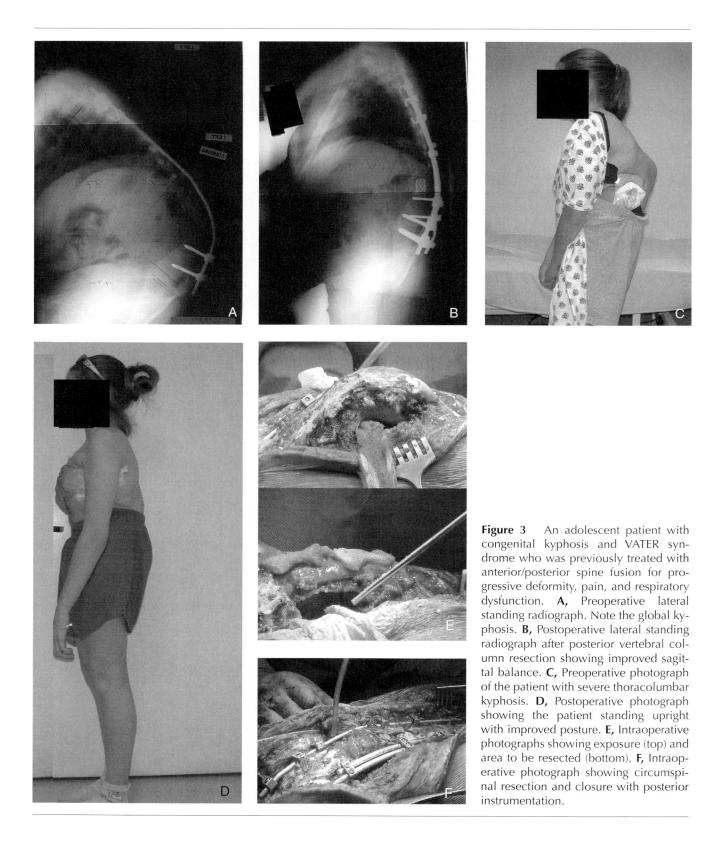

Figure 3 An adolescent patient with congenital kyphosis and VATER syndrome who was previously treated with anterior/posterior spine fusion for progressive deformity, pain, and respiratory dysfunction. **A,** Preoperative lateral standing radiograph. Note the global kyphosis. **B,** Postoperative lateral standing radiograph after posterior vertebral column resection showing improved sagittal balance. **C,** Preoperative photograph of the patient with severe thoracolumbar kyphosis. **D,** Postoperative photograph showing the patient standing upright with improved posture. **E,** Intraoperative photographs showing exposure (top) and area to be resected (bottom). **F,** Intraoperative photograph showing circumspinal resection and closure with posterior instrumentation.

which is carefully detached from the anterior vertebral body. The nerve roots in the lumbar spine must be spared; however, thoracic intercostal nerve roots are severed. To secure fixation points, pedicle screws are placed bilaterally to the osteotomy site, usually three vertebrae on each side.[11] The osteotomy consists of laminectomy and wedge-shape resection of the vertebral body. The laminectomy should be wide and include the neural arch of the apical vertebra, and one vertebra above and below. During the resection of the vertebrae, spinal stability is maintained with provisional rods connected to the fixation anchors on one side. Working on the other side, bone removal is feasible with the use of osteotomes, rongeurs, and curets. A high-speed power drill should be used for the bone that is in contact with the dura; the anterior longitudinal ligament should be preserved. At the completion of the osteotomy, the neural tube is circumferentially exposed in the surgical field. The correction of the deformity is possible either by in situ bending of the provisional rods or by sequential replacement of the provisional rods with rods precontoured to achieve the desired correction. Alternatively, the spine can be manipulated through two correction rods placed unilaterally, fixed cranially and caudally to the osteotomy site, and held with rod holders. To avoid distraction of the neural elements, a compression force is applied to shorten the spinal column and partially close the osteotomy site before any correction is attempted. If necessary, the laminectomy should be extended to avoid impingement of the spinal cord that buckles posteriorly. Autologous cancellous bone graft is used for the anterior fusion at the resected area. For a substantial ante-

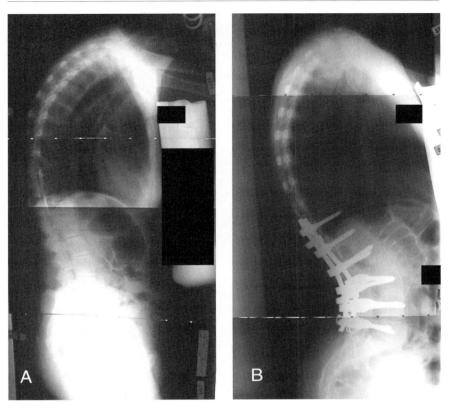

Figure 4 Radiographs of a 45-year-old woman with ankylosing spondylitis and global sagittal imbalance. The patient underwent a pedicle subtraction osteotomy at L3 with segmental transpedicular instrumentation. **A,** Preoperative radiograph showing loss of lumbar lordosis with thoracic hyperkyphosis. **B,** Postoperative radiograph showing reconstruction of lumbar lordosis and improved global sagittal balance.

rior intervertebral gap (more than 5 mm), a structural graft (preferably a titanium mesh cage filled with autograft) should be used. Compression should be performed over the cage to secure it in place. Posterior bone graft may be used at the resection area; however, the use of such a graft has been reported to cause complications such as wound hematoma. The reported anticipated mean correction in the sagittal plane ranged from 52.9% to 61.9% and from 45% to 52% in the coronal plane (Figure 4). The technical details outlined for pedicle subtraction osteotomy concerning lumbar root preservation, temporary rod application, adequate number of fixation

points proximally and distally, and the performance of the cantilever corrective force maneuver with the four-rod technique will also apply.

Postoperative Treatment
Fixed sagittal imbalance leads to a disabling crouched posture with compensatory hip and knee flexion. Treatment requires rebalancing the spine with one or more osteotomies. Depending on the stability of the construct, patients may be immobilized in a thoracolumbosacral orthosis for additional support or comfort (Figure 5).

There are few reports documenting results and complications of correction of fixed sagittal imbal-

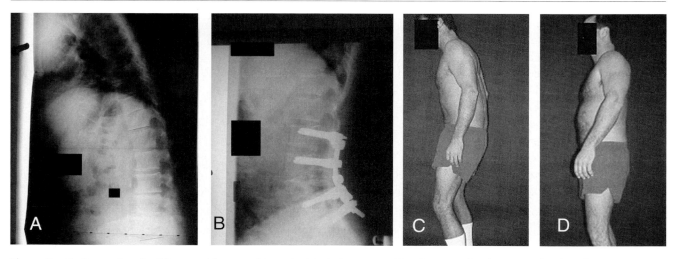

Figure 5 Radiographs of a 33-year-old-man with sagittal imbalance resulting from postlaminectomy lumbar decompensation and kyphosis. **A,** Preoperative lateral radiograph. Note lumbar kyphosis. **B,** Postoperative radiograph after treatment with a pedicle subtraction osteotomy. Note the improvement in lumbar lordosis. **C,** Photograph of the patient showing preoperative standing posture. **D,** Postoperative photograph showing improved standing posture.

ance[12-15] (Boachie-Adjei and associates, Quebec City, Canada, unpublished data, 2003). Because of the cancellous bone contact at the vertebral body level, pseudarthroses are uncommon. Pseudarthroses may occur at levels adjacent to fusion extensions, such as the thoracic spine in lumbar pedicle subtraction osteotomies.[2,14] Complications related to instrumentation, such as failure of fixation or prominent screws, can occur. Proximal degeneration with recurrence of the deformity can occur in patients who have had realignment for sagittal imbalance. If proximal degeneration is related to compression fractures, it potentially can be treated conservatively. Overall, the complication rate in patients with a complex deformity who have revision surgery is equivalent to the complication rate in patients who undergo primary anteroposterior surgery for adult spinal deformity.

Reported Outcomes

Various validated instruments have been used to assess patient outcome and identify predictive factors. Im-provements in pain, function, and self-image were highly rated in studies that included outcome assessments, although ratings were generally below population norms. Satisfaction reported with the surgery varied from 73% to 86%[2,14] (Boachie-Adjei and associates, Quebec City, Canada, unpublished data, 2003). The level of satisfaction was not related to postoperative complications, but was related to the development of pseudarthrosis. Although Booth and associates[14] found satisfaction relative to radiographic parameters such as sagittal correction and coronal balance, other investigators found the improvement of lumbar lordosis to be the sole predictive factor of the overall patient satisfaction outcome score[1,12,13] (Boachie-Adjei and associates, Quebec City, Canada, unpublished data, 2003). Few reports have dealt with the outcomes of using posterior vertebral column resection for treating sagittal imbalance. Acceptable results using vertebral column resection to treat rigid and severe scoliosis were found. Excessive blood loss and complications were found in 25% of patients (Suk and associates, Buenos Aires, Argentina, unpublished data, 2004).

Results of Pedicle Subtraction

At the author's institution, 20 of 25 patients who underwent a posterior pedicle subtraction/decancellation osteotomy with a modern bilateral pedicle screw-hook-rod construct were evaluated using standardized upright radiographs, chart review, and questionnaire. Seven of 20 patients had augmentation with anterior interbody grafting for associated pseudarthrosis, scoliosis, or coronal decompensation. Most osteotomies were performed at the L3 level (13 patients); others occurred at the L2 (4 patients), L4 (2 patients), and L5 (1 patient) levels. There were 5 male and 15 female patients in the study with an average age of 49 years (range, 33 to 74 years). The average length of follow-up was 4 years (range, 2 to 8.2 years). All patients had at least one prior surgical procedure. Diagnostic categories included 15 patients with postoperative iatrogenic flatback, 3 with posttraumatic deformities, 1 with congenital scoliosis, and 1 with severe lumbar spondylosis leading to sagittal decompensation. All patients reported back pain and deformity, and 10 of 20 patients had a preoperative neurologic deficit. Standardized lateral upright radiographs showed mean preoperative thoracic kyphosis of 27°, which improved to 41° ($P = 0.006$) after surgery. Preoperative measurements of lumbar lordosis averaged 10° (range, 55° to −65° [kyphosis]) and improved to an average of 51° (range, 20° to 99°). The average lumbar lordosis correction was 41° ($P < 0.0001$). Coronal balance did not significantly change. The sagittal vertical axis measured from C7-S1 showed a preoperative sagittal decompensation averaging 10.7 cm (range, 6 to 23 cm) with correction to 2 cm (average correction of 8.7 cm, $P < 0.0001$). Intraoperative complications included three dural tears and one nerve root injury. Early and late postoperative complications occurred frequently. Revision surgery was required for 10 patients to treat complications that included pseudarthroses with instability (3 patients), coronal decompensation treated with reinstrumentation (1 patient), epidural hematomas (2 patients), pain caused by hardware (2 patients), deep infection (1 patient), and residual stenosis (1 patient). One patient had a superficial wound infection successfully treated with antibiotics; another patient with pedicle screw pull-out was treated nonsurgically. Outcome satisfaction was determined with a simple questionnaire. Most patients were either satisfied or somewhat satisfied and would elect to undergo the same procedure.

Summary

Pedicle subtraction osteotomy and posterior vertebral column resection are effective procedures for correcting fixed sagittal imbalance and providing spinal stability. Most patients are satisfied with the outcome of the treatment, particularly when balance is achieved[2,12-14] (Suk and associates, Buenos Aires, Argentina, unpublished data, 2004). Because of the high complication rate, a careful assessment of the potential risks and benefits should be done before using these major reconstructive procedures.

There is a paucity of information in the literature regarding patients with hyperkyphosis. These limited studies are encouraging in terms of achieving correction of deformity without major neurologic complications. Long-term follow-up on a large number of patients will be needed to document the efficacy of such complex procedures used in such a select patient population.

References

1. Bradford DS, Tribus CB: Current concepts and management of patients with fixed decompensated spinal deformity. *Clin Orthop* 1994;306:64-72.

2. Bridwell KH, Lewis SJ, Lenke LG, Baldus C, Blanke K: Pedicle subtraction osteotomy for the treatment of fixed sagittal imbalance. *J Bone Joint Surg Am* 2003;85-A:454-463.

3. Hening CF, Chewning SJ Jr: Eggshell procedure, in Bradford DS (ed): *Master Techniques in Orthopaedic Surgery: The Spine*. Media, PA, Lippincott-Raven, 1996.

4. La Chapelle EH: Osteotomy of the lumbar spine for correction of kyphosis in a case of ankylosing spondylitis. *J Bone Joint Surg Br* 1945;28:851-858.

5. Boachie-Adjei O, Bradford DS: Vertebral column resection and arthrodesis for complex spinal deformities. *J Spinal Disord* 1991;4:193-202.

6. Doherty JH: News notes: Complications of fusion in lumbar scoliosis: Proceedings of The Scoliosis Society. *J Bone Joint Surg Am* 1973;55:438.

7. LaGrone MO, Bradford DS, Mo JH, Loenstein JE, Winter RB, Oglivie JW: Treatment of symptomatic flatback after spine fusion. *J Bone Joint Surg Am* 1988;70:569-580.

8. Sarwahi V, Boachie-Adjei O, Backus SI, Taira G: Characterization of gait function in patients with postsurgical sagittal (flatback) deformity. *Spine* 2002;27:2328-2337.

9. Michelle A, Krueger FA: A surgical operation of the vertebral body. *J Bone Joint Surg Am* 1949;31:873-878.

10. Thomasen E: Vertebral osteotomy for correction of kyphosis in ankylosing spondylitis. *Clin Orthop Relat Res* 1985;194:142-152.

11. Boachie-Adjei O, Girardi FP, Bansal M, Rawlins BA: Safety and efficacy of pedicle screw placement for adult spinal deformity with a pedicle-probing conventional anatomic technique. *J Spinal Disord* 2000;13:496-500.

12. Berven SH, Deviren V, Smith JA, Emami A, Hu SS, Bradford DS: Management of fixed sagittal plane deformity: Results of the transpedicular wedge resection osteotomy. *Spine* 2001;26:2036-2043.

13. Berven SH, Deviren V, Smith JA, Hu SS, Bradford DS: Management of fixed sagittal plane deformity: Outcome of combined anterior and posterior surgery. *Spine* 2003;28:1710-1715.

14. Booth KC, Bridwell KH, Lenke LG, Baldus CR, Blanke KM: Complications and predictive factors for the successful treatment of flatback deformity (fixed sagittal imbalance). *Spine* 1999;24:1712-1720.

15. Smith Petersen, Larson CB, Aufranc OE: Osteotomy of the spine for correction of flexion deformity in rheumatoid arthritis. *J Bone Joint Surg Am* 1945;27:1-11.

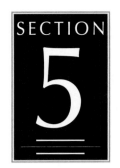

SECTION 5

Low Back Pain and Radiculopathy

Low Back Pain and Radiculopathy

Enhanced by the clinical acumen and experience of the authors, the four chapters in this section provide in-depth, comprehensive, fair, and objective reviews of the literature-based evidence on low back pain and radiculopathy. For the typical spine surgeon, the information in these four chapters provides a blueprint for managing most patients who present for spinal care. The presentations are interesting and range from all-inclusive "soup to nuts" discussions of epidemiology, natural history, patient assessment, and the treatment of single-entity disorders to detailed discussions of a single form of treatment that can be used for a variety of degenerative lumbar conditions.

Brodke and Ritter present an excellent discussion of the nonsurgical management of low back pain and lumbar disk degeneration. Despite developments in instrumentation, fusion techniques, and disk arthroplasty, nonsurgical management is the mainstay treatment modality for patients with nonspecific, nonradicular low back pain that is not associated with a neurologic deficit.

The authors review the classic literature from which most of the current understanding (and misunderstanding) originates concerning the incidence, prevalence, and natural history of low back pain. They describe a systematic method for assessing patients with low back pain that will be helpful to all orthopaedic surgeons who treat patients with spinal conditions. The authors support the belief that the choice of the most appropriate nonsurgical treatment should be based on information from the patient's clinical history, physical examination, and the judicious use of diagnostic imaging studies.

The chapter concludes with succinct discussions of a full array of nonsurgical treatment modalities, including bed rest, medication, therapy, manipulation, bracing, injections, and controversial minimally invasive procedures such as intradiskal electrothermal therapy. For each modality, Brodke and Ritter provide an unbiased and objective analysis of the evidence available at the time their chapter was written. Although the chapter was published in 2005, prior to the widely quoted European randomized controlled trials comparing nonsurgical treatment with fusion for treating low back pain, the authors' conclusions are remarkably consistent with the information learned from those later studies.

There are few topics in modern spine surgery that are as controversial and hotly debated as the role of spinal fusion for treating nonradicular, nonspecific, low back pain. Glaser and associates provide the readers with the information and components needed to understand the controversy and to formulate their own conclusions. The chapter begins with a brief history of the first methods and indications for lumbar arthrodeses. The evidence supporting the different types of lumbar fusions are then critically reviewed.

Beginning with their discussion of uninstrumented posterolateral fusion, the authors highlight the findings concerning this procedure from both classic and modern studies. Based on the quality of the reviewed literature, the authors are unable to make definitive, diagnosis-based conclusions concerning the value of the fusion procedure. For example, the body of literature regarding uninstrumented lumbar fusions was derived from randomized controlled trials of patients with degenerative spondylolisthesis, isthmic spondylolisthesis, and so-called discogenic low back pain. This same pattern of trying to compare studies involving patients with a range of spinal conditions is also problematic in discussions of outcomes after instrumented fusions.

The bulk of the literature regarding fusion for degenerative disorders deals with the evaluation or comparison of different interbody fusion techniques. Glaser and associates provide an excellent discussion of the rationale, application, advantages, disadvantages, and complications of these techniques. The chapter's summary offers an excellent decision-making algorithm for selecting the ideal method of lumbar fusion for a patient with a lumbar degenerative disorder.

Because disk herniations are common in the lumbar spine, the chapter by Rhee and associates should be considered requisite reading for all surgeons who treat patients with this condition. This is one of the most comprehensive, well-planned, and superbly executed discussions of lumbar disk herniations that I have read.

Rhee and associates begin by relating pertinent anatomic and structural details of the intervertebral disk with its propensity for the development of herniations. They provide the reader with an exact understanding of why and how a herniated disk produces symptoms and/or neural dysfunction. They exquisitely integrate biomechanical, biochemical, and imaging data in a way that is logical and easy to understand.

Many articles have been published about the treatment of lumbar disk herniations, but few articles offer an understanding of the natural history of this condition. Rhee and associates detail the findings of classic, often quoted (and sometimes misquoted) studies and provide the backdrop for counseling patients and discussing the most recent data regarding treatment outcomes. Appropriately and astutely, the authors make the important distinction between the natural history of the condition and nonsurgical treatment. Various nonsurgical modalities are discussed in detail and supporting evidence is presented for each treatment option.

A truthful interpretation of the current body of literature regarding the surgical treatment of lumbar disk herniation also is presented. For example, they emphasize the data regarding the equivalence of recovery of stable neurologic deficits (excluding cauda equina syndrome) with surgical treatment compared with nonsurgical treatment. This information is crucial for the surgeon who reads this chapter and later must answer patients' queries on whether their weakness and numbness will improve. Unfortunately, lacking this knowledge, mild deficits are often used as leverage to convince patients that surgery is required.

There have been many studies published in recent years regarding predictors of surgical and nonsurgical outcomes in patients with radiculopathy from lumbar disk herniations. Rhee and associates present an excellent review of these data in a systematic and usable manner. In mentioning the Spine Patient Outcome Research Trial (SPORT) study, the findings of which had not yet been presented at the time this chapter was published, Rhee and associates forecasted that it would help "provide clearer guidelines" for treating lumber disk herniations. In my opinion, Rhee and associates provide a very clear and thoughtful discussion of treatments for this common condition. In stating that "nonsurgical treatment is the initial 'default' pathway for most patients with lumbar radiculopathy due to disk herniation," the authors reinforce the idea that surgery is only one treatment option, usually initiated after failure of conservative management, and not commonly viewed as a competitive modality with nonsurgical care.

The fourth chapter in this section, written by Hu and associates, is another excellent discussion focused on a specific degenerative disorder; in this case, spondylolisthesis. As with lumbar disk herniations, any orthopaedic surgeon caring for spine patients will encounter many individuals with this condition. The chapter primarily discusses isthmic spondylolisthesis—slips that occur because of a stress fracture in the pars interarticularis. A brief discussion of degenerative spondylolisthesis also is included.

Isthmic defects can be both a diagnostic and treatment challenge. Hu and associates present a current analysis of the role of advanced imaging, nonsurgical management, and nonfusion surgical techniques, such as pars repair.

The authors touch on nearly every treatment decision-making dilemma associated with the care of low- and high-grade slips. Is decompression always warranted? Is instrumentation indicated if fusion is to be performed? What is the role of interbody fusion when the decision to fuse has been made? Perhaps the most controversial questions concern the indications for reduction and its necessity and clinical benefit.

Among the four chapters in this section, this chapter is unique in that it provides a description of key and critical surgical steps. As the authors are leaders in the field of spine surgery, these pearls were penned by learned hands and minds. Although evidence-based medicine and the critical appraisal of available data will guide general decisions, the insight of these authors is of considerable benefit to the orthopaedic surgeon who treats patients with disorders of the spine.

Christopher M. Bono, MD
Chief, Orthopedic Spine Service
Brigham and Women's Hospital
Assistant Professor
Department of Orthopedic Surgery
Harvard Medical School
Boston, Massachusetts

Dr. Bono or an immediate family member serves as a board member, owner, officer, or committee member for the North American Spine Society, the Spine Arthroplasty Society, and the American Academy of Orthopaedic Surgeons; is a member of a speakers' bureau or has made paid presentations on behalf of Stryker Spine and DePuy Spine; is a paid consultant for or is an employee of DePuy Spine, Life Spine, and Stryker; has received research or institutional support from DePuy Spine and Synthes Spine; and has received nonincome support (such as equipment or services), commercially derived honoraria, or other non–research-related funding (such as paid travel) from Stryker.

15

Nonsurgical Management of Low Back Pain and Lumbar Disk Degeneration

Darrel S. Brodke, MD
Stephen M. Ritter, MD

Abstract

Lumbar disk degeneration is a ubiquitous and complex phenomenon. The etiology varies widely and may be difficult to identify. Many techniques have been proposed to manage the pain and disability resulting from disk degeneration. Medicines, bed rest, orthotics, physical therapy, chiropractics, selective injections, and intradiskal electrothermal therapy have been used. Some of these therapies have been more successful than others, but most have at least some role in the current techniques of helping patients deal with this syndrome. How best to use these tools in conjunction with patient education is critical to success.

The approach to the management of low back pain has undergone substantial change in recent decades. Low back pain can often present as a difficult problem to solve. It is a loosely defined diagnosis that may refer to multiple patterns of pain with complex issues surrounding its pathoanatomic diagnosis and treatment. There is a paucity of evidence from the health professional literature regarding its cause, management, and prognosis. The difficulty of managing patients with low back pain stems from the fact that there often is very little association between any pathologic physical findings and the patient's pain and disability. The professional must then find ways of clinically treating a syndrome that betrays the principles of basic science.

In recent years, the advancement in diagnostic modalities and therapies has led to the belief that there are precise and treatable organic causes of low back pain. The quickly evolving fields of radiology, electrodiagnostics, and injection techniques have yielded advances in diagnostic reliability and more directed treatment plans. Many who routinely treat axial low back pain favor the idea that identification of a particular pain generator should be aggressively pursued and identified. Only after a thorough attempt has been made to provide a focused pathoanatomic diagnosis should the diagnosis of a nonspecific low back disorder be accepted by the patient or physician.

With the understanding that there are still many difficulties in the management of low back syndromes, some of the available nonsurgical modes of low back pain treatment are reviewed, which can be applied regardless of whether a particular pain mediator has been identified.

Epidemiology and Natural History

Currently, low back pain is epidemic in the United States. Its annual incidence has been projected to be 5% per year, with an associated prevalence of 60% to 90%.[1] The 1-month prevalence of low back pain is estimated to be 43% of the population.[2] Only visits for the common cold have outnumbered presentations of low back pain to primary care physicians.[3] The medical costs and vocational disabilities that occur with low back pain are substantial. The length of time that a patient is absent from work because of low back pain correlates with a decreasing chance of return to work. A patient who has missed work for more than 6 months has a 50% chance of returning to work, one who has missed more than 1 year has a 25% chance of returning, and a patient who has missed 2 years or more has less than a 5% chance of returning.[4] Low back pain is the leading cause of disability in the largest working population, which is persons younger than 45 years.

In addition to causing substantial morbidity, low back pain is expensive. It has been estimated that between $33 and $55 billion is spent yearly in direct medical costs for the treatment of low back pain.[5,6] The indirect costs to society, such as lost work days and productivity, are even higher. Indirect costs for musculoskeletal diseases as a group have been estimated to be $90 billion,[7] and low back pain is the major contributor to this cost. This problem is not isolated to the United States. Seitz and associates[8] estimated that in Germany in 2001 low back pain led to €5 billion (euro) in direct medical costs and €13 billion (euro) in indirect costs. Both direct and indirect costs continue to rise.

Most studies have suggested that low back pain is usually a self-limited disease, with dramatic improvement in 1 week or longer. Improvement can be seen in up to 80% of people in the first 2 weeks.[9] Furthermore, many studies have shown that observation is as good as active treatment of low back pain. Thus, it behooves the physician to manage this syndrome effectively to limit its negative impact.

Low back pain has many different causes. Frymoyer[10] suggested that nearly 85% of low back conditions cannot be diagnosed on the basis of the history, findings of the physical examination, or diagnostic testing. In fact, the rapid resolution of most back pain often prevents a diagnosis from ever being made. Confounding the problems with diagnosis is the difficulty in understanding the motive of the patient seeking help. Psychologic and emotional factors, particularly depression, can play a role.[11] There may be unknown social pressures, and it may not be possible or effective to manipulate work accommodations.

Smoking deserves mention. There is an increased incidence of both low back pain and disk herniations in smokers.[1,2,13] An and associates[14] found a threefold higher risk of lumbar disk herniations and a 3.9-fold higher risk of cervical disk herniations in smokers. Nicotine appears to interfere with bone metabolism through induced calcitonin resistance and decreased osteoblastic function.[15,16] Disk nutrition is impaired by a decreased exchange capacity, with progressive disk degeneration.[17] An autoimmune response may also be involved in progressive disk degeneration in smokers.[14] Furthermore, oxygen levels are reduced in smokers, leading to hyalinization and necrosis of the nucleus pulposus.[18] Outcomes of treatment, surgical or nonsurgical, are less successful in patients who smoke than they are in those who do not smoke. There is a higher incidence of persistent back pain after treatment and of progressive osteoporosis with associated complications, and surgical healing rates are lower.[19-23] Therefore, cessation of smoking is an important aspect of the treatment of patients with low back pain.

Clinical Presentation

In the past, there has been variability in the understanding of the clinical presentation of lumbar disk disease. Low back pain with radiation to one or both buttocks and posterior aspects of the thighs in combination with exacerbation while coughing or sneezing is suggestive of lumbar disk disease. A positive straight leg raising test or a decreased Achilles tendon reflex is a characteristic finding associated with disk herniation. Radicular sensory deficits, unilateral pain, and tension signs with or without reflex alterations all suggest nerve root impingement. Paraspinous muscle tenderness probably indicates a myofascial component to the pain. Pain with standing that improves with short walks, and pain with back flexion and with no substantial muscle tenderness suggest a discogenic etiology. Focal night pain without associated tenderness may be consistent with a tumor. Nonspinal causes of low back pain may include systemic diseases, intraperitoneal lesions, and particularly retroperitoneal lesions. Low back pain also could be a physical manifestation of a psychologic malady.

Psychosocial and occupational risk factors often cloud the diagnosis and make it difficult to establish an organic cause of low back pain. Smoking, as stated earlier, as well as obesity may contribute to the incidence of low back pain.[24] Repetitive bending and twisting can increase the risk of low back pain and disk herniation.[25] Additionally, job dissatisfaction or involvement in a workers' compensation lawsuit portends a poorer prognosis for recovery.[26]

Nonmusculoskeletal causes of low back pain should be considered during the workup phase. The most common causes are renal and vascular pathology, such as a kidney stone or an abdominal aortic aneurysm. Tenderness and pain with percussion over the dorsal twelfth rib region lateral to the midline suggest kidney involvement. Laboratory studies, including urinalysis and a blood metabolic panel, should be performed. A patient with cardiovascular disease who has back pain that is unresponsive to early treatment and no back tenderness should have an abdominal examination to palpate for an aneurysm. An aneurysm may also be detected on MRI or CT scans of the lumbar spine made to look for spinal pathology. Finally, tumors may manifest as back pain. Pain at night and without response to activity or rest, unexplained weight loss, and fatigue should be red flags during the workup for low back pain.

Imaging

A diagnosis can be confirmed with radiographic imaging. AP and lateral plain radiographs of the lumbar spine are conventionally the first radiographic images made, and they are useful for the evaluation of osseous anatomy and alignment (Figure 1). Benefits of myelography include the dynamic assessment of nerve compression with the ability to obtain standing flexion and extension views. With the refinement of MRI, however, myelography is performed less frequently, but it has a useful application when it is followed by a CT scan. The CT scan adds the clarity of osseous anatomy and the ability to reformat in sagittal and coronal planes. CT is helpful for the assessment of fractures and spondylolysis or in preoperative planning, and it is an important alternative for assessing a patient with instrumentation in place.

MRI has had a dramatic impact on the diagnosis and treatment of spinal disease (Figure 2). It is the most accurate and sensitive modality for the diagnosis of subtle spinal pathology, making it the test of choice.[27]

Bone scanning with single-photon emission CT allows physiologic assessment of bone by identifying increased osteoblastic activity. It is a highly sensitive study with a low specificity, making it a good screening test for degenerative changes or metastatic disease. It may be useful for localizing a pain generator when multiple radiographic abnormalities are identified.

Diskography is an invasive, provocative, painful procedure done under fluoroscopic guidance. Contrast medium is injected to pressurize the disk and mimic the pressure of prolonged sitting or standing.[28] When an abnormal appearance (with fissuring and leakage of the contrast medium) is seen on fluoroscopy and CT scanning, the patient's pain response is the most important determinant of the result. Diskography, although possibly the best study for identifying the pain generator in some patients, remains a subjective study and should be thought of as a part of the entire diagnostic workup. It should not be given excessive importance.

Treatment Options

The best strategy for nonsurgical management of low back pain combines active intervention with education and rehabilitation. The patient should be an active participant in the healing process. There are many treatment options for patients with low back pain; however, although there is a plethora of reports in the literature regarding these treatment options, there is very little conclusive evidence for any of them. The treatment options are often used in combination.

Bed Rest

Bed rest is a common treatment of low back pain. As is the case for many of the other treatment options discussed below,

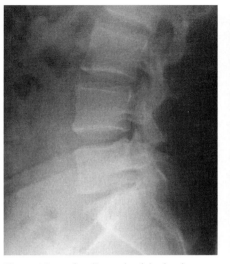

Figure 1 Lateral radiograph of the lumbar spine. Note the disk space narrowing at the L5-S1 level. No other abnormalities are seen.

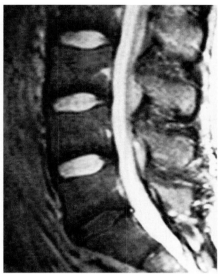

Figure 2 T2-weighted MRI scan of the lumbar spine. The L5-S1 disk is desiccated (loss of water signal) with a high-intensity zone lesion in the posterior portion of the anulus fibrosus consistent with an annular tear.

there are conflicting reports in the literature regarding the benefits. Although some authors have shown that bed rest can provide a benefit with regard to alleviating overall pain, others have shown a quicker return to work with little or no bed rest.[29-31] The general consensus seems to be that bed rest should be short term (2 days) if used at all.

Medications

Although no analgesic should be promoted as a cure for pain or a replacement for nonpharmacologic interventions, medications are frequently used in the nonsurgical care of low back pain. The different pharmacologies of various medicines can be applied more effectively when a particular pain generator has been diagnosed.

Nonsteroidal anti-inflammatory drugs are commonly used to treat inflammation, but they also have a role as analgesics.[32] They are recognized for their ability to limit inflammation by interfering with prostaglandin synthesis and cyclooxygenase (COX) activity. Dyspepsia is common, and complications such as gastric erosion, ulceration, and hemorrhage can develop. COX-1 regulates con-

stitutive cellular processes, whereas COX-2 activity is induced by mediators of inflammation. Newer, selective COX-2 inhibitors provide anti-inflammatory benefits while limiting the disruption of cellular homeostasis and thus decreasing some adverse effects on the gastrointestinal system. Other risks, such as renal toxicity, are associated with COX-1 and COX-2-regulating nonsteroidal anti-inflammatory drugs. Prescribing nonsteroidal anti-inflammatory drugs on an as-needed basis is more likely to take advantage of their analgesic effects than to provide the anti-inflammatory benefit that comes with scheduled administration.[33]

Acetaminophen and opioids are commonly used analgesics, but they are associated with substantial risks. Although hepatotoxicity is a risk with overdosing, acetaminophen is generally very well tolerated. Although opioid use is on the rise and can be effective for symptom control, these drugs do not work over the long term, and they can lead to other problems. They often are associated with adverse effects including drowsiness, dizziness, fatigue, nausea, respiratory depression, and constipation. Tolerance to some adverse effects occurs within days after the initiation of therapy. Other effects, such as constipation, may persist longer. Tolerance to the analgesic effect of opioids begins to occur when the drugs have been continuously used for longer than several weeks. However, tolerance to respiratory and sedative effects occurs much more quickly. Opioids produce analgesia by binding to receptors that are normally bound by endogenous compounds in the central nervous system. Short-acting narcotics can cause sleep deprivation despite their use to help people with pain to sleep. They are also more likely to encourage overuse. Long-acting opioids have less addictive potential and are, therefore, better tolerated.[34] Combining acetaminophen with oxycodone yields analgesia superior to that produced by either drug alone.[35] All narcotics are best avoided if possible.

Steroids should play a minimal role in the treatment of low back pain. They are associated with substantial gastrointestinal risks. Long-term use is known to lead to osteopenia and an increased risk of infection. Concerns about osteonecrosis of the proximal part of the femur and humerus should prompt judicious use.

Muscle relaxants play a role in acute back pain and appear to be more effective than a placebo alone. Paraspinous muscle spasm is commonly associated with acute back injuries of various etiologies and can respond well to these medications. Muscle relaxants work for only a limited period and should be considered for the acute treatment of back pain rather than for long-term treatment.

Antidepressants also have a role in the management of low back pain, especially when there is a comorbid mood disorder. Their concomitant effects as analgesics and antidepressants are particularly useful for individuals in whom back pain would otherwise be increased by depression. Likewise, when anxiety predomi-

nates, the threshold for pain perception is lowered.[36] Although antidepressants may be effective when used alone, they may be extremely effective compared with a placebo when they are part of combination therapy.

Antiseizure medications are useful in the treatment of neurologic pain, particularly in the lower extremities. Their effectiveness in the treatment of low back pain is in question.

Recommendations with regard to the use of medications for the treatment of low back pain are fairly individualized. The authors' preference is to treat acute low back pain with a nonsteroidal anti-inflammatory drug, starting with an inexpensive generic medication or one with which the patient has had prior success. If the patient has a history of gastritis or ulcer disease, a COX-2-selective nonsteroidal anti-inflammatory drug is chosen. Muscle relaxants are occasionally prescribed for a short duration as well. For subacute or more chronic low back pain, an antidepressant is often added with other treatment modalities as outlined below. Muscle relaxants and opioids should be avoided in patients with chronic pain.

Physical Therapy

Physical therapy can be used as a broad term to refer to stretching and strength training, back school for the education of patients, and other modalities to address low back pain. It has been shown to be better than medical care alone over a 6-month period, especially when the program is medically supervised.[37,38] It is also better than chiropractic manipulation for the treatment of chronic pain.[39] Specific types of back flexion and extension stretching have been thought to have beneficial effects for patients with low back pain.[40] Flexion-based isometric exercises appear to have the most support in the literature, although extension-based exercises, progressive-resistance exercises, and dynamic stabilization

training are useful adjuncts.[30,41] They may offer benefit by decreasing local muscle spasm and stabilizing the spine. Stand-alone strengthening programs have also shown benefit.[42] Currently, however, it is unclear whether one form of exercise therapy is more effective than another, but all seem to provide benefits.[43] A comparison of McKenzie extension exercises with an intensive strengthening program showed no difference in the reduction of disability or pain at the time of follow-up.[44] In a systematic review of the available literature on the effectiveness of massage in the management of low back pain, massage was shown to decrease symptoms and improve function in patients with nonspecific low back pain, especially when the massage was coupled with exercise and education.[45] The ultimate goal should be to involve patients in their back pain management.

Exercise can be supplemented with other modalities, such as transcutaneous electrical nerve stimulation, which is electrotherapy applied to the low back. Hypotheses to explain how this treatment works have ranged from the suggestion that there is a release of endogenous analgesic endorphins to the implication of a central nervous system process in which a control center is altered to block transmission of pain.[46] The best study to date showed that the effects of transcutaneous electrical nerve stimulation are no different than those of a placebo.[47]

Traction is another modality used during therapy. The goal of lumbar traction is to distract the lumbar vertebrae. There are many potential effects, such as enlargement of the intervertebral foramen, creation of a vacuum to reduce herniated disks, placement of the posterior longitudinal ligament under tension to aid in reduction of herniated disks, relaxation of muscle spasm, and freeing of adherent nerve roots.[48] Intradiskal pressure can be decreased by 20% to 30%.[49] Prospective studies have shown, however, that traction is not a means with which to definitively manage low back pain and that it does change its natural history.[30]

Chiropractic Manipulation

Chiropractic manipulation is the most common alternative therapy for managing low back pain. It has been estimated that nearly 15% of the US population seeks chiropractic help each year.[50] The majority of visits are for the treatment of neck and low back pain. How chiropractic manipulation provides relief is not fully understood, but it has been shown to have a role in the treatment of acute low back pain. Chiropractic manipulation and physical therapy have equivalent success in the management of acute low back pain, and both are better than medical care alone.[37] Skargren and associates[51] compared cost and effectiveness of chiropractic and physical therapy and found chiropractic treatment to be more effective for acute low back pain (less than 1 week in duration) and physical therapy to be more effective for pain of longer duration. More patients in the chiropractic group had recurrent symptoms and repeat treatments of low back pain. There is no evidence to support the use of long-term manipulation for the treatment of chronic back pain.

Lumbosacral Orthotic Devices

The purpose of a lumbosacral orthosis is to stabilize or immobilize. Conditions such as vertebral body fracture and spondylolysis with spondylolisthesis as well as the need for postoperative support are all possible indications for prescribing an orthosis. There is no evidence in the literature to support long-term use of orthotic devices for the treatment of low back pain. Reasons for not prescribing orthoses may include concerns about a lack of compliance on the part of the patient, creating psychologic dependence, and validating the disability. Although weakening of postural back and abdominal muscles has also been a con-

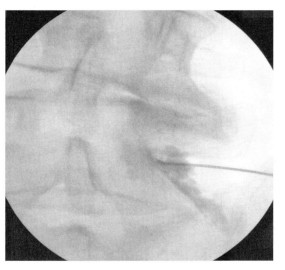

Figure 3 PA fluoroscopic radiograph of a selective L5 nerve-root block. Note the contrast medium tracking along the path of the nerve root.

cern, it has been shown not to occur to any substantial extent.[52] The ability of orthoses to limit motion is in doubt, with conflicting reports in the literature. Axelsson and associates[53] found no limitation of sagittal translation in patients who wore a thoracolumbosacral orthosis. Corset-type orthoses have been shown to decrease intersegmental motion at all levels by 30%.[54] Although they are commonly prescribed, orthoses do not appear to change the natural history of low back pain.

Selective Injections

Selective spinal injections produce focused and controlled anesthesia of particular anatomic structures to help define loci of pain. In addition to this diagnostic benefit, the addition of the potent anti-inflammatory effects of glucocorticoids to the local anesthetic offers a potential therapeutic benefit as well. The epidural space is probably the most common location for selective injections. With fluoroscopic guidance, an interlaminar, caudal, or transforaminal approach can be used[55] (Figure 3). Epidural steroid injections are most useful in the treatment of nerve root irritation. Their benefit in the treatment of low back pain is in doubt, although they are possibly useful for the

treatment of low back pain secondary to sacroiliac joint dysfunction. An injection into the sacroiliac joint may provide both diagnostic information and some therapeutic benefit.[56] The joint is a difficult pain generator to implicate because it has diffuse regional innervation. Schwarzer and associates[56] reviewed the results of intra-articular injections in patients who, when their history had been elicited, had localized their pain specifically to the sacroiliac joint region. Only 30% of the patients had substantial relief, indicating that the sacroiliac joint was probably not the source of the pain in the majority of the patients. Positive findings on physical examination, with pain in the medial aspect of the buttock reproduced with the Patrick test, are suggestive. Treatment should focus on physical therapy.

Facet or zygapophyseal joints can be generators of low back pain with referred buttock and lower limb pain. Use of a controlled injection technique has shown that facet joints can produce low back pain.[57] The patient's history, physical examination, and imaging studies have each been shown to be unreliable when used alone for the diagnosis of symptomatic facet joints. CT scans of the lumbar spines of asymptomatic individuals older than 40 years frequently show

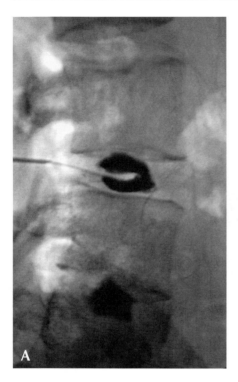

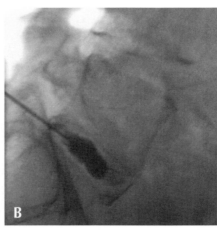

Figure 4 A, Lateral fluoroscopic radiograph of a two-level diskogram. The L3-4 level is normal, whereas the L4-5 level shows degeneration of the disk and some leakage of contrast medium posteriorly. **B,** Lateral fluoroscopic radiograph of an L5-S1 diskogram (made with the levels in A). The L5-S1 level shows severe degeneration with substantial leakage of contrast medium.

degenerative changes of the facet joints, so such studies alone are not diagnostic.[58] Extension-based back pain, as opposed to worse pain with flexion, along with radiographic evidence of arthropathy suggest the presence of facet-mediated pain. A bone scan may be used to help to confirm the presence of facet arthritis. Correlating radiographic evidence of contrast medium-laden local anesthetic injected into a facet joint with pain relief may be considered diagnostic evidence of a pathologic facet joint.

An alternative to injecting the facet joint directly is addressing the medial branch nerve, which carries afferent pain fibers from the facet joint. The nerve branches from the dorsal ramus of the exiting nerve root, and it innervates the immediately caudal two facets. For example, the L3 medial branch nerve innervates the L3-4 and L4-5 facet joints. Relief of back pain with selective blockade of this nerve can help to diagnose painful facet joints, but it is rarely long lasting. When a medial branch block is effective but temporary, more permanent

relief may be afforded by radiofrequency dorsal rhizotomy. This technique denervates the facet joint by the localized insertion of a probe that destroys the afferent fibers with a radiofrequency current.[59] The results of dorsal rhizotomy have been variable. Modest success has been shown with single-level rhizotomy. Multilevel rhizotomy may have better outcomes.[60] Studies have yet to consistently show clinical efficacy, however.

Intradiskal Electrothermal Therapy
Intradiskal electrothermal therapy has become popular in recent years for the treatment of low back pain thought to be of discogenic origin. Internal disk derangement is used specifically for internal disk derangement, but not classic degenerative disk disease. Radiographic changes are not characteristic of internal disk derangement, and radiculopathy is not typically associated with it. It is diagnosed with diskography and MRI, the latter of which often shows a high-intensity zone or internal tear in the posterior portion of the anulus fibrosus (Figure 2).

Pain is caused by chemical and mechanical mediation of nociceptors. The procedure involves the posterolateral placement of a probe around the inner circumference of the anulus fibrosus followed by heating of the probe. The exact mechanism by which intradiskal electrothermal therapy provides relief is unknown. Alteration in collagen has been hypothesized, as has neuronal deafferentation of the anulus fibrosus.[61,62] However, studies of cadavers have suggested that there is no change in the stability of the spine after intradiskal electrothermal therapy.[63]

The indications for intradiskal electrothermal therapy are somewhat similar to those for spine arthrodesis, although intradiskal electrothermal therapy is performed for patients who, because of their age or other reasons, are not ideal surgical candidates. The developers of the treatment suggested that the indications should include persistent low back pain for more than 6 months after failure of a program of back education, activity modification, nonsteroidal anti-inflammatory medications, physical therapy, and progressive intensive exercises.[64] Frequently, an epidural steroid injection has been tried and has failed. The findings on physical examination should include normal results of a neurologic examination with a negative straight leg raising sign. The absence of compressive lesions on MRI and a positive concordant diskogram with negative findings at an asymptomatic control level are essential for proper patient selection (Figure 4). Reports on the results of intradiskal electrothermal therapy have been criticized because of the lack of a concrete understanding of the mechanism of action of the therapy, the lack of peer review, and the lack of long-term follow-up. Recent double-blinded randomized sham-controlled trials have shown conflicting outcomes.[6,65] With further refinement of indications, outcomes may improve.

Back Pain Treatment Algorithm

Early Interventions

1. Medicines: NSAIDs
                  Acetaminophen
                  Muscle relaxants
                  Narcotics (short duration)

2. Short-term bed rest (2 days maximum)

3. Physical therapy

4. Chiropractics

Later Alternatives

1. Medicines: Antidepressants

2. Orthotic devices

3. Physical therapy–Back school

4. Therapeutic injections: Epidural
                              Nerve root
                              Medial branch

5. Dorsal root neurotomy

6. Intradiskal electrothermal therapy

Figure 5 A stepwise algorithm for management of lumbar disk degeneration. NSAIDs = nonsteroidal anti-inflammatory drugs.

Summary

The treatment of low back pain is a challenge faced by most practitioners in the medical community. Acute back pain is generally a self-limited process that is likely to get better in the short term no matter what treatment is undertaken. Supportive care is key to early pain relief, with therapeutic stretching and strengthening exercises used to promote patient involvement in the process and to allow resumption of normal activities. Chronic low back pain is far more difficult to treat or even to define in terms of etiology. Multiple diagnostic modalities and treatment options exist because of the very nature of this problem. A specific treatment program must be customized to the patient's specific findings, and all patients must be active participants in their return to health and activity (Figure 5). For the initial treatment of acute low back pain, a nonsteroidal anti-inflammatory drug and a muscle relaxant combined with no more than 2 days of bed rest are recommended. Use of the nonsteroidal anti-inflammatory drug should be continued, and physical therapy should be started within 1 week if possible. The therapy should include stretching, strengthening, and trunk stabilization exercises. Modalities to relieve symptoms should be used only initially, if at all, to enable the patient to start the exercises. Patient education is an integral part of this active treatment program. The patient should be given the tools with which to continue long-term self-treatment, with injury avoidance and a home therapeutic exercise program. Empowering the patient with the responsibility for self-care is the most effective means of treating low back pain.

References

1. Frymoyer JW, Pope MH, Clements JH, Wilder DG, MacPherson B, Ashikaga T: Risk factors in low-back pain: An epidemiological survey. *J Bone Joint Surg Am* 1983;65:213-218.

2. Papageorgiou AC, Croft PR, Ferry S, Jayson MI, Silman AJ: Estimating the prevalence of low back pain in the general population: Evidence from the South Manchester Back Pain Survey. *Spine* 1995;20:1889-1894.

3. Cypress BK: Characteristics of physician visits for back symptoms: A national perspective. *Am J Public Health* 1983;73:389-395.

4. Bergquist-Ullman M, Larsson U: Acute low back pain in industry: A controlled prospective study with special reference to therapy and confounding factors. *Acta Orthop Scand* 1977;170:1-117.

5. Waddell G: Low back pain: A twentieth century health care enigma. *Spine* 1996;21:2820-2825.

6. Pauza KJ, Howell S, Dreyfuss P, Peloza JH, Dawson K, Bogduk N: A randomized, placebo-controlled trial of intradiscal electrothermal therapy for the treatment of discogenic low back pain. *Spine J* 2004;4:27-35.

7. Yelin E: Cost of musculoskeletal diseases: Impact of work disability and functional decline. *J Rheumatol Suppl* 2003;68:8-11.

8. Seitz R, Schweikert B, Jacobi E, Tschirdewahn B, Leidl R: Economic rehabilitation management among patients with chronic low back pain. *Schmerz* 2001;15:448-452.

9. Quinet RJ, Hadler NM: Diagnosis and treatment of backache. *Semin Arthritis Rheum* 1979;8:261-287.

10. Frymoyer JW: Back pain and sciatica. *N Engl J Med* 1988;318:291-300.

11. Pincus T, Burton AK, Vogel S, Field AP: A systematic review of psychological factors as predictors of chronicity/disability in prospective cohorts of low back pain. *Spine* 2002;27: E109-E120.

12. Deyo RA, Bass JE: Lifestyle and low-back pain: The influence of smoking and obesity. *Spine* 1989;14:501-506.

13. Svensson HO, Vedin A, Wilhelmsson C, Andersson GB: Low-back pain in relation to other diseases and cardiovascular risk factors. *Spine* 1983;8:277-285.

14. An HS, Silveri CP, Simpson JM, et al: Comparison of smoking habits between patients with surgically confirmed herniated lumbar and cervical disc disease and controls. *J Spinal Disord* 1994;7:369-373.

15. de Vernejoul MC, Bielakoff J, Herve M, et al: Evidence for defective osteoblastic function: A role for alcohol and tobacco consumption in osteoporosis in middle-aged men. *Clin Orthop* 1983;179:107-115.

16. Hollo I, Gergely I, Boross M: Smoking results in calcitonin resistance. *JAMA* 1977;237:2470.

17. Holm S, Nachemson A: Nutrition of the intervertebral disc: Acute effects of cigarette smoking. An experimental animal study. *Ups J Med Sci* 1988;93:91-99.

18. Iwahashi M, Matsuzaki H, Tokuhashi Y, Wakabayashi K, Uematsu Y: Mechanism of intervertebral disc degeneration caused by nicotine in rabbits to explicate intervertebral disc disorders caused by smoking. *Spine* 2002;27:1396-1401.

19. Hanley EN Jr, Shapiro DE: The development of low-back pain after excision of a lumbar disc. *J Bone Joint Surg Am* 1989;71:719-721.

20. McDermott MT, Witte MC: Bone mineral content in smokers. *South Med J* 1988;81: 477-480.

21. Hopper JL, Seeman E: The bone density of female twins discordant for tobacco use. *N Engl J Med* 1994;330:387-392.

22. Theiss SM, Boden SD, Hair G, Titus L, Morone MA, Ugbo J: The effect of nicotine on gene expression during spine fusion. *Spine* 2000;25:2588-2594.

23. Glassman SD, Anagnost SC, Parker A, Burke D, Johnson JR, Dimar JR: The effect of cigarette smoking and smoking cessation on spinal fusion. *Spine* 2000;25:2608-2615.

24. Heliovaara M: Body height, obesity, and risk of herniated lumbar intervertebral disc. *Spine* 1987;12:469-472.

25. Mundt DJ, Kelsey JL, Golden AL, et al: An epidemiologic study of non-occupational lifting as a risk factor for herniated lumbar intervertebral disc: The Northeast Collaborative Group on Low Back Pain. *Spine* 1993;18:595-602.

26. Milhous RL, Haugh LD, Frymoyer JW, et al: Determinants of vocational disability in patients with low back pain. *Arch Phys Med Rehabil* 1989;70:589-593.

27. Sluming VA, Scutt ND: The role of imaging in the diagnosis of postural disorders related to low back pain. *Sports Med* 1994;18:281-291.

28. Sachs BL, Spivey MA, Vanharanta H, et al: Techniques for lumbar discography and computed tomography/discography in clinical practice. *Orthop Rev* 1990;19:775-778.

29. Wiesel SW, Cuckler JM, Deluca F, Jones F, Zeide MS, Rothman RH: Acute low back pain: An objective analysis of conservative therapy. *Spine* 1980;5:324-330.

30. Deyo RA: Conservative therapy for low back pain. Distinguishing useful from useless therapy. *JAMA* 1983;250:1057-1062.

31. Deyo RA, Diehl AK, Rosenthal M: How many days of bed rest for acute low back pain? A randomized clinical trial. *N Engl J Med* 1986;315:1064-1070.

32. Abramowicz M: Drugs for pain. *Med Lett* 1993;35:1-6.

33. Brooks PM, Day RO: Nonsteroidal antiinflammatory drugs: Differences and similarities. *N Engl J Med* 1991;324:1716-1725.

34. Holmquist GL. Pain management: Drug decisions for patients with chronic non-cancer pain syndromes. *Drug Benefit Trends*. 2001; May.

35. Cooper SA, Engel J, Ladove M, Rauch D, Prechaun H, Rosenheck A: An evaluation of oxycodone and acetaminophen in the treatment of postoperative dental pain. *Clin Pharm Ther* 1979;25:219.

36. Marcus DA: Treatment of nonmalignant chronic pain. *Am Fam Physician* 2000;61:1331-1338.

37. Hurwitz EL, Morgenstern H, Harber P, et al: A randomized trial of medical care with and without physical therapy and chiropractic care with and without physical modalities for patients with low back pain: 6-month follow-up outcomes from the UCLA low back pain study. *Spine* 2002;27:2193-2204.

38. Torstensen TA, Ljunggren AE, Meen HD, Odland E, Mowinckel P, Geijerstam S: Efficiency and costs of medical exercise therapy, conventional physiotherapy, and self-exercise in patients with chronic low back pain: A pragmatic, randomized, single-blinded, controlled trial with 1-year follow-up. *Spine* 1998;23:2616-2624.

39. Postacchini F, Facchini M, Palieri P: Efficacy of various forms of conservative treatment in low back pain: A comparative study. *Neuroorthopedics* 1988;6:28-35.

40. Jackson CP, Brown MD: Analysis of current approaches and a practical guide to prescription of exercise. *Clin Orthop* 1983;179:46-54.

41. Kendall PH, Jenkins JM: Exercises for backache: A double-blind controlled trial. *Physiotherapy* 1968;54:154-157.

42. Rissanen A, Kalimo H, Alaranta H. Effect of intensive training on the isokinetic strength and structure of lumbar muscles in patients with chronic low back pain. *Spine* 1995;20:333-340.

43. van Tulder M, Malmivaara A, Esmail R, Koes B: Exercise therapy for low back pain: A systematic review within the framework of the Cochrane Collaboration Back Review Group. *Spine* 2000;25:2784-2796.

44. Petersen T, Kryger P, Ekdahl C, Olsen S, Jacobsen S: The effect of McKenzie therapy as compared with that of intensive strengthening training for the treatment of patients with subacute or chronic low back pain: A randomized controlled trial. *Spine* 2002;27:1702-1709.

45. Furlan AD, Brosseau L, Imamura M, Irvin E: Massage for low-back pain: a systematic review within the framework of the Cochrane Collaboration Back Review Group. *Spine* 2002;27:1896-1910.

46. Sjolund BH, Eriksson MB: The influence of naloxone on analgesia produced by peripheral conditioning stimulation. *Brain Res* 1979;173:295-301.

47. Deyo RA, Walsh NE, Martin DC, Schoenfeld LS, Ramamurthy S: A controlled trial of transcutaneous electrical nerve stimulation (TENS) and exercise for chronic low back pain. *N Engl J Med* 1990;322:1627-1634.

48. White AA III, Panjabi MM: *Clinical Biomechanics of the Spine,* ed 2. Philadelphia, PA, Lippincott, 1990.

49. Scientific approach to the assessment and management of activity-related spinal disorders: A monograph for clinicians: Report of the Quebec Task Force on Spinal Disorders. *Spine* 1987;12(suppl 7):S1-S59.

50. Coulter ID, Hurwitz EL, Adams AH, Genovese BJ, Hays R, Shekelle PG: Patients using chiropractors in North America: Who are they, and why are they in chiropractic care? *Spine* 2002;27:291-298.

51. Skargren EI, Carlsson PG, Oberg BE: One-year follow-up comparison of the cost and effectiveness of chiropractic and physiotherapy as primary management for back pain: Subgroup analysis, recurrence, and additional health care utilization. *Spine* 1998;23:1875-1884.

52. Walsh NE, Schwartz RK: The influence of prophylactic orthoses on abdominal strength and low back injury in the workplace. *Am J Phys Med Rehabil* 1990;69:245-250.

53. Axelsson P, Johnsson R, Stromqvist B: Effect of lumbar orthosis on intervertebral mobility: A roentgen stereophotogrammetric analysis. *Spine* 1992;17:678-681.

54. Fidler MW, Plasmans CM: The effect of four types of support on the segmental mobility of the lumbosacral spine. *J Bone Joint Surg Am* 1983;65:943-947.

55. Weiner BK, Fraser RD: Foraminal injection for lateral lumbar disc herniation. *J Bone Joint Surg Br* 1997;79:804-807.

56. Schwarzer AC, Aprill CN, Bogduk N: The sacroiliac joint in chronic low back pain. *Spine* 1995;20:31-37.

57. Schwarzer AC, Aprill CN, Derby R, Fortin J, Kine G, Bogduk N: Clinical features of patients with pain stemming from the lumbar zygapophysial joints: Is the lumbar facet syndrome a clinical entity? *Spine* 1994;19:1132-1137.

58. Wiesel SW, Tsourmas N, Feffer HL, Citrin CM, Patronas N: A study of computer-assisted tomography: I. The incidence of positive CAT scans in an asymptomatic group of patients. *Spine* 1984;9:549-551.

59. Gallagher J, Petriccioni di Vadi P, Wedley J: Radiofrequency of facet joint denervation in the treatment of low back pain: A prospective, double blind study to assess its efficacy. *Pain Clin* 1994;7:193-198.

60. Strait TA, Hunter SE: Intraspinal extradural sensory rhizotomy in patients with failure of lumbar disc surgery. *J Neurosurg* 1981;54:193-196.

61. Saal JS, Saal JA: Management of chronic discogenic low back pain with a thermal intradiscal catheter: A preliminary report. *Spine* 2000;25:382-388.

62. Biyani A, Andersson GB, Chaudhary H, An HS: Intradiscal electrothermal therapy: A treatment option in patients with internal disc disruption. *Spine* 2003;28(15 suppl):S8-S14.

63. Lee J, Lutz GE, Campbell D, Rodeo SA, Wright T: Stability of the lumbar spine after intradiscal electrothermal therapy. *Arch Phys Med Rehabil* 2001;82:120-122.

64. Saal JA, Saal JS: Intradiscal electrothermal treatment for chronic discogenic low back pain: Prospective outcome study with a minimum 2-year follow-up. *Spine* 2002;27:966-974.

65. Freeman B, Chapple D, Fraser RD, Cain C, Hall DJ: *A Randomized Double Blind Efficacy Study: IDET Versus Placebo.* Prague, Czech Republic, European Spine Society, 2003.

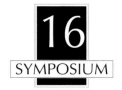

16
SYMPOSIUM

Lumbar Arthrodesis for Degenerative Conditions

John A. Glaser, MD
Mark Bernhardt, MD
Ernest M. Found, MD
Gregory S. McDowell, MD
F. Todd Wetzel, MD

Abstract

There is significant disagreement among spine surgeons regarding the optimal technique of arthrodesis for treatment of degenerative disorders of the lumbar spine.

Degenerative conditions of the lumbar spine include degenerative disk "disease," post-decompression degeneration, degenerative spondylolisthesis, junctional degeneration, spondylolyis, and low-grade lytic spondylolisthesis. Although it is impossible to develop strict evidence-based criteria for the selection of one surgical approach over another, some generalizations are possible based on empiric process, anecdotal experience, and published surgical series. Patient selection, cessation of nicotine use, and use of autologous bone graft are factors that influence clinical outcome after lumbar arthrodesis.

Arthrodesis was first described in 1911 and is one of the oldest and most commonly performed reconstructive spinal procedures.[1-3] Since that time, arthrodesis has become an accepted and recommended treatment of numerous conditions of the lumbar spine. The rationale for arthrodesis was well described more than 50 years ago by Hallock in an *Instructional Course Lecture*. "Lumbosacral spine fusion is a rational procedure, for it eliminates mobility and creates stability in a joint that is mechanically inadequate and strained. It is indicated when nonsurgical methods have failed or when the structural changes disclosed by the x-ray are so great as to preclude the possibility of otherwise achieving a satisfactory and lasting result."[4]

The techniques have changed considerably but the basic concept of immobilizing a painful motion segment remains. The indications, contraindications, techniques, and results for the commonly performed types of arthrodesis are discussed.

Uninstrumented Posterolateral Fusion

The first arthrodesis performed was a direct posterior fusion. Bone was harvested from the tibia and placed over denuded laminae and spinous processes; local bone graft from the spinous processes was used. The technique became more popular during the 1940s and 1950s, and the indications were expanded to include degenerative conditions. After this time, there was a gradual trend toward a posterolateral arthrodesis (Figure 1). Satisfactory results from posterolateral grafting for such indications as spondylolisthesis and failure of previous fusion were subsequently reported.[5-10] Both a midline and paraspinal approach were described. In a review of two groups of patients, operated on in separate decades, Prothero and associates[11] noted a gradual modification of technique to include more of the lateral elements. No increase in complications was noted using this approach, along with a higher success rate when using autograft and a lower rate of arthrodesis with increasing number of levels fused.

The posterolateral technique has several advantages over the posterior technique, including (1) less adjacent segment stress and more surgical segment stiffness;[12] (2) a more extensive vascular supply from decorticated transverse processes; [13,14](3) soft-tissue coverage of the bone graft is more reliable in the posterolateral region, and the soft

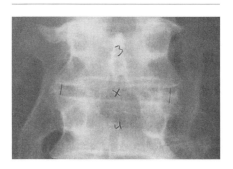

Figure 1 Coronal plane radiograph of uninstrumented posterolateral fusion at L3-4.

tissue has been shown to be a good source of nutrition to the fusion mass;[15] (4) physical separation of the bone graft from the dura and spinal nerves; and (5) the posterolateral technique can be performed if the posterior elements are absent or mechanically disconnected from the rest of the spine, such as occurs with isthmic spondylolisthesis.

For the past two decades, discussion has centered less on the type of posterior arthrodesis and more on the indications for instrumentation. Spinal instrumentation was actually described before arthrodesis and some forms of instrumentation have been available for many years.[5,16] Probably the most common form of spinal instrumentation in recent decades has been the insertion of screws through the pedicle with some form of posterior connector, such as a rod or plate.

Literature has been published that argues both for and against the use of supplemental instrumentation with lumbar arthrodesis.[17-19] In a prospective comparative study of 68 patients published in 1991, Lorenz and associates[20] found that fusion rate, return to work rate, and level of pain relief were higher in patients who had undergone supplemental instrumentation. Zdeblick[21] performed a prospective random-

ized study looking at three groups: those without instrumentation, those with semirigid, and those with rigid instrumentation, with generally better results found in those with rigid instrumentation, followed by semirigid, and then those without instrumentation. In a study of patients with degenerative spondylolisthesis, Bridwell and associates[22] reported a higher rate of satisfaction with instrumentation and a high rate of progressive deformity without. The largest study to date was a historical cohort analysis comparing instrumented and uninstrumented arthrodesis performed by Yuan and associates.[23] A surgeon survey was done, with radiographic analysis and case report forms completed by the surgeon. There were 3,498 cases assessed from 303 surgeons. Diagnoses included degenerative spondylolisthesis and trauma. The authors found a moderately higher rate of radiographic arthrodesis and slightly higher function in patients with instrumentation compared with those without.[23]

Fischgrund and associates[24] performed a prospective randomized trial in 47 patients with degenerative spondylolisthesis. They found a higher fusion rate in those with instrumentation when compared with uninstrumented but no significant differences in clinical outcome.

Other studies have concluded there is little benefit to supplemental instrumentation. In 1992, Bernhardt and associates[25] did a retrospective study on 47 patients treated for "clinical instability" with instrumented and uninstrumented arthrodesis and found no significant difference between the two groups. In a study of three military medical centers, 71 patients were prospectively evaluated. No statistically significant differences in radiographic rate of arthrodesis or

patient-based outcomes were observed.[26] Moller and Hedlund[27] studied patients with isthmic spondylolisthesis and found that surgery did improve their symptoms, but no differences in pain, rate of arthrodesis, or disability rating were noted when comparing those with instrumentation to those without. Fritzell and associates[28,29] studied patients with chronic low back pain and degenerative changes. They found that surgical treatment had more favorable results when compared with nonsurgical treatment, but no difference in pain reduction and disability were reported between different types of arthrodesis. They did find a higher radiographic rate of fusion as well as a higher complication rate in the patients with instrumentation. Christensen and associates[30] and Thomsen and associates[31] reported on a group of 130 patients with a diagnosis of spondylolisthesis or disk degeneration treated in a randomized manner. In the study by Thomsen and associates, the only difference found between groups was that patients with instrumentation reported a higher daily activity scale score. In the study by Christensen and associates, patients who were thought to have instability generally did better with instrumentation and those with spondylolisthesis generally did better without.[30,31]

Based on the literature and clinical experience, the general indications for uninstrumented posterolateral arthrodesis include (1) one- and occasionally two-level procedures; (2) nonsmoking patients; (3) degenerative spondylolisthesis with no evidence of instability; (4) degenerative disk disease with no indication for restoration of disk height; and (5) spondylolysis/ low-grade spondylolisthesis.

The deleterious effect of nicotine on spinal fusion has been shown in both the clinical and laboratory setting.[32-34] As was stated earlier, cessation of nicotine use is strongly recommended. Instrumentation and/or biologic methods to attempt to increase the success rate in smokers are indicated. Whether these measures are necessary in the reformed smoker is not completely known. In patients with degenerative spondylolisthesis, there is literature showing both low and high success rates for arthrodesis without instrumentation.[22,35] Instability, demonstrated by supraphysiologic motion on dynamic radiographs, is generally an indication for instrumentation. Isthmic spondylolysis and low-grade spondylolisthesis, in the absence of significant neurologic compromise, have been treated successfully with uninstrumented arthrodesis, particularly when decompression is not included.[10,36]

Although not well studied, obesity may be a relative indication for instrumentation. Regarding technique, the approach to the lumbar spine can be through a midline or paraspinal approach. The midline approach is more familiar to many surgeons but may cause more muscle injury.[37] The paraspinal approach can be performed through two paraspinal skin incisions or a single midline skin incision and paraspinal fascial incisions. Figures 2 and 3 show the plane of dissection for the paraspinal approach. Although not impossible, decompression is more difficult through a paraspinal approach. If separate paraspinal muscular dissections are performed, radiographic verification of the correct level for each side is indicated.

Thorough exposure of the posterolateral region from the pars to the end of the transverse process is required to maximize the area available for grafting. Whether to remove the capsule of the facet joint is a point of debate. Removal not only increases the segmental motion but also

increases available surface area for grafting.[38]

Adequate decortication allows for access to the vascular supply of the transverse process, and in an animal model, it has been shown that arthrodesis does not regularly occur without decortication.[14] This can be performed with power or hand instruments.

Although many different graft materials have been used and there is significant promise in many biologic enhancements, autologous iliac crest graft remains the gold standard graft material. Postoperative bracing remains controversial. Little benefit has been demonstrated in terms of fusion rate, but bracing may restrict motion and provide some pain relief.[39] Although it may take up to 1 year to obtain solid arthrodesis, the usual period of postoperative brace wear is 6 to 12 weeks.[40]

Instrumented Posterolateral Fusion

Degenerative conditions affecting the lumbar spine include disk herniation, degenerative spondylolisthesis, spinal stenosis, degenerative scoliosis, and degenerative disk disease. Most patients with these conditions are treated successfully with nonsurgical means; however, a significant percentage will undergo surgical treatment that involves decompression and/or lumbar fusion.

Spinal fusion is considered the standard treatment of progressive spinal deformity such as scoliosis and instability resulting from trauma. Its use to treat many degenerative conditions of the lumbar spine, however, remains controversial. Turner and associates[41,42] performed a meta-analysis of outcomes after lumbar fusion for degenerative conditions of the lumbar spine that included studies with more than 30 patients and 1 year or more of follow-up. Their meta-analysis showed a mean satisfactory outcome rate of 68% with a range from 16% to 95%. Relief of back pain was described as good or excellent in 61% and fair or poor in 35%. They concluded that the literature did not support the superiority of any specific fusion procedure over others when assessing clinical outcomes.

In a larger review of randomized controlled studies of spine surgery performed by the Cochrane group, no scientific evidence of the effectiveness of any form of surgical decom-

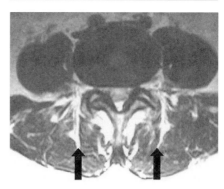

Figure 2 Axial MRI scan with arrows showing plane of dissection for paraspinal approach.

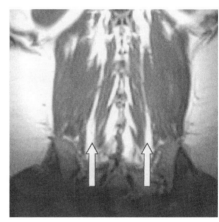

Figure 3 Coronal MRI scan with arrows showing plane of dissection for paraspinal approach.

pression or fusion for degenerative lumbar spondylosis was found.[43] As a result, the role of lumbar arthrodesis continues to be controversial.

A multicenter randomized control trial involving 19 centers in Sweden was designed to compare nonsurgical treatment to fusion for chronic low back pain. It was concluded that lumbar fusion improves both pain and disability and compares favorably with nonsurgical treatments.[28] However, there are several variations and uncertainties that must be considered when reviewing these studies. (1) The determination of the fusion integrity can be problematic and lacks the sensitivity and specificity that most studies require. Short of fusion exploration, there is no entirely reliable method for determination of fusion integrity. (2) There is a high degree of variability in the methods used to determine what the outcomes measures are. (3) It is well known that the deformity per se may not be at all related to pain. (4) Functional outcomes do not always correlate with patient satisfaction and pain relief. Because of these uncertainties, it can be quite difficult to decide which surgical procedure, if any, would be best suited for each individual patient. The meta-analysis data by Turner and associates[41,42] confirmed that lumbar fusion is associated with a definite complication rate and that, therefore, the risk-benefit ratio must be considered carefully before performing spinal arthrodesis as an adjunct after decompressive lumbar surgery or as a primary procedure for low back pain. The reasons for failure of lumbar fusion operations include improper diagnosis, poor patient selection, psychosocial factors, inadequate surgical technique, incorrect indications, and complications inherent to the surgical procedure. Of these, patient selection remains the single most important factor in minimizing the risk of failure of lumbar fusion. It is incumbent upon the surgeon to serve first as conscientious physician and second as a surgeon when making decisions.

The goals of instrumentation, when compared with uninstrumented fusion, are to augment the fusion, correct deformities, increase the rate and degree of fusion, enhance stabilization, hasten recovery, and lead to less postoperative immobilization and earlier return to activities. Various systems for posterior stabilization have been described using wire, hook, and pedicle screw-based constructs. Their efficacy has been described in the literature.[20,44,45] Pedicle screw instrumentation has become the most popular modality for internal fixation and was reported in a meta-analysis of the literature of 1970 through 1993 by Mardjetko and associates.[46] These authors reviewed 25 acceptable articles comprising a total of 889 patients with degenerative spondylolisthesis. The results indicated that posterolateral spinal fusion rates are enhanced by adjunctive spinal instrumentation ($P = 0.08$) with no significant differences detectable between control devices and pedicle screw devices. The complications related to pedicle screw instrumentation versus the control devices were very similar, with specific types of complications unique to each device.

Yuan and associates[23] retrospectively analyzed the outcomes for 2,684 patients with degenerative spondylolisthesis who had been managed with pedicle screw fixation compared with the results for patients who had not had pedicle screw instrumentation at the time of their index operation. There were two control groups consisting of 456 patients who had an arthrodesis without instrumentation and 51 who had instrumentation with nonpedicle screw devices. Intraoperative events related to the pedicle screw fixation occurred infrequently; the rate of breakage of the implant was 0.2%, and the rate of root, spinal cord, and vascular injuries was less than 0.5%. Dural tears were rare (0.1%) and the rates of tears that were not associated with placement of the screws were comparable between the groups that were managed with and without instrumentation. The rate of revision in patients who had pedicle screw instrumentation was higher than in those who did not (18% versus 15%). Most of these procedures were related to removal of the device, and the rates of repeat arthrodesis were similar among the groups. At 2-year follow-up, patients who had undergone pedicle screw instrumentation had a statistically significant higher rate of fusion than the uninstrumented group (83% compared with 75%). The patients who had pedicle screw instrumentation tended to have a more rapid rate of consolidation of the fusion and more often were able to maintain spinal alignment. Their clinical outcomes were better with regard to pain, function, and neurologic recovery as compared with the control group that was managed without instrumentation. Yuan and associates concluded that the benefits associated with pedicle screw use were substantially greater than the potential risks.[23] In a prospective randomized study of patients who had degenerative conditions of the lumbar spine, Zdeblick[21] evaluated the results of posterolateral arthrodesis with and without pedicle screw instrumentation. Superior results were noted with rigid internal fixation. The rate of fusion in patients managed with pedicle screw instrumentation was 86% compared with 64% for those in whom no instrumentation was used.

Complications associated with the many types of implants available for spine surgery are cause for concern. Survivorship analysis and complication rates of pedicle screw instrumentation are described in the literature.[47-50] West and associates[50] describe their experience with 124 consecutive cases of posterior spinal fusion with variable screw-plate fixation during the early phases of pedicle screw instrumentation. Complications, including those not related to pedicle screws, occurred in approximately 27% (33 patients). Dural tear occurred in seven patients. Neurologic deficits occurred in seven patients, but only two of seven were believed to be caused by misplaced pedicle screws. Reported rates of screw breakage can be summarized to occur in the range of 3% to 5.7%.[47-51] Many of these reports relate to early instrumentation systems, and as pedicle screw technology has developed, the rates of screw breakage have significantly decreased. Screw breakage is often associated with pseudarthrosis, and if discovered, nonunion should be suspected. McAfee and associates[52] described their early survivorship analysis of pedicle screw instrumentation used in 120 consecutive spinal reconstruction procedures. Of those patients, 21% required additional procedures (24 procedures were performed). Of 526 pedicle screws placed, only 22 (4.2%) were considered likely to cause a problem. They concluded that the probability of avoiding instrumentation difficulty within the first 20 months was 90%, and at 10 years, the probability was 80%.

Instrumentation can theoretically result in stress shielding. Myers and associates[53] used absorptiometry to compare vertebral body density in patients undergoing posterolateral fusion with and without instrumentation. Patients who had undergone instrumented fusion had decreased vertebral body bone mineral density compared with that of matched controls. Kanayama and associates[54-56] extensively studied the effect of spinal-impaired rigidity on vertebral bone density in a canine model. They discovered a linear correlation between decreasing volumetric density of bone and increased rigidity of the spinal implant. The likelihood of obtaining fusion at 6 months after surgery was increased if rigid instrumentation was used, and the authors concluded that vertebral osteoporosis secondary to instrumentation is not deleterious.[54-56]

Anterior Interbody Fusion

Anterior lumbar interbody fusions have been performed for more than 70 years. A wide range of techniques have been explored, including structural autogenous bone graft, impacted femoral ring allograft, impacted machined femoral ring allograft, and more recently, various threaded titanium interbody devices, both cylindrical and lordotic as well as threaded allograft bone dowels. The earliest reports of anterior lumbar interbody fusions to treat spondylolisthesis appear in 1932 and 1933.[57] Sporadic reports that appeared in the literature in the 1930s and 1940s further explored the use of autogenous bone in treating lumbar pathology, with many reports appearing in the late 1940s, 1950s, and 1960s pertaining to the treatment of degenerative disk disease.[58-60]

In 1972, Stauffer and Coventry[61] reviewed the Mayo Clinic experience. In this retrospective study, the authors reviewed the results of 83 surgeries performed by 7 surgeons. Fifty of these surgeries were for pseudarthrosis, 17 for failed previous laminectomy, 8 for spondylolysis, and 3 for degenerative disk disease. In this difficult group of patients, 64% had a fair or poor outcome. The technique involved cavitation of the end plate and creation of a trough. Overall, fusion success rates were 56% to 68% for one-level, 53% for two-level, and 36% for three-level fusions.[61,62] The use of autogenous iliac crest bone has in some series shown promising results. Linson and Williams[63] in 1991 and Newman and Grinstead[64] in 1992 reported on their use of hybrid grafting techniques incorporating allograft and autograft struts in the same intersperse. The fusion success rates were 76% and 89%, respectively. Moon and associates[65] in 1994 reported their experience using a Bailey-Badgley fusion technique with one strut of structural iliac crest bone graft and chips of cancellous graft around it. In their series of 26 patients, 10 of whom had isthmic lesions, a 94% fusion success rate was seen in the degenerative conditions and a 60% fusion rate was seen in spondylolisthesis or lytic conditions. Christensen and associates[30] in 1996 reported on the use of impacted structural autograft. A single strut of bone was used, with a fusion success rate of 76%. Crock[66] reported the results of a two-bone dowel technique used over a 20-year period, harvested with a Hudson drill, and placed transversely in the affected degenerative disk space. No specific mention of functional or surgical outcome was made.

The use of femoral ring allografts supplemented with autogenous bone or allograft bone has also been reported. Holte and associates[67] in 1994 described the use of femoral ring allograft plus autogenous iliac crest bone graft packed centrally. In 40 patients, half of whom had had previous surgery, a 98% fusion rate was observed when a femoral ring was used in association with posterior fixation. In the eight patients who did not have posterior fixation, union was achieved in only six. Sarwat and associates[68] later reported in 2001 on the use of femoral ring allograft with cancellous allograft chips packed centrally in a group of 43 patients, 41 of whom also had posterior fixation. This report also argued in favor of supplemental posterior fixation. Buttermann and associates[69] in 1996 wrote favorably of femoral ring allograft as an anterior spacer with biologic ingrowth potential. They did, however, express a preference for the use of posterior fixation as well.

Contemporary devices have been modeled after the Bagby basket.[70,71] Threaded titanium cylindrical and lordotically tapered titanium devices are now available. By 1999, McAfee and associates[72] estimated that US surgeons were implanting 5,000 such devices per month. Two-year results suggest a 91% fusion rate in a group of 947 patients operated on by 42 surgeons in 19 centers; 591 of these patients were treated with anterior approaches. The first device was implanted in 1992. Food and Drug Administration (FDA) approval for this device was offered in 1996. Twenty-six percent of the patients in the multicenter trial were smokers, and 36% had a previous laminectomy. Fifty-seven percent of the patients were seen through the worker's compensation system. Based on the high reported fusion rate, high return to work rate, a one third reduction in functional outcome scores, and a fall in the Prolo pain score from 5 to 2.9 at 24 months, the technique appeared

promising.[71] In 2002, McAfee and associates[73] subsequently reported that a complete en bloc diskectomy before cage insertion led to a higher fusion rate than did a partial reaming of the disk space. In 100 patients randomized to two groups, a 100% fusion rate was seen in the complete diskectomy group contrasted to eight pseudarthroses in the 50 patients treated with partial channel reaming and minimal disk space preparation. Fourteen percent of the patients in the latter group required revision surgery, and no revisions were required in the complete diskectomy group.

Ray's economic comparison of interbody cages with anterior/posterior fusions also suggested that there were time savings and cost savings associated with the stand-alone devices.[74] Mixed results have been seen in patients treated with laparoscopic threaded interbody fusion devices, however, presumably as a result of difficulties in preparing the end plate, higher rates of retrograde ejaculation, longer surgical times, and greater costs associated with treatment.[75]

Little has been published thus far on the clinical efficacy of lordotic tapered cylindrical fusion devices. Klemme and associates[76] reported favorable results with the use of a tapered cage supplemented with 1.5 mg of bone morphogenetic protein (BMP) impregnated in a collagen sponge. Clinical enthusiasm for the use of bone morphogenetic protein remains high after a variety of well-designed human and experimental studies suggesting a high fusion rate with the BMP impregnated collagen sponge. At present, FDA approval only exists for the use of the BMP collagen sponge with one particular design of cage.

Impacted machined femoral ring allograft spacers have also been commercially marketed but general-

ly are not intended for stand-alone use. In Janssen and associates'[77] study of 179 patients, most were treated with central autograft, although some had allograft placed. Thirty-three of these patients were treated with stand-alone impacted femoral ring allografts, and five of these developed a pseudarthrosis. There is a risk of graft fracture during insertion. Threaded allograft bone dowels have been used for interbody fusion in the last decade. Long-term clinical results are somewhat lacking at this time.

Contemporary fusion technology is associated with a higher cost of implants. In October 2002, the *Orthopaedic Network News* reported that the hospital costs for threaded bone dowels and threaded fusion cylinders ranged between $4,590 and $5,440.[78] Commercially available femoral rings and machined femoral ring allografts are less costly. The cost associated with the use of autogenous iliac crest bone is determined primarily by the surgical time and treatment of complications associated with harvesting. Fiscal year 2003 hospital Diagnosis Related Group reimbursement for spinal fusions without complications and comorbidities is $11,523. With complications and comorbidities, the reimbursement rises to $15,809. At present market cost, there is little residual revenue once implant costs are covered to manage patient hospitalizations.

There are many potential and actual advantages of anterior interbody fusions. Surgical time and blood loss are reduced in most series. The device or devices are placed in the load-bearing column anteriorly where they are able to load share or load bear. The interbody construct theoretically allows for annular tensioning, foraminal distraction, and some degree of reconstitution of sagittal balance. Based on the reports published to date, there are no reports of mechanical failure of titanium cylindrical devices. Unlike some posterior fusion constructs, adjacent segments are not violated. There is no posterior pain associated with the dissection, denervation, or devitalization of the paraspinous musculature. Anterior interbody fusion constructs have a proven track record for anterior cervical arthrodesis, thoracolumbar burst fractures, and anterior deformity surgery. For these reasons, it makes sense that this type of reconstruction technique would have merit in the lumbar spine for degenerative applications as well.

Interbody fusions performed with autogenous or allograft bone alone are at risk for graft collapse, graft extrusion, or graft subsidence. Stability may be difficult to achieve through the anterior column alone, particularly in the presence of a posterior destabilizing lesion such as a laminectomy or pars insufficiency. Regarding titanium devices, undersizing the devices can lead to instability. Asymmetric positioning of the devices can lead to root irritation, and use of the devices in osteoporotic bone can lead to subsidence. The cage creates image artifact, and radiographic assessment of fusion integrity is difficult. Inadequate diskectomy and a limited preparation of the disk space increase the risk of nonunion. Anterior stand-alone techniques do address foraminal stenosis but not central and posterolateral stenotic lesions. For those with perineural scar, distraction of the perineural scar about a root can lead to an aggravation or precipitation of nerve root pain. Togawa and associates[79] have reported on their experience with retrieving cages that look to be biologically ingrown but were

painful. Their work suggests that some cages that appear to be mechanically stable are not biologically ingrown. This emphasizes the need for critical evaluation of any fusion rate determined solely by radiographic criteria.

The work of Janssen and associates[77] indicates that femoral ring and machined femoral ring allograft ultimate strength exceeds vertebral body strength by a factor of two or three, but that iliac crest bone graft is weaker than vertebral body strength and may not stand up to in vivo loads. Dennis and associates[80] in 1989 suggested that structural autogenous bone impacted into a disk space anteriorly leads only to a temporary improvement in disk height. In 31 patients studied, 100% had lost height at follow-up, with 46% having disk spaces that were actually more narrow than their preoperative height. In 2001, Vamvanij and associates[81] suggested that, with threaded interbody instrumentation, improvements of 40% could be seen in foraminal volume. Chen and associates[82] had suggested earlier that foraminal cross-sectional area improvements of more than 20% can be expected with such a device and that disk height posteriorly might be increased 37% to 45%.

McAfee[83] has shown that most threaded cages and impacted devices have very similar stiffness but that intracage pressures are lower in threaded devices than they are in the impacted devices. As such, some greater degrees of stress shielding may be seen in the threaded devices. Oxland and Lund[84] established that supplemental posterior spinal fixation substantially increased the stability of an anterior cage construct. Chow and associates[85] suggested that segments above a fusion tested in vitro show intradiskal pressure and hypermobil-

ity, signifying stress transfer. Studies by Penta and associates[86] suggested that 10 years after a stand-alone anterior lumbar interbody fusion, one third of patients had developed disk abnormalities, by MRI assessment, adjacent to the fusion. In contrast, studies by Van Horn and Bohnen[87] suggested that rates of degeneration adjacent to interbody fusions were similar to age-matched controls without fusions at 16 years in 46 patients. In a study of 40 patients followed for 30 years, 85% had a satisfactory outcome. Most of the patients, however, who had had fusions to L4 showed radiographic adjacent segment degenerative problems at L3-4 by 15 years, regardless of age.[88,89]

Arguably, the best indication for stand-alone anterior interbody fusion is degenerative disk disease associated with loss of height and moderately severe or severe foraminal stenosis, especially at L5-S1. Such patients usually will report long-standing severe axial pain and leg pain localizing to a single root. Another indication for anterior interbody fusion is the treatment of degenerative disk disease alone without foraminal stenosis in the setting of intractable or severe low back pain recalcitrant to conservative measures. The technique may be useful in treating severe low back pain following previous decompression or diskectomy in which stability has been maintained. Good outcomes have been observed anecdotally in the treatment of spondylolysis and grade 1 spondylolisthesis in adults. In patients who have had multiple failed previous surgeries or pseudarthrosis, better surgical options exist than with a stand-alone fusion anteriorly. Although international reports suggest that good outcomes can be seen in degenerative spondylolisthesis and in treating disk herniation, these indications are not common in the United States.[65,90-93]

Patients with significant central and posterolateral stenosis, and those with facet enlargement or some degree of significant underlying congenital stenosis are not well suited for this technique. There is also little indication for higher-grade spondylolisthesis and spondylolysis in children. Patients with vascular anomalies or calcifications present greater technical challenges. The technique is contraindicated in males with fertility concerns because of the risk of retrograde ejaculation. Elderly patients with osteoporotic spines are at risk for subsidence. Arthrodesis involving more than two levels is also a relative contraindication.

Complications associated with anterior interbody fusions include pseudarthrosis, ileus, vascular injury, retrograde ejaculation, or sexual dysfunction. Neurogenic leg pain, wound infection, or hematoma, as well as deep venous thrombosis and problems with cage migration or malposition can occur. McAfee and associates[72] reported on their experience in revising 20 cages in 1999. A variety of technical and clinical factors contributed to the need for revision. One of the more common complications is adynamic ileus; the risk of developing this condition may be significantly reduced by limited open exposures, particularly when retroperitoneal. Christensen and Bunger[94] reported an incidence of retrograde ejaculation of approximately 8% in 50 men. Kleeman and associates[95] reported a 16% incidence in males treated laparoscopically and a 63% incidence in two-level laparoscopic fusions. Tiusanen and associates[96] also reported a high rate of retrograde ejaculation in patients

undergoing two-level anterior interbody fusion procedures to L4 in their cohort of 40 patients. Seven of nine patients developed retrograde ejaculation. Published reports of females experiencing sexual dysfunction following anterior interbody fusion procedures are lacking.

The measure of success of fusion requires a multifaceted look at the patient's response. Reduction in pain scores, improvement in functional scores, the need for revision, patient satisfaction, cost analysis, return to work issues and radiographic evaluation are all potential measures. The sentinel sign is the presence of bridging bone in the disk space anterior to the devices. Although never fully validated, this sign is believed to reliably reflect successful arthrodesis. Also important may be the presence of bridging posterior lateral or between the devices. A thin cut CT scan with sagittal and coronal reconstruction may be useful as well. The presence of subsidence does not denote pseudarthrosis. Some devices may subside to a point of stability. In one author's experience, a high patient satisfaction can be seen with interbody fusion (3% of 71 patients studied from 1998 to 2001 were dissatisfied at a mean 2-year follow up; GS McDowell, MD, unpublished data, 2003). The average estimated blood loss was 175 mL, and surgical time averaged approximately 2 hours. Length of stay averaged 4 days. Patients reported an average graft site analog pain score at final follow-up of 2.0 (range, 0 to 10). Preoperative analog pain scores averaged 6.6 and were reduced to a final analog pain score of 2.5. Ten revisions were performed. Indications included unrecognized posterolateral stenosis, subsidence leading to recurrent foraminal stenosis, pseudarthrosis, and root aggravation. Six patients experienced altered sexual function. Three

females reported decreased frequency of orgasm, one male reported retrograde ejaculation, and two reported fewer erections and less ejaculate. Eighty-three percent of patients eligible to return to work did so with an average time off work of 5.5 months. Fifty percent improvement in the Oswestry score was noted. A higher rate of clinical failures was seen in patients with two previous disk surgeries or pseudarthrosis. Higher failure rates were also noted in patients who smoked and those with workers' compensation histories, disability, or chronic pain.

Posterior and Transforaminal Interbody Fusion

Fusion of the lumbar spine from the posterior surgical approach has a long record of success and is the most common approach used by surgeons. Historically, anterior lumbar fusion has been used to treat anterior spinal column infections, but anterior lumbar fusions have also been used for treating other conditions such as fractures, tumors, scoliotic deformities, kyphotic deformities, and painful degenerative disks. Fusion of the anterior column of the lumbar spine from a posterior approach provides mechanical support of the anterior column and avoids an anterior surgical approach. Techniques of interbody fusion performed from a posterior approach include the posterior lumbar interbody fusion (PLIF) and the transforaminal lumbar interbody fusion (TLIF). PLIFs and TLIFs are useful techniques to treat several degenerative conditions, including discogenic low back pain, spondylolisthesis, and recurrent disk herniation.

Cloward[97,98] advocated PLIF more than 40 years ago. PLIFs originally were performed with bone graft alone, without structural implant. In the United States, the traditional PLIF never became a popular fusion technique. Nonstructural grafts with the traditional PLIF technique typically collapsed into kyphosis because of the tremendous compressive forces on the anterior portion of the functional spinal unit. However, with recent outcomes studies showing the efficacy of fusion as a treatment of severe, isolated degenerative disk disease and with the introduction of threaded interbody fusion cages in the mid 1990s, stand-alone PLIF, as well as stand-alone anterior lumbar interbody fusion with cages, have been done in increasing numbers.[28,71,99] Interbody fusion cages are capable of withstanding the large compressive forces on the anterior aspect of the functional spinal unit.

Traditional PLIF and contemporary PLIF with stand-alone cages are fusions of the anterior column only. In performing a contemporary PLIF, specialized tools and implants are used to distract and hold the anterior column of the spine in a lengthened position with a porous structural spacer capable of carrying bone graft materials or substitutes. In performing the approach for a PLIF, the midline bony-ligamentous tether (that is, the contiguous laminae, spinous processes, and supraspinous and intraspinous ligaments) is sacrificed. A wide, destabilizing laminectomy and essentially bilateral facetectomies are required to make room for the implantation of screw-in cages. The extensive posterior column resection required of the PLIF procedure provides for a direct decompression of the dural sac and the exiting and traversing nerve roots bilaterally. Thus, a PLIF may be used for patients with large recurrent herniated disks or spinal stenosis at a single level when a fusion is

also indicated. Although specialized instruments are used to protect the dural sac and nerve roots from injury during the reaming, tapping, and cage implantation procedure, significant retraction of the dural sac is necessary to perform a PLIF with a threaded fusion cage. Additionally, epidural bleeding can be a problem because of the wide laminectomy and the bilateral annulectomies.

Some of the problems reported with contemporary PLIFs using stand-alone threaded fusion cages include pseudarthrosis, implant loosening, implant subsidence into the adjacent vertebrae, and extrusion of the cages into the spinal canal. Combining instrumented posterolateral fusions and PLIFs with fusion cages is a way to minimize these potential complications.

Steffee and Sitkowski[19] in the late 1980s and 1990s advocated PLIF in combination with posterolateral fusion and pedicle screw fixation, thus providing for an anterior and posterior column fusion in one stage. This type of spine-implant construct can maintain or restore lordosis of the functional spinal unit by means of a force couple; that is, simultaneous distraction of the anterior column and compression of the posterior column. As with stand-alone PLIFs, wide laminectomy and bilateral facetectomies are usually required and the midline bony-ligamentous tether is sacrificed. The extensive posterior element resection, additional dissection out to the transverse processes for posterolateral fusion, and pedicle screw instrumentation lead to longer surgical time and greater risk of complications. Epidural bleeding can be a significant problem. Significant retraction of the dural sac is usually necessary to insert the cages.

Although metal interbody fusion cages provide adequate structure to the anterior column of the spine, these radiopaque implants interfere with determining the radiographic fusion status of the anterior column. CT is helpful in visualizing the fusion inside the cages. On the other hand, if radiolucent cages or structural allografts are used for the PLIF, the anterior column fusion usually can be visualized and monitored on plain radiographs. The use of pedicle screw fixation interferes with determining the fusion status of the posterior column but does not obstruct visualization of the anterior fusion.

The TLIF is a modification of the PLIF.[100] TLIFs are always performed in combination with pedicle screw fixation and usually a posterolateral fusion as well. Like PLIF, TLIF involves anterior and posterior column fusions. The spine-implant construct with a TLIF also causes lordosis by distracting the anterior column and compressing the posterior column. In contrast to PLIF, TLIF only requires a hemilaminectomy and unilateral facetectomy, usually performed on the side of the predominant symptoms or the most significant neural compression. Thus, the midline bony-ligamentous tether is preserved. The transforaminal approach to the disk is lateral to the dural sac, between the exiting and traversing nerve roots. Minimal traction of the neural elements is required. From this unilateral approach, a combination of morcellized autograft and structural allograft (commercially available in many sizes) is usually inserted into the disk space after a thorough diskectomy is performed with specialized tools. Some surgeons insert obliquely oriented threaded fusion cages through this approach rather than structural allograft. Other surgeons insert wire mesh cages from the unilateral approach. Because of their smaller size and radiographic opacity, wire mesh cages do not obstruct radiographic assessment of the healing fusion as much as threaded cages.

Because TLIF is done via a hemilaminectomy, direct decompression of the neural elements is unilateral. An indirect decompression via ligamentotaxis may be accomplished on the contralateral side. A unilateral TLIF is contraindicated if bilateral direct neural decompression is necessary (such as in severe spinal stenosis). A top-loading pedicle screw instrumentation system is preferred to perform a TLIF. Rods medial to the pedicle screws obstruct the transforaminal approach to the disk.

Techniques to fuse the anterior column of the lumbar spine from a posterior approach have several advantages over the anterior approach and the combined anterior/posterior (circumferential) approach in treating degenerative conditions of the spine. (1) The posterior surgical approach is familiar to all spinal and orthopaedic surgeons. (2) Both the anterior and posterior columns of the spine can be fused, reducing the risk of pseudarthrosis. (3) The inherent risks of the anterior approach to the spine are avoided: great vessel injury, ureter injury, retrograde ejaculation, bowel injury, abdominal muscle denervation, and abdominal wall herniation. (4) The anterior approach is left undisturbed and can be used in the future for salvage procedures if needed, without the risk of dissecting about great vessels adherent to the spine. (5) Pedicle screw instrumentation can be used to immobilize both columns of the spine. (6) Total surgical and anesthetic times are reduced with a posterior approach when compared with circumferential fusion.

TLIF does have advantages when compared with PLIF. The TLIF technique is less destructive to the posterior elements. TLIF requires only a unilateral laminectomy and unilateral facetectomy. TLIF preserves the midline bony-ligamentous tether. There is less epidural bleeding with TLIF compared with PLIF and less retraction on the dural sac and nerve roots with the transforaminal approach to the disk.

Suggested Sequence of Surgical Technique

Performing a two-column fusion through a posterior approach is a major spinal reconstructive procedure. Therefore, TLIF and PLIF should be performed in a planned, logical sequence. The following sequence is suggested for TLIF and PLIF. The pedicle screws should be placed first. Obtaining sturdy pedicle screw fixation is required before performing the radical diskectomy. These destructive procedures of the anterior column should not be performed if the spine cannot be safely stabilized. The bone graft should be harvested next. If autogenous iliac crest is being used, the bone graft should be harvested and prepared before performing the diskectomy, so it is ready to use when needed. If morcellized autograft harvested from the laminectomy is to be used, the laminectomy should be done next. If significant epidural bleeding is encountered during the diskectomy portion of the TLIF or PLIF, the interbody fusion can be abandoned, the bone graft placed between the transverse processes quickly, and the wound closed. The diskectomy and interbody fusion are done last.

Circumferential Fusion

Circumferential fusion has been described predominantly for patients with deformity, disabling degenerative disk disease, or as salvage for prior failed surgery. In the last category especially, it seems intuitively plausible that anterior and posterior column support should yield the best outcomes, at least from a purely biomechanical point of view. Many articles have documented successful outcomes; most were retrospective in study design, lacked patient-based outcomes, and did not necessarily correlate results with diagnosis. In 1986, O'Brien and associates[101] reported on circumferential fusion in 150 patients whose diagnoses included failed back surgery syndrome and discogenic back pain. Clinical improvement was reported in 86% of patients. In 1990, Kozak and O'Brien[102] reported on 69 patients who underwent anterior and posterior fusion for discogenic low back pain. This group included some patients who underwent previous surgery as well. A radiographic fusion rate of greater than 90% was reported, with 77% of patients judged to have successful outcomes. Subsequent studies have suggested that circumferential fusion is a dependable way to obtain arthrodesis.[103-112] The advantages include elimination of any anterior or posterior mechanical source of pain, a concept that may be particularly germane to discogenic pain, maximization of the surface area for the fusion bed, and increased mechanical stability. For the purposes of this review, anterior column support with posterior column fixation without supplemental posterior grafting (sometimes referred to as a "270") will be considered to be a variant of the circumferential fusion.[110,113]

Circumferential fusions are indicated for a specific subset of patients with failed previous surgery, or severe discogenic back pain that will respond to immobilization. The anterior column is predominantly load bearing and has an increased surface area compared with the posterolateral fusion bed. In general, the posterior column may be thought of, in this instance, as load sharing.

Arthrodesis for discogenic pain syndromes continues to be widely studied, albeit controversial. In fact, there was little randomized prospective evidence in the literature until the study of Fritzell and associates [28,29] to suggest that arthrodesis was of benefit for degenerative lumbar disk disease. In this study, patients were enrolled into one of four groups in a randomized prospective manner: one nonsurgical and three surgical. The surgical groups, encompassing three different fusion techniques, were not analyzed separately. The nonsurgical group (72 patients) was treated with various sorts of physical therapy. At 2-year follow-up, back pain was reduced in the surgical group by 33%, compared with 7% in the nonsurgical group ($P = 0.0002$). Disability, as determined by the Oswesty disability questionnaire, was reduced by 25% in the surgical group compared with 6% in the nonsurgical group ($P = 0.015$). Overall, 63% of patients in the surgical group rated themselves as "much better" or "better," compared with 29% in the nonsurgical group ($P < 0.0001$). The overall return to work rate was disappointing in both groups, albeit statistically significant; 36% in the surgical group versus 13% in the nonsurgical group. Arguably, one of the flaws of this study was the surgical indication, with levels for fusion being guided on the basis of radiographic degenerative change only. Given the high incidence of asymptomatic degenerative changes with virtually all noninvasive imaging

techniques, a study such as diskography could have improved patient selection.

In the literature, there is a suggestion that discogenic pain syndromes may be treated more efficaciously by the anterior column support. Wetzel and associates [114] reported on 48 patients who underwent fusion for discogenic pain syndrome and found that radiographic fusion correlated with outcome; several patients in this cohort were treated with circumferential fusions. A trend toward better clinical outcomes was evident in this subgroup. Subsequent studies, however, although continuing to report a high rate of fusion for circumferential surgeries, did not necessarily report high rates of patient satisfaction with functional improvement. Gertzbein and associates [106] retrospectively reviewed 62 patients who underwent circumferential fusion. They reported a radiographic fusion rate of 100% but a satisfactory clinical outcome only slightly higher than 50%, based on pain scores (standard visual analog scale), use of pain medication, and return to work. Slosar and associates [111] reported on 131 patients who underwent anterior interbody fusion with femoral allograft and posterior instrumented fusion; 92 of these patients had previous back surgery. The authors found that 81% of patients reported improved outcomes after surgery, although only 62% were satisfied with the procedure and 37% were able to return to work. Carpenter and associates [115] distributed a postoperative questionnaire to assess pain, functional status, and work history after surgery. Eighty-six patients who had at least one previous attempt for pseudarthrosis were studied, and 94% of the fusions in the group were judged to be solid radiographically; only 26% of the patients reported good or excellent results.

This is in contrast to other reports, one of which suggested that the conversion of a posterolateral fusion to a circumferential fusion may improve clinical outcome and diskogenic pain. Barrick and associates [103] performed repeat discography in patients with solid posterolateral fusions that were confirmed at the time of repeat surgery. In this cohort, 89% of patients expressed satisfaction at the functional outcome, with a 100% fusion rate noted.

Various techniques have been described for anterior and posterior fusion, including anterior transperitoneal, anterior extraperitoneal, anterolateral (predominantly useful for approaching L2-L4), and both open and laparoscopic techniques for L4-5 and L5-S1. Various grafts have also been described including autograft, allograft, and interbody devices. As noted previously, autograft is the most widely accepted graft material, although certain biologics, specifically bone morphogenetic protein, have been shown to be highly promising. Posterior fusions are usually augmented with interpedicular or translaminar instrumentation, although fusion in situ has been described as well. The fate of the posterior column bone graft remains controversial, with some suggesting that reabsorption may occur because of load sharing. If in fact this is the case, the "270" may be particularly attractive.

Major complications have been reported in 4% to 29% of patients. Less than 2% of complications relate to the anterior approach per se.[104] The most severe are deep venous thromboses and retrograde ejaculation.[106,107] The incidence of iliac vessel injury is less than 1%. Retrograde ejaculation, perhaps the most feared complication, has been reported in 0% to 16% of patients. A high incidence was noted with early laparoscopic approaches as a result of disruption of the sympathetic trunk that fimbriates at L4-5 and passes behind or on top of the iliac vessels. With more limited dissection of the iliac vessels and use of bipolar electrocautery, the risk of retrograde ejaculation has diminished. Ileus is ubiquitous in most series, with a rate of approximately 70%. This typically resolves within 48 hours.

Concern has been raised regarding the risk of transitional syndromes with the more rigid fixation afforded by circumferential fusions. Lehmann and associates[116] reported 30% incidence in spinal stenosis rostral to posterior surgery, whereas Frymoyer and associates,[117] at 10-year follow-up, noted a 45% incidence of radiographic disk degeneration above posterolateral fusions. For anterior procedures, Penta and Fraser[118] noted a 10.5% incidence of disk bulging, 0.01% incidence of herniated nucleus pulposus, and a 2.5% incidence of stenosis in a group of 81 patients assessed 10 years after interbody fusion. Overall, the 32% incidence of degenerative disk disease above a solid fusion was comparable to the incidence adjacent to a floating fusion or pseudarthosis. The authors suggested that the incidence is more strongly related to age and other factors than the types of arthrodesis.

Although the increased degree of risk for transitional syndromes, if any, associated with anterior and posterior fusion is unclear, prudence certainly dictates that certain factors be considered, particularly sagittal alignment. For every 10° decrease in lordosis within a lumbar fusion, lordosis in the adjacent rostral unfused segment will increase by 2°. This will increase the load across posterior instrumentation, posterior shear

force, and laminar strain. Umehara and associates[119] noted an increase of 192 N for every 2° change in lordosis in an upright posture. With every 2° loss of lordosis, posterior strain can increase up to 98%. Thus, preservation of lordosis would certainly appear to be important in designing an appropriate construct.

Overall, circumferential fusion appears to be a reasonable approach to salvage surgery or, particularly in the context of less invasive techniques, primary discogenic disease. Based on the literature to date, radiographic success does not strictly correlate with clinical success. Certainly, however, the anterior and posterior fusion appears to be a viable way to achieve stability.

A final note of caution regarding fusion rates must be sounded. Except for the study of Barrick and associates,[103] all studies reported radiographic fusion rates. Brodsky and associates[120] found the incidence of discordance between radiographic fusion and surgical reexploration to be 36% based on plain radiographs, 46% based on tomography, 38% based on flexion extension views, and 43% based on CT. Thus, given the possibility of significant false-negatives and false-positives with radiographic fusion rates, most correlations with fusion and pain relief should be made cautiously. Nevertheless, a circumferential fusion may be the most efficacious way to achieve stability in the specific diagnostic groups discussed.

Summary

Although strict evidence-based guidelines do not exist for the surgical treatment of degenerative disorders of the lumbar spine, the following general guidelines may be helpful. Uninstrumented posterolateral spinal fusion has been seen to be well suited to treating adolescent patients with spondylolysis and grade I degenerative spondylolisthesis and no evidence of segmental instability. Instrumented posterolateral fusion is a rational approach in patients with central and posterolateral stenosis or previous decompressive or disk surgery who have degenerative instability, low back pain, and neurogenic leg pain and who would benefit from a direct posterior decompression and fusion. Instrumented posterior lumbar interbody fusion is best suited for patients with degenerative instability and posterior stenosis with collapsed disks and high-grade foraminal stenosis not well addressed with a direction decompression only. Therefore, this technique is useful with restoration of disk and foraminal height is indicated in conjunction with decompression.

An anterior-posterior fusion is indicated when patients have higher degrees of acquired instability and central and foraminal stenosis. Indirect and direct decompression techniques may need to be coupled to achieve a reasonable outcome. When restoration of height and stability cannot safely be achieved posteriorly, a circumferential approach should be strongly considered. Stand-alone anterior interbody fusion should be considered for patients who have single-level disk degeneration with significant foraminal stenosis but without posterolateral or central stenosis or significant degenerative facet disease. Posterior direct decompression should not be required to achieve a good result.

References

1. Albee FH: Transplantation of a portion of the tibia into the spine for the treatment of pott's disease. *JAMA* 1911;57:885-887.

2. Hibbs RA: An operation for progressive spinal deformities. *New York Medical J* 1911;93:1013-1036.

3. Mixter WJ, Barr JS: Rupture of the intervertebral disc with involvement of the spinal canal. *N Engl J Med* 1934;211:210.

4. Hallock H: The surgical treatment of low back pain. *Instr Course Lect* 1947;2:95-102.

5. Bosworth DM: Techniques of spinal fusion. *Instr Course Lect* 1948;3:295-313.

6. Cleveland M, Bosworth DM, Thompson FR: Pseudarthrosis in the lumbosacral spine. *J Bone Joint Surg Am* 1948;30:302-312.

7. Watkins MB: Posterolateral fusion of the lumbar and lumbosacral spine. *J Bone Joint Surg Am* 1953;35:1014-1020.

8. Watkins MB: Posterolateral bone grafting for fusion of the lumbar and lumbsacral spine. *J Bone Joint Surg Am* 1959;41:388-396.

9. Watkins MB: Posterolateral fusion in pseudarthrosis and posterior element defects of the lumbosacral spine. *Clin Orthop* 1964;35:80-85.

10. Wiltse LL, Hutchinson RH: Surgical treatment of spondylolisthesis. *Clin Orthop* 1964;35:116-135.

11. Prothero SR, Parkes JC, Stinchfield FE: Complications after low-back fusion in 1000 patients: A comparison of two series one decade apart: 1966. *Clin Orthop* 1994;306:5-11.

12. Lee CK, Langrana NA: Lumbosacral spinal fusion: A biomechanical study. *Spine* 1984;9:574-581.

13. Toribatake Y, Hutton WC, Tomita K, Boden SD: Vascularization of the fusion mass in a posterolateral intertransverse process fusion. *Spine* 1998;23:1149-1154.

14. Boden SD, Schimandle JH, Hutton WC: An experimental lumbar intertransverse process spinal fusion model: Radiographic, histologic, and biomechanical healing characteristics. *Spine* 1995;20:412-420.

15. Hurley LA, et al: The Role of soft tissues in osteogenesis: An experimental study of canine spine fusions. *J Bone Joint Surg Am* 1959;41:1243-1254.

16. Hadra BE: The classic: Wiring of the vertebrae as a means of immobilization in fracture and Potts' disease: Berthold E. Hadra: Med Times and Register, Vol 22, May 23, 1891. *Clin Orthop* 1975;112:4-8.

17. Roy-Camille R, Benazet JP,Desauge JP, Kuntz F: Lumbosacral fusion with pedicular screw plating instrumentation: A 10-year follow-up. *Acta Orthop Scand Suppl* 1993;251:100-104.

18. Louis R: Fusion of the lumbar and sacral spine by internal fixation with screw plates. *Clin Orthop* 1986;203:18-33.

19. Steffee AD, Sitkowski DJ: Posterior lumbar interbody fusion and plates. *Clin Orthop* 1988;227:99-102.

20. Lorenz M, Zindrick M, Schwaegler P, et al: A comparison of single-level fusions with and without hardware. *Spine* 1991;16(suppl 8):S455-S458.

21. Zdeblick TA: A prospective, randomized study of lumbar fusion: Preliminary results. *Spine* 1993;18:983-991.

22. Bridwell KH, Sedgewick TA, O'Brien MF, Lenke LG, Baldus C: The role of fusion and instrumentation in the treatment of degenerative spondylolisthesis with spinal stenosis. *J Spinal Disord* 1993;6:461-472.

23. Yuan HA, Garfin SR, Dickman CA, Mardjetko SM: A historical cohort study of pedicle screw fixation in thoracic, lumbar, and sacral spinal fusions. *Spine* 1994;19(suppl 20):2279S-2296S.

24. Fischgrund JS, Mackay M, Herkowitz HN, Brower R, Montgomery DM, Kurz LT: Degenerative lumbar spondylolisthesis with spinal stenosis: A prospective, randomized study comparing decompressive laminectomy and arthrodesis with and without spinal instrumentation. *Spine* 1997;22: 2807-2812.

25. Bernhardt M, Swartz DE, Clothiaux PL, Crowell RR, White AA III: Posterolateral lumbar and lumbosacral fusion with and without pedicle screw internal fixation. *Clin Orthop* 1992;284:109-115.

26. France JC, Yaszemski MJ, Lauerman WC: A randomized prospective study of posterolateral lumbar fusion: Outcomes with and without pedicle screw instrumentation. *Spine* 1999;24:553-560.

27. Moller H, Hedlund R: Instrumented and noninstrumented posterolateral fusion in adult spondylolisthesis: A prospective randomized study. Part 2. *Spine* 2000;25:1716-1721.

28. Fritzell P, Hagg O, Wessberg P, Nordwall A, Swedish Lumbar Spine Group: Lumbar fusion versus nonsurgical treatment for chronic low back pain: A multicenter randomized controlled trial from the Swedish Lumbar Spine Study Group. *Spine* 2001;26:2521-2534.

29. Fritzell P, Hagg O, Wessberg P, Nordwall A, Swedish Lumbar Spine Study Group: Chronic low back pain and fusion: A comparison of three surgical techniques. A prospective multicenter randomized study from the Swedish lumbar spine study group. *Spine* 2002;27:1131-1141.

30. Christensen FB, Karlsmose B, Hansen ES, Bunger CE: Radiological and functional outcome after anterior lumbar interbody spinal fusion. *Eur Spine J* 1996;5:293-298.

31. Thomsen K, Christensen FB, Eiskjaer SP, Hansen ES, Fruensgaard S, Bunger CE: The effect of pedicle screw instrumentation on functional outcome and fusion rates in posterolateral lumbar spinal fusion: A prospective, randomized clinical study. *Spine* 1997;22:2813-2822.

32. Hadley MN, Reddy SV: Smoking and the human vertebral column: A review of the impact of cigarette use on vertebral bone metabolism and spinal fusion. *Neurosurgery* 1997;41:116-124.

33. Brown CW, Orme TJ, Richardson HD: The rate of pseudarthrosis (surgical nonunion) in patients who are smokers and patients who are nonsmokers: A comparison study. *Spine* 1986;11:942-943.

34. Andersen T, Christensen FB, Laursen M, Hoy K, Hansen E, Bunger C: Smoking as a predictor of negative outcome in lumbar spinal fusion. *Spine* 2001;26: 2623-2628.

35. McCulloch JA: Microdecompression and uninstrumented single-level fusion for spinal canal stenosis with degenerative spondylolisthesis. *Spine* 1998;23: 2243-2252.

36. Carragee EJ: Single-level posterolateral arthrodesis, with or without posterior decompression, for the treatment of isthmic spondylolisthesis in adults: A prospective, randomized study. *J Bone Joint Surg Am* 1997;79:1175-1180.

37. Weber BR, Grob D, Dvorak J, Muntener M: Posterior surgical approach to the lumbar spine and its effect on the multifidus muscle. *Spine* 1997;22: 1765-1772.

38. Boden SD, Martin C, Rudolph R, Kirkpatrick JS, Moeini SM, hutton WC: Increase of motion between lumbar vertebrae after excision of the capsule and cartilage of the facets: A cadaver study. *J Bone Joint Surg Am* 1994;76:1847-1853.

39. Connolly PJ, Grob D: Bracing of patients after fusion for degenerative problems of the lumbar spine: Yes or no? *Spine* 1998;23:1426-1428.

40. Johnsson R, Selvik G, Stromqvist B, Sunden G: Mobility of the lower lumbar spine after posterolateral fusion determined by roentgen stereo-photogrammetric analysis. *Spine* 1990;15:347-350.

41. Turner JA, Ersek M, Herron L: Patient outcomes after lumbar spinal fusions. *JAMA* 1992;268:907-911.

42. Turner JA, Herron L, Deyo RA: Meta-analysis of the results of lumbar spine fusion. *Acta Orthop Scand* 1993:251 (suppl):120-122.

43. Gibson JN, Grant IC, Waddell G: The Cochrane review of surgery for lumbar disc prolapse and degenerative lumbar spondylosis. *Spine* 1999;24:1820-1832.

44. Grubb SA, Lipscomb HJ: Results of lumbosacral fusion for degenerative disc disease with and without instrumentation: Two- to five-year follow-up. *Spine* 1992;17:349-355.

45. Wood GW II, Boyd RJ, Carothers TA: The effect of pedicle screw/plate fixation on lumbar/lumbosacral autogenous bone graft fusions in patients with degenerative disc disease. *Spine* 1995;20:819-830.

46. Mardjetko SM, Connolly PJ, Shott S: Degenerative lumbar spondylolisthesis: A meta-analysis of literature 1970-1993. *Spine* 1994;19(suppl 20):2256S-2265S.

47. Cotler JM, Star AM: Complications of spine fusions, in Cotler JM, Cotler HB (eds): *Spinal Fusions: Science and Technique.* New York, NY, Springer-Verlag, 1990, pp 361-387.

48. Matsuzaki H, Tokuhashi Y, Matsumoto F, Hoshino M, Kiuchi T, Toriyama S: Problems and solutions of pedicle screw plate fixation of lumbar spine. *Spine* 1990;15:1159-1165.

49. Ohlin A, Karlsson M, Duppe H, Hasserius R, Redlund-Johnell I: Complications after transpedicular stabilization of the spine: A survivorship analysis of 163 cases. *Spine* 1994; 19:2774-2779.

50. West JL III, Ogilvie JW, Bradford DS: Complications of the variable screw plate pedicle screw fixation. *Spine* 1991; 16:576-579.

51. Davne SH, Myers DL: Complications of lumbar spinal fusion with transpedicular instrumentation. *Spine* 1992;17(suppl 6):S184-S189.

52. McAfee PC, Weiland DJ, Carlow JJ: Survivorship analysis of pedicle spinal instrumentation. *Spine* 1991;16(suppl 8):S422-S427.

53. Myers MA, Casciani T, Whitbeck MG Jr, Puzas JE: Vertebral body osteopenia associated with posterolateral spine fusion in humans. *Spine* 1996;21:2368-2371.

54. Kanayama M, Cunningham BW, Weis JC, Parker LM, Kaneda K, McAfee PC: Maturation of the posterolateral spinal fusion and its effect on load-sharing of spinal instrumentation: An in vivo sheep model. *J Bone Joint Surg Am* 1997;79:1710-1720.

55. Kanayama M, Cunningham BW, Sefter JC: Does spinal instrumentation influence the healing process of posterolateral spinal fusion?: An in vivo animal model. *Spine* 1999;24:1058-1065.

56. Kanayama M, Cunningham BW, Haggerty CJ, Abumi K, Kaneda K, McAfee PC: In vitro biomechanical investigation of the stability and stress-shielding effect of lumbar interbody fusion devices. *J Neurosurg* 2000;93(suppl 2):259-265.

57. Burns BH: An operation for spondylolisthesis. *Lancet* 1933;1: 1233-1239.

58. Lane JD, Moore ES: Transperitoneal approach to the intervertebral disc in the lumbar area. *Ann Surg* 1948;127:537-551.

59. Harmon PH: Anterior excision and vertebral body fusion operation for intervertebral disc syndromes of the lower lumbar spine. *Clin Orthop* 1963;26:107-127.

60. Sacks S: Anterior interbody fusion of the lumbar spine: Indications and results in 200 cases. *Clin Orthop* 1966;44:163-170.

61. Stauffer RN, Coventry MB: Posterolateral lumbar-spine fusion: Analysis of Mayo Clinic series. *J Bone Joint Surg Am* 1972;54:1195-1204.

62. Stauffer RN, Coventry MB: Anterior interbody lumbar spine fusion: Analysis of Mayo Clinic series. *J Bone Joint Surg Am* 1972;54:756-768.

63. Linson MA, Williams H: Anterior and combined anteroposterior fusion for lumbar disc pain: A preliminary study. *Spine* 1991;16:143-145.

64. Newman MH, Grinstead GL: Anterior lumbar interbody fusion for internal disc disruption. *Spine* 1992;17:831-833.

65. Moon MS, Kim SS, Sun DH, Moon YW: Anterior spondylodesis for spondylolisthesis: Isthmic and degenerative types. *Eur Spine J* 1994;3:172-176.

66. Crock HV: Anterior lumbar interbody fusion: Indications for its use and notes on surgical technique. *Clin Orthop* 1982;165:157-163.

67. Holte DC, O'Brien JP, Renton P: Anterior lumbar fusion using a hybrid interbody graft: A preliminary radiographic report. *Eur Spine J* 1994;3:32-38.

68. Sarwat AM, O'Brien JP, Renton P, Sutcliffe JC: The use of allograft (and avoidance of autograft) in anterior lumbar interbody fusion: a critical analysis. *Eur Spine J* 2001;10:237-241.

69. Buttermann GR, Glazer PA, Bradford DS: The use of bone allografts in the spine. *Clin Orthop* 1996;324:75-85.

70. Bagby G: The Bagby and Kuslich (BAK) method of lumbar interbody fusion. *Spine* 1999;24:1857.

71. Kuslich SD, Ulstrom CL, Griffith SL, Ahern JW, Dowdle JD: The Bagby and Kuslich method of lumbar interbody fusion: History, techniques, and 2-year follow-up results of a United States prospective, multicenter trial. *Spine* 1998;23:1267-1279.

72. McAfee PC, Cunningham BW, Lee GA: Revision strategies for salvaging or improving failed cylindrical cages. *Spine* 1999;24:2147-2153.

73. McAfee PC, Lee GA, Fedder IL, Cunningham BW: Anterior BAK instrumentation and fusion: Complete versus partial discectomy. *Clin Orthop* 2002;394:55-63.

74. Ray CD: Threaded titanium cages for lumbar interbody fusions. *Spine* 1997;22:667-680.

75. Regan JJ, Yuan H, McAfee PC: Laparoscopic fusion of the lumbar spine: Minimally invasive spine surgery: A prospective multicenter study evaluating open and laparoscopic lumbar fusion. *Spine* 1999;24:402-411.

76. Klemme WR, Owens BD, Dhawan A, Zeidman S, Polly DW Jr: Lumbar sagittal contour after posterior interbody

fusion: Threaded devices alone versus vertical cages plus posterior instrumentation. *Spine* 2001;26:534-537.

77. Janssen ME, Lam C, Beckham R: Outcomes of allogenic cages in anterior and posterior lumbar interbody fusion. *Eur Spine J* 2001;10(suppl 2):S158-S168.

78. Mendenhall S (ed): Bone grafts and bone substitutes, in *Orthopedic Network News*. Ann Arbor, MI, Mendenhall Associates, 1999, vol 10, pp 10-17.

79. Togawa D, Bauer TW, Brantigan JW, Lowery GL: Bone graft incorporation in radiographically successful human intervertebral body fusion cages. *Spine* 2001;26:2744-2750.

80. Dennis S, Watkins R, Landaker S, Dillin W, Springer D: Comparison of disc space heights after anterior lumbar interbody fusion. *Spine* 1989;14:876-878.

81. Vamvanij V, Ferrara LA, Hai Y, Zhao J, Kolata R, Yuan HA: Quantitative changes in spinal canal dimensions using interbody distraction for spondylolisthesis. *Spine* 2001;26:E13-E18.

82. Chen D, Fay LA, Lok J, Yuan P, Edwards WT, Yuan HA: Increasing neuroforaminal volume by anterior interbody distraction in degenerative lumbar spine. *Spine* 1995;20:74-79.

83. McAfee PC: Interbody fusion cages in reconstructive operations on the spine. *J Bone Joint Surg Am* 1999;81:859-880.

84. Oxland TR, Lund T: Biomechanics of stand-alone cages and cages in combination with posterior fixation: A literature review. *Eur Spine J* 2000;9 (suppl 1):S95-101.

85. Chow DH, Luk KD, Evans JH, Leong JC: Effects of short anterior lumbar interbody fusion on biomechanics of neighboring unfused segments. *Spine* 1996;21:549-555.

86. Penta M, Sandhu A, Fraser RD: Magnetic resonance imaging assessment of disc degeneration 10 years after anterior lumbar interbody fusion. *Spine* 1995;20:743-747.

87. Van Horn JR, Bohnen LM: The development of discopathy in lumbar discs adjacent to a lumbar anterior interbody spondylodesis: A retrospective matched-pair study with a postoperative follow-up of 16 years. *Acta Orthop Belg* 1992;58:280-286.

88. Takahashi K, Kitahara H, Yamagata M, et al: Long-term results of anterior interbody fusion for treatment of degenerative spondylolisthesis. *Spine* 1990;15:1211-1215.

89. Miyamoto K: Long-term follow-up results of anterior discectomy and interbody fusion for lumbar disc herniation. *Nippon Seikeigeka Gakkai Zasshi* 1991;65:1179-1190.

90. Inoue S, Watanabe T, Hirose A, et al: Anterior discectomy and interbody fusion for lumbar disc herniation: A review of 350 cases. *Clin Orthop* 1984;183:22-31.

91. Inoue S, Watanabe T, Goto S, Takhashi K, Takata K, Sho E: Degenerative spondylolisthesis: Pathophysiology and results of anterior interbody fusion. *Clin Orthop* 1988;227:90-98.

92. Kim NH: Anterior interbody fusion in the treatment of the lumbar herniated nucleus pulposus. *Yonsei Med J* 1999;40:256-264.

93. Vishteh AG, Dickman CA: Anterior lumbar microdiscectomy and interbody fusion for the treatment of recurrent disc herniation. *Neurosurgery* 2001;48:334-338.

94. Christensen FB, Bunger CE: Retrograde ejaculation after retroperitoneal lower lumbar interbody fusion. *Int Orthop* 1997;21:176-180.

95. Kleeman TJ, Michael Ahn U, Clutterbuck WB, Campbell CJ, Talbot-Kleeman A: Laparoscopic anterior lumbar interbody fusion at L4-L5: An anatomic evaluation and approach classification. *Spine* 2002;27:1390-1395.

96. Tiusanen H, Seitsalo S, Osterman K, Soini J: Retrograde ejaculation after anterior interbody lumbar fusion. *Eur Spine J* 1995;4:339-342.

97. Cloward RB: Spondylolisthesis: Treatment by laminectomy and posterior interbody fusion. *Clin Orthop* 1981;154:74-82.

98. Cloward RB: Posterior lumbar interbody fusion updated. *Clin Orthop* 1985;193:16-19.

99. Kuslich SD, Danielson G, Dowdle JD, et al: Four-year follow-up results of lumbar spine arthrodesis using the Bagby and Kuslich lumbar fusion cage. *Spine* 2000;25:2656-2662.

100. Pitzen T, Caspar W, Matthis D, et al: Primary stability of 2 PLIF (posterior lumbar interbody fusion): A biomechanical in vitro comparison. *Z Orthop Ihre Grenzgeb* 1999;137:214-218.

101. O'Brien JP, Dawson MH, Heard CW, Mombergr G, Speck G, Weathery CR: Simultaneous combined anterior and posterior fusion: A surgical solution for failed spinal surgery with a brief review of the first 150 patients. *Clin Orthop* 1986;203:191-195.

102. Kozak JA, O'Brien JP: Simultaneous combined anterior and posterior fusion: An independent analysis of a treatment for the disabled low-back pain patient. *Spine* 1990;15:322-328.

103. Barrick WT, Schofferman JA, Reynolds JB, et al: Anterior lumbar fusion improves discogenic pain at levels of prior posterolateral fusion. *Spine* 2000;25:853-857.

104. Buttermann GR, Garvey TA, Hunt AF: Lumbar fusion results related to diagnosis. *Spine* 1998;23:116-127.

105. Fraser RD: Interbody, posterior, and combined lumbar fusions. *Spine* 1995;20(suppl 24):167S-177S.

106. Gertzbein SD, Hollopeter M, Hall SD: Analysis of circumferential lumbar fusion outcome in the treatment of degenerative disc disease of the lumbar spine. *J Spinal Disord* 1998;11:472-478.

107. Gertzbein SD, Hollopeter MR, Hall S: Pseudarthrosis of the lumbar spine: Outcome after circumferential fusion. *Spine* 1998;23:2352-2357.

108. Grob D, Scheier HJ, Dvorak J: Circumferential fusion of the lumbar and lumbosacral spine: Comparison of two techniques of anterior spinal fusion. *Chir Organi Mov* 1991;76:123-131.

109. Grob D, Scheier HJ, Dvorak J, Siegrist H, Rubeli M: Circumferential fusion of the lumbar and lumbosacral spine. *Arch Orthop Trauma Surg* 1991;111:20-25.

110. Schofferman J, Slosar P, Reynold J, Goldthwaite N, Koestler M: A prospective randomized comparison of 270 degrees fusions to 360 degrees fusions (circumferential fusions). *Spine* 2001;26:E207-E212.

111. Slosar PJ, Reynolds JB, Schofferman J, Goldthwaite N, White AH, Keaney D: Patient satisfaction after circumferential lumbar fusion. *Spine* 2000;25:722-726.

112. Albert TJ, Pinto M, Denis F: Management of symptomatic lumbar pseudarthrosis with anteroposterior fusion: A functional and radiographic outcome study. *Spine* 2000;25:123-130.

113. Slosar PJ, Reynolds JB, Goldthwaite ND: The "270" Lumbar Fusion: An Alternative to the Circumferential Fusion. *Proceedings of the North American*

Spine Society Annual Meeting. San Francisco, CA, North American Spine Society, 1998.

114. Wetzel FT, LaRocca SH, Lowery GL, Aprill CN: The treatment of lumbar spinal pain syndromes diagnosed by discography: Lumbar arthrodesis. *Spine* 1994;19:792-800.

115. Carpenter CT, Dietz JW, Leung KY, Hanscom DA, Wagner TA: Repair of a pseudarthrosis of the lumbar spine: A

functional outcome study. *J Bone Joint Surg Am* 1996;78:712-720.

116. Lehmann TR, Spratt KF, Tozzi JE, et al: Long-term follow-up of lower lumbar fusion patients. *Spine* 1987;12:97-104.

117. Frymoyer JW, Hanley EN Jr, Howe J, Kuhlmann D, Matteri RE: A comparison of radiographic findings in fusion and nonfusion patients ten or more years following lumbar disc surgery. *Spine* 1979;4:435-440.

118. Penta M, Fraser RD: Anterior lumbar interbody fusion: A minimum 10-year follow-up. *Spine* 1997;22:2429-2434.

119. Umehara S, Zindrick MR, Patwardhan AG, et al: The biomechanical effect of postoperative hypolordosis in instrumented lumbar fusion on instrumented and adjacent spinal segments. *Spine* 2000;25:1617-1624.

120. Brodsky AE, Kovalsky ES, Khalil MA: Correlation of radiologic assessment of lumbar spine fusions with surgical exploration. *Spine* 1991;16(suppl 6):S261-S265.

17

Radiculopathy and the Herniated Lumbar Disk: Controversies Regarding Pathophysiology and Management

John M. Rhee, MD
Michael K. Schaufele, MD
William A. Abdu, MD, MS

Abstract

Lumbar disk herniation is one of the most common problems encountered in orthopaedic practice. Despite the frequency of its occurrence, however, much about lumbar disk herniation is poorly understood. It is important to review the basic and clinical science underlying the pathophysiology and treatment, surgical and nonsurgical, of this disorder.

Lumbar disk herniations remain among the most common diagnoses encountered in clinical spine practice. The incidence of symptomatic lumbar disk herniations in the American population has been estimated to be 1% to 2%,[1] for which approximately 200,000 lumbar diskectomies are performed annually.[2] Yet despite the frequency with which lumbar disk herniation occurs, there is substantial controversy regarding its pathophysiology and treatment. For example, from the standpoint of basic science, mounting evidence suggests that biochemical factors—in addition to the mechanical effects of the disk material on the nerve root—underlie the development of symptomatic radiculopathy, but those factors remain to be clearly elucidated. On the clinical

end of the spectrum, large (fivefold to fifteenfold) variations[3] in the rates of lumbar surgery in geographically adjacent areas suggest radical heterogeneity in the application of surgical criteria to this diagnosis. In this chapter, the available basic science regarding the anatomy and pathophysiology of lumbar disk herniations is examined as well as the clinical evidence supporting nonsurgical compared with surgical management of this common, yet surprisingly poorly understood, orthopaedic disorder.

Anatomy of Lumbar Disk Herniation

Structurally, the lumbar disk has three components: the anulus fibrosus, which forms the circumferential rim of the disk; the nucleus pulposus,

which comprises its central core; and the cartilaginous end plates on the adjacent vertebral bodies. The anulus fibrosus has a multilayer lamellar architecture made of collagen fibers. Within each layer, the collagen is oriented at approximately 30° to the horizontal. Each successive layer is oriented at 30° to the horizontal in the opposite direction, leading to a "crisscross" type pattern. This composition allows the anulus fibrosus, and in particular the outer anulus fibrosus, which has the highest tensile modulus, to resist torsional, axial, and tensile loads. The nucleus pulposus provides resistance to axial compression and is the principal determinant of disk height because of its unique composition consisting of large, highly charged proteoglycan macromolecules within a collagen matrix. These macromolecules are hydrophilic and are contained within the confines of the anulus fibrosus peripherally and the end plates above and below. Thus, imbibed water causes the nucleus to swell and to generate large hydrostatic pressures within the disk. A healthy nucleus consists of approximately 70% water. The nucleus also contains a cellular component of both fibroblast-like and chondrocyte-like cells. These cells maintain the matrix in which they exist, and they also receive metabolic nutrients that diffuse through the matrix.

The intervertebral disk is anatomically unique for several reasons. First, it is mostly avascular—it is the largest avascular structure in the body. Blood vessels lie on the surface of the anulus fibrosus but penetrate only a very short distance into the outer portions of the anulus fibrosus. Similarly, blood vessels from the vertebral body lie against the cartilaginous end plates but do not enter the central regions of the disk. As a result, disk cells derive their nutrition from diffusion through the end plates and connective tissue transport from one part of the matrix to the other. Second, the disk is only minimally innervated. Nerve endings are present only on the surface of the disk, and they penetrate a very short distance into the outer anulus fibrosus. The normal inner anulus fibrosus and nucleus completely lack innervation. In contrast, the posterior and anterior longitudinal ligaments are innervated. The anterior longitudinal ligament receives nerve branches from the segmental ventral ramus and sympathetic trunk. The posterior longitudinal ligament is innervated by a branch of the dorsal root ganglion known as the sinuvertebral nerve. Experimental studies of patients undergoing diskectomy with local anesthetic have demonstrated that surgical stimulation of the posterior longitudinal ligament can cause low back pain.[4] Thus, stimulation of the sinuvertebral nerve may be one mediator of the low back pain component associated with lumbar disk hernia-

tions and annular tears.

The terminology used to describe the spectrum of lumbar disk herniations varies and is often confusing; however, when properly applied, it provides useful descriptive information. One useful method of classifying disk herniations is according to whether the herniated fragments are "contained" or "noncontained" by the anulus fibrosus.[5] A protrusion is a focal bulging of nuclear material contained by the anulus fibrosus (that is, the annular fibers remain continuous and attached to the vertebral bodies). Subannular extrusions occur when the anulus fibrosus remains intact but the fragment has migrated behind the body either above or below the disk while maintaining continuity with the disk. Transannular extruded disk herniations occur when the fragments have ruptured through the anulus fibrosus but maintain continuity with the disk space of origin. A sequestration arises when the material has not only broken through the anulus fibrosus but has also migrated away from the disk space of origin and is no longer in contact with it. Any of the three components of the intervertebral disk (the nucleus, anulus fibrosus, or end plate), alone or in combination, may be the offending material when a disk herniates.

Pathophysiology of Lumbar Disk Herniation

The origins of the modern era of lumbar disk surgery can be traced to the seminal work of Mixter and Barr[6] 70 years ago. Those authors found that sciatic pain could be relieved by removing herniated disk material compressing a nerve root. Logically, the association was made between lumbar disk herniation and the clinical entity of sciatica. That finding led to the general assump-

tion that mechanical compression of the nerve root is the primary pathogenic factor inducing radiculopathy. Several lines of evidence support this notion. First, the structure of the nerve root renders it relatively poorly resistant to compression. Like peripheral nerves, nerve roots have an endoneurium. However, the layers equivalent to the perineurium and epineurium are cerebrospinal fluid and dural lining, respectively. Thus, the nerve root is a comparatively delicate structure that is not well insulated to resist compressive forces. Second, because nerve roots are tethered to the vertebral body at their takeoff from the common dural sac and to the subjacent pedicle within the foramen by ligamentous attachments, a disk herniation ventral to the root is poised to generate high tensile forces. The situation is analogous to the tension generated in a bowstring by the pull of an archer's hand. Third, animal models of cauda equina compression have demonstrated that compression of a nerve root impairs its nutrition. In a series of experiments, Olmarker and associates[7,8] showed that mechanical compression on nerve roots within the porcine cauda equina led to decreased nutrient delivery by reducing both blood flow and nutrient diffusion from cerebrospinal fluid. Histologically, compressed nerve roots demonstrate evidence of intraneural edema, which can directly lead to nerve fibrosis and injury. Alternatively, intraneural edema can secondarily lead to an intraneural "compartment syndrome," as pressures within the nerve root overcome perfusion pressures, resulting in nerve root ischemia and injury.[9]

Although this and other studies suggest that the mechanical effect of a herniated disk is the main factor in the genesis of radiculopathy, other lines of evidence indicate that mechanical compression alone may not be a sufficient cause for the radiculopathy associated with herniated disks. First, MRI studies have shown that nerve root compression is often asymptomatic (Figure 1). Boden and associates[10] found that, in a group of people who had never had radicular pain, 20% of those under the age of 60 years and 36% of those over the age of 60 years had evidence of a herniated disk on MRI. Second, other reports have suggested that, although irritated nerve roots demonstrate susceptibility to mechanical compression, normal (nonsensitized) roots do not. Smyth and Wright[11] found that, when sutures placed around nerve roots at the time of surgery were tugged postoperatively, only those roots that had been noted at surgery to be compressed by a herniated disk generated a radicular pain response. When there had been no intraoperative evidence of root compression by a herniated disk, tugging on the suture and creating tension in the root postoperatively did not elicit radicular symptoms. Kuslich and associates[4] performed lumbar diskectomy, using local anesthesia, on awake patients and found that surgical stimulation of compressed roots caused pain 90% of the time, whereas manipulation of normal roots provoked pain only 9% of the time. These observations suggest that a nerve root needs to be sensitized to be mechanically susceptible and that mechanical compression alone is not the sine qua non of radiculopathy.

A growing body of evidence has implicated bioactive molecules within the disk as important in sensitizing nerve roots and participating in the pathogenesis of radiculopathy. Olmarker and associates[12] re-

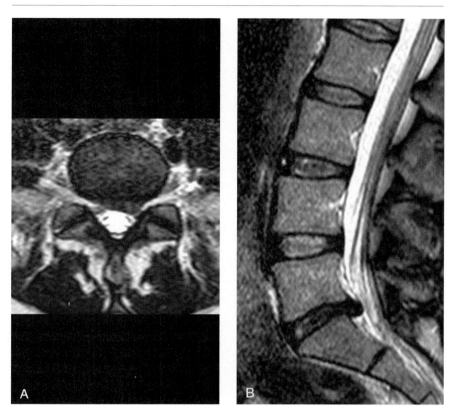

Figure 1　Asymptomatic posterolateral disk herniation in a 45-year-old woman with pain in the right leg. She had absolutely no symptoms in the left leg, despite the axial **(A)** and sagittal **(B)** T2-weighted MRI scans demonstrating an extruded left L5-S1 disk herniation. Asymptomatic disk herniations are not uncommon, underlying the need to treat symptoms rather than MRI findings per se.

ported that, when autogenous nucleus pulposus was applied to the porcine cauda equina, physiologic and anatomic evidence suggestive of radiculopathy was noted, even in the absence of any nerve root compression. Compared with control animals in which autologous fat had been applied epidurally, those in which nucleus pulposus had been applied demonstrated a decrease in nerve conduction velocity and histologic evidence of nerve fiber degeneration (axonal swelling and demyelination). This study suggested that nuclear material could itself lead to neural injury in the absence of mechanical compression. Authors of later studies attempted to deter-

mine whether the observed changes in nerve structure and electrophysiology correlated with a clinical syndrome of radiculopathy. In one such study, rats underwent laminectomy and were randomized to one of three groups: (1) incision of the disk such that nuclear contents could come into contact with, but not displace, the nerve root; (2) displacement of the nerve root by placement of a pin into the vertebral body that deflected the course of the root but no incision of the disk; or (3) incision of the disk and displacement of the nerve root with the vertebral body pin.[13] Only the animals that had both disk incision and root displacement displayed behaviors consistent with pain and radiculopathy.

The picture emerging is that disk herniation-associated radiculopathy is both a biochemical and a mechanical disorder. Several bioactive molecules known to be present in the nucleus pulposus, including interleukins and other inflammatory factors,[14-16] have been purported to be biochemical "sensitizers" capable of making nerve roots susceptible to the mechanical effect of the herniated mass. Tumor necrosis factor-α (TNF-α) has received considerable attention in this regard. In the porcine model, TNF-α caused reductions in nerve conduction velocity similar to those seen with autologous nucleus pulposus, whereas interleukin 1β (IL-1β) and interferon gamma (INF-γ) did not.[17] Furthermore, TNF-α inhibition with infliximab (a monoclonal antibody to TNF-α) blocked the pain behaviors noted above after the performance of disk incision and root displacement in rats.[18] Overall, the roles of TNF-α and other bioactive agents in herniated disk-associated radiculopathy remain poorly undiagnosed.

Epidemiology and Natural History

Various studies have shown that the lifetime prevalence of a major episode of low back pain ranges from 60% to 80%, but only 10% of these episodes are accompanied by sciatica. Sciatica lasting longer than 2 weeks is even less common, with a lifetime prevalence of 1.6%.[19] The highest prevalence (23.7 per 100 persons) is in individuals between the ages of 45 and 64 years.[20] A sedentary lifestyle, frequent driving, chronic cough, pregnancy, smoking, and frequent lifting of heavy objects are considered risk factors.[19,21,22]

It is commonly agreed that lumbar disk herniation has a favorable natural history (that is, the clinical course of the disease without therapeutic intervention). Hakelius[23] examined essentially a natural history cohort, in that the patients were treated with only bed rest and a corset for 2 months, and he observed a marked reduction in pain and improvement in function over time: 80% of the patients had major improvements after 6 weeks; 90%, after 12 weeks; and 93%, after 24 weeks. Other studies have revealed less favorable results in that, although most patients without surgical treatment had improvement, 30% had persistent pain and restrictions at work and leisure activities after 1 year.[24] Most disk herniations diminish in size over time, with 80% decreasing by more than 50% in one study.[25] Larger disk herniations tend to regress more, most likely because of their higher water content. A positive correlation has been noted between regression of lumbar disk herniations and resolution of symptoms,[25,26] and regression is thought to occur as the herniated tissue dehydrates and immunologic responses help to resorb the disk material. In terms of motor function, Hakelius did not find a significant advantage to surgical treatment of patients with stable motor deficits (excluding those with cauda equina syndrome): 45% of such patients had improvement with nonsurgical treatment, and 53% had improvement after surgery.

Evidence Regarding Nonsurgical Treatment

Currently accepted indications for nonsurgical treatment of lumbar disk herniations include the absence of a progressive neurologic deficit or cauda equina syndrome. Thus, nonsurgical treatment is the initial "default" pathway for most patients with lumbar radiculopathy due to disk herniation. It is not clear, however, whether nonsurgical treatment offers improvement over the natural history of the disorder. Although there have been numerous studies of nonsurgical treatments of low back pain, there have been few randomized controlled trials specifically comparing the various nonsurgical regimens (physical therapy, medications, traction, manipulation, immobilization, and spinal injections) with the natural history (no treatment at all). However, predictors of favorable outcomes of nonsurgical care have been reported to include a negative result on the crossed straight leg-raising test, absence of leg pain with spinal extension, absence of stenosis on imaging studies, favorable response to steroids, return of neurologic deficits within 12 weeks, a motivated physically fit patient with more than 12 years of education, no workers' compensation claim, and a normal psychological profile.[27] Nonsurgical treatment of noncontained disk herniations may also have a favorable outcome.[28]

Medications

Commonly used medications for pain associated with lumbar disk herniations include nonsteroidal anti-inflammatory drugs, corticosteroids, muscle relaxants, and opioid pain medications. Nonsteroidal anti-inflammatory drugs have been shown to be helpful for the management of acute low back pain,[29] but a meta-analysis of the literature demonstrated that they had no benefit in the treatment of radiculopathy compared with controls (odds ratio = 0.99).[30] Corticosteroids are administered orally or by injection. Although oral steroids are commonly prescribed in clinical practice, only one study on their use for the treatment of lumbosacral radicular pain was found.[31] In that study, dexamethasone was not superior to a placebo for either early or long-term relief of lumbosacral radicular pain, but it helped patients who had presented with a positive result on the straight leg raising test. The use of intramuscular corticosteroid injections for acute sciatica was examined in two randomized controlled trials. One trial showed no benefit (odds ratio = 0.8),[32] and the other trial showed a modest benefit (odds ratio = 2.0).[33] We are not aware of any randomized clinical trials that tested the effectiveness of opioid analgesics for patients with lumbar disk herniations, although such analgesics are commonly used in clinical practice for the treatment of acute and chronic radiculopathies. Muscle relaxants have been shown to be effective for the treatment of acute low back pain,[34] but we found no data from well-controlled studies of their use for pain associated with lumbar disk herniations. Antiepileptics such as gabapentin and tricyclic antidepressants such as amitriptyline are commonly used to treat the neuropathic pain component associated with lumbar disk herniations. Again, we are not aware of any controlled trials of the use of those medications for patients who have lumbar disk herniation with radiculopathy, but one open, uncontrolled trial of lamotrigine showed a significant improvement in patients with chronic sciatica ($P < 0.05$).[35]

Physical Medicine

When a patient has incapacitating pain, a period of bed rest is often unavoidable. Immobilization presumably diminishes inflammation around an irritated nerve root. However, there are no data to suggest that bed rest alters the natural history of lumbar disk herniations or improves outcomes. Because of the potentially harmful effects of prolonged bed rest, it is best to advise patients to limit bed rest to a short term only and to resume activities as soon as possible.[36] Bracing is another method of immobilizing the lumbar spine, but there is a lack of good evidence to support the use of braces and corsets for patients with lumbar disk herniations. These devices have not been shown to be effective for primary or secondary prevention of low back pain; however, the Cochrane review found "limited" evidence favoring lumbar supports compared with no treatment.[37]

Traction remains of unproven benefit in the treatment of lumbar disk herniations. A meta-analysis of pooled data from four randomized controlled trials showed some benefit of traction therapy compared with a placebo (odds ratio = 1.2).[38] In one controlled trial, traction with physical therapy resulted in a greater reduction in the sizes of disk herniations than did physical therapy alone.[39] Vertebral axial decompression (VAX-D) therapy was developed according to the principles of traction and is popular among chiropractors. One randomized clinical trial, in which one of the authors was the medical director for a VAX-D manufacturer, demonstrated greater than 50% relief of chronic low back pain in 68.4% of patients treated with VAX-D therapy compared with 0% of patients treated with transcutaneous electrical nerve stimulation.[40] However, we are not aware of any studies of VAX-D therapy for patients with isolated lumbar disk herniation. The Cochrane Review in 2005 concluded that "traction is probably not effective" on the basis of the finding that neither continuous nor intermittent traction was more effective for decreasing pain, disability, or work absence than were placebo, sham, or other treatments of patients with low back pain, with or without sciatica.[41]

Physical therapy in general has not been proven to be beneficial for patients with acute low back pain, but it may be helpful for those with chronic low back pain.[42] We are not aware of any randomized trials examining the outcomes of physical therapy alone for the treatment of lumbar radiculopathy. Active exercises are more appropriate than passive modalities, particularly for patients with subacute or chronic pain.[27] Hofstee and associates[43] showed that bed rest and physiotherapy are not more effective for the treatment of acute sciatica than is continuation of activities of daily living. McKenzie therapy is commonly advocated for treatment of lumbar disk herniations. However, in one study on the management of low back pain, there was no difference among the results of McKenzie therapy, manipulation, and providing the patient with an educational booklet.[44] Another common physical therapy technique involves the spectrum of lumbar stabilization exercises. Although randomized trials have not been performed, to our knowledge, outcomes of nonsurgical treatment have been better in studies employing active lumbar stabilization exercises[45] than they were in older controlled trials that used passive treatment modalities.[46]

Acupuncture is another physical medicine modality that might be applied to the treatment of lumbar disk herniations. Although anecdotal stories of success are extant in popular culture, the available literature has not demonstrated the efficacy of acupuncture in treating low back pain.[47] Manipulation and chiropractic are similarly unproven. Burton and associates[48] compared chemonucleolysis with manipulation in the treatment of symptomatic lumbar disk herniations in a controlled trial. After 12 months, there was no significant difference in overall outcome between the treatments, but manipulation did result in a greater decrease in back pain and disability during the first weeks. At a minimum, manipulation is relatively unlikely to cause harm: it has been estimated that less than 1 in 3.7 million treatments with spinal manipulation results in clinical worsening of disk herniation.[49] Other modalities that are commonly used in clinical practice include massage therapy, transcutaneous electrical nerve stimulation, and biofeedback. These methods have not been evaluated for the treatment of lumbar disk herniations and radiculopathy in well-controlled trials. Cognitive behavioral therapy has shown efficacy for the treatment of chronic low back pain,[50] but we are not aware of any studies of its effectiveness for patients with lumbar disk herniation.

Epidural Steroid Injections

Epidural steroid injections have been used for decades for the treatment of spinal pain, particularly radiculopathy. In a review of four older randomized trials, epidural steroid injections were found to be more beneficial than the control treatment, especially with respect to short-term outcomes, for the treatment of acute radiculopathy (odds ratio = 2.2).[38] A more recent study of interlaminar epidural steroid injections demonstrated a transient decrease in sciatic symptoms at 3 weeks but no sustained benefits in

terms of pain relief, function, or avoidance of surgery.[51] Epidural steroid injections also do not appear to change the rate at which lumbar disk herniations regress.[52]

Fluoroscopically guided transforaminal injection techniques, which have the theoretic advantage of delivering the injectate to the site of the disk herniation in the anterior epidural space, have been more commonly used in modern studies. Although the traditional, more dorsal interlaminar approaches may allow the injectate to flow to the site of the lesion by seeping around the thecal sac and into the ventral epidural space, a transforaminal route is presumably more reliable for delivering the steroid to the affected area, where the herniated disk comes into contact with the nerve root. One study showed transforaminal injections to be superior to trigger-point injections, with "successful" outcomes following 84% of the former procedures and 48% of the latter.[53] Other studies have suggested that transforaminal epidural steroid injections may actually change the natural history of radiculopathy by decreasing the need for surgery. In one study of 55 patients with lumbar radiculopathy who were all considered surgical candidates, 71% of those who received a steroid nerve-root injection and 33% of those who received a control injection of local anesthetic only decided not to have surgery.[54] Another study compared pain scores on a visual analog scale and the need for surgery between patients who had received transforaminal steroid injections and those who had received interlaminar epidural steroid injections.[55] The patients treated with the transforaminal injections had a 46% reduction in the pain score, and 10% went on to need surgery. In contrast, the pa-

tients treated with the interlaminar injections had a 19% reduction in the pain score, and 25% required surgery. These findings indicated that the short-term outcomes were better following transforaminal injections.

It is impossible to directly compare the literature on outcomes of surgical diskectomy with reports on outcomes of epidural injections because of the numerous differences in surgical technique (open, "minimally invasive," microdiskectomy, and aggressive disk-space curettage); injection technique (transforaminal or interlaminar, fluoroscopically guided or not); dose, timing, and type of steroid delivered; and patient selection criteria (in many studies, those with severe pain or progressive neurologic deficits were not considered candidates for nonsurgical treatment). In a recent study that provided level I evidence, 100 patients who had had failure of 6 weeks of noninvasive treatment of a disk herniation measuring at least 25% of the cross-sectional area of the spinal canal were randomized to be treated with interlaminar epidural injections or surgical diskectomy.[56] The success rates, which were 92% to 98% in the surgically treated group and 42% to 56% in the group treated with epidural injection, were significantly different. Twenty-seven patients crossed over from the epidural injection group to the surgical group because of persistent pain, but their outcomes were not adversely affected by the delay in surgery because of the trial of the epidural injection. Whether the transforaminal approach would have led to better outcomes of the epidural injections remains unclear, but, on the basis of this study, surgery appears to be more effective than injections, at least in patients with large disk herniations. Although informative, this finding does not change the commonly accepted indications for surgery, as surgery is associated with not only greater benefit but also with higher risk than epidural injections. Data from the United States National Institutes of Health-funded multicenter randomized trial comparing surgical with nonsurgical treatment of lumbar disk herniations, spinal stenosis, and spondylolisthesis (the Spine Patient Outcome Research Trial [SPORT] study) will hopefully provide clearer guidelines when they become available.

Novel Treatments

On the basis of the understanding that the mechanisms underlying herniated disk-associated radiculopathy are both biochemical and mechanical, novel treatments have been developed to attenuate biochemical sensitization of the nerve root by factors within the nucleus pulposus. As mentioned previously, TNF-α appears to play a role in the pathogenesis of radiculopathy associated with disk herniations. In a very small pilot trial in which 10 patients received a single intravenous injection of infliximab (a monoclonal antibody to TNF-α) for treatment of acute sciatica (lasting 2 to 12 weeks) due to disk herniation, 8 patients had no leg pain at 12 months, compared with 43% of a historical control population who had received saline solution nerve root blocks.[57] However, when a subsequent randomized controlled trial was performed by the same authors on the basis of these promising pilot data, they noted no difference in the reduction of leg pain or the need for surgery at 3 months between patients who had received a single dose of infliximab and controls.[58] Other authors reported success with medical ozone injections into the disk and around the nerve root,[59] although the

study lacked a control group treated without ozone. Various percutaneous, intradiskal treatments, such as electrothermal disk decompression, percutaneous disk decompression, and nucleoplasty, have been developed and marketed by manufacturers. However, the efficacy of these methods is yet to be demonstrated in properly controlled trials.

Overview of Nonsurgical Treatment

The available literature indicates that effective nonsurgical treatments of lumbar disk herniations include observation only as the condition has a favorable natural history, and probably epidural steroid injection, at least for short-term relief. Intramuscular injections of steroids may provide some benefit. Nonsteroidal anti-inflammatory drugs are effective for low back pain only, and traction is probably not effective. There are insufficient data to provide recommendations regarding the role of oral steroids, physical therapy, transcutaneous electrical stimulation, corsets, and manual therapy. On the horizon are medications to suppress reactive nerve root inflammation and medications to inhibit cytokine production, which may improve the pharmacologic treatment options for lumbar disk herniations.

Evidence Regarding Surgical Treatment

Despite the facts that more than $90 billion per year is spent on the management of spine conditions and more than seven decades have passed since Mixter and Barr reported on the surgical management of disk herniations, there remains little level I evidence regarding the effectiveness of surgery for symptomatic lumbar disk herniations. Although many retrospective studies have

suggested a benefit, these studies have the common weakness of inadequate design. The lack of level I data leads to widespread uncertainty with regard to the selection of patients for surgery, as reflected in the varied rates of disk excision surgery: there was a nearly twentyfold difference between high and low surgery rate regions in an otherwise controlled population analysis in the United States.[60,61] However, these statements should not be misconstrued as a condemnation of diskectomy surgery. Much to the contrary, under the right circumstances, surgery clearly "works" very well: any surgeon who has seen a patient suffer for months before surgery and then wake up from a diskectomy with immediate relief of leg pain, numbness, and weakness can attest to that fact. Instead, the question that remains unanswered by the available literature is that, given that not every patient has an excellent result from surgery, surgery has the potential for complications, and the natural history of lumbar disk herniation tends to be favorable in most patients, when and in whom should surgery be recommended?

Neurologic Variables

Although one might expect surgery to be superior to nonsurgical care of patients with stable neurologic deficits, this has not been supported by the available literature. Hakelius,[23] Weber,[46] the Maine Lumbar Spine Study,[60] and Saal[27,45] demonstrated that stable radicular weakness resolves equally well regardless of treatment. In a more recent pilot study of 60 patients with stable paresis associated with lumbar disk herniation, Dubourg and associates[62] also found no difference between neurologic recovery following surgical management and that following medical management. This finding is in contrast to the situation for a patient with a progressive neurologic deficit and cauda equina syndrome, for whom, the evidence suggests, urgent decompression provides the best functional improvement.[63]

Surgical Volume

Increased surgical volume has been correlated with improved outcomes of several operations, including joint arthroplasty, cardiac surgery, and cancer surgery, suggesting that a surgeon's experience and skill as well as the hospital's overall experience play important roles in outcomes. Paradoxically, the same may not be true for lumbar diskectomy. The Maine Lumbar Spine Study showed that patients who had surgery in the highest utilization regions actually had worse outcomes than those treated in the lowest utilization area.[64] The authors concluded that these paradoxically inferior results may be related to the application of more stringent criteria for surgery in regions with lower surgical rates and expanded indications beyond what might be considered the standard in the higher rate regions. Thus, patient selection and patient factors may have a greater influence than surgical technique on the results of spine surgery, for which the indications are not as clear-cut as they are for the types of surgery listed above.

Anatomic Features of the Herniation

Although the size of a disk herniation correlates poorly with pain, there is evidence to suggest that other anatomic characteristics of the herniated disk may be predictive of clinical outcome following diskectomy. In one study,[65] patients who had extruded disk fragments with a

largely intact anulus fibrosus and those who had extruded fragments contained within an intact anulus fibrosus had the best postoperative outcome scores and the lowest reherniation rates. The scores were poorer for those who had extruded disk fragments with a massive annular defect as well as for those who had no identifiable fragment within an intact anulus fibrosus. Those with a massive annular defect had the highest rate of reherniation, whereas those without identifiable fragments had a high rate of persistent symptoms postoperatively despite the absence of clear structural abnormalities to account for them. This last group of patients had a clinical profile (for example, with regard to compensation status and psychometric abnormalities) that was similar to that of patients with chronic low back pain: both had pain behavior that was out of proportion to the anatomic pathologic findings.

Contrary to popular opinion, the size of a disk herniation does not appear to correlate with the need for eventual surgical intervention. Natural history studies[27,66-68] have shown that the largest disk herniations actually demonstrate the greatest degree of resorption, whereas contained herniations demonstrate the least. Thus, the disk abnormality that seems to be best suited for surgery—a large extruded fragment—also has the greatest likelihood of natural regression; this means that size cannot be used reliably as a criterion for surgery.

Variations in Surgical Technique

Although various surgical techniques have been used to decompress symptomatic nerves, the data suggest that the choice of surgical technique is less critical to a good

outcome than proponents of various techniques have suggested.[69] To date, there has been no proven difference in outcomes regardless of whether the root is decompressed by means of a traditional ("large incision") laminotomy-diskectomy, an endoscopic diskectomy, or a micro-diskectomy (Figure 2).

The optimal amount of disk that should be removed during surgery is not clear. Although it has been established that the primary goal of surgery is neural decompression, competing considerations remain: too little removal seemingly raises the specter of increased recurrence, whereas too much removal raises concerns about accelerated disk degeneration and increased back pain. The available evidence, based largely on case reports and retrospective studies, suggests no benefit to more aggressive disk removal in terms of recurrence; to the contrary, it may be deleterious with respect to the later development of back pain.[70-73] Lumbar disk herniations recur at about equal rates (approximately 5%) regardless of treatment, and neither surgical intervention nor medical management can prevent reherniation.

Patient Factors Affecting Surgical Outcome

Although traditionally, spinal research has focused on physician-determined outcomes—such as a physician's assessment of relief of symptoms (for example, according to Odom's criteria),[74] radiographic evidence of a successful fusion, and the magnitude of deformity correction—it has become increasingly evident that the most useful measure of a given operation's success is whether the patient perceives it to be successful, regardless of what the physician-determined outcomes

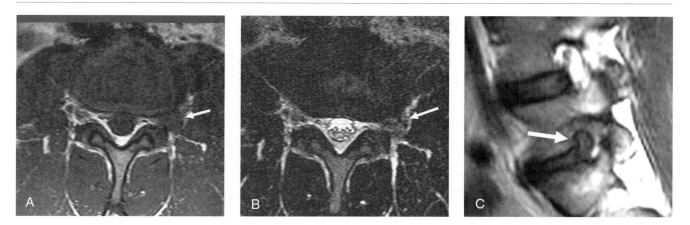

Figure 2   Axial T1-weighted **(A)** and T2-weighted **(B)** MRI scans of a patient with an extraforaminal disk herniation (arrows). This type of herniation is more readily removed by an extraforaminal approach rather than from inside the spinal canal. Extraforaminal herniations are often better seen on T1-weighted images and are more likely to be missed on T2-weighted images. Posterolateral disk herniations, in contrast, are generally well demonstrated on T2-weighted images (see Figure 1). **C,** The sagittal T1-weighted image of a different patient demonstrates that the exiting nerve root is pinned cephalad against the undersurface of the pedicle by the foraminal portion of the disk herniation.

may demonstrate. The patient's perception of successful treatment, in turn, appears to be influenced at least as much by psychosocial and other patient factors as it is by the specific type of disk lesion or the design and execution of a proper operation by the treating surgeon. Patient-reported health surveys, which allow self-evaluation of function, are useful tools for assessing these patient factors preoperatively and postoperatively.[75-77] The health surveys include both condition-specific surveys, such as the Roland-Morris Disability Questionnaire and the Oswestry Disability Index (ODI), and the commonly used general health survey, the Short Form-36 (SF-36).[78-80] Although the outcomes measured by the SF-36 are not specific to the spine, it is useful for measuring the outcomes of spine surgery because spinal disorders have been shown to impart a substantial negative effect on self-reported physical function. As demonstrated in one study by the Physical Component Score (PCS) of the SF-36, spinal stenosis had a greater

negative effect on physical function than all other medical conditions studied with use of the SF-36,[81] including cancer, chronic obstructive pulmonary disease, and congestive heart failure.

Studies of self-reported health surveys have identified several patient factors with significant effects on patient-determined outcomes after spine surgery. In one such study, smoking had a significant negative effect ($P < 0.05$) on self-reported function at baseline as measured by all eight subscales of the SF-36.[82] One year after spinal surgery, smokers did not have significant improvement in the scores on any subscale of the SF-36, whereas their non-smoking counterparts had significantly improved scores on six subscales ($P < 0.05$). In another study, a low education level was an independent predictor of poor self-reported function at baseline as measured with both the condition-specific ODI and the SF-36 general health survey.[83] It was also noted that the major drivers of physical function as measured by the SF-36 and ODI were psychoso-

cial variables rather than traditional medical conditions. In addition to low education level, these other variables included poor self-reported health, work and disability status, legal status, body mass index, and smoking. In a related study, self-reported health was also found to be an independent predictor of functional outcome following surgery.[84] Of 1833 patients who had undergone surgical intervention for lumbar disk herniation, those reporting "good" health and "poor" health both had improvement following surgical intervention. However, there was a significant difference ($P < 0.05$) between the groups with respect to scores on the SF-36 bodily pain and physical function components as well as the ODI scores, with those reporting good health faring better. Other studies have also demonstrated a negative effect of patient factors such as depression, frequent headaches, compensation status, low education level, and unemployment on both the ODI and the PCS of the SF-36.[85]

Taken together, these studies

demonstrate that proper selection of patients for lumbar diskectomy should include a thorough assessment of patient factors as such factors have important effects on function and on the response to treatment independent of the specifics regarding the disk lesion. Identifying these factors can assist providers and patients in decision-making as well as guide reasonable expectations from surgery. In certain patient populations, the effect of low back problems may be a greater reflection of psychosocial distress than anatomic dysfunction, which may explain why the traditional surgical model of treating spinal problems fails in many patients. If patients and surgeons are not aware of this association between patient factors and functional outcome, both may be disappointed with the results.

Medical Comorbidities Affecting Surgical Outcome

The presence of comorbidities also has a significant effect on surgical outcomes. In one study, the presence of four comorbidities was noted to significantly ($P < 0.05$) and independently lower the improvement in the ODI score by almost five points and the improvement in the SF-36 score by more than four points at 1 year after lumbar spine surgery.[86] In another study, of 15,974 patients, obesity had a negative influence on self-reported function, as measured by both the SF-36 and the ODI, and obese patients reported a greater degree of pain than nonobese patients.[87]

Surgical Compared With Nonsurgical Treatment

There is a dearth of level I evidence comparing surgical with nonsurgical management of lumbar disk herniations. In 1983, Weber's classic work, "Lumbar Disc Herniation. A Controlled, Prospective Study with Ten Years of Observation,"[46] included a randomized trial (the first randomized trial in spinal surgery) in which 60 patients had surgery and 66 continued to be treated with conservative measures. Weber found that those treated with surgery had a significantly better result at 1 year postoperatively ($P < 0.05$). At 4 years postoperatively, the surgically treated patients had a trend toward better results, but that difference was not present at 10 years. The surgically treated patients had far fewer relapses than the nonsurgically treated group in the first 4 years. Motor weakness improved equally in both groups, as did sensory dysfunction. Thirty-five percent of the patients, equally distributed in the two groups, had demonstrable sensory dysfunction 10 years after the hospitalization for the herniated lumbar intervertebral disk. Although it was a breakthrough study, it did have flaws. Not all of the patients were randomized: 67 additional patients had "symptoms and signs that beyond doubt required surgical therapy" and 87 others were treated "conservatively as there was no indication for operative intervention." Furthermore, a large number of nonsurgically treated patients crossed over into the surgical group, the study lacked adequate statistical power, the outcome assessment was not blinded, and the outcome measurement was relatively insensitive.[88]

More recently, the Maine Lumbar Spine Study, an observational (nonrandomized) study of 507 patients (with follow-up data available for 400 of them), compared the 10-year results of surgical and nonsurgical treatment.[60] As would be expected with an observational study, the surgically treated patients had had worse baseline symptoms and functional status than the nonsurgically treated patients. Despite that fact, over the 10-year period, the proportion of patients who reported that their low back pain and leg pain were greatly decreased or completely gone was larger in the surgically treated group than in the nonsurgically treated group (56% compared with 40%, $P = 0.006$), and more surgically treated patients than nonsurgically treated patients were satisfied with their current status (71% compared with 56%, $P = 0.002$). The greatest improvement in the surgically treated group occurred in the first 2 years after the operation. There was smaller but continued improvement in both groups through the 10-year period.

Overview of Surgery for Lumbar Disk Herniations

Regardless of treatment, lumbar disk herniations usually have a favorable natural history with improvement over time, but it may take 1 to 2 years for functional improvement to plateau. In the absence of a cauda equina syndrome or progressive weakness, the best indication for surgical management is refractory radicular pain. Surgical decision-making should not be based on the size of the disk herniation, as large extruded herniations tend to resolve more predictably, or on either stable motor weakness or numbness, as the ultimate resolution of weakness and sensory deficits is similar following either nonsurgical or surgical management, although surgery hastens the process. When intractable radicular pain is the strict indication for surgery, surgical intervention provides substantial and more rapid pain relief than does nonsurgical treatment.

The specific method of surgical intervention probably contributes little to the overall success of the intervention as long as the root is properly decompressed.

The treatment should be chosen by the patient—after proper education through a process of shared decision-making—rather than reflect the "surgical signature" of the surgeon. Health surveys can provide additional assessment of psychosocial comorbidities that are not otherwise evident during the usual clinical evaluation. Such comorbidities should be identified preoperatively as they are not likely to resolve with surgical intervention but may have greater impact than the diskal pathoanatomy on the ultimate outcome.

Summary
Both mechanical and biomechanical factors play roles in the development of lumbar radiculopathy with disk herniation. In most instances, symptoms resolve with time. Nonsurgical treatments such as physical therapy, medications, and spinal injections may provide symptom relief, but none have been demonstrated to conclusively alter the natural history of the condition. When pain persists despite time and conservative care, surgical decompression of the nerve root provides predictable relief of radicular leg pain.

References
1. Deyo RA, Tsui-Wu YJ: Descriptive epidemiology of low-back pain and its related medical care in the United States. *Spine* 1987;12:264-268.

2. Taylor VM, Deyo RA, Cherkin DC, Kreuter W: Low back pain hospitalization: Recent United States trends and regional variations. *Spine* 1994;19:1207-1213.

3. Atlas SJ, Deyo RA, Keller RB, et al: The Maine Lumbar Spine Study, Part II: 1-year outcomes of surgical and nonsurgical management of sciatica. *Spine* 1996;21:1777-1786.

4. Kuslich SD, Ulstrom CL, Michael CJ: The tissue origin of low back pain and sciatica: A report of pain response to tissue stimulation during operations on the lumbar spine using local anesthesia. *Orthop Clin North Am* 1991;22:181-187.

5. McCulloch JA, Young PH: Pathophysiology and clinical syndromes in lumbar disc herniation, in McCulloch JA, Young PH (eds): *Essentials of Spinal Microsurgery*. Philadelphia, PA, Lippincott-Raven, 1998, pp 219-247.

6. Mixter WJ, Barr JS: Rupture of the intervertebral disk with involvement of the spinal canal. *N Engl J Med* 1934;211:210-215.

7. Olmarker K, Rydevik B, Holm S, Bagge U: Effects of experimental graded compression on blood flow in spinal nerve roots: A vital microscopic study on the porcine cauda equina. *J Orthop Res* 1989;7:817-823.

8. Olmarker K, Rydevik B, Hansson T, Holm S: Compression-induced changes of the nutritional supply to the porcine cauda equina. *J Spinal Disord* 1990;3:25-29.

9. Rydevik BL, Myers RR, Powell HC: Pressure increase in the dorsal root ganglion following mechanical compression: Closed compartment syndrome in nerve roots. *Spine* 1989;14:574-576.

10. Boden SD, Davis DO, Dina TS, Patronas NJ, Wiesel SW: Abnormal magnetic-resonance scans of the lumbar spine in asymptomatic subjects: A prospective investigation. *J Bone Joint Surg Am* 1990;72:403-408.

11. Smyth MJ, Wright V: Sciatica and the intervertebral disc: An experimental study. *J Bone Joint Surg Am* 1958;40:1401-1418.

12. Olmarker K, Rydevik B, Nordborg C: Autologous nucleus pulposus induces neurophysiologic and histologic changes in porcine cauda equina nerve roots. *Spine* 1993;18:1425-1432.

13. Olmarker K, Larsson K: Tumor necrosis factor alpha and nucleus-pulposus-induced nerve root injury. *Spine* 1998;23:2538-2544.

14. Brisby H, Byrod G, Olmarker K, Miller VM, Aoki Y, Rydevik B: Nitric oxide as a mediator of nucleus pulposus-induced effects on spinal nerve roots. *J Orthop Res* 2000;18:815-820.

15. Kang JD, Georgescu HI, McIntyre-Larkin L, Stefanovic-Racic M, Donaldson WF III, Evans CH: Herniated lumbar intervertebral discs spontaneously produce matrix metalloproteinases, nitric oxide, interleukin-6, and prostaglandin E2. *Spine* 1996;21:271-277.

16. Miyamoto H, Saura R, Doita M, Kurosaka M, Mizuno K: The role of cyclooxygenase-2 in lumbar disc herniation. *Spine* 2002;27:2477-2483.

17. Aoki Y, Rydevik B, Kikuchi S, Olmarker K: Local application of disc-related cytokines on spinal nerve roots. *Spine* 2002;27:1614-1617.

18. Murata Y, Olmarker K, Takahashi I, Takahashi K, Rydevik B: Effects of selective tumor necrosis factor-alpha inhibition to pain-behavioral changes caused by nucleus pulposus-induced damage to the spinal nerve in rats. *Neurosci Lett* 2005;382:148-152.

19. Kelsey JL, White AA III: Epidemiology and impact of low-back pain. *Spine* 1980;5:133-142.

20. Praemer A, Furner S, Rice DP: *Musculoskeletal Conditions in the United States*, ed 2. Rosemont, IL, American Academy of Orthopaedic Surgeons, 1999.

21. Kelsey JL: An epidemiological study of the relationship between occupations and acute herniated lumbar intervertebral discs. *Int J Epidemiol* 1975;4:197-205.

22. Kelsey JL, Githens PB, O'Conner T, et al: Acute prolapsed lumbar intervertebral disc: An epidemiologic study with special reference to driving automobiles and cigarette smoking. *Spine* 1984;9:608-613.

23. Hakelius A: Prognosis in sciatica: A clinical follow-up of surgical and non-surgical treatment. *Acta Orthop Scand Suppl* 1970;129:1-76.

24. Weber H: The natural history of disc herniation and the influence of intervention. *Spine* 1994;19:2234-2238.

25. Saal JA, Saal JS, Herzog RJ: The natural history of lumbar intervertebral disc extrusions treated nonoperatively. *Spine* 1990;15:683-686.

26. Bush K, Cowan N, Katz DE, Gishen P: The natural history of sciatica associated with disc pathology: A prospective study with clinical and independent radiologic follow-up. *Spine* 1992;17:1205-1212.

27. Saal JA: Natural history and nonoperative treatment of lumbar disc herniation. *Spine* 1996;21(24 suppl):2S-9S.

28. Ito T, Takano Y, Yuasa N: Types of lumbar herniated disc and clinical course. *Spine* 2001;26:648-651.

29. van Tulder MW, Scholten RJ, Koes BW, Deyo RA: Nonsteroidal anti-inflammatory drugs for low back pain: A systematic review within the framework of the Cochrane Collaboration Back Review Group. *Spine* 2000;25:2501-2513.

30. Vroomen PC, De Krom MC, Slofstra PD, Knottnerus JA: Conservative treatment of sciatica: A systematic review. *J Spinal Disord* 2000;13:463-469.

31. Haimovic IC, Beresford HR: Dexamethasone is not superior to placebo for treating lumbosacral radicular pain. *Neurology* 1986;36:1593-1594.

32. Porsman O, Friis H: Prolapsed lumbar disc treated with intramuscularly administered dexamethasonephosphate: A prospectively planned, double-blind, controlled clinical trial in 52 patients. *Scand J Rheumatol* 1979;8:142-144.

33. Hofferberth B, Gottschaldt M, Grass H, Buttner K: The usefulness of dexamethasonephosphate in the conservative treatment of lumbar pain: A double-blind study. *Arch Psychiatr Nervenkr* 1982;231:359-367

34. van Tulder MW, Touray T, Furlan AD, Solway S, Bouter LM, Cochrane Back Review Group: Muscle relaxants for nonspecific low back pain: A systematic review within the framework of the Cochrane Collaboration. *Spine* 2003;28:1978-1992.

35. Eisenberg E, Damunni G, Hoffer E, Baum Y, Krivoy N: Lamotrigine for intractable sciatica: Correlation between dose, plasma concentration and analgesia. *Eur J Pain* 2003;7:485-491.

36. Hagen KB, Hilde G, Jamtvedt G, Winnem MF: The Cochrane review of bed rest for acute low back pain and sciatica. *Spine* 2000;25:2932-2939.

37. Van Tulder MW, Jellema P, van Poppel MN, Nachemson AL, Bouter LM: Lumbar supports for prevention and treatment of low back pain. *Cochrane Database Syst Rev* 2000;3:CD001823.

38. Vroomen PC, de Krom MC, Slofstra PD, Knottnerus JA: Conservative treatment of sciatica: a systematic review. *J Spinal Disord* 2000;13:463-469.

39. Ozturk B, Gunduz OH, Ozoran K, Bostanoglu S: Effect of continuous lumbar traction on the size of herniated disc material in lumbar disc herniation. *Rheumatol Int* 2006;26:622-626.

40. Sherry E, Kitchener P, Smart R: A prospective randomized controlled study of VAX-D and TENS for the treatment of chronic low back pain. *Neurol Res* 2001;23:780-784.

41. Clarke JA, van Tulder MW, Blomberg SE, de Vet HC, van der Heijden GJ, Bronfort G: Traction for low-back pain with or without sciatica. *Cochrane Database Syst Rev* 2005;4:CD003010.

42. van Tulder MW, Malmivaara A, Esmail R, Koes BW: Exercise therapy for low back pain. *Cochrane Database Syst Rev* 2000;2:CD000335.

43. Hofstee DJ, Gijtenbeek JM, Hoogland PH, et al: Westeinde sciatica trial: Randomized controlled study of bed rest and physiotherapy for acute sciatica. *J Neurosurg* 2002;96(1 suppl):45-49.

44. Cherkin DC, Deyo RA, Battie M, Street J, Barlow W: A comparison of physical therapy, chiropractic manipulation, and provision of an educational booklet for the treatment of patients with low back pain. *N Engl J Med* 1998;339:1021-1029.

45. Saal JA, Saal JS: Nonoperative treatment of herniated lumbar intervertebral disc with radiculopathy: An outcome study. *Spine* 1989;14:431-437.

46. Weber H: Lumbar disc herniation. A controlled, prospective study with ten years of observation. *Spine* 1983;8:131-140.

47. van Tulder MW, Cherkin DC, Berman B, Lao L, Koes BW: The effectiveness of acupuncture in the management of acute and chronic low back pain: A systematic review within the framework of the Cochrane Collaboration Back Review Group. *Spine* 1999;24:1113-1123.

48. Burton AK, Tillotson KM, Cleary J: Single-blind randomised controlled trial of chemonucleolysis and manipulation in the treatment of symptomatic lumbar disc herniation. *Eur Spine J* 2000;9:202-207.

49. Oliphant D: Safety of spinal manipulation in the treatment of lumbar disk herniations: A systematic review and risk assessment. *J Manipulative Physiol Ther* 2004;27:197-210.

50. van Tulder MW, Ostelo R, Vlaeyen JW, Linton SJ, Morley SJ, Assendelft WJ: Behavioral treatment for chronic low back pain: A systematic review within the framework of the Cochrane Back Review Group. *Spine* 2000;25:2688-2699.

51. Arden NK, Price C, Reading I, et al; WEST Study Group.: A multicentre randomized controlled trial of epidural corticosteroid injections for sciatica: The

WEST study. *Rheumatology (Oxford)* 2005;44:1399-1406.

52. Buttermann GR: Lumbar disc herniation regression after successful epidural steroid injection. *J Spinal Disord Tech* 2002;15:469-476.

53. Vad VB, Bhat AL, Lutz GE, Cammisa F: Transforaminal epidural steroid injections in lumbosacral radiculopathy: A prospective randomized study. *Spine* 2002;27:11-16.

54. Riew KD, Yin Y, Gilula L, et al: The effect of nerve-root injections on the need for operative treatment of lumbar radicular pain: A prospective, randomized, controlled, double-blind study. *J Bone Joint Surg Am* 2000;82:1589-1593.

55. Schaufele M, Hatch L: Interlaminar versus transforaminal epidural injections in the treatment of symptomatic lumbar intervertebral disc herniations. *Arch Phys Med Rehabil* 2002;83:1661.

56. Buttermann GR: Treatment of lumbar disc herniation: epidural steroid injection compared with discectomy: A prospective, randomized study. *J Bone Joint Surg Am* 2004;86:670-679.

57. Korhonen T, Karppinen J, Malmivaara A, et al: Efficacy of infliximab for disc herniation-induced sciatica: One-year follow-up. *Spine* 2004;29:2115-2119.

58. Korhonen T, Karppinen J, Paimela L, et al: The treatment of disc herniation-induced sciatica with infliximab: Results of a randomized, controlled, 3-month follow-up study. *Spine* 2005;30:2724-2728.

59. Andreula CF, Simonetti L, De Santis F, Agati R, Ricci R, Leonardi M: Minimally invasive oxygen-ozone therapy for lumbar disk herniation. *AJNR Am J Neuroradiol* 2003;24:996-1000.

60. Atlas SJ, Keller RB, Wu YA, Deyo RA, Singer DE: Long-term outcomes of surgical and nonsurgical management of sciatica secondary to a lumbar disc herniation: 10 year results from the Maine Lumbar Spine Study. *Spine* 2005;30:927-935.

61. Weinstein JN, Birkmeyer JD: *The Dartmouth Atlas of Musculoskeletal Health Care.* Chicago, IL, American Hospital Association Press, 2000.

62. Dubourg G, Rozenberg S, Fautrel B, et al: A pilot study on the recovery from paresis after lumbar disc herniation. *Spine* 2002;27:1426-1431.

63. Ahn UM, Ahn NU, Buchowski JM, Garrett ES, Sieber AN, Kostuik JP:

Cauda equina syndrome secondary to lumbar disc herniation: A meta-analysis of surgical outcomes. *Spine* 2000;25:1515-1522.

64. Keller RB, Atlas SJ, Singer DE, et al: The Maine Lumbar Spine Study, Part 1: Background and concepts. *Spine* 1996;21:1769-1776.

65. Carragee EJ, Han MY, Suen PW, Kim D: Clinical outcomes after lumbar discectomy for sciatica: The effects of fragment type and anular competence. *J Bone Joint Surg Am* 2003;85:102-108.

66. Bush K, Cowan N, Katz DE, Gishen P: The natural history of sciatica associated with disc pathology: A prospective study with clinical and independent radiologic follow-up. *Spine* 1992;17:1205-1212.

67. Reyentovich A, Abdu WA: Multiple independent, sequential, and spontaneously resolving lumbar intervertebral disc herniations: A case report. *Spine* 2002;27:549-553.

68. Ahn SH, Ahn MW, Byun WM: Effect of the transligamentous extension of lumbar disc herniations on their regression and the clinical outcome of sciatica. *Spine* 2000;25:475-480.

69. Gibson JN, Grant IC, Waddell G: The Cochrane review of surgery for lumbar disc prolapse and degenerative lumbar spondylosis. *Spine* 1999;24:1820-1832.

70. Faulhauer K, Manicke C: Fragment excision versus conventional disc removal in the microsurgical treatment of herniated lumbar disc. *Acta Neurochir (Wien)* 1995;133:107-111.

71. Spengler DM: Lumbar discectomy. Results with limited disc excision and selective foraminotomy. *Spine* 1982;7:604-607.

72. Striffeler H, Groger U, Reulen HJ: "Standard" microsurgical lumbar discectomy vs. "conservative" microsurgical discectomy: A preliminary study. *Acta Neurochir (Wien)* 1991;112:62-64.

73. Balderston RA, Gilyard GG, Jones AA, et al: The treatment of lumbar disc herniation: Simple fragment excision versus disc space curettage. *J Spinal Disord* 1991;4:22-25.

74. Odom GL, Finney W, Woodhall B: Cervical disk lesions. *JAMA* 1958;166:23-28.

75. Nelson EC, Batalden PB, Homa K, et al: Microsystems in health care: Part 2. Creating a rich information environment. *Jt Comm J Qual Saf* 2003;29:5-15.

76. Nelson EC, Batalden PB, Huber TP, et al: Microsystems in health care: Part 1. Learning from high-performing front-line clinical units. *Jt Comm J Qual Improv* 2002;28:472-493.

77. Weinstein JN, Brown PW, Hanscom B, Walsh T, Nelson EC: Designing an ambulatory clinical practice for outcomes improvement: From vision to reality—the Spine Center at Dartmouth-Hitchcock, year one. *Qual Manag Health Care* 2000;8:1-20.

78. Roland M, Morris R: A study of the natural history of back pain. Part I: Development of a reliable and sensitive measure of disability in low-back pain. *Spine* 1983;8:141-144.

79. Fairbank JC, Couper J, Davies JB, O'Brien JP: The Oswestry low back pain questionnaire. *Physiotherapy* 1980;66:271-273.

80. Ware JE Jr: SF-36 health survey update. *Spine* 2000;25:3130-3139.

81. Fanuele JC, Birkmeyer NJ, Abdu WA, Tosteson TD, Weinstein JN: The impact of spinal problems on the health status of patients: Have we underestimated the effect? *Spine* 2000;25:1509-1514.

82. Vogt MT, Hanscom B, Lauerman WC, Kang JD: Influence of smoking on the health status of spinal patients: The National Spine Network database. *Spine* 2002;27:313-319.

83. Abdu WA, Weinstein JN, Hanscom B, Fanuele J: The impact of education on the health status of lumbar spine patients. Read at the Annual Meeting of the North American Spine Society; 2001 Oct 31-Nov 3; Seattle, WA.

84. Abdu W, Mitchell B, Hanscom B, Weinstein J: Self-reported health as a predictor of lumbar surgical outcomes. Read at the Annual Meeting of the International Society for the Study of the Lumbar Spine; 2004 May 30-June 5; Porto, Portugal.

85. Slover J, Abdu WA, Hanscom B, Lurie J, Weinstein JN: Can condition-specific health surveys be specific to spine disease? An analysis of the effect of comorbidities on baseline condition-specific and general health survey scores. *Spine* 2006;31:1265-1271.

86. Slover J, Abdu W, Hanscom B, Lurie J, Weinstein J: The impact of comorbidities on the change in SF-36 and Oswestry scores following lumbar spine surgery. *Spine* 2006;31:1974-1980.

87. Fanuele JC, Abdu WA, Hanscom B, Weinstein JN: Association between obesity and functional status in patients with spine disease. *Spine* 2002;27:306-312.

88. Bessette L, Liang MH, Lew RA, Weinstein JN: Classics in Spine: Surgery literature revisited. *Spine* 1996;21:259-263.

Spondylolisthesis and Spondylolysis

*Serena S. Hu, MD
*Clifford B. Tribus, MD
Mohammad Diab, MD
*Alexander J. Ghanayem, MD

Abstract

Spondylolisthesis is a common condition that can be managed both nonsurgically and surgically. More than 80% of children treated nonsurgically have resolution of symptoms. For those patients requiring surgical treatment, fusion in situ may provide adequate treatment for young patients. Patients with neural compression may require decompression to relieve symptoms, and fusion is also usually indicated. High-grade and degenerative spondylolisthesis require care that is unique to those conditions.

Spondylolysis is a defect in the pars interarticularis that occurs in approximately 5% of the general population. Approximately 15% of individuals with a pars interarticularis lesion have progression to spondylolisthesis.

The term spondylolisthesis refers to slipping, or olisthesis, of a vertebra (spondylos in Greek) relative to an adjacent vertebra. The term spondylolysis refers to dissolution of, or a defect in, the pars interarticularis of a vertebra. To these original terms has been added spondyloptosis, from the Greek "ptosis" (falling off or down) to indicate a vertebra that is completely or essentially completely dislocated.

There are five types of spondylolisthesis: dysplastic, isthmic, degenerative, traumatic, and pathologic.[1] In the dysplastic type, facet joints allow anterior translation of one vertebra on another. Because the neural arch of the olisthetic vertebra is intact, it can compress the cauda equina as it translates. This type accounts for the only reported case of spondylolisthesis at birth.[2] "Isthmic" is from the Greek, meaning "narrow." The isthmic type involves a lesion of the pars interarticularis (the narrow part of bone between the superior and inferior articular processes) (Figure 1). There are three subclasses: type A, which is caused by a stress fracture of the pars interarticularis; type B, an elongation of the pars interarticularis; and type C, which is caused by an acute fracture of the pars interarticularis. Dysplastic and isthmic are the two subtypes found in children, with the latter accounting for approximately 85% of cases.

Degenerative spondylolisthesis is secondary to osteoarthritis leading to facet incompetence and disk degeneration. This condition allows anterior translation of one vertebra on another. Traumatic spondylolisthesis is caused by a fracture of the posterior elements, other than the pars interarticularis, leading to instability and olisthesis. A pathologic spondylolisthesis is caused by a tumor or another primary disease of bone affecting the pars interarticularis or the facet joints and leads to instability and olisthesis.

The dysplastic and isthmic patterns can be classified as congenital, whereas the degenerative, traumatic, and pathologic patterns are considered acquired.[3] The dysplastic type is considered to be high if L5 is abnormal and low if L5 is normal. The low types are higher-grade deformities, with domed-shaped S1 end plates and a trapezoidal L5 vertebral body. The severity of spondylolisthesis is graded on the basis of the percentage of translation of one vertebra relative to the caudal vertebra.[4] Grade I is translation of up to 25%; grade II, 26% to 50%; grade III, 51% to 75%; grade IV, 76% to 100%; and grade V, more than 100% (spondyloptosis). Most cases of spondylolis-

Serena S. Hu, MD or the department with which she is affiliated has received research or institutional support from Medtronic and DePuy. Clifford B. Tribus, MD or the department with which he is affiliated has received research or institutional support from Medtronic and St. Francis; miscellaneous nonincome support, commercially-derived honoraria, or other nonresearch-related funding from Medtronic, Stryker, St. Francis, and Kyphon; royalties from Stryker; holds stock or stock options in St. Francis; and is a consultant or employee for Kyphon and Stryker. Alexander J. Ghanayem, MD or the department with which he is affiliated has received research or institutional support from DePuy, Synthes, and Medtronic.

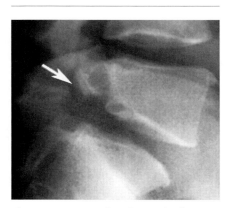

Figure 1 Lateral radiograph showing isthmic spondylolisthesis. The arrow points to the pars interarticularis defect.

thesis (75%) are grade I, and 20% are grade II. A simpler classification system divides spondylolisthesis into cases with translation of 50% or less (stable) and those with translation of more than 50% (unstable).[5]

Pathophysiology
When the lumbar spine extends, the inferior articular process of the cranial vertebra impacts the pars interarticularis of the caudal vertebra.[6,7] Repeated impacts can produce a stress or fatigue fracture of the pars interarticularis. Lumbar hyperextension activities, such as gymnastics and American football, and lumbar hyperextension secondary to spinal deformity, such as Scheuermann disease, are associated with spondylolysis, findings that support the traumatic mechanism.[8-10] This mechanism is consistent with the observation that spondylolysis never has been reported in individuals who cannot walk and the fact that up to 40% of athletes with spondylolysis recall a specific back injury.[11,12] This direct compression by means of a "nutcracker" mechanism is one explanation, but another is that the pars interarticularis fails in tension through a traction mechanism.[13,14]

Which of the two mechanisms is more likely to be present in a given individual is believed to be determined by the lordosis of the spine and the lumbosacral relationship. More recently, reviews of surgical and radiographic findings in patients with high-grade spondylolisthesis as well as biomechanical studies have suggested that abnormalities of the sacral growth plate may be an etiology of high-grade slippage. Yue and associates[15] found that the only constant abnormal anatomic feature in 27 patients treated for spondyloptosis was rounding of the proximal sacral end plate. Biomechanical studies of immature calf spines placed under shear loads showed the growth plate to be the site of failure in all patients.[16] These studies have raised the question of which of these abnormalities, the pars interarticularis defect or the sacral growth plate, is the primary cause of spondylolysis and spondylolisthesis.

Genetics
Family history, gender, and race all are implicated. Spondylolysis occurs in 15% to 70% of first-degree relatives of individuals with the disorder.[17-19] Lysis is two to three times more frequent in boys than girls, but slippage affects girls two to three times more often than boys.[20] The prevalence of spondylolysis is approximately 6% in the white population, a rate that is two to three times higher than that in the black population.[21,22] In the Inuit population, the rate is as high as 25%.[23]

Natural History
The prevalence of a defect in the pars interarticularis is approximately 5% in the general population. Fredrickson and associates[22] started a prospective study of 500 first-grade

children in 1955. The prevalence of spondylolysis was 4.4% at 6 years of age and 6% in adulthood. It was twice as common in males. Pain was not associated with the development of the pars interarticularis defect. Approximately 15% of individuals with a pars interarticularis lesion had progression to a spondylolisthesis. The slip was seen predominantly during the growth spurt, with minimal change after age 16 years. Progression to a slip did not cause pain. After these individuals had been followed for 45 years, 30 had a pars interarticularis defect (22 of the 30 individuals had final lumbar radiographs).[24] No slip was greater than 40%. Slip progression also appeared to slow with each decade and, of particular note, the results from a back pain questionnaire and a Medical Outcomes Study 36-Item Short Form survey were no different from those for an age-matched general population control group.

Patients with low dysplastic spondylolisthesis have a lower prevalence of progression than those with high dysplastic spondylolisthesis. Patients with higher grades of spondylolisthesis and higher slip angles, a measure of lumbosacral kyphosis, have a higher risk of progression.[25-27] Low-grade isthmic spondylolisthesis can progress in an adult, but the progression is believed to be secondary to progressive degeneration of the L5-S1 intervertebral disk.[28]

Clinical Presentation
In most children with back pain (75%), the cause is idiopathic or so-called overuse.[29,30] The most common identifiable cause of back pain in a child is spondylolysis. The child typically describes a history of activity-related pain, and 40% recall a specific traumatic event.[12]

The child may have lumbar hyperlordosis, which may be the cause of the spondylolysis, or lumbar flattening if he or she has severe pain or a high-grade spondylolisthesis. A high-grade spondylolysis in a child is characterized by a palpable lumbosacral step-off as well as lumbosacral kyphosis with a retroverted sacrum that results in a heart-shaped buttocks. Hyperextension of the lumbar spine may cause pain, particularly during single-limb stance. Hamstring contracture is common, although its mechanism is unknown, but it resolves with spinal fusion. In severe cases, the child has a gait disturbance characterized by crouching, a short stride length, and an incomplete swing phase, as described by Phalen and Dickson.[31]

The child may have a radiculopathy that manifests as changes in sensation, a motor deficit, or tension signs distinct from the hamstring contracture. When a child has high-grade olisthesis (translation of > 50%), a rectal examination should be performed. An abnormal finding suggests compromise of the sacral roots. The importance of this finding is highlighted by reports of cauda equina syndrome after surgery, presumably caused by the loss of reflex protection under anesthesia, which makes the patient more vulnerable to nerve root injury.[32-34]

Scoliosis may be associated with spondylolysis.[35] When the scoliosis is caused by pain, the scoliosis usually resolves spontaneously following successful treatment of the spondylolysis.

When an adult with low-grade isthmic spondylolisthesis seeks medical attention, pain, usually lower limb pain, is invariably the chief symptom.[36] It is important to correlate the pain pattern with the findings of the diagnostic work up, because adults may have other spinal disease that is causing the pain.

Imaging

Radiography

Collimated lateral and angled (according to the inclination of the L5-S1 intervertebral disk) AP radiographs of the lumbosacral spine reduce parallax and provide the best detail.[27,28,31] Oblique lumbar views highlight the "Scotty dog," the ear of which is the superior articular process, the eye is the pedicle, the nose is the transverse process, the neck is the pars interarticularis, and the front limb is the inferior articular process. Spondylolysis is seen as a broken neck or a collar (Figure 2). Full-length radiographs of the spine are essential to determine spinal balance, especially in the sagittal plane, and to evaluate for associated deformity. Flexion and extension lateral radiographs help to determine how much postural reduction of the lumbosacral angulation and translation can be obtained.

The degree of slip, slip angle, sacral inclination, chronicity of the slip, and pelvic incidence are all seen on the lateral radiograph.[13,14,37-39] The degree of slip is the percentage of displacement, with a slip of more than 50% considered unstable and associated with progression and lumbosacral kyphosis. The slip angle is the angle between a perpendicular drawn along the posterior aspect of the sacrum and a line drawn along the inferior end plate of L5, and a positive value is defined as lumbosacral lordosis. The sacral inclination is the angle between the posterior aspect of the sacrum and the vertical, and a value of more than 60° is associated with progression. The chronicity of the slip is reflected by blunting of the osseous margins; a trapezoidal L5 and a

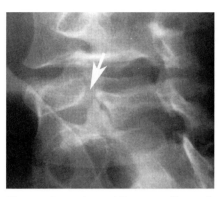

Figure 2 An oblique radiograph showing a "collar" (*arrow*), or "broken neck," of the "Scotty dog." The nose of the Scotty dog is the transverse process, the eye is the pedicle, the neck is the pars interarticularis, the ear is the superior articular facet, the front leg is the inferior articular facet, and the body is the lamina.

domed shape or rounding of the superior end plate of S1 indicates long-standing alterations. The pelvic incidence is the angle between a line drawn between the center of the femoral head to the midpoint of the sacral end plate and a line perpendicular to the center of the sacral end plate; it is increased in patients with spondylolisthesis, and it correlates with the slip angle.[13,14] There is controversy about the relevance of this measurement.[40-42]

Single-Photon Emission CT

Tomography of a scintigram enables localization of the signal to the posterior vertebral elements, specifically the pars interarticularis.[43] In addition to facilitating a diagnosis, the study may aid in the treatment of spondylolysis. Increased signal intensity suggests osseous activity and healing potential, whereas absence of an increased signal suggests a nonunion and diminished healing potential.[44]

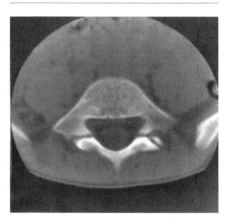

Figure 3 CT scan showing a right pars interarticularis defect.

Computed Tomography

CT scans may play several roles.[45-47] When the pars interarticularis appears normal on the CT scan but there is increased activity on the single-photon emission CT scan, a stress response, or "prelysis" defect, is the diagnosis. This is akin to the "preslip" condition in slipped capital femoral epiphysis. Prelysis may be evaluated further with MRI. On the other hand, when the pars interarticularis is seen to have a defect on the CT scan and there is no increased activity on the single-photon emission CT scan, the patient probably has a nonunion with little healing potential. CT scans are also excellent for the follow-up evaluation of healing, to rule out another lesion (such as osteoid osteoma) when there is an atypical presentation, and for surgical planning in patients with dysplastic vertebrae or associated anomalies (Figure 3).

Magnetic Resonance Imaging

MRI is useful to evaluate an atypical presentation, including prelysis, when the CT scan shows normal findings.[48] MRI is indicated for patients with high-grade spondylolisthesis and for those with a radiculopathy.[49,50]

Medical Treatment

Activity modification, including cessation of inciting sports activities, and nonsteroidal anti-inflammatory agents are combined with an exercise regimen aimed principally at the reduction of lumbar lordosis as well as the treatment of hip flexion and hamstring contracture.[51] This is sufficient for a child in whom it alleviates symptoms or reduces them to an acceptable level. The child should be evaluated annually through maturity because of the risk of progression during adolescent growth acceleration.[52]

Physical therapy should be the first line of treatment for adults with symptoms from spondylolisthesis. Hamstring stretching, trunk strengthening, and avoidance of inciting activities are beneficial for adults. Steroid injections, at the nerve root and/or the pars interarticularis, can be both diagnostic and therapeutic in adults.

The key role of spinal orthotics in the treatment of spondylolysis is reduction of the lumbar lordosis. The orthotic device is typically molded at 15° of flexion of the lumbar spine.[53,54] It is indicated for a child with unacceptable symptoms and for one with positive findings on a single-photon emission CT scan, which suggests healing potential. The typical recommendation is 3 months of full-time wear (more than 20 hours per day) with no sports activities followed by 3 months of full-time wear with sports activities allowed.[55] The patient is evaluated at the conclusion of each phase, principally to confirm that the pain has been alleviated. If the pain persists, surgical intervention should be considered.

Nonsurgical Management

More than 80% of children treated nonsurgically have resolution of symptoms. There is no consensus in the literature on the healing rate of spondylolysis, but it has been estimated that 75% to 100% of acute lesions heal, all unilateral acute lesions heal, 50% of bilateral acute lesions heal, but no chronic defects heal. There is an intermediate defect, with MRI findings only, that has a variable healing rate.[48] Cephalad lumbar defects heal more often than do L5 lesions. Even with these numbers, most children (≥ 90%) return to their previous levels of activity.[56] This suggests that the stability of a fibrous union can be acceptable.

Surgical Options

An L5-S1 in situ fusion with an autogenous posterior iliac crest bone graft is the standard of care for patients with a symptomatic L5 spondylolysis.[57-60] Instrumentation is not necessary because the spine is inherently stable. The procedure may be performed through a midline approach or a paraspinous muscle-splitting approach.[61] The former approach has the advantages of familiarity to surgeons and a greater surface area for fusion, whereas the latter approach is associated with less blood loss and preserves the soft-tissue stabilizers. Postoperative protocols vary widely, from no immobilization to the use of a lumbosacral orthotic with unilateral hip immobilization. We are not aware of any data supporting the efficacy of one bracing protocol over another, but we prefer to use at least a lightweight rigid brace for most patients, with a greater degree of immobilization for younger patients who have a greater slip and a lesser degree of immobilization for older adolescents or young adults with a lesser degree of slip.

A repair of the pars interarticularis is recommended for adolescents and young adults with L4 or

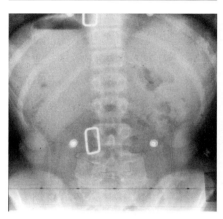

Figure 4 AP plain radiograph made after a bilateral lateral fusion to treat a spondylolysis between L5 and L6.

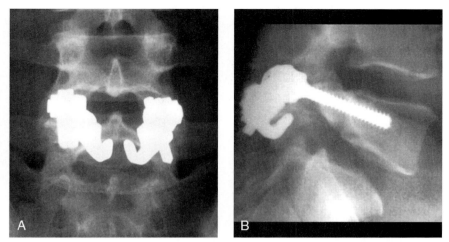

Figure 5 AP **(A)** and lateral **(B)** radiographs made following internal fixation of a pars interarticularis defect.

more cephalad spondylolysis and a normal intervertebral disk. The transverse process, which may serve as an anchor site or a site for fusion, is sufficiently large compared with a relatively small L5 transverse process (Figure 4). In addition, loss of motion from a fusion cephalad to L4 is more relevant clinically than a loss between L5 and S1. Instrumentation techniques include placement of a screw across the lytic defect in the pars interarticularis, placement of a wire between the transverse process and the spinous process, or attachment of a pedicle screw to the spinous process with a rod and hook or a wire[62-68] (Figure 5).

Kakiuchi[66] reported on 16 patients treated with bilateral L5 transpedicular fixation with rod and sublaminar hook fixation. Preoperatively, the patients had persistent pain and a positive response to lidocaine infiltrated into the pars interarticularis defect. Thirteen patients reported having no back pain after healing, and the other three had only occasional back pain without limitations in their activity.

In adults with a potentially reparable pars interarticularis defect, it is important to establish that the defect

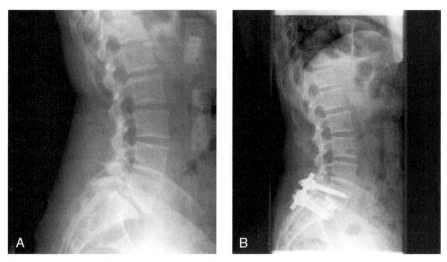

Figure 6 An adult with severe lower limb pain secondary to spondylolisthesis and a herniated disk at L5-S1. **A,** Preoperative lateral radiograph. **B,** Postoperative lateral radiograph made after posterior spinal fusion with transforaminal interbody fusion performed because removal of the herniated disk had increased the instability of the spine.

is the source of pain.[69] Pain relief after a lidocaine injection at the pars interarticularis supports the concept that the defect is the cause of the pain. When the L5-S1 intervertebral disk appears normal on an MRI scan and there is minimal dynamic instability, a pars interarticularis repair can be considered. The most com-

mon technique is excision of the nonunion site, placement of a pedicle screw, bone grafting, placement of a sublaminar hook with connection of each hook by means of a rod to the ipsilateral pedicle screw (Figure 6).

Surgical decompression is indicated when the patient has neural

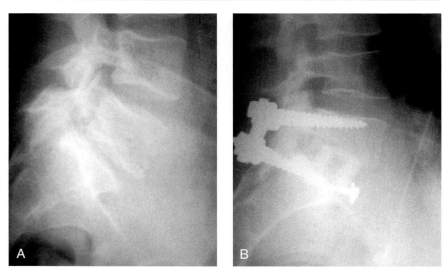

Figure 7   A patient with spondylolisthesis and a degenerated disk between L5 and S1. **A,** Preoperative lateral radiograph. **B,** Postoperative radiograph. Stability has been obtained with posterior instrumentation, and the disk height has been restored with a bone graft placed from an anterior approach.

compromise, with a radiculopathy or bowel or bladder dysfunction.[34,70,71] Decompression must be wide and bilateral with removal of the loose lamina (a Gill procedure) and a foraminotomy, possibly including a facetectomy. Decompression increases the rate of pseudarthrosis and increases instability, which can result in progression of deformity if instrumentation is not used.[72] In the literature, there is both support for and advice against concomitant decompression and fusion for patients with spondylolisthesis.[70-76] Decompression with instrumentation at the time of fusion if there is any lower-limb pain or neural compression.

Carragee[72] enrolled 46 adults with symptomatic low-grade isthmic spondylolisthesis into a randomized prospective study to evaluate the effect of decompression. All smokers were treated with transpedicular instrumentation, whereas the non-smokers had no instrumentation. Patients were randomized with regard to whether or not they underwent a formal decompression. Only one of the 24 patients without decompression had an unsatisfactory result. Obtaining fusion was more important than the decompression, and use of instrumentation was found to improve the fusion rate.

Instrumentation

The use of instrumentation in the treatment of low-grade isthmic spondylolisthesis in adults increased with the widespread use of pedicle screws and the belief that a fusion is necessary to obtain a good result. Transpedicular fixation increases the rate of fusion, and there is a positive correlation between successful fusion and clinical outcome.[77-83] On the other hand, it was found that instrumentation offered no advantage when a comparison was made between patients treated with in situ fusion with transpedicular fixation and those treated with in situ fusion without transpedicular fixation.[84,85] Furthermore, the patients who were treated with instrumentation had

greater blood loss and a longer surgical time.[84,85] Therefore, an in situ arthrodesis without instrumentation remains a reasonable option, particularly in patients with osteoporotic bone. Despite this, and because of better fusion rates and at least a suggestion of better outcomes with a solid fusion, we recommend instrumentation with transpedicular fixation, especially when a decompression is done.

Interbody Fusion

There are several theoretic advantages to adding anterior column support to the standard posterolateral fusion. These include providing a larger surface area for bone graft incorporation, placing the bone graft under compression, obtaining an indirect reduction of foraminal stenosis by using the graft to restore the height of the intervertebral disk, improving lumbar lordosis, and ablating the degenerated disk (a potential source of pain) (Figure 7). The interbody device or bone graft may be placed through a transforaminal lumbar interbody fusion approach or a posterolateral approach. The disadvantages of performing the interbody fusion through a posterolateral approach are the additional surgical time compared with that needed for posterior-only surgery and the risk of injury to the neural elements with the retraction required for disk excision and placement of the interbody device.[86-90]

The interbody fusion can be done through an anterior approach without a posterior fusion. This is called an anterior lumbar interbody fusion. Proponents of this approach prefer it because it provides the same treatment advantages of the interbody fusion while avoiding disruption of the posterior paraspinal muscles and the exposure of the neural elements.[91-93] An anterior-only interbody fusion in a patient with spondylolisthesis must achieve inherent stability or it will displace. One of the authors (CBT) had encouraging results in a small group of patients after using an anterior plate and an interbody component to fuse the site of an isthmic spondylolisthesis with an anterior-only approach. The anterior approach adds the risk of retrograde ejaculation in males and vascular complications. Aunoble and associates[92] reported successful outcomes of anterior lumbar interbody fusion in a series of 20 patients.

Combining both posterior and anterior approaches in the treatment of low-grade isthmic spondylolisthesis in an adult has both advantages and disadvantages compared with the single approaches. The anterior approach allows better reduction of the deformity than is possible with the posterior approach, whereas the posterior approach allows a direct decompression of compressed nerve roots, and transpedicular fixation increases the rigidity of the construct. The combined approach addresses the pars interarticularis defect, foraminal stenosis, degenerative disk disease, a "loose lamina," and dynamic instability. The disadvantage is that this technique requires two separate procedures, with increased surgical time and morbidity. In a prospective study, patients who had undergone the combined approach had better outcome measures in all categories at 6 and 12 months postoperatively compared with patients treated with posterior fusion only.[94] The differences were less pronounced at 2 years.

The treatment approach for a high-grade spondylolisthesis should differ from that for a low-grade spondylolisthesis (Figure 8). The

management of patients with more than 50% slippage (grade III or higher) or lumbosacral kyphosis is more complex. High-grade spondylolisthesis can be associated with dysplastic L5-S1 facets without a pars interarticularis defect and therefore is more likely to cause severe stenosis. With the displacement of the vertebral body, the posterior lamina is pulled forward rather than remaining posteriorly (separated from the vertebral body), as occurs if there is a pars interarticularis defect. Although the preferred surgical treatment is fusion in situ, that procedure is associated with a higher rate of slip progression, pseudarthrosis, neurologic injury, and, if instrumentation is used, failure of the hardware even in young patients.[95-98]

Even without reduction, management of a high-grade spondylolisthesis presents risks.[32,34] The management of an adult with a high-grade spondylolisthesis should start with nonsurgical methods that include physical therapy and epidural steroids. A child with a high-grade spondylolisthesis or an adult who does not respond to nonsurgical care should have surgical stabilization. An in situ fusion can be successful in many young patients. Because these patients often have a dysplastic L5 transverse process and an L5-S1 fusion would place the fusion bed under tension, inclusion of L4 is generally required to achieve a successful fusion. A paramedian Wiltse approach is preferred to maintain the integrity of the midline structures. An external brace is usually applied until the fusion site heals. Patients followed over the long term after an in situ fusion generally have good function and pain relief, although the surgery does not affect their appearance.[99,100] Although the ham-

string tightness that many of these patients exhibit is suspected to be related to neurologic compression, it usually resolves without decompression when a successful fusion has been achieved. This may take up to 18 months, however, and some authors believe that a subtle gait abnormality persists.[59]

Reduction of high-grade spondylolisthesis has become more common, probably because of the availability of smaller implants, which are needed in these patients, as well as the higher prevalence of unsuccessful fusion in patients with high-grade spondylolisthesis.[100] A patient who is considered for a reduction of a spondylolisthesis should have substantial angulation of L5 over S1 (a slip angle of > 45°, lumbosacral kyphosis, or an inability to stand upright with the head balanced over the pelvis), require a decompression, have demonstrated progression of the slip angle, have demonstrated progression after an attempted fusion, or have an unacceptable clinical appearance. It is important that the patient and his or her family understand and accept the risks associated with a reduction.

Reduction can be done with external cast techniques, particularly in very young patients in whom pedicle screw fixation may not be possible.[101] The reduction is performed after the bone graft is placed and the wound is closed. The patient is placed on a spica table or Stryker frame and should be awake so that he or she can report any neurologic changes. A padded support is placed over the sacrum, and the spine is allowed to extend to reduce the lumbosacral kyphosis. The trunk and at least one thigh are then incorporated into a spica cast. A brace with a thigh extension can be used when early healing is apparent on radiographs, usually at 6 to 12 weeks.

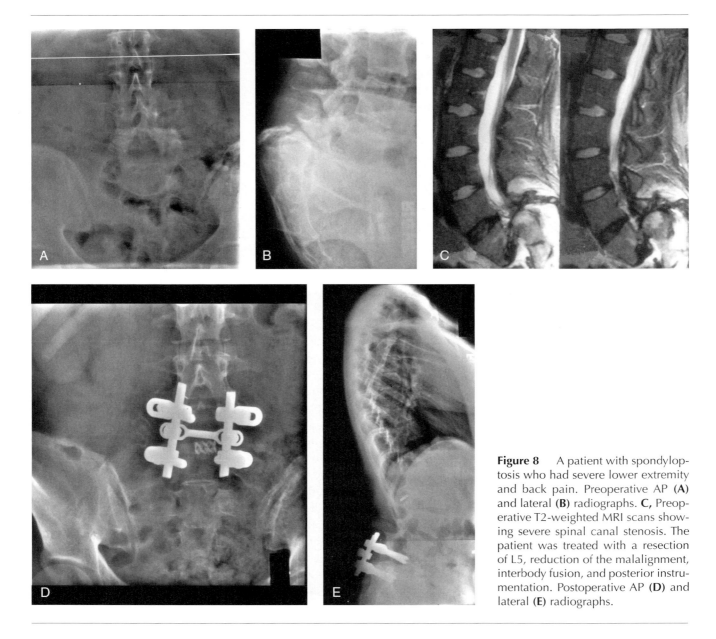

Figure 8 A patient with spondyloptosis who had severe lower extremity and back pain. Preoperative AP (**A**) and lateral (**B**) radiographs. **C,** Preoperative T2-weighted MRI scans showing severe spinal canal stenosis. The patient was treated with a resection of L5, reduction of the malalignment, interbody fusion, and posterior instrumentation. Postoperative AP (**D**) and lateral (**E**) radiographs.

Open reduction with instrumentation is used for patients who require a decompression or for whom a fusion attempt without instrumentation has failed, with progression of the slip. A wide surgical decompression is performed, with care taken to adequately decompress the nerve roots (usually L5). A temporary distraction rod is applied from L3 to the sacrum, usually with temporary hooks. Pedicle screws are then placed in L4 and L5, and sacral screws are directed to the sacral promontory, where maximal purchase in the sacrum is achieved, or the sacral screws can be drilled through the sacrum into L5. Neurophysiologic monitoring is advised. We have found that it helps to monitor several muscle groups, both motor and sensory, as well as electromyographic activity and sphincter activity. Removal of the L5-S1 disk and/or osteotomy of the sacral dome can be done to improve the reduction. The reduction maneuvers of distraction and translation should be performed slowly. The final millimeters of translation and the final degrees of angular reduction are the most risky, and partial reduction is an option.[102] Care should be taken during the reduction, not only because of the neurologic risk but also because of the risk of pedicle screw pullout. This is particularly true for the caudal fixation. Transsacral screws, iliac screws, and Jackson intrasacral buttress rods have all been used to improve the strength of the caudal fixation with varying degrees of success. Once correction has been achieved, a decision regarding whether to perform an interbody fusion is made. A standard interbody cage filled with bone or a transsacral fibular graft provides additional stability during the posterior approach.[103-105] An alternative surgical option is combined anterior and posterior fusion, with the anterior fusion done first to release the anterior structures and thus make the reduction and placement of the interbody spacer easier.[106,107]

The long-term results of the different treatment options for high-grade spondylolisthesis are relatively good. In one study of 67 children and adolescents, the results of posterolateral, anterior, and circumferential fusion were compared at an average of 17 years postoperatively, and the best clinical outcome, as measured with the Oswestry Disability Index, was found after circumferential fusion.[108] A review of the results of posterolateral decompression and fusion with transsacral placement of a fibular graft in 14 patients demonstrated complete neurologic recovery in patients in whom neurologic deficits had developed after surgery, and incorporation of the fibular graft and achievement of a solid fusion in all but one of the patients.[105] In a similar series, one patient was not satisfied with the cosmetic result and one patient had a nonunion and continued back pain.[109] The results after reduction of high-grade spondylolisthesis are generally good.[103,110-113]

When a patient has complete spondyloptosis, particularly with L5

below the level of the sacral end plate, resection of L5 and reduction of L4 onto the sacrum, through a combined anterior and posterior approach (the Gaines procedure), can be considered.[114] Although this is a spine-shortening procedure and thus intended to be associated with decreased neurologic injury in this particularly high-risk patient group, the rate of neurologic injury was 76% in Gaines' original series;[114] however, only 2 of the 30 patients in that series required lower-extremity bracing at the time of long-term follow-up.[115]

Degenerative Spondylolisthesis

Unlike isthmic spondylolisthesis, degenerative spondylolisthesis occurs most often (in 85% of patients) at L4-L5. The L3-L4 level is the next most common level (Figure 9), with L5-S1 rarely being involved. Degenerative spondylolisthesis is most common in the sixth decade of life and is more common in females than in males (a ratio of 6:1).

The pathophysiology of this type of spondylolisthesis has been postulated to be a combination of disk and facet joint degeneration. Patients with degenerative spondylolisthesis have more sagittally oriented facet joints than do patients without degenerative spondylolisthesis; however, it is unclear whether the facet orientation is a primary cause or a secondary effect.[116,117] The slip rarely progresses beyond grade I.

Patients usually present with neurogenic claudication or radicular symptoms from the spinal stenosis, and some patients recount a long history of back pain prior to the development of lower extremity symptoms. Evaluation of a patient with degenerative spondylolisthesis is similar to that of any patient with a

back condition, with a careful neurologic examination and evaluation of the spine, including the patient's stance and sagittal balance. Vascular insufficiency and peripheral neuropathy need to be considered as alternative causes of the symptoms. Patients whose symptoms do not correspond to the level of the stenosis should have a complete neurologic work-up or electromyographic studies. Patients who do not have palpable peripheral pulses, do not have relief of pain with sitting, or do not need to sit to relieve the claudication are more likely to have vascular insufficiency. Spinal tumors, infection, and nonspinal etiologies also need to be considered. As is the case with isthmic spondylolisthesis, upright radiographs are necessary to determine the degree of degenerative spondylolisthesis.[118] MRI scans are ideal for assessing the severity of spinal canal and foraminal narrowing.

Conservative management may help many patients with symptoms of degenerative spondylolisthesis. Nonsteroidal anti-inflammatory medications, physical therapy, and cardiovascular conditioning, as well as alternative treatments such as acupuncture, may relieve symptoms to the point where surgery is not necessary. Patients with substantial radicular or claudication symptoms often benefit from epidural steroid injections or selective nerve root blocks.

Surgical management is offered when nonsurgical options have not adequately relieved symptoms. Although both nonsurgical and surgical treatment can substantially decrease symptoms, surgery seems to provide faster and greater improvement for patients with severe symptoms and associated severe stenosis.[119] The most common surgical treatment options are a limited decompression (laminoforaminotomy

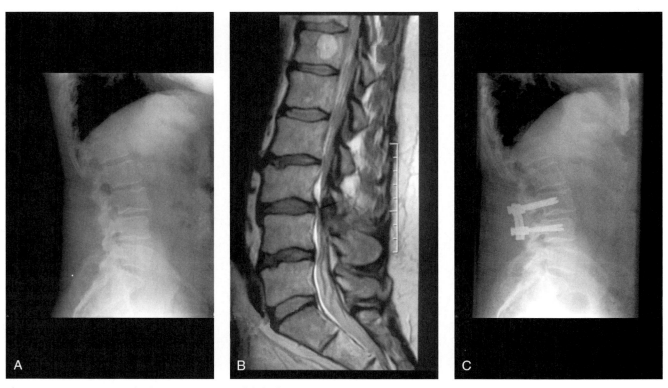

Figure 9 A patient with degenerative spondylolisthesis at L3-L4 and severe lower extremity and low back pain refractory to conservative treatment. **A,** Preoperative lateral radiograph. **B,** Preoperative T2-weighted sagittal MRI scan showing moderately severe stenosis at L3-L4. **C,** Postoperative lateral radiograph.

or interlaminar decompression), laminectomy, or laminotomy with fusion (with or without instrumentation). The severity of the stenosis and where it is located (foraminal, lateral recess, central, or, most commonly, a combination of these sites) determine the extent of decompression required and, therefore, the likelihood of slip progression without fusion. A limited decompression may be considered for patients who have unilateral disease without evidence of motion on flexion-extension radiographs.[120] At least 50% of the facet joints and the interspinous ligaments need to be preserved during the decompression to maintain inherent stability.

Most patients who undergo surgery should have a laminectomy and fusion. Studies have shown that patients who have a laminectomy and

fusion do significantly better than patients who have a laminectomy alone.[121-125] Short-term follow-up did not show an advantage to using instruments with the fusion, which increased the prevalence of complications. However, longer follow-up showed that patients did better if a fusion had been achieved, and fusion was achieved more reliably with internal fixation. Patients with substantial comorbidities or with osteoporosis and/or substantial disk space narrowing may be better treated by fusion without internal fixation. Most symptomatic patients with degenerative spondylolisthesis who are in reasonable health and for whom nonsurgical treatment has failed should have a laminectomy and fusion with instrumentation. Such an approach has resulted in a

high fusion rate and excellent clinical success.[124,126]

To improve the fusion rate and patient outcomes, some surgeons are including interbody fusion in their surgical approach. Posterior-based transforaminal interbody fusion or posterolateral interbody fusion may improve restoration of disk and foraminal height.[127,128] However, to our knowledge there are no published studies that demonstrate improved outcomes with the addition of posterior-based transforaminal interbody fusion or posterolateral interbody fusion to the surgical procedure in patients with degenerative spondylolisthesis.

Currently, motion-preservation and nonfusion devices are receiving tremendous attention in the lay press. While early, preclinical investigational device exemption studies have shown favorable results,[129,130] the use of these devices in patients with degenerative spondylolisthesis has yet to be validated in independent, randomized prospective studies. Because of the selection criteria used in the preclinical studies, only a small number of cases of degenerative spondylolisthesis were included.

Summary

Spondylolisthesis is a common condition and most patients are successfully treated without surgery. Patients for whom surgery is indicated usually have good outcomes. Young patients may require only a fusion in situ; however, patients who have evidence of neural compression may need a decompression to relieve symptoms, and fusion is usually also indicated in these patients. Additional adjuncts have been proposed to improve outcomes, but there are few randomized, prospective trials to demonstrate superiority of one technique over another.

References

1. Wiltse LL, Newman PH, MacNab I: Classification of spondylolysis and spondylolisthesis. *Clin Orthop Relat Res* 1976;117:23-29.

2. Borkow SE, Kleiger B: Spondylolisthesis in the newborn. A case report. *Clin Orthop Relat Res* 1971;81:73-76.

3. Marchetti PG, Bartolozzi P: Classification of spondylolisthesis as a guideline for treatment, in Bridwell KH, DeWald RL (eds): *The Textbook of Spinal Surgery*, ed 2. Philadelphia, PA, Lippincott-Raven, 1997, p 1212.

4. Meyerding H: Spondylolisthesis. *Surg Gynecol Obstet* 1932;54:371-377.

5. Taillard WF: Les spondylolisthesis chez l'enfant et l'adolescent. (Etude de 50 cas). *Acta Orthop Scand* 1955;24: 115-144.

6. Farfan HF, Osteria V, Lamy C: The mechanical etiology of spondylolysis and spondylolisthesis. *Clin Orthop Relat Res* 1976;117:40-55.

7. Wiltse LL, Widell EH Jr, Jackson DW: Fatigue fracture: The basic lesion in isthmic spondylolisthesis. *J Bone Joint Surg Am* 1975;57:17-22.

8. Ferguson RJ, McMaster JH, Stanitski CL: Low back pain in college football linemen. *J Sports Med* 1974;2: 63-69.

9. Jackson DW, Wiltse LL, Cirincoine RJ: Spondylolysis in the female gymnast. *Clin Orthop Relat Res* 1976; 117:68-73.

10. Ogilvie JW, Sherman J: Spondylolysis in Scheuermann's disease. *Spine* 1987;12:251-253.

11. Rosenberg NJ, Bargar WL, Friedman B: The incidence of spondylolysis and spondylolisthesis in nonambulatory patients. *Spine* 1981;6: 35-38.

12. el Rassi G, Takemitsu M, Woratanarat P, Shah SA: Lumbar spondylolysis in pediatric and adolescent soccer players. *Am J Sports Med* 2005;33: 1688-1693.

13. Labelle H, Roussouly P, Berthonnaud E, Dimnet J, O'Brien M: The importance of spino-pelvic balance in L5-S1 developmental spondylolisthesis: A review of pertinent radiologic measurements. *Spine* 2005; 30(suppl 6):S27-S34.

14. Labelle H, Roussouly P, Berthonnaud E, et al: Spondylolisthesis, pelvic incidence, and spinopelvic balance: A correlation study. *Spine* 2004; 29:2049-2054.

15. Yue WM, Brodner W, Gaines RW: Abnormal spinal anatomy in 27 cases of surgically corrected spondyloptosis: Proximal sacral endplate damage as a possible cause of spondyloptosis. *Spine* 2005;30(6 suppl):S22-S26.

16. Kajiura K, Katoh S, Sairyo K, Ikata T, Goel VK, Murakami RI: Slippage mechanism of pediatric spondylolysis: Biomechanical study using immature calf spines. *Spine* 2001;26:2208-2213.

17. Albanese M, Pizzutillo PD: Family study of spondylolysis and spondylolisthesis. *J Pediatr Orthop* 1982;2: 496-499.

18. Friberg S: Studies on spondylolisthesis. *Acta Chir Scand* 1939;(suppl):55.

19. Wynne-Davies R, Scott JH: Inheritance and spondylolisthesis: A radiographic family survey. *J Bone Joint Surg Br* 1979;61:301-305.

20. Roche MB, Rowe GG: The incidence of separate neural arch and coincident bone variations: A summary. *J Bone Joint Surg Am* 1952;34:491-494.

21. Baker DR, McHolick W: Spondyloschisis and spondylolisthesis in children. *J Bone Joint Surg Am* 1956; 38:933-934.

22. Fredrickson BE, Baker D, McHolick WJ, Yuan HA, Lubicky JP: The natural history of spondylolysis and spondylolisthesis. *J Bone Joint Surg Am* 1984;66:699-707.

23. Stewart TD: The incidence of neural-arch defects in Alaskan natives, considered from the standpoint of etiology. *J Bone Joint Surg Am* 1953;35: 937-950.

24. Beutler WJ, Fredrickson BE, Murtland A, Sweeney CA, Grant WD, Baker D: The natural history of spondylolysis and spondylolisthesis: 45-year follow-up evaluation. *Spine* 2003;28:1027-1035.

25. Frennered AK, Danielson BI, Nachemson AL: Natural history of symptomatic isthmic low-grade spondylolisthesis in children and adolescents: A seven-year follow-up study. *J Pediatr Orthop* 1991;11: 209-213.

26. Saraste H: Long-term clinical and radiological follow-up of spondylolysis and spondylolisthesis. *J Pediatr Orthop* 1987;7:631-638.

27. Seitsalo S, Osterman K, Hyvarinen H, Tallroth K, Schlenzka D, Poussa M: Progression of spondylolisthesis in children and adolescents: A long term follow-up of 272 patients. *Spine* 1991;16:417-421.

28. Floman Y: Progression of lumbosacral isthmic spondylolisthesis in adults. *Spine* 2000;25:342-347.

29. Feldman DS, Hedden DM, Wright JG: The use of bone scan to investigate back pain in children and adolescents. *J Pediatr Orthop* 2000;20: 790-795.

30. Feldman DS, Straight JJ, Badra MI, Mohaideen A, Madan SS: Evaluation of an algorithmic approach to pediatric back pain. *J Pediatr Orthop* 2006;26: 353-357.

31. Phalen GS, Dickson JA: Spondylolisthesis and tight hamstrings. *J Bone Joint Surg Am* 1961;43:505-512.

32. Maurice HD, Morley TR: Cauda equina lesions following fusion in situ and decompressive laminectomy for severe spondylolisthesis: Four case reports. *Spine* 1989;14:214-216.

33. Newman PH: A clinical syndrome associated with severe lumbo-sacral subluxation. *J Bone Joint Surg Br* 1965; 47:472-481.

34. Schoenecker PL, Cole HO, Herring JA, Capelli AM, Bradford DS: Cauda equina syndrome after in situ arthrodesis for severe spondylolisthesis at the lumbosacral junction. *J Bone Joint Surg Am* 1990;72:369-377.

35. Seitsalo S, Osterman K, Poussa M: Scoliosis associated with lumbar spondylolisthesis: A clinical survey of 190 young patients. *Spine* 1988;13: 899-904.

36. Möller H, Sundin A, Hedlund R: Symptoms, signs, and functional disability in adult spondylolisthesis. *Spine* 2000;25:683-690.

37. Lowe RW, Hayes TD, Kaye J, Bagg RJ, Leukens CA: Standing roentgenograms in spondylolisthesis. *Clin Orthop Relat Res* 1976;117:80-84.

38. Wiltse LL, Guyer RD, Spencer CW, Glenn WV, Porter IS: Alar transverse process impingement of the L5 spinal nerve: The far-out syndrome. *Spine* 1984;9:31-41.

39. Wiltse LL, Winter RB: Terminology and measurement of spondylolisthe-

sis. *J Bone Joint Surg Am* 1983;65: 768-772.

40. Legaye J, Duval-Beaupere G, Hecquet J, Marty C: Pelvic incidence: A fundamental pelvic parameter for three-dimensional regulation of spinal sagittal curves. *Eur Spine J* 1998;7: 99-103.

41. Mac-Thiong JM, Labelle H: A proposal for a surgical classification of pediatric lumbosacral spondylolisthesis based on current literature. *Eur Spine J* 2006;15:1425-1435.

42. Huang RP, Bohlmann HH, Thompson GH, Poe-Kochert C: Predictive value of pelvic incidence in progression of spondylolisthesis. *Spine* 2003; 28:2381-2385.

43. Read MT: Single photon emission computed tomography (SPECT) scanning for adolescent low back pain: A sine qua non? *Br J Sports Med* 1994;28:56-57.

44. van den Oever M, Merrick MV, Scott JHS: Bone scintigraphy in symptomatic spondylolysis. *J Bone Joint Surg Br* 1987;69:453-456.

45. Gregory PL, Batt ME, Kerslake RW, Scammell BE, Webb JF: The value of combining single photon emission computerised tomography and computerised tomography in the investigation of spondylolysis. *Eur Spine J* 2004;13:503-509.

46. Grogan JP, Hemminghytt S, Williams AL, Carrera GF, Haughton VM: Spondylolysis studied with computed tomography. *Radiology* 1982;145: 737-742.

47. McAfee PC, Yuan HA: Computed tomography in spondylolisthesis. *Clin Orthop Relat Res* 1982;166:62-71.

48. Sairyo K, Katoh S, Takata Y, et al: MRI signal changes of the pedicle as an indicator for early diagnosis of spondylolysis in children and adolescents: A clinical and biomechanical study. *Spine* 2006;31:206-211.

49. Birch JG, Herring JA, Maravilla KR: Splitting of the intervertebral disc in spondylolisthesis: A magnetic resonance imaging finding in two cases. *J Pediatr Orthop* 1986;6:609-611.

50. Szypryt EP, Twining P, Mulholland RC, Worthington BS: The prevalence of disc degeneration associated with neural arch defects of the lumbar spine assessed by magnetic resonance imaging. *Spine* 1989;14:977-981.

51. Pizzutillo PD, Hummer CD III: Nonoperative treatment for painful adolescent spondylolysis or spondylolisthesis. *J Pediatr Orthop* 1989;9: 538-540.

52. Sairyo K, Katoh S, Ikata T, Fujii K, Kajiura K, Goel VK: Development of spondylytic olisthesis in adolescents. *Spine J* 2001;1:171-175.

53. Bell DF, Ehrlich MG, Zaleske DJ: Brace treatment for symptomatic spondylolisthesis. *Clin Orthop Relat Res* 1988;236:192-198.

54. Blanda J, Bethem D, Moats W, Lew M: Defect of pars interarticularis in athletes: A protocol for nonoperative treatment. *J Spinal Disord* 1993;6: 406-411.

55. Steiner ME, Micheli LJ: Treatment of symptomatic spondylolysis and spondylolisthesis with the modified Boston brace. *Spine* 1985;10:937-943.

56. Sys J, Michielsen J, Bracke P, Martens M, Verstreken J: Nonoperative treatment of active spondylolysis in elite athletes with normal X-ray findings: Literature review and results of conservative treatment. *Eur Spine J* 2001; 10:498-504.

57. Hensinger RN, Lang JR, MacEwen GD: Surgical management of spondylolisthesis in children. *Spine* 1976;1:207-217.

58. Lenke LG, Bridwell KH, Bullis D, Betz RR, Baldus C, Schoenecker PL: Results of in situ fusion for isthmic spondylolisthesis. *J Spinal Disord* 1992;5:433-442.

59. Pizzutillo PD, Mirenda W, MacEwan GD: Posterolateral fusion for spondylolisthesis in adolescence. *J Pediatr Orthop* 1986;6:311-316.

60. Sherman FC, Rosenthal RK, Hall JE: Spine fusion for spondylolysis and spondylolisthesis in children. *Spine* 1979;4:59-66.

61. Wiltse LL, Jackson DW: Treatment of spondylolisthesis and spondylolysis in children. *Clin Orthop Relat Res* 1976; 117:92-100.

62. Buck JE: Direct repair of the defect in spondylolisthesis: Preliminary report. *J Bone Joint Surg Br* 1970;52:432-437.

63. Buck JE: Further thoughts on direct repair of the defect in spondylolysis. *J Bone Joint Surg Br* 1979;61:123.

64. Bradford DS, Iza J: Repair of the defect in spondylolysis or minimal degrees of spondylolisthesis by segmental wire fixation and bone grafting. *Spine* 1985;10:673-679.

65. Scott JHS: The Edinburgh repair of isthmic (Group II) spondylolysis. *J Bone Joint Surg Br* 1987;69:491.

66. Kakiuchi M: Repair of the defect in spondylolysis: Durable fixation with pedicle screws and laminar hooks. *J Bone Joint Surg Am* 1997;79:818-825.

67. Morscher E, Gerber B, Fasel J: Surgical treatment of spondylolisthesis by bone grafting and direct stabilization of spondylolysis by means of a hook screw. *Arch Orthop Trauma Surg* 1984; 103:175-178.

68. Songer MN, Rovin R: Repair of the pars interarticularis defect with a cable-screw construct: A preliminary report. *Spine* 1998;23:263-269.

69. Suh PB, Esses SI, Kostuik JP: Repair of pars interarticularis defect: The prognostic value of pars infiltration. *Spine* 1991;16(suppl 8):S445-S448.

70. Gill GG: Long-term follow-up evaluation of a few patients with spondylolisthesis treated by excision of the loose lamina with decompression of the nerve roots without spinal fusion. *Clin Orthop Relat Res* 1984;182: 215-219.

71. Gill GG, Manning JG, White HL: Surgical treatment of spondylolisthesis without spine fusion: Excision of the loose lamina with decompression of the nerve roots. *J Bone Joint Surg Am* 1955;37:493-520.

72. Carragee EJ: Single-level posterolateral arthrodesis, with or without posterior decompression, for the treatment of isthmic spondylolisthesis in adults: A prospective, randomized study. *J Bone Joint Surg Am* 1997;79: 1175-1180.

73. Davis IS, Bailey RW: Spondylolisthesis: Long-term follow-up study of treatment with total laminectomy. *Clin Orthop Relat Res* 1972;88:46-49.

74. McGuire RA, Amundson GM: The use of primary internal fixation in spondylolisthesis. *Spine* 1993;18: 1662-1672.

75. Peek RD, Wiltse LL, Reynolds JB, Thomas JC, Guyer DW, Widell EH: In situ arthrodesis without decompression for grade III or IV isthmic spondylolisthesis in adults who have severe sciatica. *J Bone Joint Surg Am* 1989;71:62-68.

76. de Loubresse CG, Bon T, Deburge A, Lassale B, Benoit M: Posterolateral fusion for radicular pain in isthmic spondylolisthesis. *Clin Orthop Relat Res* 1996;323:194-201.

77. Zdeblick TA: A prospective, randomized study of lumbar fusion: Preliminary results. *Spine* 1993;18:983-991.

78. Yuan HA, Garfin SR, Dickman CA, Mardjetko SM: A historical cohort study of pedicle screw fixation in thoracic, lumbar, and sacral spinal fusions. *Spine* 1994;19(20 suppl): 2279S-2296S.

79. Bjarke Christensen F, Stender Hansen E, Laursen M, Thomsen K, Bünger CE: Long-term functional outcome of pedicle screw instrumentation as a support for posterolateral spinal fusion: Randomized clinical study with a 5-year follow-up. *Spine* 2002;27:1269-1277.

80. Deguchi M, Rapoff AJ, Zdeblick TA: Posterolateral fusion for isthmic spondylolisthesis in adults: Analysis of fusion rate and clinical results. *J Spinal Disord* 1998;11:459-464.

81. Ricciardi JE, Pflueger PC, Isaza JE, Whitecloud TS III: Transpedicular fixation for the treatment of isthmic spondylolisthesis in adults. *Spine* 1995;20:1917-1922.

82. Chang P, Seow KH, Tan SK: Comparison of the results of spinal fusion for spondylolisthesis in patients who are instrumented with patients who are not. *Singapore Med J* 1993;34: 511-514.

83. Bono CM, Lee CK: Critical analysis of trends in fusion for degenerative disc disease over the past 20 years: Influence of technique on fusion rate and clinical outcome. *Spine* 2004;29: 455-463.

84. Möller H, Hedlund R: Surgery versus conservative management in adult isthmic spondylolisthesis: A prospective randomized study. Part 1. *Spine* 2000;25:1711-1715.

85. Möller H, Hedlund R: Instrumented and noninstrumented posterolateral fusion in adult spondylolisthesis: A prospective randomized study. Part 2. *Spine* 2000;25:1716-1721.

86. Dehoux E, Fourati E, Madi K, Reddy B, Segal P: Posterolateral versus interbody fusion in isthmic spondylolisthesis: Functional results in 52 cases with a minimum follow-up of 6 years. *Acta Orthop Belg* 2004;70: 578-582.

87. Harris BM, Hilibrand AS, Savas PE, et al: Transforaminal lumbar interbody fusion: The effect of various instrumentation techniques on the flexibility of the lumbar spine. *Spine* 2004;29:E65-E70.

88. Kwon B, Zaremski J, Kim D, Tromanhauser S, Banco R, Jenis L: Surgical outcomes after treatment of spondylolytic spondylolisthesis: Analysis of three techniques. The Spine Journal Website. Available at: http://www.thespinejournalonline.com/article/PIIS1529943006004396/abstract. Accessed January 2008.

89. Suk SI, Lee CK, Kim WJ, Lee JH, Cho KJ, Kim HG: Adding posterior lumbar interbody fusion to pedicle screw fixation and posterolateral fusion after decompression in spondylolytic spondylolisthesis. *Spine* 1997; 22:210-220.

90. Holly LT, Schwender JD, Rouben DP, Foley KT: Minimally invasive transforaminal lumbar interbody fusion: Indications, technique, and

complications. *Neurosurg Focus* 2006;20:E6.

91. Cheng CL, Fang D, Lee PC, Leong JC: Anterior spinal fusion for spondylolysis and isthmic spondylolisthesis: Long term results in adults. *J Bone Joint Surg Br* 1989;71:264-267.

92. Aunoble S, Hoste D, Donkersloot P, Liquois F, Basso Y, Le Huec JC: Video-assisted ALIF with cage and anterior plate fixation for L5-S1 spondylolisthesis. *J Spinal Disord Tech* 2006;19:471-476.

93. Pavlov PW, Spruit M, Havinga M, Anderson PG, van Limbeek J, Jacobs WC: Anterior lumbar interbody fusion with threaded fusion cages and autologous bone grafts. *Eur Spine J* 2000;9:224-229.

94. Swan J, Hurwitz E, Malek F, et al: Surgical treatment for unstable low-grade isthmic spondylolisthesis in adults: A prospective controlled study of posterior instrumented fusion compared with combined anterior-posterior fusion. *Spine J* 2006;6: 606-614.

95. Boxall D, Bradford DS, Winter RB, Moe JH: Management of severe spondylolisthesis in children and adolescents. *J Bone Joint Surg Am* 1979;61: 479-495.

96. Matthiass HH, Heine J: The surgical reduction of spondylolisthesis. *Clin Orthop Relat Res* 1986;203:34-44.

97. Molinari RW, Bridwell KH, Lenke LG, Ungacta FF, Riew KD: Complications in the surgical treatment of pediatric high-grade isthmic dysplastic spondylolisthesis: A comparison of three surgical techniques. *Spine* 1999; 24:1701-1711.

98. Newton PO, Johnston CE II: Analysis and treatment of poor outcomes following in situ arthrodesis in adolescent spondylolisthesis. *J Pediatr Orthop* 1997;17:754-761.

99. Johnson JR, Kirwan EO: The long-term results of fusion in situ for severe spondylolisthesis. *J Bone Joint Surg Br* 1983;65:43-46.

100. Seitsalo S, Osterman K, Hyvarinen J, Schlenzka D, Poussa M: Severe spondylolisthesis in children and adolescents: A long-term review of fusion in situ. *J Bone Joint Surg Br* 1990; 72:259-265.

101. Burkus JK, Lonstein JE, Winter RB, Denis F: Long-term evaluation of adolescents treated operatively for spondylolisthesis: A comparison of in situ arthrodesis only with in situ arthrodesis and reduction followed by immobilization in a cast. *J Bone Joint Surg Am* 1992;74:693-704.

102. Petraco DM, Spivak JM, Cappadona JG, Kummer FJ, Neuwirth MG: An anatomic evaluation of L5 nerve stretch in spondylolisthesis reduction. *Spine* 1996;21:1133-1139.

103. Shufflebarger HL, Geck MJ: High-grade isthmic dysplastic spondylolisthesis: Monosegmental surgical treatment. *Spine* 2005;30(6 suppl): S42-S48.

104. Bohlman HH, Cook SS: One-stage decompression and posterolateral and interbody fusion for lumbosacral spondyloptosis through a posterior approach: Report of two cases. *J Bone Joint Surg Am* 1982;64:415-418.

105. Hanson DS, Bridwell KH, Rhee JM, Lenke LG: Dowel fibular strut grafts for high-grade dysplastic isthmic spondylolisthesis. *Spine* 2002;27: 1982-1988.

106. Bradford DS, Boachie-Adjei O: Treatment of severe spondylolisthesis by anterior and posterior reduction and stabilization: A long-term follow-up study. *J Bone Joint Surg Am* 1990;72:1060-1066.

107. Muschik M, Zippel H, Perka C: Surgical management of severe spondylolisthesis in children and adolescents: Anterior fusion in situ versus anterior spondylodesis with posterior transpedicular instrumentation and reduction. *Spine* 1997;22: 2036-2043.

108. Remes V, Lamberg T, Tervahartiala P, et al: Long-term outcome after posterolateral, anterior, and circumferential fusion for high-grade isthmic spondylolisthesis in children and adolescents: Magnetic resonance imaging findings after average of 17-year follow-up. *Spine* 2006;31:2491-2499.

109. Roca J, Ubierna MT, Cáceres E, Iborra M: One-stage decompression and posterolateral and interbody fusion for severe spondylolisthesis: An analysis of 14 patients. *Spine* 1999;24: 709-714.

110. Ruf M, Koch H, Melcher RP, Harms J: Anatomic reduction and monosegmental fusion in high-grade developmental spondylolisthesis. *Spine* 2006; 31:269-274.

111. Bartolozzi P, Sandri A, Cassini M, Ricci M: One-stage posterior decompression-stabilization and trans-sacral interbody fusion after partial reduction for severe L5-S1 spondylolisthesis. *Spine* 2003;28: 1135-1141.

112. Fabris DA, Costantini S, Nena U: Surgical treatment of severe L5-S1 spondylolisthesis in children and adolescents: Results of intraoperative reduction, posterior interbody fusion, and segmental pedicle fixation. *Spine* 1996;21:728-733.

113. Smith JA, Deviren V, Berven S, Kleinstueck F, Bradford DS: Clinical outcome of trans-sacral interbody fusion after partial reduction for high-grade L5-S1 spondylolisthesis. *Spine* 2001;26:2227-2234.

114. Gaines RW, Nichols WK: Treatment of spondyloptosis by two stage L5 vertebrectomy and reduction of L4 onto S1. *Spine* 1985;10:680-686.

115. Gaines RW: L5 vertebrectomy for the surgical treatment of spondyloptosis: Thirty cases in 25 years. *Spine* 2005;30 (6 suppl):S66-S70.

116. Boden SD, Riew KD, Yamaguchi K, Branch TP, Schellinger D, Wiesel SW: Orientation of the lumbar facet joints: Association with degenerative disc disease. *J Bone Joint Surg Am* 1996;78:403-411.

117. Love TW, Fagan AB, Fraser RD: Degenerative spondylolisthesis: Developmental or acquired? *J Bone Joint Surg Br* 1999;81:670-674.

118. Bendo JA, Ong B: Importance of correlating static and dynamic imaging

studies in diagnosing degenerative lumbar spondylolisthesis. *Am J Orthop* 2001;30:247-250.

119. Weinstein JN, Lurie JD, Tosteson TD, et al: Surgical versus nonsurgical treatment for lumbar degenerative spondylolisthesis. *N Engl J Med* 2007; 356:2257-2270.

120. Epstein NE: Decompression in the surgical management of degenerative spondylolisthesis: Advantages of a conservative approach in 290 patients. *J Spinal Disord* 1998;11:116-123.

121. Fischgrund JS, Mackay M, Herkowitz HN, Brower R, Montgomery DM, Kurz LT: Degenerative lumbar spondylolisthesis with spinal stenosis: A prospective, randomized study comparing decompressive laminectomy and arthrodesis with and without spinal instrumentation. *Spine* 1997;22:2807-2812.

122. Herkowitz HN, Kurz LT: Degenerative lumbar spondylolisthesis with spinal stenosis: A prospective study comparing decompression with decompression and intertransverse process arthrodesis. *J Bone Joint Surg Am* 1991;73:802-808.

123. Kornblum MB, Fischgrund JS, Herkowitz HN, Abraham DA, Berkower DL, Ditkoff JS: Degenerative lumbar spondylolisthesis with spinal stenosis: A prospective long-term study comparing fusion and pseudarthrosis. *Spine* 2004;29: 726-734.

124. France JC, Yaszemski MJ, Lauerman WC, et al: A randomized prospective study of posterolateral lumbar fusion: Outcomes with and without pedicle screw instrumentation. *Spine* 1999; 24:553-560.

125. Mardjetko SM, Connolly PJ, Shott S: Degenerative lumbar spondylolisthesis: A meta-analysis of literature 1970-1993. *Spine* 1994;19(20 suppl): 2256S-2265S.

126. Nork SE, Hu SS, Workman KL, Glazer PA, Bradford DS: Patient outcomes after decompression and instrumented posterior spinal fusion for degenerative spondylolisthesis. *Spine* 1999;24:561-569.

127. Lauber S, Schulte TL, Liljenqvist U, Halm H, Hackenberg L: Clinical and radiologic 2-4-year results of transforaminal lumbar interbody fusion in degenerative and isthmic spondylolisthesis grades 1 and 2. *Spine* 2006;31: 1693-1698.

128. Potter BK, Freedman BA, Verwiebe EG, Hall JM, Polly DW Jr, Kuklo TR: Transforaminal lumbar interbody fusion: Clinical and radiographic results and complications in 100 consecutive patients. *J Spinal Disord Tech* 2005;18:337-346.

129. Zigler J, Delamarter R, Spivak JM, et al: Results of the prospective, randomized, multicenter Food and Drug Administration investigation device exemption study of the ProDisc-L total disc replacement versus circumferential fusion for the treatment of 1-level desenerative disc disease. *Spine* 2007;32:1155-1163.

130. Kondrashov DG, Hannibal M, Hsu KY, Zucherman JF: Interspinous process decompression with X-STOP device for lumbar spinal stenosis: A 4-year follow-up study. *J Spinal Disord Tech* 2006;19:323-327.

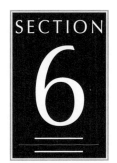

SECTION 6

Degenerative Lumbar Stenosis

Degenerative Lumbar Stenosis

Spinal stenosis is a very common radiographic finding in elderly patients. Although this condition is frequently asymptomatic, patients with symptoms report tightness, cramping, heaviness, or a drawing sensation in the buttocks and thighs. As symptoms progress, patients may notice a decrease in their quality of life resulting from a reduced ability to ambulate for prolonged distances. Often, this limitation is ignored in elderly patients and is viewed as a function of normal aging. However, accurate diagnosis and treatment of spinal stenosis can often lead to significant improvement in the patient's symptoms.

The three chapters in this section describe the evaluation and treatment options for patients with symptomatic spinal stenosis. The first chapter, authored by Daffner and Wang, describes the pathophysiology and nonsurgical treatment of lumbar spinal stenosis. The second chapter by Knaub and associates explains the indications for arthrodesis and spinal instrumentation for patients with symptomatic spinal stenosis. The section concludes with a chapter by Crawford and Glassman describing the treatment of patients with lumbar spinal stenosis associated with adult scoliosis. Together, these three chapters provide an excellent overview of the available diagnosis and treatment options for patients with lumbar spinal stenosis.

The chapter by Daffner and Wang begins with the definition and classification of lumbar spinal stenosis. Although this information is typically well known by spinal surgeons, this succinct review is helpful in determining the etiology of a patient's symptoms. The pathophysiology of this disease is a result of a series of changes in the bone and soft-tissue anatomy resulting in decreased space for the neural elements. A combination of intervertebral disk degeneration, facet joint changes, and ligamentum hypertrophy contribute to the crowding of nerve roots in the spinal canal. These changes are frequently referred to as degenerative changes. Recent studies highlighted in the chapter explain the molecular changes that occur secondary to the inflammatory mediators.

A variety of nonsurgical options are described in the first section of the Daffner and Wang chapter. Although patients may occasionally present to the spine surgeon having completed a nonsurgical course of treatment, it is incumbent for the practitioner to discuss nonsurgical options for those patients who have not yet received treatment. Although they have not been found to be clinically effective, some historic treatment recommendations include bed rest, activity modification, bracing, chiropractic manipulation, traction therapy, and acupuncture. Frequently prescribed medications include nonsteroidal antiinflammatory drugs, muscle relaxants, analgesics, and occasionally, antidepressant drugs in low doses. Although medications are often prescribed, their use should be carefully monitored because this patient population often has significant medical comorbidities with the potential for adverse side effects caused by the prolonged use of these drugs.

The Daffner and Wang chapter highlights the conflicting evidence in the published literature concerning the use of epidural steroids to treat patients with spinal stenosis. Although complications are rare, patients should be counseled on the potential morbidities of epidural steroid treatment. Patients will often enjoy short-term relief, which may be adequate for those who are acutely symptomatic after a flare-up. However, patients should be discouraged from long-term steroid treatments if they are ineffective, comorbidities exist such as diabetes that can be affected by extrinsic corticosteroid, or if long-term treatment with anticoagulants is required.

Daffner and Wang conclude that nonsurgical treatment is appropriate for patients with mild symptoms, and that surgical treatment is appropriate for patients with severe stenosis and long-term unrelenting pain. An overview of the Spine Outcomes Research Trial (SPORT) also is discussed. The important result from this trial is found in the "as-treated" analysis, which concluded that patients with spinal stenosis (and degenerative spondylolisthesis) had significant improvement with surgery compared with patients who elected nonsurgical treatment.

The chapter by Knaub and associates focuses on the important question regarding the indications for fusion in a patient receiving surgical treatment for lumbar spinal stenosis. It is well known that simple decompression alone, such as a laminectomy, will often lead to excellent relief of leg pain in a symptomatic patient. However, many prospective randomized trials have clearly shown that function in some patients will quickly deteriorate if an arthrodesis is not performed at the time of the initial surgery.

This chapter outlines the indications for fusion and instrumentation, and reviews the pertinent literature from the past 20 years on this subject.

Degenerative spondylolisthesis is perhaps the most common indication for fusion with instrumentation in a patient with spinal stenosis. The chapter accurately reviews the history of study results and how they have changed our practice patterns. Patients with degenerative spondylolisthesis have better long-term outcomes if fusion is performed at the time of the initial decompression. Several other studies have clearly shown that the addition of instrumentation improves the fusion rate. Based on a review of the literature, Knaub and associates conclude that patients with spinal stenosis and degenerative spondylolisthesis will have a significantly improved outcome if fusion and instrumentation are performed at the time of the index procedure.

Other less common situations, such as the development of recurrent spinal stenosis at the same segment or at an adjacent level, may also require the addition of a fusion for patients undergoing a decompression. As life expectancy continues to improve, the prevalence for the development of stenosis above a previous posterolateral fusion will increase. This situation usually requires fusion in addition to standard decompression.

The authors also discuss intraoperative findings that may indicate the need for fusion. An example is a radical diskectomy, which may be necessary in patients with lumbar spinal stenosis and a concomitant disk herniation. Fusion may also be needed to prevent the development of iatrogenic instability in patients who require excessive resection of the facet joints to adequately decompress the nerve root.

As surgical techniques continue to evolve, many surgeons have recommended the addition of a transforaminal lumbar interbody fusion for patients treated with instrumented fusion after decompression for spinal stenosis. In theory, the addition of an interbody fusion has significant benefits, including restoration of disk height, an increase in foraminal height, and an increased fusion rate. However, these benefits must be weighed against the increased surgical time, blood loss, and possible postoperative radicular pain. More long-term prospective studies are needed before interbody fusion can be routinely recommended for patients with spinal stenosis and degenerative spondylolisthesis.

The chapter by Crawford and Glassman focuses on the functional limitations experienced by patients with axial back pain and neurogenic leg pain resulting from progressive degenerative spinal deformity with nerve compression. The etiology of this disease can result from the development of degenerative scoliosis or curve progression in patients with a preexisting deformity. The authors point out that scoliotic deformity can develop as degeneration advances, even in patients with no prior abnormal curvature of the spine. When evaluating clinical and radiographic characteristics, it is mandatory to determine the magnitude of the curve in both the coronal and sagittal planes. Although coronal deformities are easily identified on radiographs, significant sagittal imbalance often leads to an increase in pain and deterioration in function.

Numerous classification schemes for adult degenerative scoliosis are reviewed by Crawford and Glassman. Although independent authors have proposed various classification schemes, they have not been widely adopted. Recently, the Scoliosis Research Society adopted and validated a comprehensive classification system for adult deformity including degenerative scoliosis. Because this classification system is relatively new, it has not yet been widely adopted.

The authors observe that high-quality, evidence-based recommendations to support surgical treatment options are lacking. As with all spinal conditions, the pros and cons of various surgical procedures should be discussed with the patient preoperatively to allow the patient to make an informed decision regarding treatment.

Surgical options discussed in the chapter include anterior versus posterior or combined procedures, anterior and posterior instrumentation, and the use of transforaminal lumbar interbody grafts. The chapter also includes a discussion of the outcomes of surgical treatment over the past 10 years. Important tools for the postoperative assessment of patients include the Scoliosis Research Society Instrument and the Oswestry Disability Index.

Newer surgical techniques such as the lateral approach to the thoracolumbar and lumbar spine may ultimately prove to be a less invasive method for treating these complex pathologies. Proponents of this technology claim that significant reduction in deformity can be obtained through this minimally invasive approach.[1] The placement of an interbody graft theoretically enlarges the canal diameter, reducing the need for decompression. It remains to be seen if these evolving techniques can replace the more standard techniques described in this chapter.

The three chapters in this section will provide the clinician with an excellent outline of the clinical presentation, natural history, and treatment options for patients with spinal stenosis, with or without spinal deformity. Although many new surgical techniques have been introduced over the past several years, it is recommended that successful controlled clinical trials be completed before these techniques are adopted.

Jeffrey S. Fischgrund, MD
Clinical Professor, Department of
     Orthopaedic Surgery at Oakland
     University William Beaumont School
     of Medicine
Rochester, Michigan
Michigan Orthopaedic Institute
Southfield, Michigan

Reference

1. Ozgur BM, Aryan HE, Pimenta L, Taylor WR: Extreme lateral interbody fusion (XLIF): A novel surgical technique for anterior lumbar interbody fusion. *Spine J* 2006;6:435-443.

Dr. Fischgrund or an immediate family member serves as a board member, owner, officer, or committee member for the Cervical Spine Research Society, Spine Arthroplasty Society, Spine Study Group, Lumbar Spine Research Society, and North American Spine Society; has received royalties from DePuy and Stryker; is a member of a speakers' bureau or has made paid presentations on behalf of DePuy, Smith & Nephew, and Stryker; serves as a paid consultant for or is an employee of DePuy, Smith & Nephew, Stryker, and Apatech; serves as an unpaid consultant for Fziomed; has received research or institutional support from DePuy, Smith & Nephew, and Stryker; and has received nonincome support (such as equipment or services), commercially derived honoraria, or other non–research-related funding from the *Journal of the American Academy of Orthopaedic Surgeons.*

The Pathophysiology and Nonsurgical Treatment of Lumbar Spinal Stenosis

Scott D. Daffner, MD
*Jeffrey C. Wang, MD

Abstract

Lumbar spinal stenosis, which affects an ever-increasing number of patients, is best defined as a collection of clinical symptoms that includes low back pain, bilateral lower extremity pain, paresthesias, and other neurologic deficits that occur concomitantly with anatomic narrowing of the neural pathway through the spine. The narrowing may be centrally located in the spinal canal or more laterally in the lateral recesses or neuroforamina. Lumbar spinal stenosis can have a congenital or acquired etiology, and the origin of acquired lumbar stenosis is classified as degenerative, posttraumatic, or iatrogenic. In degenerative lumbar stenosis, the anatomic changes result from a cascade of events that includes intervertebral disk degeneration, facet joint arthrosis, and hypertrophy of the ligamentum flavum. The altered biomechanical characteristics of the spinal segment perpetuate a cycle of degenerative changes, and the resulting stenosis produces radicular pain through a combination of direct mechanical compression of nerve roots, restriction of microvascular circulation and axoplasmic flow, and inflammatory mediators.

The initial treatment of lumbar spinal stenosis is nonsurgical. The most effective nonsurgical treatment is a comprehensive combination of oral anti-inflammatory drugs, physical therapy and conditioning, and epidural steroid injections. A significant number of patients improve after nonsurgical treatment, although most studies have found that patients treated surgically have better clinical results. Delaying surgical treatment until after a trial of nonsurgical treatment does not affect the outcome. Surgical intervention should be considered only if a comprehensive program of nonsurgical measures fails to improve the patient's quality of life.

Lumbar spinal stenosis is best defined as a constellation of clinical symptoms that occur with anatomic narrowing of the neural pathway through the spine, which can be caused by decreased diameter of the central spinal canal, the lateral recess, or neuroforamen. Patients typically report an insidious onset of low back and sciatic pain, occasionally with lower extremity paresthesias. The symptoms usually are bilateral and worsen with walking or other activity. Sitting rapidly relieves the pain. Many patients report that symptoms improve during activities that place the spine in a relatively flexed position, such as walking uphill or pushing a shopping cart. Clinical examination may reveal objective weakness, most frequently in the tibialis anterior and extensor hallucis longus. A careful history and physical examination are necessary to distinguish between neurogenic and vascular claudication, which can have similar symptoms.

Lumbar spinal stenosis can cause significant pain and disability,[1] and it has become a leading diagnosis among older patients undergoing spinal surgery.[2] Zanoli and associates[3] reported significantly decreased health-related quality of life, as measured using the Medical Outcomes Study Short Form-36 Health Survey, among patients scheduled for lumbar surgery. For most patients, the initial treatment of lumbar spinal stenosis is nonsurgical.

Jeffrey C. Wang, MD or the department with which he is affiliated has received royalties from Biomet, Medtronic, Aesculap, DePuy, and Stryker and is a consultant for or employee of Synthes, Zimmer, Amedica, FzioMed, and Facet Solutions.

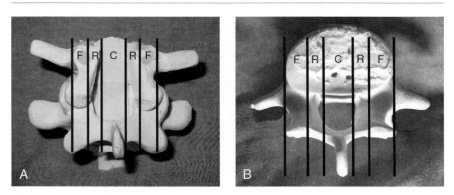

Figure 1 Coronal (**A**) and axial (**B**) photographs of a lumbar vertebral motion segment, showing the central (C), lateral recess (R), and foraminal (F) regions of lumbar spinal stenosis.

Definition and Classification

The classification systems for lumbar spinal stenosis are based on etiology (acquired or congenital) or location (central, lateral recess, or foraminal).[4] In the useful etiologic scheme proposed by Arnoldi and associates,[5] congenital or developmental stenosis is classified either as caused by achondroplasia or other dwarfism or as idiopathic (in patients with normal stature). Idiopathic stenosis is usually caused by a congenitally narrow canal (short pedicles or narrow lamina). Acquired stenosis is usually degenerative in nature, but it also can have a spondylolisthetic, iatrogenic, posttraumatic, or metabolic cause. It can occur in combination with congenital stenosis.[5]

Lumbar spinal stenosis also can be classified based on the primary location of the stenotic lesion (Figure 1). Central stenosis involves the region bordered anteriorly by the vertebral body and intervertebral disk and posteriorly by the lamina and ligamentum flavum; this region extends laterally to the edge of the thecal sac, where the nerve root exits the dura. Central stenosis most commonly occurs around the level of the intervertebral disk. It can result from disk bulges or herniation,

vertebral body osteophyte formation, ligamentum flavum hypertrophy or infolding, or hypertrophic changes of the inferior facets. As defined by Verbiest,[6] relative stenosis is a midsagittal lumbar canal diameter of less than 13 mm, and absolute stenosis is a diameter of less than 10 mm.

The lateral recess encompasses the initial portion of the nerve root canal, from the point at which the root leaves the dura medially until it runs under the medial border of the pedicle. This area is bordered anteriorly by the vertebral body and intervertebral disk and posteriorly by the pars interarticularis and facet joint. Compression usually is caused by posterolateral disk bulging, vertebral body or superior facet osteophytes, ligamentum flavum hypertrophy, or facet cysts. Lateral recess stenosis tends to affect the traversing nerve root at the level of the stenosis. It has been suggested that narrowing to less than 3 or 4 mm between the superior facet and the posterior vertebral body results in symptomatic stenosis.[4]

Foraminal stenosis occurs in an area bordered anteriorly by the vertebral body and disk, posteriorly by the lateral border of the pars interarticu-

laris, and superiorly and inferiorly by the pedicles. Superior disk margin osteophytes, a far lateral disk herniation, or substantial facet joint hypertrophy can impinge on the nerve root as it exits the neuroforamen. Stenosis frequently occurs centrally as well as in the lateral recess and neuroforamen.

Pathophysiology

Degenerative lumbar spinal stenosis does not develop from a single inciting event. Instead, it is the result of a series of changes in the bony or soft-tissue anatomy that decrease the anatomic space for the neural elements. The pathologic changes leading to lumbar spinal stenosis typically begin with degeneration of the intervertebral disk, which causes a loss of disk height and bulging of the anulus fibrosus into the spinal canal. This event alters the forces across the facet joints, leading to sclerosis, osteophyte formation, and facet capsule hypertrophy. As the disk space decreases and micromotion of the spinal segment increases, infolding and hypertrophy of the ligamentum flavum occurs. The result is compression of the neural elements centrally and, more commonly, laterally as they traverse the lateral recess and foramen (Figure 2). The compression of nerve roots causes symptoms of neurogenic claudication through ischemia, venous congestion, or localized release of inflammatory mediators.[7,8]

Intervertebral Disk Degeneration

The composition of the lumbar intervertebral disk changes with increasing age. Alterations in the ratio of proteoglycans within the disk lead to an overall decrease in the disk's affinity for water. As hydration decreases, the disk's resistance to loading stresses also decreases. Increased loads applied to the disk can further decrease disk hydration.[9]

Vascular changes about the disk occur with aging and degeneration. By the time a person reaches adulthood, the intervertebral disk is largely avascular and derives its nutritional support through diffusion.[10] Kauppila[11] found that disk degeneration is preceded by significant vascular changes characterized by obliteration of the anastomosing arteries in the posterior longitudinal ligament and neovascularization of the anterolateral anulus fibrosus. This finding suggests that decreased nutrition also contributes to disk degeneration.

These changes cause increased biomechanical demand on a structure no longer able to respond to it. Posterior bulging and decreased disk height are the result of changes in the proteoglycan content, water content, collagen cross-linking, vasculature, and nutrition of the disk.[10]

Facet Joint Changes

The functional unit of spinal motion comprises a three-joint complex consisting of the intervertebral disk and the two facet joints. Decreasing disk height alters the biomechanical stresses on the facet joints of the lumbar spine, shifting the load posteriorly from the disk to the facet joints and altering spinal motion.[12,13] Abnormal motion as the result of degenerative changes in the facet joints can further contribute to degeneration of the intervertebral disk, perpetuating the cycle.[12]

Abnormal motion or loading of the facet joints triggers degenerative morphologic changes in the joint structures as the joint structures attempt to compensate. These changes include bony hypertrophy and osteophyte formation as well as thickening of the facet joint capsule, and they can

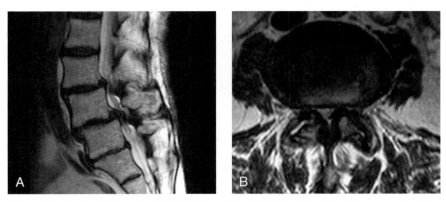

Figure 2 Sagittal (**A**) and axial (**B**) T2-weighted MRI studies showing severe lumbar spinal stenosis. **A**, Decreased disk height, disk bulging, posterior infolding and thickening of the ligamentum flavum, and spondylolisthesis at L3-4 and L4-5. **B**, Bilateral hypertrophy of the facets with thickening of the ligamentum flavum at the L3-4 level, causing severe central, lateral recess, and foraminal stenosis. The dural sac is almost completely collapsed because of compression from these changes.

result in impingement of the nerve root, leading to symptoms of neurogenic claudication. Lateral recess and foraminal stenosis is further increased by the loss of foraminal height due to disk degeneration. Localized inflammatory responses secondary to facet joint degeneration contribute to the development of radicular symptoms.[14,15]

Ligamentum Flavum Hypertrophy

As the disk space narrows and the intervertebral height decreases, the ligamentum flavum folds in on itself, becoming redundant and contributing to compression of the thecal sac. In addition, the ligamentum flavum thickens, becomes more fibrotic, and stiffens, encroaching the neural elements.[16,17]

Histologically, the ligamentum flavum has greater thickness, an increased rate of calcification, and increased fibrosis (as evidenced by a decreased ratio of elastic to collagenous fibers) in patients with lumbar spinal stenosis.[16] Mechanical and biochemical influences may be responsible for these changes. Sairyo and

associates[17] found that not only did the thickness and degree of fibrosis increase with advancing age among patients with spinal stenosis but also that the dorsal fibers of the ligamentum flavum experienced greater biomechanical stresses than the dural-side fibers. Histologically, the degree of fibrosis and loss of elastic fibers were found to be much more pronounced in the dorsal fibers. These changes may be caused by molecular changes secondary to inflammatory mediators. Expression of transforming growth factor-β, known to occur during the early stages of scar formation and fibrosis, was found to decrease as the thickness of the ligamentum flavum increased. Transforming growth factor-β was localized in the endothelial cells of the blood vessels of the ligamentum, rather than in the fibroblasts themselves.[17] Tissue inhibitors of metalloproteinase (TIMPs) are implicated in the development of other fibrotic conditions, and Park and associates[18] examined the potential role of TIMPs on pathologic changes in the ligamentum flavum. The expression of TIMP-2 in the hypertrophied ligamentum flavum was found to be increased in patients with lumbar spinal stenosis in comparison with control subjects. The TIMP was expressed by the fibroblasts themselves. These findings suggest a complex interplay of mechanical stresses and molecular signaling in the development of ligamentum flavum hypertrophy. Sairyo and associates[17] hypothesized that altered biomechanics lead to increased stress and tissue damage of the primarily dorsal fibers in the ligamentum flavum, initiating scar formation as part of a reparative effort, as mediated by TGF-β expression, and leading to further fibrosis and hypertrophy. Other molecular mediators also may be at work.

Neurogenic Claudication

Multiple factors have been cited in the development of leg pain resulting from spinal stenosis. Chronic compression of the lumbar nerve roots leads to dysfunction through a combination of mechanical compression, vascular changes, and inflammatory mediators. Direct compression of the nerve root often is the starting point. As the degree and duration of compression increase, nerve conduction decreases.[19] A threshold of approximately 50% reduction in the cross-sectional area of the canal and 50 to 75 mm Hg of pressure on the nerve root appears to be required before changes in conduction can be observed.[8,20] The relationship of posture and onset of symptoms can be partly explained by the exacerbation of compression and increased epidural pressure that occurs during activities requiring extension of the spine or axial loading, such as standing or walking.[21-23]

Compression of lumbar nerve roots has been shown to impair microvascular circulation as well as axoplasmic flow. Delamarter and associates[20] found that compression of the exiting nerve root led to wallerian degeneration in motor roots distal to the site of compression and proximally in sensory roots and the posterior column. Mechanical compression of the nerve roots can lead to central sensitization and centralized mediation of pain perception. Hunt and associates[24] found that repetitive injury to nerve roots could cause allodynia in a rodent model. Mechanical allodynia worsened bilaterally following unilateral nerve root injury, and this finding suggests a centralized modulation of radicular pain. Because the bilateral response was greater after repeated injury, Hunt and associates suggested that central sensitization occurs after the initial injury. The increased levels of the inflammatory cytokine interleukin-β found in the spinal cord after injury further suggest a central sensitization involvement in the development of chronic radicular pain.

The dorsal root ganglion probably plays a major role in the development of radicular pain. The dorsal root ganglion is known to produce nociceptive neuropeptides such as substance P, calcitonin gene-related peptide, and somatostatin.[8,25] Transmission of these, and probably other, neurotransmitters from the sensory neurons of the dorsal root ganglion to cells of the dorsal horn via axonal flow may contribute to the stimulus of pain caused by nerve root compression.[26] Physical compression of the nerve root may cause changes in axoplasmic flow, resulting in impaired cellular nutrition, decreased concentrations of neurotransmitters in the cells of the dorsal root ganglion, and accumulation of nociceptive neuropeptides distal to the site of compression.[25,27]

In addition to restriction of axoplasmic flow, compression can lead to vascular changes around the nerve root.[8,20] Constriction initially leads to venous congestion and edema of the root and dorsal root ganglion. With prolonged compression or greater pressures, arteriolar narrowing occurs. As edema increases, endoneural pressure also increases, essentially causing a compartment syndrome of the dorsal root ganglion and ultimately leading to cell death.[8] Ikawa and associates[28] found that in rodents with experimentally created lumbar spinal stenosis, venous congestion contributed to ectopic firing of the dorsal root ganglion; no such firing was seen with induced venous congestion in control animals. This finding suggests an interplay of venous stasis and dorsal root ganglion firing in the etiology of neurogenic claudication symptoms.

Inflammatory mediators arising in both the nerve root and the associated spinal structures also may contribute to the development of leg pain. In a canine model, Kobayashi and associates[29] found that compression of lumbar nerve roots produced intraradicular inflammation and wallerian degeneration. Tachihara and associates[15] found that when inflammation was stimulated in the facet joints of rats to simulate facet arthritis, increased levels of inflammatory cytokines (specifically, tumor necrosis factor-α) were found in the epidural space and were correlated with increased radicular symptoms. This finding suggests that inflammatory mediators released from degenerative facets have a role in the generation of neurogenic claudication. Igarashi and associates[14] found that in humans, inflammatory cytokines originating within a degenerative facet joint can leak into the intraspinal space through the facet capsule, producing radicular pain. They noted that patients with degenerative lumbar spinal stenosis who had higher levels of interleukin-1β in their facet joint cartilage reported worse leg pain and disability.

The development of radicular pain is multifactorial. Inflammatory mediators arising within the axon secondary to mechanical compression, as well as those leaking from an arthritic facet or the degenerative disk, can induce chemical radiculitis. These inflammatory mediators contribute to the development of radicular pain, in combination with impaired axoplasmic flow and microcirculatory compromise, wallerian degeneration, altered synthesis and transport of neuropeptides, ectopic discharges, and central sensitization.

Nonsurgical Treatment Options

Initial nonsurgical treatment of lumbar spinal stenosis is appropriate for patients with mild or moderate symptoms and may improve or limit the progression of symptomatic neurogenic claudication and back pain.[30,31] Delaying surgical intervention until after a trial of nonsurgical treatment appears to have little or no negative effect on clinical outcome.[32] Nonsurgical treatment may be the only option for a patient who refuses surgery or has medical comorbidities that preclude surgical intervention. A nonsurgical treatment plan should focus on counteracting the biomechanical and inflammatory pathologic changes associated with lumbar spinal stenosis. To alleviate pain and improve function, an optimal plan should include multiple modalities and active patient involvement.[33]

Nonsurgical treatment is described as having passive and active phases.[34] Among the passive phase treatments are activity modification, medications, chiropractic manipulation, acupuncture, and epidural steroid injections. The active phase includes formal physical therapy and exercise.

Bed Rest and Activity Modification

There is no significant evidence that prolonged bed rest improves the symptoms associated with degenerative lumbar spinal stenosis.[35,36] A short period of rest (no more than 2 days) can alleviate an acute exacerbation of back or leg pain; the patient should be encouraged to resume most normal activities as soon as they can be tolerated. The patient should be instructed to avoid activities that exacerbate the symptoms, particularly activities that place the spine in excess extension, such as heavy lifting.[34]

Bracing

No evidence exists to support the use of spinal bracing to prevent episodes of low back pain.[37] A rigid orthotic device tends to place the lumbar spine in extension and therefore may exacerbate symptoms. However, an elastic binder can provide effective short-term relief by reducing strain across the lumbar spine and acting as a counterforce to posterior spinal muscular contracture.[7] Long-term use can lead to deconditioning and weakening of the paraspinal muscles and is discouraged.[7,34] Although one study reported that patients who wore a lumbosacral corset had an increased walking distance and decreased pain, these benefits were not sustained when the brace was removed.[38]

Chiropractic Manipulation and Traction Therapy

Increasing numbers of patients are seeking alternative treatments, of which chiropractic manipulation is among the most common. There is insufficient evidence that chiropractic manipulation offers significant improvement of symptoms caused by lumbar spinal stenosis.[30] A randomized trial of medical care with and without physical therapy versus chiropractic care with and without physical modalities found no significant difference in symptom improvement between patients managed medically and those who underwent chiropractic manipulation.[39] A recent review found no evidence to support the clinical efficacy of manual traction in treating back pain or sciatica.[40]

Acupuncture

Acupuncture is also popular as an alternative treatment. In an animal model, Inoue and associates[41] found that blood flow to the sciatic nerve was increased as a result of acupuncture needle placement in 57% of specimens. Although their results provide a physiologic explanation for the relief some patients experience following acupuncture, the clinical evidence is inconclusive. A review of the literature on the clinical efficacy of acupuncture and dry needling in the treatment of low back pain[42] found a short-term benefit only, although these treatments were more effective than no treatment. Acupuncture and dry needling may be useful adjuncts to other therapies.

Medications

Nonsteroidal Anti-inflammatory Drugs

Nonsteroidal anti-inflammatory drugs (NSAIDs) are among the

mainstays of the initial treatment of degenerative lumbar spinal stenosis.[7,34] The use of NSAIDs is based on the theory that the pathomechanical changes associated with the disease cause inflammation, which leads to pain. NSAIDs have been found effective in treating acute low back pain; however, studies are lacking to determine their efficacy in treating lumbar spinal stenosis.[33,43] Although judicious use of NSAIDs may help improve symptoms, they should be used with caution because of their adverse effects and because lumbar spinal stenosis typically affects older patients. Renal insufficiency, antiplatelet effects, and gastrointestinal bleeding are among the most serious potential adverse effects of NSAID use. To counteract the gastrointestinal adverse effects, especially if long-term NSAID use is anticipated, the drug should be used in conjunction with an H_2-receptor antagonist, proton pump inhibitor, or other prophylaxis. Patients also should undergo routine screening to detect renal insufficiency.

Muscle Relaxants

The direct application of muscle relaxants may be somewhat effective in the treatment of low back pain, but data are lacking as to their efficacy in treating lumbar spinal stenosis.[33,43] Muscle relaxants may help to relieve an acute exacerbation of symptoms related to lumbar spinal stenosis, especially muscle spasm, but long-term use is not recommended.

Analgesic Drugs

Physicians frequently prescribe opioids to relieve pain from chronic low back pain or neurogenic claudication. These drugs act centrally to alter the reception of painful stimuli. Because of their potential adverse effects, including sedation, constipation, and habituation or addiction, narcotics should be used only for brief periods and usually in patients who cannot tolerate NSAIDs or other nonsurgical measures.[7,34]

Antidepressant Drugs and Other Pharmacologic Therapies

Antidepressant drugs are frequently used in patients with chronic pain. They can have a beneficial effect on subclinical depression, and the sedative effect can improve the ability to sleep. However, clinical trials of antidepressant drugs for the treatment of low back pain have had conflicting results.[43]

Several other pharmacologic agents have been used in treating lumbar spinal stenosis. Currently, there is no strong evidence available to show significant long-term benefit of using intranasal or intramuscular calcitonin or methylcobalamin, or intravenous lipoprostaglandin E1.[30]

Epidural Steroid Injections

An epidural injection of steroids, frequently combined with local anesthetics, may relieve lower extremity pain caused by spinal stenosis. This treatment frequently is considered for patients whose radicular symptoms have been unresponsive for a prolonged time to other nonsurgical measures, such as drugs and therapy, and whose imaging studies document nerve root compression that is clinically correlated with the symptoms.[44] Only sparse literature is available on the use of epidural steroids in patients with spinal stenosis, and the available results are conflicting. A single epidural steroid injection may provide significant short-term relief, but the long-term benefits and the results of multiple injections are less predictable.[30] In a double-blinded, placebo-controlled prospective study, Cuckler and associates[45] administered epidural injections of procaine and either methylprednisolone or saline to patients with lumbar radicular symptoms caused by spinal stenosis or disk herniation. Patients in the two groups had no significant difference in symptom improvement at either 24-hour follow-up or an average 20-month follow-up. Hoogmartens and Morelle[46] retrospectively reviewed 49 patients with symptomatic lumbar spinal stenosis and reported that only 32% had good or excellent pain relief and functional outcome 2 years after an injection of a local anesthetic and a steroid. Fukusaki and associates[47] randomly assigned 53 patients with neurogenic claudication to receive an epidural injection of methylprednisolone and mepivacaine, mepivacaine alone, or saline alone. At 1-week follow-up, the patients who received the placebo had poorer results than the other patients. However, there was no significant difference between the two groups of patients who received medication. This finding suggests that the steroid added no benefit to the local anesthetic. At 3-month follow-up, only one patient in each of the three groups reported a good or excellent result. On the other hand, Riew and associates[48] reported favorable results when a steroid (betamethasone) was added to a local anesthetic (bupivacaine) for selective nerve root injection in patients with symptomatic stenosis. A double-blinded, randomized prospective study of 55 patients who had initially requested surgery found that 71% of those who received the combined betamethasone-bupivacaine injection had avoided surgery at a minimum 13-month follow-up, compared with 33% of those who had received bupivacaine only. Of the 21 patients who initially avoided surgery, 17 (81%) had continued to do so at a minimum 5-year follow up.[49] After 5 years, there was no significant difference in symptom improvement between the two groups. These results suggest that in most patients a favorable response to a selective nerve root injection after 1 year will be sustained over the long term. Evidence supports the short-term benefit of a single fluoroscopically-guided transforaminal epidural steroid injection, but few studies have shown a long-term benefit of a multiple injection protocol.[30]

It might be intuitively expected that patients whose radiographic studies show more severe stenosis would be less responsive to epidural steroid injection than patients with less severe stenosis. However, the efficacy of injections, as determined by avoidance of surgery, was found to be unrelated to the dimensions of the spinal canal.[50] Campbell and associates[50] retrospectively reviewed 84 patients who had epidural steroid injection for lumbar spinal stenosis and found that 34 had improved after injection, and 50 required surgical intervention. The dimensions of the central spinal canal, as measured from a preinjection CT scan, was not significantly different in patients who required surgery and those whose symptoms improved after the injection. In a study of patients who had symptoms for more than 1 year, Derby and associates[51] found that a good response to epidural steroid injection can predict a good outcome in patients who ultimately undergo surgical decompression. Among patients who had a good response to selective nerve root injec-

tion, 85% had a positive surgical outcome; in contrast, 95% of those who had a minimal response to injection had a poor surgical outcome.

Epidural injections may be administered via either a translaminar or transforaminal approach. To achieve the best result, an epidural injection should be performed under fluoro-

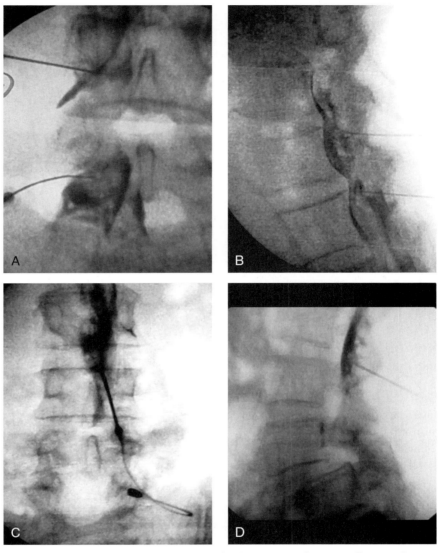

Figure 3 Fluoroscopic images show epidural injections that typically are administered through a transforaminal **(A, B)** or translaminar **(C, D)** approach. **A** and **C,** AP views. **B** and **D,** Lateral views. For patients with pain localized to a specific nerve root distribution, a transforaminal selective nerve root injection is suggested. Injections performed under fluoroscopic guidance yield superior results. (Courtesy of David Fish, MD, Santa Monica, CA.)

scopic guidance[30,33,34] (Figure 3). A transforaminal selective nerve root injection is recommended for patients who have pain in a specific nerve root distribution. Epidural steroid injections may be a valuable adjunct to other nonsurgical measures in patients who refuse surgical treatment or for whom surgical intervention is contraindicated. At the very least, epidural steroid injections facilitate the progress or resumption of active treatment, including physical therapy.[7,34] Epidural injection is an invasive procedure with associated risks, including but not limited to infection (including a potential epidural abscess), dural puncture, bleeding (including epidural hematoma), intravascular injection, and local or systemic reaction to the injected drug.[44] However, these complications are rare.

Physical Therapy and Exercise

The active phase of nonsurgical treatment comprises formal physical therapy and exercise. This aspect of care may be underused; in an evaluation of a large national database, Freburger and associates[52] found that only 38% of patients were given a physical therapy referral during their first appointment with a spine care physician. Of the patients with a diagnosis of spinal stenosis, only 22% were referred for physical therapy.

Although it is widely believed among physicians that physical therapy provides a significant benefit to patients with lumbar spinal stenosis, a recent review found insufficient evidence to recommend physical therapy as a stand-alone treatment.[30] Instead, it is of benefit as part of a comprehensive treatment plan including epidural steroid injection or other medications. A physical therapy program for patients with lumbar spinal stenosis should emphasize core strengthening and aerobic conditioning.

Comparison of Surgical and Nonsurgical Outcomes

There is continuing debate as to whether nonsurgical or surgical treatment is preferable for degenerative lumbar spinal stenosis. No randomized studies are available comparing any nonsurgical measure to simple observation of the natural course of the disease. As a result, it is unclear whether nonsurgical treatment offers benefits.[30] To better define the natural history of the condition, Johnsson and associates[53] followed 32 patients with lumbar spinal stenosis who received no treatment. After an average of 45 months, 70% of patients rated their symptoms as unchanged, 15% as improved, and 15% as worse. On objective clinical examination, 41% of the patients were found to have unchanged symptoms, 41% had improved symptoms, and 18% had worse symptoms.

Simotas and associates[54] reported the results of 49 patients with lumbar spinal stenosis who were treated with varied combinations of limited bed rest, NSAIDs, oral corticosteroids, epidural steroid injections, and physical therapy. At an average 33-month follow-up, 18% required surgical intervention for worsening symptoms, 24% reported significant and sustained improvement in symptoms, 22% reported mild improvement, 24% reported no change, and 10% reported worsening symptoms (a total of 28% had worsening symptoms, including those who required surgery). Because almost half of the patients improved with nonsurgical treatment, aggressive nonsurgical treatment was recommended as an alternative to surgery.

In a prospective study of 100 patients with symptomatic lumbar spinal stenosis, Amundsen and associates[32] randomly assigned 13 patients with moderate spinal stenosis to surgical treatment and 18 patients with moderate stenosis who were considered suitable for surgery to nonsur-

gical treatment. Two nonrandomized cohorts included 50 patients with mild symptoms who were treated nonsurgically and 19 patients with severe symptoms who were surgically treated. At 4-year follow-up, 11 of the patients (92%) randomly assigned to surgical treatment and 8 of the patients (47%) randomly assigned to nonsurgical treatment reported a good result; 28 of those (57%) who were nonrandomly assigned to nonsurgical treatment and 16 of those (84%) who were nonrandomly assigned to surgical treatment reported a good result. At 10-year follow-up, only 75 patients remained; the rest had died or undergone reoperation. Ten of the 18 patients (56%) who were randomly assigned to nonsurgical treatment had received surgical treatment; of the remaining 8 patients, 6 (75%) reported moderate pain, and 2 (25%) reported mild or minimal pain. Of the 50 patients who were nonrandomly assigned to nonsurgical treatment, 19 (56%) had moderate or severe pain, and 15 (44%) had mild or minimal pain at 10-year follow-up. No difference was found in the outcomes of the patients who were initially treated with surgery and those whose surgery was delayed. Although the overall outcomes of surgical treatment were more favorable, initial nonsurgical treatment was found to be appropriate. A patient who does not respond to nonsurgical treatment can be surgically treated and expect a good outcome.[32]

The Maine Lumbar Spine Study, a prospective observational cohort study of patients with lumbar spinal stenosis,[55] found that, although at 1- and 4-year follow-up the outcomes favored surgical treatment, at 8- to 10-year follow-up surgically and nonsurgically treated patients reported similar improvement in back pain (53% and 50%, respectively), relief of their predominant symptom (54% and 42%, respectively, for back or leg pain), and overall satisfaction (55% and 49%, respectively). At 10-year follow-up, 39% of patients who initially received nonsurgical treatment had undergone at least one lumbar spine surgical procedure, and 23% of patients who initially received surgical treatment had undergone at least one additional lumbar spine surgical procedure; however, the treatment received was not correlated with a statistical or clinical difference in outcome.[56]

Many authors agree that nonsurgical treatment is appropriate for patients with mild symptoms and that surgical treatment is appropriate for patients with severe stenosis and long-term, unrelenting pain. There is debate as to the optimal treatment of the many patients whose condition is between these two extremes. Malmivaara and associates[57] randomly assigned 50 such patients to surgical decompression and 44 to nonsurgical treatment with NSAIDs and physical therapy. Although both groups of patients had improvement in back pain, leg pain, and disability, the improvement was significantly greater in the surgically treated patients at all time points within 2 years.

In a prospective study evaluating the effect of nonsurgical treatment in patients who would otherwise be considered candidates for surgery, Athiviraham and Yen[58] found better results in patients who were treated surgically. All 125 patients were offered surgery after unsuccessful nonsurgical treatment; 54 underwent decompression alone, 42 underwent decompression and fusion, and 29 declined surgery in favor of various combinations of physical therapy, bracing, pharmacotherapy, weight management, manipulation, and epidural steroid injections. After 2 years, the surgically treated patients in both groups had similar results: 34 (63%) of the patients treated with decompression alone reported feeling better, 2 (4%) reported feeling worse, and 18 (32.7%) reported no change. Of the patients treated with decompression and fusion, 26 (61.5%) felt better, 1 (2.6%) felt worse, and 15 (35.9%) reported no change. Of the patients treated nonsurgically, 7 (25%) felt better, 4 (12.5%) felt worse, and 18 (62.5%) reported no change.

The Spine Outcomes Research Trial[59] evaluated the roles of surgical and nonsurgical treatment in patients with lumbar spinal stenosis and degenerative spondylolisthesis. Patients who had undergone at least 3 months of unsuccessful nonsurgical treatment were randomly assigned to continue nonsurgical treatment or undergo surgical decompression, with or without fusion. A nonrandomized observational cohort was also followed. The investigators did not dictate the types of nonsurgical treatments to be used; they included (in order of decreasing frequency) NSAIDs, epidural steroid injections, physical therapy, and opioid analgesics. There was significant crossover between the two groups; only 64% of those randomly assigned to surgical treatment ultimately underwent a procedure, and 49% of those randomly assigned to nonsurgical treatment elected to undergo surgery. An intention-to-treat analysis revealed no significant difference in the primary outcome measures of the two groups. The large number of crossover patients necessitated an as-treated analysis including both the randomized and nonrandomized cohorts; this analysis found a significant difference for all outcomes in favor of surgical treatment.

Clinical evidence, primarily from level II and level IV studies, suggests that one third to one half of patients with mild or moderate degenerative lumbar spinal stenosis have a favorable outcome after nonsurgical treatment or observation.[30] Patients with mild or moderate symptoms may benefit from long-term nonsurgical treatment, whereas patients with moderate or severe symptoms are more likely to benefit from surgery.[60]

Summary

Lumbar spinal stenosis is degenerative in most patients. A cascade of spondylotic changes induces narrowing of the central spinal canal, the lateral recesses, or neuroforamina. These changes probably begin with degeneration of the intervertebral disk, leading to alterations in biomechanical loads throughout the lumbar spinal segment and causing changes in the facet joints and ligamentum flavum, which further destabilize the segment. Posterior disk bulging, loss of disk height, osteophytes, redundant and hypertrophied ligamentum flavum, and arthritic facet joints all contribute to the development of stenosis. Impingement on the neural elements results in the development of neurogenic claudication and radicular symptoms through a combination of direct mechanical compression, alterations in microvascular circulation, impaired axoplasmic flow, and inflammatory mediators.

The initial treatment of a symptomatic patient with lumbar spinal stenosis should be a comprehensive nonsurgical program of anti-inflammatory medication, physical therapy and conditioning, and epidural steroid injections. As many as

50% of patients experience long-term relief after nonsurgical treatment, and delaying surgical treatment does not alter the clinical outcome. Therefore, surgical intervention should be considered only after conscientious nonsurgical treatment has failed to restore the patient's quality of life.

References

1. Lin SI, Lin RM, Huang LW: Disability in patients with degenerative lumbar spinal stenosis. *Arch Phys Med Rehabil* 2006;87:1250-1256.

2. Turner JA, Ersek M, Herron L, Deyo R: Surgery for lumbar spinal stenosis: Attempted meta-analysis of the literature. *Spine* 1992;17:1-8.

3. Zanoli G, Jonsson B, Stromqvist B: SF-36 scores in degenerative lumbar spine disorders: Analysis of prospective data from 451 patients. *Acta Orthop* 2006;77:298-306.

4. Hai Y: Classification, natural history, and clinical evaluation, in Herkowitz HN, Dvorak J, Bell GR, Nordin M, Grob D (eds): *The Lumbar Spine*, ed 3. Philadelphia, PA, Lippincott Williams & Wilkins, 2004, pp 464-471.

5. Arnoldi CC, Brodsky AE, Chauchoix J, et al: Lumbar spinal stenosis and nerve root entrapment syndromes: Definition and classification. *Clin Orthop Relat Res* 1976;115:4-5.

6. Verbiest H: The significance and principles of computerized axial tomography in idiopathic developmental stenosis of the bony lumbar vertebral canal. *Spine* 1979;4:369-378.

7. Hilibrand AS, Rand N: Degenerative lumbar stenosis: Diagnosis and management. *J Am Acad Orthop Surg* 1999;7:239-249.

8. Truumees E: Spinal stenosis: Pathophysiology, clinical and radiologic classification. *Instr Course Lect* 2005;54:287-302.

9. Urban JP, McMullin JF: Swelling pressure of the lumbar intervertebral discs: Influence of age, spinal level, composition, and degeneration. *Spine* 1988;13:179-187.

10. Martin MD, Boxell CM, Malone DG: Pathophysiology of lumbar disc degeneration: A review of the literature. *Neurosurg Focus* 2002;13:E1.

11. Kauppila LI: Ingrowth of blood vessels in disc degeneration: Angiographic and histological studies of cadaveric spines. *J Bone Joint Surg Am* 1995;77:26-31.

12. Berven S, Tay BB, Colman W, Hu SS: The lumbar zygapophyseal (facet) joints: A role in the pathogenesis of spinal pain syndromes and degenerative spondylolisthesis. *Semin Neurol* 2002;22:187-196.

13. Panjabi MM, Krag MH, Chung TQ: Effects of disc injury on mechanical behavior of the human spine. *Spine* 1984;9:707-713.

14. Igarashi A, Kikuchi S, Konno S: Correlation between inflammatory cytokines released from the lumbar facet joint tissue and symptoms in degenerative lumbar spinal disorders. *J Orthop Sci* 2007;12:154-160.

15. Tachihara H, Kikuchi S, Konno S, Sekiguchi M: Does facet joint inflammation induce radiculopathy? An investigation using a rat model of lumbar facet joint inflammation. *Spine* 2007;32:406-412.

16. Schrader PK, Grob D, Rahn BA, Cordey J, Dvorak J: Histology of the ligamentum flavum in patients with degenerative lumbar spinal stenosis. *Eur Spine J* 1999;8:323-328.

17. Sairyo K, Biyani A, Goel V, et al: Pathomechanism of ligamentum flavum hypertrophy: A multidisciplinary investigation based on clinical, biomechanical, histologic, and biologic assessments. *Spine* 2005;30:2649-2656.

18. Park JB, Lee JK, Park SJ, Riew KD: Hypertrophy of ligamentum flavum in lumbar spinal stenosis associated with increased proteinase inhibitor concentration. *J Bone Joint Surg Am* 2005;87:2750-2757.

19. Pedowitz RA, Garfin SR, Massie JB, et al: Effects of magnitude and duration of compression on spinal nerve root conduction. *Spine* 1992;17:194-199.

20. Delamarter RB, Bohlman HH, Dodge LD, Biro C: Experimental lumbar spinal stenosis: Analysis of the cortical evoked potentials, microvasculature, and histopathology. *J Bone Joint Surg Am* 1990;72:110-120.

21. Takahashi K, Kagechika K, Takino T, Matsui T, Miyazaki T, Shima I: Changes in epidural pressure during walking in patients with lumbar spinal stenosis. *Spine* 1995;20:2746-2749.

22. Takahashi K, Miyazaki T, Takino T, Matsui T, Tomita K: Epidural pressure measurements: Relationship between epidural pressure and posture in patients with lumbar spinal stenosis. *Spine* 1995;20:650-653.

23. Willén J, Danielson B, Gaulitz A, Niklason T, Schönström N, Hansson T: Dynamic effects on the lumbar spinal canal: Axially loaded CT-myelography and MRI in patients with sciatica and/or neurogenic claudication. *Spine* 1997;22:2968-2976.

24. Hunt JL, Winkelstein BA, Rutkowski MD, Weinstein JN, DeLeo JA: Repeated injury to the lumbar nerve roots produces enhanced mechanical allodynia and persistent spinal neuroinflammation. *Spine* 2001;26:2073-2079.

25. Kobayashi S, Yoshizawa H, Yamada S: Pathology of lumbar nerve root compression: Part 2. Morphological and immunohistochemical changes of dorsal root ganglion. *J Orthop Res* 2004;22:180-188.

26. Hasue M: Pain and the nerve root: An interdisciplinary approach. *Spine* 1993;18:2053-2058.

27. Kobayashi S, Kokubo Y, Uchida K, et al: Effect of lumbar nerve root compression on primary sensory neurons and their central branches: Changes in the nociceptive neuropeptides substance P and somatostatin. *Spine* 2005;30:276-282.

28. Ikawa M, Atsuta Y, Tsunekawa H: Ectopic firing due to artificial venous stasis in rat lumbar spinal canal stenosis model: A possible pathogenesis of neurogenic intermittent claudication. *Spine* 2005;30:2393-2397.

29. Kobayashi S, Yoshizawa H, Yamada S: Pathology of lumbar nerve root compression: Part 1. Intraradicular inflammatory changes induced by mechanical compression. *J Orthop Res* 2004;22:170-179.

30. North American Spine Society: *Clinical Guidelines for Multidisciplinary Spine Care: Diagnosis and Treatment of Degenerative Lumbar Spinal Stenosis.* Burr Ridge, IL, North American Spine Society, 2007.

31. Benoist M: The natural history of lumbar degenerative spinal stenosis. *Joint Bone Spine* 2002;69:450-457.

32. Amundsen T, Weber H, Nordal HJ, Magnaes B, Abdelnoor M, Lilleâs F: Lumbar spinal stenosis: Conservative or surgical management? A prospective 10-year study. *Spine* 2000;25:1424-1435.

33. Herno A: Spinal stenosis without deformity: Nonoperative treatment, in Herkowitz HN, Dvorak J, Bell GR, Nordin M, Grob D (eds): *The Lumbar Spine,* ed 3. Philadelphia, PA, Lippincott Williams & Wilkins, 2004, pp 490-494.

34. Yuan PS, Booth RE Jr, Albert TJ: Nonsurgical and surgical management of lumbar spinal stenosis. *Instr Course Lect* 2005;54:303-312.

35. Coomes EN: A comparison between epidural anaesthesia and bed rest in sciatica. *BMJ* 1961;1:20-24.

36. Pal B, Mangion P, Hossain MA, Diffey BL: A controlled trial of continuous lumbar traction in the treatment of back pain and sciatica. *Br J Rheumatol* 1986;25:181-183.

37. van Poppel MN, Koes BW, van der Ploeg T, Smid T, Bouter LM: Lumbar supports and education for the prevention of low back pain in industry: A randomized controlled trial. *JAMA* 1998;279:1789-1794.

38. Prateepavanich P, Thanapipatsiri S, Santisatisakul P, Somshevita P. Charoensak T: The effectiveness of lumbosacral corset in symptomatic degenerative lumbar spinal stenosis. *J Med Assoc Thai* 2001;84:572-576.

39. Hurwitz EL, Morgenstern H, Harber P, et al: A randomized trial of medical care with and without physical therapy and chiropractic care with and without physical modalities for patients with low back pain: 6-month follow-up outcomes from the UCLA low back pain study. *Spine* 2002;27:2193-2204.

40. Chou R, Huffman LH: Nonpharmacologic therapies for acute and chronic low back pain: A review of the evidence for an American Pain Society/American College of Physicians clinical practice guideline. *Ann Intern Med* 2007;147:492-504.

41. Inoue M, Hojo T, Yano T, Katsumi Y: Effects of lumbar acupuncture stimulation on blood flow to the sciatic nerve trunk: An exploratory study. *Acupunct Med* 2005;23:166-170.

42. Furlan AD, van Tulder M, Cherkin D, et al: Acupuncture and dry-needling for low back pain: An updated systematic review within the framework of the Cochrane collaboration. *Spine* 2005;30:944-963.

43. Deyo RA: Drug therapy for back pain: Which drugs help which patients? *Spine* 1996;21:2840-2849.

44. Young IA, Hyman GS, Packia-Raj LN, Cole AJ: The use of lumbar epidural/transforaminal steroids for managing spinal disease. *J Am Acad Orthop Surg* 2007;15:228-238.

45. Cuckler JM, Bernini PA, Wiesel SW, Booth RE Jr, Rothman RH, Pickens GT: The use of epidural steroids in the treatment of lumbar radicular pain: A prospective, randomized, double-blind study. *J Bone Joint Surg Am* 1985;67:63-66.

46. Hoogmartens M, Morelle P: Epidural injection in the treatment of spinal stenosis. *Acta Orthop Belg* 1987;53:409-411.

47. Fukusaki M, Kobayashi I, Hara T, Sumikawa K: Symptoms of spinal stenosis do not improve after epidural steroid injection. *Clin J Pain* 1998;14:148-151.

48. Riew KD, Yin Y, Gilula L, et al: The effect of nerve-root injections on the need for operative treatment of lumbar radicular pain: A prospective, randomized, controlled, double-blind study. *J Bone Joint Surg Am* 2000;82-A:1589-1593.

49. Riew KD, Park JB, Cho YS, et al: Nerve root blocks in the treatment of lumbar radicular pain: A minimum five-year follow-up. *J Bone Joint Surg Am* 2006;88:1722-1725.

50. Campbell MJ, Carreon LY, Glassman SD, McGinniss MD, Elmlinger BS: Correlation of spinal canal dimensions to efficacy of epidural steroid injection in spinal stenosis. *J Spinal Disord Tech* 2007;20:168-171.

51. Derby R, Kine G, Saal JA, et al: Response to steroid and duration of radicular pain as predictors of surgical outcome. *Spine* 1992;17:S176-S183.

52. Freburger JK, Carey TS, Holmes GM: Physician referrals to physical therapists for the treatment of spine disorders. *Spine J* 2005;5:530-541.

53. Johnsson KE, Rosen I, Uden A: The natural course of lumbar spinal stenosis. *Clin Orthop Relat Res* 1992;279:82-86.

54. Simotas AC, Dorey FJ, Hansraj KK, Cammisa F Jr: Nonoperative treatment for lumbar spinal stenosis: Clinical and outcome results and a 3-year survivorship analysis. *Spine* 2000;25:197-203.

55. Atlas SJ, Keller RB, Wu YA, Deyo RA, Singer DE: Long-term outcomes of surgical and nonsurgical management of lumbar spinal stenosis: 8 to 10 year results from the Maine Lumbar Spine Study. *Spine* 2005;30:936-943.

56. Chang Y, Singer DE, Wu YA, Keller RB, Atlas SJ: The effect of surgical and nonsurgical treatment on longitudinal outcomes of lumbar spinal

stenosis over 10 years. *J Am Geriatr Soc* 2005;53:785-792.

57. Malmivaara A, Slatis P, Heliovaara M, et al: Surgical or nonoperative treatment for lumbar spinal stenosis? A randomized controlled trial. *Spine* 2007;32:1-8.

58. Athiviraham A, Yen D: Is spinal stenosis better treated surgically or nonsurgically? *Clin Orthop Relat Res* 2007;458:90-93.

59. Weinstein JN, Lurie JD, Tosteson TD, et al: Surgical versus nonsurgical treatment for lumbar degenerative

spondylolisthesis. *N Engl J Med* 2007; 356:2257-2270.

60. Snyder DL, Doggett D, Turkelson C: Treatment of degenerative lumbar spinal stenosis. *Am Fam Physician* 2004;70:517-520.

Lumbar Spinal Stenosis: Indications for Arthrodesis and Spinal Instrumentation

Mark A. Knaub, MD
Douglas S. Won, MD
Robert McGuire, MD
Harry N. Herkowitz, MD

Abstract

Surgical indications for simple decompression in patients with lumbar spinal stenosis are well established. Following these guidelines, surgeons can expect good and excellent outcomes in 75% to 90% of patients. Despite the publication of many studies pertaining to the addition of arthrodesis and instrumentation, the indications for adding these procedures to a decompression are much less clear. Preoperative and intraoperative factors must be carefully considered when contemplating the addition of arthrodesis in the setting of spinal stenosis. In patients with preoperative degenerative spondylolisthesis, scoliosis, or kyphosis, and those in whom stenosis develops at a previously decompressed segment, serious consideration should be given for inclusion of an arthrodesis. Fusion should also be considered for those patients with stenosis adjacent to a previously fused lumbar segment. Excision of a significant portion of the facet joints or radical excision of the intervertebral disk during the course of the decompression predispose the patient to postoperative instability. The addition of an arthrodesis will likely benefit these patients. Relative indications for the use of spinal instrumentation in the setting of spinal stenosis include correction of deformity, recurrent spinal stenosis with instability, degenerative spondylolisthesis, adjacent segment stenosis with instability, and multiple level fusions.

The surgical indications for patients with clinical symptoms of spinal stenosis and a confirming imaging study to undergo decompression are well defined. The clinical success rate of the decompression is between 75% to 90%.[1-6]

The indications for the addition of an arthrodesis and spinal instrumentation following decompressive laminectomy remain controversial. The following factors should be considered when deciding whether or not arthrodesis should be performed at the time of a decompression: the preoperative structural integrity of each functional spinal unit in the lumbar spine, the preoperative coronal and sagittal plane alignment of the lumbar spine, and the alterations of the structural integrity that occur secondary to the decompression.

The significant preoperative structural alterations that occur in the clinical setting with spinal stenosis include the presence of degenerative spondylolisthesis or scoliosis and/or kyphosis. Other preoperative considerations include the development of recurrent spinal stenosis at a previously decompressed level and the presence of spinal stenosis adjacent to a previously fused lumbar segment (adjacent segment degeneration/stenosis).

The decision to perform an arthrodesis following a decompressive laminectomy may also be affected by issues that arise during the course of the decompression. Significant removal of the lumbar facet joints or radical excision of the intervertebral disk at the decompressed levels may destabilize the decompressed segments and lead to postoperative instability.

Preoperative Structural Alterations
Degenerative Spondylolisthesis

There has been controversy regarding the role of arthrodesis and spinal instrumentation following decompressive laminectomy in patients with degenerative spondylolisthesis. Some authors have advocated decompressive laminectomy alone, whereas others have recommended arthrodesis with or without spinal instrumentation. Several prospective and retrospective studies comparing decom-

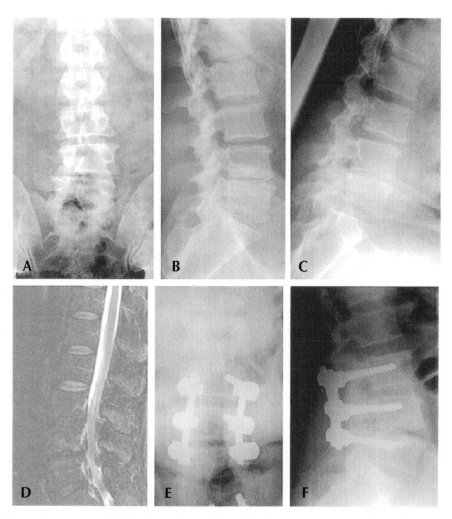

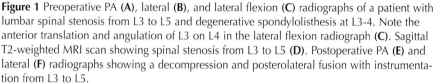

Figure 1 Preoperative PA (**A**), lateral (**B**), and lateral flexion (**C**) radiographs of a patient with lumbar spinal stenosis from L3 to L5 and degenerative spondylolisthesis at L3-4. Note the anterior translation and angulation of L3 on L4 in the lateral flexion radiograph (**C**). Sagittal T2-weighted MRI scan showing spinal stenosis from L3 to L5 (**D**). Postoperative PA (**E**) and lateral (**F**) radiographs showing a decompression and posterolateral fusion with instrumentation from L3 to L5.

pression with and without arthrodesis have shown that patients who undergo a concomitant fusion have improved clinical results. Herkowitz and Kurz[7] prospectively compared 50 patients with single-level spinal stenosis associated with degenerative spondylolisthesis who underwent decompressive laminectomy alone versus decompressive laminectomy with intertransverse process arthrodesis with autogenous bone graft. Clinical outcomes in the arthrodesis group were sig-

nificantly better than those in the decompression alone group. Subsequently, other studies have reported similar results.[8-11]

Mardjetko and associates[12] performed a meta-analysis of the literature concerning surgery for degenerative spondylolisthesis from 1970 to 1993. The study compared the results of patients who underwent decompressive laminectomy alone, decompressive laminectomy with bone graft, and decompressive laminec-

tomy with bone graft and spine instrumentation. Satisfactory outcomes were found in 69%, 90%, and 86% of patients, respectively. The rate of solid arthrodesis between instrumented and noninstrumented fusions was not significant (86% versus 93%).

Postacchini and Cinotti[13] reported on the occurrence of laminar regrowth following decompressive laminectomy for spinal stenosis. They reviewed 40 patients with an average follow-up of 8.6 years. Sixteen of the 40 patients had degenerative spondylolisthesis along with their spinal stenosis. Six of these 16 patients had decompressive laminectomy alone, and 10 had decompression and fusion. Patients who had decompression alone had greater bone regrowth and significantly poorer clinical outcomes than those with decompression and fusion.

Bridwell and associates[14] compared patients with spinal stenosis associated with degenerative spondylolisthesis who underwent decompression alone, decompression with fusion, and decompression with fusion and instrumentation. The group that had fusion and instrumentation had a statistically significantly higher fusion rate and less progression of spondylolisthesis than the other two groups. The authors recommended fusion and instrumentation in patients undergoing decompression for spinal stenosis associated with degenerative spondylolisthesis (Figure 1).

Zdeblick[15] prospectively studied 124 patients who underwent lumbar fusion for degenerative disorders. Fifty-six of 124 patients had degenerative spondylolisthesis. Patients were randomized to one of three groups: posterolateral fusion without instrumentation, posterolateral fusion with semirigid instrumentation, and posterolateral fusion with rigid pedicle screw instrumentation. The rate of successful fusion in patients treated with rigid instrumentation was 86% compared with 65% in patients treated with noninstrumented fusion. Clinical outcomes between these two groups were also significantly different; 95% good to excellent results occurred when rigid instrumentation was used versus 71% good to excellent results in the noninstrumented group. As a result, the author recommended the use of rigid pedicle screw instrumentation in patients undergoing fusion for degenerative spondylolisthesis.

Fischgrund and associates,[16] in a prospective, randomized study, compared decompressive laminectomy and fusion with and without instrumentation in patients with degenerative spondylolisthesis. They reported an 83% fusion rate in the instrumented group whereas only 45% of those in the noninstrumented group went on to solid arthrodesis. Surprisingly, no significant difference in the clinical outcome was found between these groups at 3-year follow-up.

Kornblum and associates[17] reviewed the long-term clinical outcomes of the prospectively followed patients who were initially reported by Herkowitz and Kurz[7] and by Fischgrund and associates.[16] These patients were treated by laminectomy and fusion (both noninstrumented and instrumented) for spinal stenosis and degenerative spondylolisthesis. The clinical outcomes of those patients with a solid arthrodesis, regardless of whether instrumentation was used or not, were compared with those who were found to have a pseudarthrosis. Good to excellent results were achieved in 86% of patients with a solid fusion and 56% of patients with a pseudarthrosis. These data suggest that the long-term clinical outcomes after decompression and fusion for spinal stenosis and spondylolisthesis may be dependent on the formation of a solid arthrodesis.

In summary, the data regarding spinal stenosis in association with degenerative spondylolisthesis strongly support the addition of posterolateral arthrodesis at the time of the decompressive laminectomy. Also, strong evidence exists that supports the notion that higher fusion rates and

---

Table 1
Guidelines for Appropriate Levels of Instrumentation

Instrument all rotated vertebrae.

Do not stop proximal instrumentation at L1 or within the thoracic kyphosis. Fuse to T11 or T12 for lumbar curves and fuse to T4 or T5 for thoracic curves.

Do not include a segment only because osteoarthritis is present.

Fusion to the sacrum in the face of L5-S1 arthritis is not necessary unless the L5 vertebrae is significantly rotated.

Do not stop instrumentation at a segment where the vertebral body is tilted 15° or more because this leads to an increased incidence of adjacent level degeneration/stenosis.

Curves that cannot be brought into satisfactory balance on side bending films may require anterior releases or osteotomy in conjunction with posterior instrumentation.

---

improved long-term clinical outcomes occur when instrumentation is performed with the decompression and fusion.

Degenerative Scoliosis With Spinal Stenosis

Degenerative lumbar scoliosis develops following disk degeneration and facet joint arthritis and instability. Lateral listhesis may occur within the degenerative lumbar curve because of the instability created by the asymmetric facet degeneration. The surgical management of spinal stenosis in association with degenerative scoliosis consists of several options. Decompressive laminectomy alone is indicated for patients with primarily radiculopathy with stiff curves without significant overall sagittal or coronal imbalance.

Multiple factors must be taken into account when considering the addition of an arthrodesis following laminectomy in patients with degenerative scoliosis. The flexibility of the curve must be determined. Flexible curves have a greater propensity to progress following laminectomy; therefore, the addition of an instrumented fusion is recommended. The presence or absence of progression of the curve must be considered. Curves with documented progression are "unstable" and will continue to progress with laminectomy alone. Patients with significant coronal and/or sagittal imbalance are prone to persistent back pain in conjunction with the activity limitations created by the inability to stand erect. Finally, nerve root compression within the concavity of the curve may not respond to decompression alone because of the pedicular kinking that may be present. Therefore, distraction may be necessary to ensure adequate neural decompression.

Figure 2 shows a degenerative lumbar scoliosis with concomitant spinal stenosis. An instrumented arthrodesis was added to the decompression to allow for distraction on the concave side of the curve to alleviate right-sided radicular symptoms.

Once the decision to add instrumentation is made, the question of what levels to include in the instrumentation must be addressed. All segments with documented stenosis on imaging studies should be decompressed. The appropriate levels for instrumentation follow the guidelines as listed in Table 1.

Recurrent Spinal Stenosis at the Same Segment

Patients who previously had a decompressive laminectomy and who have recurrent spinal stenosis at the same segment may require arthrodesis in addition to revision decompression. To sufficient-

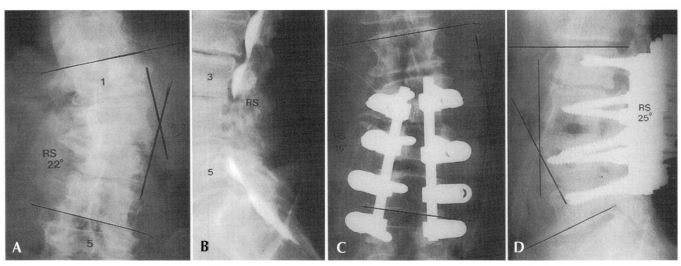

Figure 2 Preoperative PA radiograph (**A**) and lateral myelogram (**B**) showing degenerative lumbar scoliosis with lumbar spinal stenosis. This patient underwent decompressive laminectomy and posterolateral fusion with segmental instrumentation. Postoperative radiographs show partial correction of the coronal plane deformity (**C**) with maintenance of lumbar lordosis (**D**).

ly decompress the neural elements, further resection of the facet joints is usually necessary.[18-20] If more than 50% of both facet joints at a single level have been compromised, then the segment is considered unstable and the patient is a candidate for an arthrodesis.[21,22]

Recurrent spinal stenosis may also be produced by laminar regrowth following laminectomy for spinal stenosis as reported by Postacchini and Cinotti.[13] They reviewed 40 patients, and 88% of the patients treated with laminectomy or laminotomy with or without arthrodesis had some degree of regrowth of lamina. Forty percent of patients with moderate to severe bone regrowth had symptomatic recurrence. This was more common in patients who had a degenerative spondylolisthesis but only had a decompressive laminectomy. They also found that patients with either preoperative or postoperative instability were found to have greater laminar regrowth than those with no instability. As a result, the authors suggested that regrowth of the posterior arch may be stimulated by abnormal vertebral motion. The addition of an arthrodesis in this patient group lessened the magnitude of regrowth.

Adjacent Segment Stenosis

Stenosis above a previous posterolateral fusion is not infrequent. Lehmann and associates[23] reported a 42% incidence of adjacent segment stenosis in their long-term follow-up study. Only 45% of these patients exhibited segmental instability above the fusion and only 15% required revision surgery.

Patel and Herkowitz[24] retrospectively reviewed 47 consecutive patients who required a second operation because of an adjacent segment lumbar stenosis and found that instrumented fusion had an increased and accelerated rate of symptomatic adjacent segment stenosis compared with noninstrumented fusion. The instrumentation group developed symptoms from stenosis at an average of 62 months whereas the patients who underwent non-instrumented fusion developed symptoms at an average of 143 months. This difference was statistically significant. They also found that adjacent segment stenosis occurred in the proximal segment in 89% of patients who underwent floating fusions. Thirty of 47 patients required extension of the arthrodesis in addition to decompression. They recommended decompression alone in the absence of instability; otherwise, decompressive laminectomy with instrumented arthrodesis was recommended. An example of a patient with adjacent segment degeneration, stenosis, and instability is shown in Figure 3. Whitecloud and associates[25] reported 14 patients with adjacent segment stenosis who were treated with decompression and fusion. Noninstrumented fusion resulted in a pseudarthrosis rate of 80% whereas only 17% of those treated with a decompression and instrumented fusion went on to develop a pseudarthrosis. The authors recommend the addition of an instrumented fusion to the decompression at segments adjacent to a previous fusion.

Intraoperative Considerations
Radical Diskectomy

Five percent to 25% of lumbar disk herniations occur in the setting of spinal stenosis.[1,2] Many of these represent simple extrusions or free fragments of disk resulting in nerve root compression at

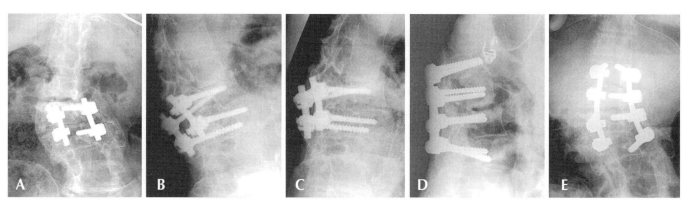

Figure 3 PA (**A**), lateral (**B**), and lateral flexion (**C**) radiographs of a patient with a previous instrumented fusion from L3-4. Degenerative changes and instability have developed above the previously fused levels. The patient underwent adjacent segment decompression and extension of the instrumented fusion. Postoperative lateral (**D**) and PA (**E**) images show adjacent segment decompression and extension of the fusion to the degenerative, adjacent level.

the level of the foramen. In this situation, removal of the herniated disk during the decompressive laminectomy will address both the central and foraminal stenosis. Aggressive diskectomy, removal of as much disk as possible, may result in destabilization of the anterior column. Iatrogenic spondylolisthesis may occur as a result of destabilization of the anterior column by the aggressive disk removal and the posterior column by the laminectomy.[26] Therefore, arthrodesis should be added when a radical diskectomy is combined with a laminectomy for the treatment of concomitant disk herniation and central stenosis. Traditionally, posterolateral arthrodesis with or without instrumentation has been used to achieve fusion in this setting. More recently, the addition of an anterior column support, via a posterior or transforaminal interbody fusion technique, to the posterolateral arthrodesis has been suggested. Although controversial, the addition of an anterior column support may help maintain disk space height and lumbar lordosis and may increase fusion rates.[27,28]

Excessive Resection of Facet Joints

The ultimate goal of surgical intervention in spinal stenosis is decompression of the

neural elements. In an attempt to meet this goal during surgery, excessive bone resection may be required. Narrow, hypertrophic facet joints may contribute to central lateral recess and foraminal stenosis, necessitating partial or complete removal during the decompression. In a cadaveric biomechanical study, Abumi and associates[21] demonstrated the importance of the lumbar facet joints in maintaining the structural integrity of the functional spinal unit. Cyclic loading of the lumbar motion segment after progressive facetectomies revealed that removal of greater than 50% of each facet joint led to unacceptable motion at that segment. Boden and associates[29] also noted increased motion with progressive removal of the facet joints in a cadaveric study. Extrapolation of these data to the clinical setting would suggest that when excessive facet removal is necessary during the decompression, posterolateral arthrodesis should be added to prevent iatrogenic instability.

Although cadaveric studies suggest that excision of larger portions of the facet joints may lead to clinical instability, some clinical reports refute this claim. Hazlett and Kinnard[30] reported on 33 patients undergoing complete unilateral or bilateral facet joint removal. Late insta-

bility developed in four of the patients and only two of those four had poor results. Some authors have reported that the morphology of the facet joints played a larger role in the progression of spondylolisthesis than did the absolute amount of facet joint resection. Preoperative and postoperative CT scans were reviewed in patients undergoing decompression for spinal stenosis. Patients who went on to develop spondylolisthesis postoperatively had facet coronal dimensions less than those patients who did not develop instability. Patients who developed postoperative spondylolisthesis also had more sagittally oriented facet joints.[22,31]

Clinical studies exist that support the findings of the above noted cadaveric studies. Mullin and associates[32] reported that 54% of patients undergoing decompressive lumbar laminectomy with medial facetectomy went on to develop instability postoperatively. Although instability did not guarantee a poor clinical outcome, those patients with radiographic instability tended to have a poor clinical course.

The exact degree of instability created by a given decompression is impossible to predict. Even patients with radiographic evidence of instability may do well clinically. Despite this, most surgeons advocate the addition of posterolateral arthrodesis when significant intraoperative removal of facet joints occurs during laminectomy.

The Role of Spinal Instrumentation

Internal fixation is used to correct deformity, to provide initial stability to the spine, to protect the neural elements, to improve the rate of successful fusion, to reduce the use of postoperative bracing, and to reduce rehabilitation time.

Prior to the use of pedicle screw systems, instrumentation of the degenerative lumbar spine in older patients was problematic. The absence of lamina in patients undergoing decompressive laminectomy precluded the use of traditional lamina and pedicle hooks. Osteopenia complicated fixation in the lumbar spine by increasing the rate of hook failure at the bone-implant interface. The use of traditional posterior distraction rods in the lumbar spine (Harrington rods) led to a loss of lumbar lordosis resulting in recurrent back and radicular symptoms.

Pedicle screw fixation offers advantages in the lumbar spine. It can be used in conjunction with a decompressive laminectomy. Fixation with these screws is obtained within the pedicle itself—the strongest part of the osteopenic vertebrae.[33] Pedicle screws allow for segmental fixation that increases the torsional rigidity of the construct, improves fusion rate, and aids in maintaining lumbar lordosis. Other potential advantages of segmental fixation include the ability to reduce the number of motion segments requiring arthrodesis.[34,35] Fixation into the sacrum and pelvis is also improved with pedicle screws.

The main goals of adding instrumentation to a decompression and fusion are to improve the ability to obtain a solid fusion and to correct preexisting deformity. Increased rates of pseudarthrosis have been documented when multiple-level fusions are done without the addition of internal fixation.[36,37] In addition, when instability is present, for example, a mobile spondylolisthesis, bone graft alone without fixation, leads to a high pseudarthrosis rate.[15,16,38-40]

Therefore, the relative indications for the addition of instrumentation following decompression of spinal stenosis and arthrodesis are deformity correction; multiple level fusions; recurrent spinal stenosis with iatrogenic instability; degenerative spondylolisthesis; and adjacent segment stenosis with instability.

Summary

The surgical indications for decompression in patients with spinal stenosis are well defined. Clinical success is expected in 75% to 90% of patients. The indications to add an arthrodesis to a decompression in the setting of spinal stenosis are less clear. Preoperative and intraoperative factors must be taken into consideration when making this decision. Instrumentation should be added following decompression and arthrodesis for multiple level fusions, deformity correction, adjacent segment spinal stenosis, and when increased translation or angular motion are present on preoperative flexion and extension radiographs.

Discussion of the details of the surgical techniques for arthrodesis and spinal instrumentation are beyond the scope of this chapter. Also, analysis of various implant systems, along with their advantages and disadvantages, has similarly been omitted from this discussion. Despite the publication of many studies addressing the controversial issues surrounding the addition of a fusion and instrumentation following decompression of spinal stenosis, many questions remain. Only prospective, randomized clinical trials will provide the information necessary to provide patients with the most effective, long-term solution to this challenging surgical problem.

References

1. Garfin SR, Glover M, Booth RE, Simeone FA, Rothman RH: Laminectomy: A review of the Pennsylvania hospital experience. *J Spinal Disord* 1988;1:116-133.

2. Herkowitz H, Garfin S: Decompressive surgery for spinal stenosis. *Semin Spine Surg* 1989;1:163-167.

3. Herron LD, Mangelsdorf C: Lumbar spinal stenosis: Results of surgical treatment. *J Spinal Disord* 1991;4:26-33.

4. Katz JN, Lipson SJ, Larson MG, McInness JM, Fossel AH, Liang MH: The outcome of decompressive laminectomy for degenerative lumbar stenosis. *J Bone Joint Surg Am* 1991;73:809-816.

5. Spengler DM: Degenerative stenosis of the lumbar spine. *J Bone Joint Surg Am* 1987;69:305-308.

6. Tile M, McNeil SR, Zarins RK, Pennal GF, Garside SH: Spinal stenosis: Results of treatment. *Clin Orthop* 1976;115:104-108.

7. Herkowitz HN, Kurz LT: Degenerative lumbar spondylolisthesis with spinal stenosis: A prospective study comparing decompression with decompression and intertransverse process arthrodesis. *J Bone Joint Surg Am* 1991;73:802-808.

8. Caputy AJ, Luessenhop AJ: Long-term evaluation of decompressive surgery for degenerative lumbar stenosis. *J Neurosurg* 1992;77:669-676.

9. Feffer HL, Wiesel SW, Cuckler JM, Rothman RH: Degenerative spondylolisthesis: To fuse or not to fuse. *Spine* 1985;10:287-289.

10. Katz JN, Lipson SJ, Chang LC, Levine SA, Fossel AH, Liang MH: Seven- to 10-year outcome of decompressive surgery for degenerative lumbar spinal stenosis. *Spine* 1996;21:92-98.

11. Postacchini F: Management of lumbar spinal stenosis. *J Bone Joint Surg Br* 1996;78:154-164.

12. Mardjetko SM, Connolly PJ, Shott S: Degenerative lumbar spondylolisthesis: A meta-analysis of literature 1970-1993. *Spine* 1994;19(suppl 20):2256S-2265S.

13. Postacchini F, Cinotti G: Bone regrowth after surgical decompression for lumbar spinal stenosis. *J Bone Joint Surg Br* 1992;74:862-869.

14. Bridwell KH, Sedgewick TA, O'Brien MF, Lenke LG, Baldus C: The role of fusion and instrumentation in the treatment of degenerative spondylolisthesis with spinal stenosis. *J Spinal Disord* 1993;6:461-472.

15. Zdeblick TA: A prospective, randomized study of lumbar fusion: Preliminary results. *Spine* 1993;18:983-991.

16. Fischgrund JS, Mackay M, Herkowitz HN, Brower R, Montgomery DM, Kurz LT: Degenerative lumbar spondylolisthesis with spinal stenosis: A prospective, randomized study comparing decompressive laminectomy and arthrodesis with and without spinal instrumentation. *Spine* 1997;22:2807-2812.

17. Kornblum MB, Fischgrund JS, Herkowitz HN, Abraham DA, Berkower DL, Ditkoff JS:

Degenerative lumbar spondylolisthesis with spinal stenosis: A prospective long-term study comparing fusion and pseudoarthrosis. *67th Annual Meeting Proceedings.* Rosemont, IL, American Academy of Orthopaedic Surgeons, 2000, pp 523-524.

18. Hansraj KK, O'Leary PF, Cammisa FP Jr, et al: Decompression, fusion, and instrumentation surgery for complex lumbar spinal stenosis. *Clin Orthop* 2001;384:18-25.

19. Herno A, Airksinen O, Saari T, Sihvonen T: Surgical results of lumbar spinal stenosis: A comparison of patients with or without previous back surgery. *Spine* 1995;20:964-969.

20. Truumees E, Herkowitz HN: Lumbar spinal stenosis: Treatment options. *Instr Course Lect* 2001;50:153-161.

21. Abumi K, Panjabi MM, Kramer KM, Duranceau J, Oxland T, Crisco JJ: Biomechanical evaluation of lumbar spinal stability after graded facetectomies. *Spine* 1990;15:1142-1147.

22. Grobler LJ, Robertson PA, Novotny JE, Ahern JW: Decompression for degenerative spondylolisthesis and spinal stenosis at L4-5: The effects on facet joint morphology. *Spine* 1993;18:1475-1482.

23. Lehmann TR, Spratt KF, Tozzi JE: Long-term follow-up of lower lumbar fusion patients. *Spine* 1987;12:97-104.

24. Patel CK, Herkowitz HN: Symptomatic spinal stenosis adjacent to a previous lumbar spinal fusion, in *Proceedings of the 17th Annual Meeting of the North American Spine Society, Montreal,*

Canada, 2002. Chicago, IL, North American Spine Society, 2002.

25. Whitecloud TS III, Davis JM, Olive PM: Operative treatment of the degenerated segment adjacent to a lumbar fusion. *Spine* 1994;19:531-536.

26. Dall BE, Rowe DE: Degenerative spondylolisthesis: Its surgical management. *Spine* 1985;10:668-672.

27. Stonecipher T, Wright S: Posterior lumbar interbody fusion with facet-screw fixation. *Spine* 1989;14:468-471.

28. Fraser RD: Interbody, posterior, and combined lumbar fusions. *Spine* 1995;20(suppl 24):167S-177S.

29. Boden SD, Martin C, Rudolph R, Kirkpatrick JS, Moeini SM, Hutton WC: Increase of motion between lumbar vertebrae after excision of the capsule and cartilage of the facets: A cadaver study. *J Bone Joint Surg Am* 1994;76:1847-1853.

30. Hazlett JW, Kinnard P: Lumbar apophyseal process excision and spinal instability. *Spine* 1982;7:171-176.

31. Robertson PA, Grobler LJ, Novotny JE, Katz JN: Postoperative spondylolisthesis at L4-5: The role of facet joint morphology. *Spine* 1993;18:1483-1490.

32. Mullin BB, Rea GL, Irsik R, Catton M, Miner ME: The effect of postlaminectomy spinal instability on the outcome of lumbar spinal stenosis patients. *J Spinal Disord* 1996;9:107-116.

33. Zindrick MR, Wiltse LL, Widell EH, et al: A biomechanical study of intrapeduncular screw fixation in the lumbosacral spine. *Clin Orthop* 1986;203:99-112.

34. Krag MH, Beynnon BD, Pope MH, Frymoyer JW, Haugh LD, Weaver DL: An internal fixator for posterior application to short segments of the thoracic, lumbar, or lumbosacral spine: Design and testing. *Clin Orthop* 1986;203:75-98.

35. Steffee AD, Biscup RS, Sitkowski DJ: Segmental spine plates with pedicle screw fixation: A new internal fixation device for disorders of the lumbar and thoracolumbar spine. *Clin Orthop* 1986;203:45-53.

36. Narayan P, Haid RW, Subach BR, Comey CH, Rodts GE: Effect of spinal disease on successful arthrodesis in lumbar pedicle screw fixation. *J Neurosurg* 2002;97(suppl 3):277-280.

37. Jackson RK, Boston DA, Edge AJ: Lateral mass fusion: A prospective study of a consecutive series with long-term follow-up. *Spine* 1985;10:828-832.

38. Johnston CE II, Ashman RB, Baird AM, Allard RN: Effect of spinal construct stiffness on early fusion mass incorporation: Experimental study. *Spine* 1990;15:908-912.

39. Luque ER: Segmental spinal instrumentation of the lumbar spine. *Clin Orthop* 1986;203:126-134.

40. McAfee PC, Weiland DJ, Carlow JJ: Survivorship analysis of pedicle spinal instrumentation. *Spine* 1991;16(suppl 8):S422-S427.

Surgical Treatment of Lumbar Spinal Stenosis Associated With Adult Scoliosis

Charles H. Crawford III, MD
*Steven D. Glassman, MD

Abstract

Lumbar spinal stenosis associated with adult scoliosis is being increasingly recognized and studied. Degenerative changes leading to spinal stenosis can precede a spinal deformity resulting in de novo scoliosis. Conversely, degenerative changes leading to spinal stenosis can occur in a preexisting deformity. Scoliosis has been shown to negatively affect the quality of life in adults studied with validated instruments. Surgical intervention can positively affect the quality of life in these patients. The optimal surgical procedure depends on a careful evaluation of involved segments and patient comorbidities. Positive sagittal imbalance is associated with significant morbidity and should be corrected when feasible. Data that continue to be collected in this patient population will guide future efforts in treating this complicated disease.

With the aging population of industrialized societies, lumber spinal stenosis is an increasingly common reason for patients to seek medical attention. In addition to the more commonly occurring spondylolisthesis, lumbar spinal stenosis can be associated with more complex spinal deformities, including variations of scoliosis.[1-3] Adults may have progressive back pain and symptoms of stenosis caused by degeneration of a preexisting deformity, or the deformity can occur de novo from degeneration of a previously straight spine.

The term de novo degenerative scoliosis is often used to differentiate curvatures of the spine secondary to spondylosis that occur or progress in adults from those that occur or progress before skeletal maturity (juvenile and adolescent idiopathic scoliosis, congenital scoliosis, neuromuscular scoliosis). The clinical picture is quite different between the two groups of patients. Older patients often have pain and functional limitations, including axial back pain and neurogenic leg pain, typically without trunk imbalance.

Younger patients typically do not have pain but instead report progressive deformities or cosmetic concerns. Some previously painless curves in young patients will progress with painful degenerative changes in adulthood, although it is not clear whether the frequency of degenerative changes is greater in these individuals than in the general population.[4]

Adult degenerative scoliosis is receiving greater attention from spine surgeons because of its increasing frequency in the aging population. Concurrent advancements in medical care, surgical techniques and instrumentation, and anesthesia make surgical treatment of this disabling disease a valuable alternative to nonsurgical treatment.[5]

Definition and Etiology

The literature and discussions of adult degenerative scoliosis can be somewhat confusing because of the inherent complexities of the disease process and the difficulties in describing and classifying the pathology. Historically, a coronal curve of more than 10° in a skeletally mature patient is considered adult scoliosis.[1-3]

*Steven D. Glassman, MD or the department with which he is affiliated has received research or institutional support, miscellaneous nonincome support, commercially derived honoraria, other nonresearch-related funding, and/or royalties from Medtronic and is a consultant for or an employee of Medtronic.

Symptoms of lumbar spinal stenosis can occur in patients with de novo degenerative scoliosis and in patients with preexisting deformities of the spine in whom degenerative changes develop later in life. The patients in the latter group have a complex combination of preexisting pelvic and lower extremity deformities with secondary scoliosis, juvenile and adolescent idiopathic scoliosis, congenital scoliosis, or other forms of preadult scoliosis. Some of these patients may have been surgically treated in the past and now present with a new constellation of symptoms related to progressive degenerative changes in the spine. An additional group of patients includes those with a developmentally normal spine who acquire deformities following a fracture. Typically, this patient is an elderly woman with osteoporosis and multiple compression fractures.

Kobayashi and associates[6] reported on the prevalence of de novo degenerative scoliosis in a recent prospective study of a community based cohort from Japan. Sixty subjects (18 men and 42 women) age 50 to 84 years without scoliosis at baseline were followed for an average of 12 years. De novo scoliosis with Cobb angles ranging from 10° to 18° developed in 22 patients (36.7%). All patients had lumbar curves associated with disk degeneration (10 single lumbar curves and 9 double thoracic and lumbar curves) except for 3 thoracic curves in women who had osteoporosis and at least one vertebral fracture within the curve. A decrease in unilateral disk height of more than 20% or an osteophyte more than 5 mm longer on one side was associated with an increased incidence of de novo degenerative scoliosis.[6]

Clinical and Radiographic Characteristics

Lui and associates[7] described the symptoms of nerve root compression associated with degenerative scoliosis. The L3 and L4 roots were typically compressed by foraminal or extraforaminal stenosis on the concave side of the curve, whereas the L5 and S1 roots were commonly affected by lateral recess stenosis on the convex side. The Cobb angle and the lateral slip in patients in whom the L3 or L4 root was affected were significantly larger than in patients in whom the L5 or S1 root was compressed.

Ploumis and associates[8] reported on 78 consecutive patients with de novo degenerative scoliosis who were studied with plain radiographs and MRI. They found that lateral translation was associated with rotation, but this finding did not correlate with dural sac area. Anteroposterior olisthesis was inversely correlated with neural canal dimensions. With increased Cobb angle, foraminal area increased on the convexity, but it did not decrease on the concavity. According to Ploumis and associates,[8] ligamentum flavum hypertrophy, posterior disk bulging, and bony overgrowth more likely contribute to stenosis, regardless of the scoliosis.

Osteoporosis and degenerative scoliosis are clinically correlated. A cause-effect relationship continues to be debated.[1-3] In a study of 454 patients at an osteoporosis clinic, Pappou and associates[9] reported that spinal bone mineral density (BMD) measurements are less valuable for monitoring osteoporosis in scoliotic patients than hip BMD measurements. Patients with scoliosis exhibited a discordantly high spinal BMD despite significant hip osteoporosis.

In 2005, Glassman and associates[10] studied 298 patients from the adult Spinal Deformity Study Group, examining the correlation between radiographic findings and clinical symptoms. Thoracolumbar and lumbar curves generated less favorable scores than thoracic curves. Significant coronal imbalance greater than 4 cm was associated with some deterioration in pain and function. Positive sagittal balance was by far the most reliable predictor of clinical symptoms in patients who had prior surgery and those who did not.

Another study by Glassman and associates[11] examined the use of nonsurgical treatment in patients with adult spinal deformity. The study reviewed 1,061 patients evaluated as part of a prospective multicenter study of adult spinal deformity. Patients were divided into high-symptom and low-symptom groups based on age-adjusted Oswestry Disability Index (ODI) scores. This division was validated by multiple regression analysis using Scoliosis Research Society (SRS) scores for pain, activity level, initial back pain, and initial leg pain and the Medical Outcomes Study 12-Item Short Form (SF-12) physical component. High-symptom patients used significantly greater resources with respect to pain management modalities, medication use, steroid injections, and referral for formal pain management. Also remarkable, however, was the extent to which low-symptom patients used nonsurgical resources.

Classification

Several classification systems for adult scoliosis have been proposed in an attempt to clarify the diagnosis and treatment of this complex condition.[2,3,12-16]

One of the first classification systems grouped adult degenerative scoliosis into two types. Type I curves have a small Cobb angle and minimal to no rotational deformity. Type II curves have greater rotational deformity and a loss of lumbar lordosis.[12]

In 2002, Schwab and associates[13] evaluated 95 patients using a visual analog scale for pain and measurements from standing radiographs and found a statistically significant correlation with pain for lateral vertebral olisthesis, L3 and L4 end-plate obliquity, loss of lumbar lordosis, and increased thoracolumbar kyphosis. The Cobb angle, patient age, level of olisthesis, sagittal pelvic tilt index, and plumb line offset were not statistically correlated with pain.

In a 2005 follow-up study, Schwab and associates[14] proposed a classification system based on the previously published findings. Patients were classified into three types based on the severity of L3 obliquity and the loss of lumbar lordosis. Self-reported pain and disability based on the Medical Outcomes Study 36-Item Short Form (SF-36) and visual analog scale increased from types I to III. This result was reflected in the treatment approach as well, with surgical rates increasing from types I to III.

Again in 2006, Schwab and associates[15] published a different classification based on clinical impact and three criteria: the location of the apex of the curve, the severity of loss of lumbar lordosis, and the severity of subluxation. The report evaluated 947 patients from the Spinal Deformity Study Group database. Patient inclusion criteria included one of the following factors: scoliotic curvature greater than 30°, sagittal or coronal imbalance greater than 5 cm, thoracic kyphosis greater than 60°, lumbar lordosis less than 30°

with scoliosis greater than 15°, thoracolumbar kyphosis greater than 20°, lumbar kyphosis of at least three levels of 10° or more, documented progression of 10° in the coronal or sagittal plane, or documented progression of 3 mm of listhesis. In this group of patients, loss of lumbar lordosis and intervertebral subluxation were associated with lower function and higher disability as measured on the SRS-22 instrument and the ODI.

The SRS has recently adopted and validated a comprehensive classification system for adult spinal deformity that includes degenerative de novo scoliosis. Adult spinal deformity is frequently characterized by associated degenerative changes including spinal stenosis, spondylolisthesis, rotational subluxation, lumbar hypolordosis, and rigidity within the deformity. The classification system has four main purposes: systemic categorization of similar disorders, prognosis regarding natural history and outcomes of care, correlation with health status or severity of deformity, and a guide for optimal care. The classification includes a major curve type, sagittal modifiers, lumbar degenerative modifiers, and global balance modifiers. Qualifications for a primary lumbar curve include de novo and idiopathic curves greater than 30° with an apical vertebral body lateral to the center sacral vertical line.[16]

In 2007, Ploumis and associates[3] introduced a new classification system for degenerative de novo scoliosis based on a review of the recent literature and personal experience. The proposed classification is based on radiographic parameters with clinical symptom modifiers. Type I curves have minimal or no rotation. Type II curves have intersegmental rotation and translation. Type III curves have coronal (more than

4 cm) or sagittal (more than 2 cm) imbalance. Clinical symptom modifiers include A for back pain without leg pain, B for sciatic nerve pain with or without back pain, and C for femoral nerve pain with or without back pain. The validity and reliability of this classification system is under investigation.

Preoperative Evaluation

A detailed history and physical examination often will alert the surgeon to areas that may require detailed imaging and diagnostic studies. Plain radiographs help determine overall balance, the degree and flexibility of the deformity, and any associated rotation or listhesis. When evaluating nerve root compression and stenosis, CT myelography may be more useful than MRI, which can be difficult to interpret with multiplanar deformities. The advantages of CT include detailed bony anatomy with two-dimensional and three-dimensional reconstructions. Provocative diskography and facet injections may be useful when evaluating pain generators. Discordant neurologic findings or dysplastic and congenital deformities should raise the suspicion of central nervous system abnormalities, which can be evaluated with MRI of the brain and spinal cord.

Careful attention to medical and psychosocial comorbidities and risk factors in the perioperative period may reduce the rate of complications, which are significant in this patient population.[17] Preoperative planning should include consideration of potential complications related to instrumentation in osteoporotic spines.[18]

Indications for Surgical Management

Deciding to proceed with surgical treatment in a patient with adult

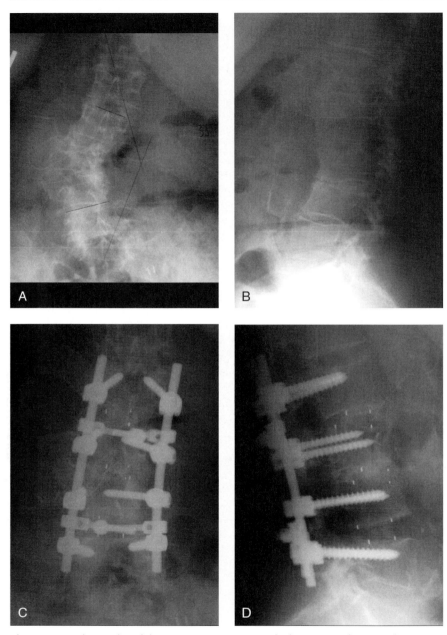

Figure 1 Radiographs of the spine or a patient with de novo scoliosis and stenosis. **A** and **B,** Radiographs demonstrating lumbar curve with lateral listhesis and rotation of L3 and L4. **C** and **D,** Postoperative radiographs demonstrating three-level decompression and transforaminal lumbar interbody fusion with posterior instrumentation and fusion.

scoliosis and spinal stenosis is a difficult and controversial topic.[19-22] Adding to the complexity of the decision-making process is a wide variety of surgical options, ranging from isolated decompression to deformity correction with osteotomy and long instrumented fusion[22-27] (Figures 1 and 2). High-quality, evidence-based recommendations to support one treatment option over another currently are lacking.[28]

A matched cohort study by Glassman and associates[21] from the Spinal Deformity Study Group examined the clinical and radiographic parameters that lead adult scoliosis patients to select surgical over nonsurgical treatment. Reports of leg pain as well as severe episodes of back pain were associated with an increased rate of surgical treatment. Significant dissatisfaction with cosmesis was also a factor in surgical decision making.

In 2001, Simmons[12] recommended decompression with short instrumented fusions for type I adult degenerative scoliosis with minimal rotational deformity. Distraction applied in the concavity of the curve helps with foraminal decompression. For type II adult degenerative scoliosis with greater rotational deformity and loss of lumbar lordosis, he recommended decompression with a longer instrumented fusion and in situ rod contouring and rotation to correct the deformity and reconstitute the sagittal plane.

In 2003, Gupta reported that decompression alone could be safely performed in patients with minor curves (less than 30°) and one- to two-level stenosis with minimal rotatory or lateral listhesis (less than 2 to 3 mm). This was especially true in men, who can have large stabilizing osteophytes and can tolerate a two-level laminectomy without fusion. Gupta noted the lack of studies documenting risks, morbidity, and reoperation rates. He also cautioned against performing limited procedures in patients with sagittal or coronal imbalance and noted that the goal of the first operation is to provide the best prognosis for the long term.[23]

In 2006, Weidenbaum[27] noted that leg pain with minimal back pain requiring a limited decompression

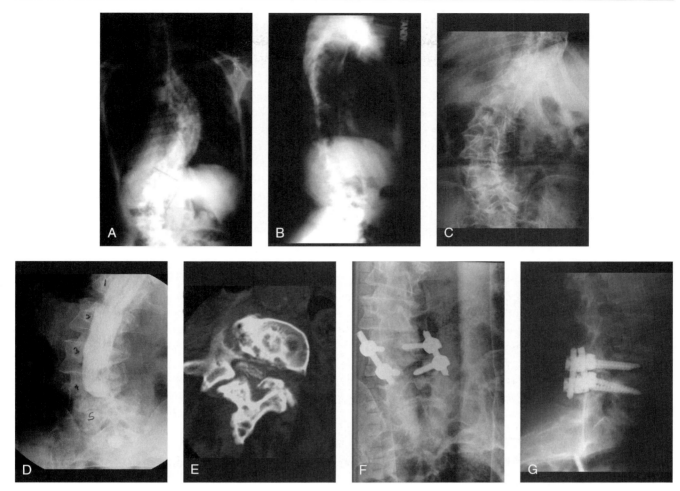

Figure 2 A patient with a history of adolescent scoliosis had degenerative changes in the lumbar spine resulting in spinal stenosis. **A** and **B,** Preoperative radiographs show thoracic and lumbar curves with good sagittal balance. **C** and **D,** Myelograms show stenosis at L4-L5. **E,** CT axial image at L4-L5 shows stenosis and facet degeneration with subluxation. **F** and **G,** Postoperative radiographs show decompression and limited instrumented fusion within the curve.

that will not destabilize the segment is a possible indication for isolated decompression. Additionally, the scoliosis should be less than 20° with less than 2 mm of listhesis. If a wide decompression is needed or if segmental instability is present, a limited fusion can be added without correcting most of the curve. If a limited procedure is chosen, preoperative coronal and sagittal balance should be acceptable, and the patient should be informed that additional surgical procedures may be necessary in the future. Long-term

follow-up studies on limited procedures are lacking.

In a 2007 review of the available literature, Ploumis and associates[3] recommended isolated decompression for patients with scoliosis less than 20° and no instability (less than 2 mm of motion on dynamic radiographs and less than 5 mm of lateral listhesis). If preoperative or postdecompression instability is present, a short instrumented fusion is recommended. Longer fusion with correction is recommended for coronal or sagittal imbalance.

Selecting the Optimal Procedure

Optimal decision making and surgical planning is a complex multifactorial process. It is imperative for the surgeon and the patient to be clear about the goals of surgery. Surgical intervention can include isolated decompression, in situ fusion with or without instrumentation, and deformity correction. Symptoms of lumbar spinal stenosis can be successfully treated with decompression at the affected areas and levels. Decision making regarding concurrent fusion and instrumentation techniques requires an assessment of instability and deformity, which may be preexisting or iatrogenic following adequate decompression. More extensive procedures are more demanding for the surgeon and the patient. Risks of complications intuitively increase with the length and complexity of the surgery. Realistic goals require careful assessment of the capacities of the patient, surgeon, and institution. Complex factors that must be considered in the decision-making process include global sagittal and coronal balance, symptoms of axial back pain, prior surgery, and bone quality.

Specific surgical techniques may include anterior, posterior, or a combination of approaches. Fusion techniques include standard posterior fusions as well as anterior, posterior, and transforaminal lumbar interbody fusions. Instrumentation options include anterior and posterior constructs, often with pedicle screw fixation. For deformity correction, anterior releases or posterior osteotomies may be required.

Irwin and associates[24] surveyed 30 spine surgeons (22 orthopaedic surgeons and 8 neurosurgeons) and found wide variations in surgical decision making. For spinal stenosis with degenerative scoliosis, orthopaedic surgeons were much more likely than neurosurgeons to recommend fusion.

Determining the optimal levels for fusion is the subject of much debate and controversy.[29-31] The goals and considerations regarding the upper instrumented vertebra include minimizing symptomatic adjacent segment degeneration while avoiding unnecessarily extensive instrumentation and fusion. Ideally, the proximal end vertebra will be "stable" with regard to neutral rotation, sagittal balance, and coronal translation.

Additionally, it will have minimal degenerative changes. The upper end vertebra typically is between T2 and L2 for correction of sagittal imbalance and can range from T10 to L2 when sagittal balance is acceptable.[29] The lower end vertebra is believed to be between L5 and S1. If the fusion is stopped at L5, symptomatic degeneration of the L5-S1 segment is a known risk. Extending the fusion to S1 introduces problems regarding instrumentation and the risk of pseudarthrosis, which may be minimized with anterior column support.[30,31]

Outcomes Measures

Surgical outcomes of adult patients with spinal deformity can be measured using clinical and radiographic parameters. Traditional radiographic parameters include deformity correction as well as complications such as pseudarthrosis, instrumentation failure, and adjacent segment degeneration. Health-Related Quality of Life (HRQOL) measures recently have been used to extensively study adults with spinal deformities. HRQOL measures include general health measures such as SF-36 and SF-12 and disease-specific measures such as the ODI and the SRS-22 instruments.

The SRS-22 was designed to be a disease-specific outcomes tool for patients with spinal deformities. The SRS-22 is sensitive to change, valid, consistent, and reliable in adults with spinal deformities.[32-34] SF-36 data have shown the significant impact of adult scoliosis on patients' perceptions of general health.[35]

Results of Surgical Treatment

In 1997, Frazier and associates[36] reported on 19 patients who had at least 15° of scoliosis before surgery. Four of the 19 patients had arthrodesis, and the remaining 15 patients had laminectomy without arthrode-

sis. A larger preoperative scoliosis was correlated with less improvement in back pain. No significant correlations could be detected between preoperative scoliosis and satisfaction or improvement in leg pain or walking capacity. The change between preoperative and postoperative scoliosis showed no correlation with outcome.

In 2003, Adachi and associates[25] reported worse outcomes for restorative lumbar laminoplasty in patients with more than 10° of scoliosis. In a 2006 review of medical complications in adult deformity surgery, Baron and Albert[37] reported that urinary tract infections were the most frequent complication, whereas pulmonary complications were the most common life-threatening complications in adult spinal deformity surgery.

In 2007, Pateder and associates[38] reported equivalent radiographic curve correction in adult lumbar scoliosis (both idiopathic and de novo) with a posterior only and with a combined anterior and posterior approach. Major complications were more frequent in patients who had staged anterior and posterior surgery (45%) than in patients who had same-day anterior and posterior (24%) or posterior-only procedures (23%). Clinical outcomes were not reported.

In 2007, Glassman and associates[39] reported clinical outcomes after decompression and posterolateral instrumented fusion in 85 patients age 65 years or older using modern HRQOL measures including the SF-36, the ODI, and Numeric Rating Scales for back and leg pain. The group included 12 patients with degenerative scoliosis. For the entire group, clinically important improvements in the HRQOL measures were seen. More limited improvement was seen in patients who had revision surgery.

In 2007, Bridwell and associates[33] showed that surgical treatment of adult scoliosis significantly improved pain, self-image, and function based on the SRS-22, the ODI, and the SF-12 HRQOL measures. The study suggested that the SRS-22 is more responsive than the ODI, which is more responsive than the SF-12 to changes in this population of patients.

In 2007, Cho and associates[40] reported the complications in 47 patients with degenerative lumbar scoliosis who had decompression with posterolateral fusion and pedicle screw instrumentation. Seven patients also had a posterior lumbar interbody fusion at the lower levels. Complications were defined as any event for which the patient required specific treatment. The overall complication rate was 68%. The mean estimated blood loss was 2,106 mL, and the mean surgical time was 197.4 minutes. The mean hospital stay was 20.7 days. Early perioperative complications were considered major when they adversely affected the patient's recovery. Major complications included one pulmonary embolism resulting in death, two instances of respiratory distress, one epidural hematoma with neurologic deficit requiring immediate reoperation, and two superficial infections requiring débridement and antibiotics. Minor complications included one urinary tract infection, three instances of ileus, and two instances of transient delirium. Estimated blood loss of more than 2,000 mL was significantly associated with an increase in early perioperative complications, whereas age, sex, smoking, medical comorbidities, and surgical time were not. Clinical outcomes based on the ODI were not adversely affected by early perioperative complications, but they were adversely affected by late complications.

Late complications included proximal adjacent segment disease in 10 patients and distal adjacent segment disease in 5 patients. Proximal adjacent segment disease was more common when the fusion ended at the thoracolumbar junction rather than T10. Two patients had pseudarthrosis and one had screw pull-out at L5-S1 when anterior column support was not used. Positive sagittal imbalance was more common in patients with late complications and poor clinical outcomes.

In 2007, Glassman and associates[41] reported the effects of perioperative complications in patients from a multicenter database of adult spinal deformity surgery. The study demonstrated that the risk for minor complications may be a less substantial obstacle than previously assumed. In contrast, major complications were reported in approximately 10% of patients and adversely affected outcome as evidenced by the deterioration in SF-12 general health scores at 1 year after surgery.

Summary

Surgical intervention can positively affect quality of life in patients with spinal stenosis and degenerative scoliosis. The optimal surgical procedure depends on a careful evaluation of involved segments and patient comorbidities. Positive sagittal imbalance is associated with significant morbidity and should be corrected when feasible. Data that continue to be collected in this patient population will guide future efforts in treating this complicated disease.

References

1. Tribus CB: Degenerative lumbar scoliosis: Evaluation and management. *J Am Acad Orthop Surg* 2003;11: 174-183.

2. Aebi M: The adult scoliosis. *Eur Spine J* 2005;14:925-948.

3. Ploumis A, Transfelt EE, Denis F: Degenerative lumbar scoliosis associated with spinal stenosis. *Spine J* 2007; 7:428-436.

4. Weinstein SL, Dolan LA, Spratt KF, Peterson KK, Spoonamore MJ, Ponseti IV: Health and function of patients with untreated scoliosis: A 50 year natural history study. *JAMA* 2003;289:559-567.

5. Everett CR, Patel RK: A systematic literature review of nonsurgical treatment in adult scoliosis. *Spine* 2007; 32 (19S):S130-S134.

6. Kobayashi T, Atsuta Y, Takemitsu M, Matsuno T, Takeda N: A prospective study of de novo scoliosis in a community based cohort. *Spine* 2006; 31: 178-182.

7. Liu H, Ishihara H, Kanamori M, Kawaguchi Y, Ohmori K, Kimura T: Characteristics of nerve root compression caused by degenerative lumbar spinal stenosis with scoliosis. *Spine J* 2003;3:524-529.

8. Ploumis A, Transfeldt EE, Gilbert TJ, Mehbod AA, Dykes DC, Perra JE: Degenerative lumbar scoliosis: Radiographic correlation of lateral rotatory olisthesis with neural canal dimensions. *Spine* 2006;31:2353-2358.

9. Pappou IP, Giraradi FP, Sandhu HS, et al: Discordantly high spinal bone mineral density values in patients with adult lumbar scoliosis. *Spine* 2006;31:1614-1620.

10. Glassman SD, Berven S, Bridwell K, Horton W, Dimar JR: Correlation of radiographic parameters and clinical symptoms in adult scoliosis. *Spine* 2005;30:682-688.

11. Glassman SD, Berven S, Kostuik JP, Dimar JR, Horton W, Bridwell K: Nonsurgical resource utilization in adult spinal deformity. *Spine* 2006;31: 941-947.

12. Simmons ED: Surgical treatment of patients with lumbar spinal stenosis with associated scoliosis. *Clin Orthop Relat Res* 2001;384:45-53.

13. Schwab FJ, Smith VA, Biserni M, Gamez L, Farcy JC, Pagala M: Adult scoliosis: A quantitative radiographic and clinical analysis. *Spine* 2002;27: 387-392.

14. Schwab F, el-Fegoun AB, Gamez L, Goodman H, Farcy JP: A lumbar classification of scoliosis in the adult patient: Preliminary approach. *Spine* 2005;30:1670-1673.

15. Schwab F, Farcy J, Bridwell K, et al: A clinical impact classification of scoliosis in the adult. *Spine* 2006;31: 2109-2114.

16. Lowe T, Berven SH, Schwab FJ, Bridwell KH: The SRS classification for adult spinal deformity: Building on the King/Moe and Lenke classification systems. *Spine* 2006;31(19S): S119-S125.

17. Hu SS, Berven SH: Preparing the adult deformity patient for spinal surgery. *Spine* 2006;31(19S):S126 -S131.

18. DeWald CJ, Stanley T: Instrumentation-related complications of multi-level fusions for adult spinal deformity patients over age 65: Surgical considerations and treatment options in patients with poor bone quality. *Spine* 2006;31(19S):S144-S151.

19. Lonstein JE: Scoliosis: Surgical versus nonsurgical treament. *Clin Orthop Relat Res* 2006;443:248-259.

20. Akbarnia BA, Ogilive JW, Hammerberg KW: Debate: Degenerative scoliosis. To operate or not to operate. *Spine* 2006;31(19S):S195-S201.

21. Glassman SD, Schwab FJ, Bridwell KH, Ondra SL, Berven S, Lenke LG: The selection of operative versus nonoperative treatment in patients with adult scoliosis. *Spine* 2007;32:93 -97.

22. Sengupta DK, Herkowitz HN: Lumbar spinal stenosis: Treatment stratigies and indications for surgery. *Orthop Clin North Am* 2003;34:281-295.

23. Gupta MC: Degenerative scoliosis: Options for surgical management. *Orthop Clin North Am* 2003;34: 269-279.

24. Irwin ZN, Hilibrand A, Gustavel M, et al: Variation in surgical decision making for degenerative spinal disorders: Part I. Lumbar spine. *Spine* 2005;30:2208-2213.

25. Adachi K, Futami T, Ebihara A, et al: Spinal canal enlargement procedure by restorative laminoplasty for the treatment of lumbar canal stenosis. *Spine J* 2003;3:471-478.

26. Bridwell KH, Lenke LG, Lewis SJ: Treatment of spinal stenosis and fixed sagittal imbalance. *Clin Orthop Relat Res* 2001;384:35-44.

27. Weidenbaum M: Considerations for focused surgical intervention in the presence of adult spinal deformity. *Spine* 2006;31(S19):S139-S143.

28. Bridwell KH, Berven S, Edwards C, Glassman S, Hamill C, Schwab F: The problems and limitations of applying evidence-based medicine to primary surgical treatment of adult spinal deformity. *Spine* 2007;32(19S): S135-S139.

29. Shufflebarger H, Suk S, Mardjetko S: Debate: Determining the upper instrumented vertebra in the management of adult degenerative scoliosis: Stopping at T10 versus L1. *Spine* 2006;31(S19):S185-S194.

30. Kuklo TR: Principles for selecting fusion levels in adult spinal deformity with particular attention to lumbar curves and double major curves. *Spine* 2006;31(19S):S132-S138.

31. Polly DW, Hamill CL, Bridwell KH: Debate: To fuse or not to fuse to the sacrum. The fate of the L5-S1 disc. *Spine* 2006;31(19S):S179-S184.

32. Bridwell KH, Cats-Baril W, Harrast J, et al: The validity of the SRS-22 instrument in an adult spinal deformity population compared with the Oswestry and SF-12: A study of response distribution, concurrent validity, internal consistency, and reliability. *Spine* 2005;30:455-461.

33. Bridwell KH, Berven S, Glassman S, et al: Is the SRS-22 instrument responsive to change in adult scoliosis patients having primary deformity surgery? *Spine* 2007;32:2220-2225.

34. Berven S, Deviren V, Demir-Deviren S, Hu SS, Bradford DS: Studies in the modified scoliosis research society outcomes instrument in adults: Validation, reliability, and discriminatory capacity. *Spine* 2003; 28:2164-2169.

35. Schwab F, Dubey A, Pagala M, Gamez L, Farcy JP : Adult scoliosis: A health assessment analysis by SF-36. *Spine* 2003;28:602-606.

36. Frazier DD, Lipson SJ, Fossel AH , Katz JN: Associations between spinal deformity and outcomes after decompression for spinal stenosis. *Spine* 1997;22:2025-2029.

37. Baron EM, Albert TJ: Medical complications of surgical treatment of adult spinal deformity and how to avoid them. *Spine* 2006;31(19S): S106-S118.

38. Pateder DB, Kebaish KM, Cascio BM, Neubaeur P, Matusz DM, Kostuik JP : Posterior only versus combined anterior and posterior approaches to lumbar scoliosis in adults: A radiographic analysis. *Spine* 2007; 32:1551-1554 .

39. Glassman SD, Carreon LY, Dimar JR, Campbell MJ, Puno RM, Johnson JR: Clinical outcomes in older patients after posterolateral lumbar fusion. *Spine J* 2007;7:547-551.

40. Cho KJ, Suk SI, Park SR, et al: Complications in posterior fusion and instrumentation for degenerative lumbar scoliosis. *Spine* 2007;32: 2232-2237.

41. Glassman SD, Hamill CL, Bridwell KH, Schwab FJ, Dimar JR, Lowe TG: The impact of perioperative complications on clinical outcome in adult deformity surgery. *Spine* 2007;32:2764-2770.

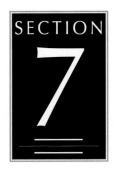

SECTION 7

The Geriatric Spine

The Geriatric Spine

Both chapters in this section should compel the orthopaedic surgeon to reflect on an increasingly important issue in spine surgery—how to approach older patients with spinal problems. Are there physiologic or mechanical disorders in these patients that require a change in perioperative care or in the surgical techniques selected? Do we need to think differently when dealing with older patients?

Hart and Prendergast provide a comprehensive overview of the physiologic concerns that should be considered when treating the elderly patient. The elderly patient does not have the cardiopulmonary reserves of a younger individual. It is well known that postoperative complications occur more frequently in older patients. A thorough understanding of the physiology of the elderly patient will help reduce the incidence of these complications. The importance of the patient's cardiac, pulmonary, renal, and nutritional status is reviewed. The concrete guidelines presented in this chapter will assist physicians in the perioperative management of these patients. The consequence of using some medications in elderly patients is carefully analyzed.

The authors review the management of degenerative stenosis, degenerative scoliosis, and degenerative spondylolisthesis in the older patient. The literature review on surgical considerations for elderly patients with these conditions will be beneficial to the reader. The role of laminectomy alone compared with laminectomy with fusion, the role of instrumentation, and the role of combined anterior-posterior fusions are discussed. The basic science of osteoporosis is presented, and a concise section on specific considerations for instrumentation of the osteoporotic spine is included. As the authors point out, despite a higher rate of complications in elderly patients, appropriate evidence-based surgical management can result in high levels of patient satisfaction and better surgical outcomes.

In their chapter, Manson and Phillips specifically discuss vertebral compression fractures in elderly patients. In a very good review of the literature, the authors present evidence of the substantial morbidity associated with these fractures in elderly patients. Whether the medical morbidity associated with these fractures is a marker of poor general health in this subset of patients or a true effect of the fracture is undetermined. The pain from these fractures can result in a rapid change in lifestyle in some elderly patients, particularly when combined with apprehension about the possibility of additional fractures and the anxiety associated with increasing dependence on family members.

The thrust of the chapter concerns the use of percutaneous cement augmentation for vertebral compression fractures. The authors review the indications, contraindications, surgical techniques, outcomes, and complications of vertebroplasty and kyphoplasty. Both procedures are similarly effective in relieving fracture pain. The use of an inflatable bone tamp during kyphoplasty prior to the injection of methylmethacrylate has been reported to achieve improved height restoration. The creation of a void by this type of bone tamp may allow the use of higher viscosity methylmethacrylate, which may reduce the incidence of cement leakage. Manson and Phillips point out that because only early results of kyphoplasty are available, additional and longer term studies are needed before definitive answers can be determined. Advantages of vertebroplasty include faster procedure times, lower costs, avoidance of general anesthesia in most patients, and the possibility of vertebral height restoration during prone positioning for the procedure. The authors have thoughtfully integrated basic science studies concerning these issues into each section of their chapter. Manson and Phillips also discuss radiation hazards incurred during vertebroplasty and kyphoplasty. This issue is important to patients and is a relevant concern for surgeons performing these procedures.

Raj D. Rao, MD
Professor of Orthopaedic Surgery
Director, Spine Surgery
Department of Orthopaedic Surgery
Medical College of Wisconsin
Milwaukee, Wisconsin

Spine Surgery for Lumbar Degenerative Disease in Elderly and Osteoporotic Patients

Robert A. Hart, MD, MA
Michael A. Prendergast, BA

Abstract

Elderly patients with lumbar spine degenerative disease present significant challenges regarding surgical decision making and management. Because osteoporosis is a particularly prevalent comorbidity in the elderly population, it must be a concern in all elderly patients with degenerative disease of the lumbar spine. Careful attention to surgical indications and surgical technique is always required for the successful treatment of this challenging patient population.

The rate of spinal stenosis surgery in the United States for patients older than 65 years has shown an eightfold increase over a 14-year period, and given the ongoing aging of the American population this trend is likely to continue.[1] This trend likely reflects several factors, including surgeons' increased ability to safely care for these patients as well as the increasing expectations of elderly patients regarding activity levels. Elective spinal surgery, especially surgical fusion, presents unique challenges to surgeons with respect to decision making, surgical tech-nique, and perioperative care.

Every organ system manifests specific changes with aging, resulting in demonstrably higher surgical morbidity and mortality among elderly patients.[2] The effect of osteoporosis is a fundamental concern for spine surgeons planning spine fusion procedures in elderly patients. The spine surgeon must be informed regarding specific surgical risk factors and work to develop an appropriate treatment plan that accommodates the specific needs of elderly and osteoporotic patients.

Physiologic Concerns in the Elderly Patient

The elderly patient has several unique considerations, including medical comorbidities, nutritional status, reduced activity demands, and osteoporosis. These factors must be

kept in mind and appropriately addressed during all phases of surgical management to optimize outcome.

Cardiac assessment should include obtaining a history of myocardial infarction, congestive heart failure, and arrhythmias. Goldman and associates[3] developed a cardiac risk assessment scale that identified several factors related to occurrence of perioperative cardiac complications. Particularly worrisome risk factors include an S3 gallop or jugular venous distension, myocardial infarction within the prior 6 months, nonsinus rhythm or premature atrial contractions, and more than five premature ventricular contractions per minute. These factors are weighted to assign a patient to one of four cardiac risk categories, a procedure that has been widely adopted among anesthesiologists.

Respiratory status also should be carefully evaluated in the elderly patient. Preoperative chest radiographs in patients older than 70 years should probably be ordered routinely, even without a more specific indication, to avoid complications and delays in treatment.[4] During the clinical evaluation, it is important to determine whether the patient has experienced

One or more of the authors or the departments with which they are affiliated have received something of value from a commercial or other party related directly or indirectly to the subject of this chapter.

Table 1
Preoperative Assessment in Elderly Patients

Organ System	Possible Tests
Cardiac	Echocardiography Stress thallium test Exercise stress test Angiography
Pulmonary	Resting o_2 saturation Arterial blood gases Forced expiratory volume in 1 second Forced vital capacity
Renal	Serum area nitrogen Creatinine clearance
Nutrition/health status	Hematocrit Total protein Albumin
Musculoskeletal	Plain radiographs DEXA scan Quantitative CT

exercise intolerance, chronic cough, or unexplained dyspnea and to look for physical findings such as wheezes or rhonchi. An assessment of arterial blood gases is useful in evaluating for hypoxia or hypercarbia.[5,6] Incentive spirometry (especially forced expiratory volume in 1 second and forced vital capacity) should be considered for patients with a history of smoking or chronic obstructive pulmonary disease and those undergoing anterior thoracic or upper abdominal spinal surgery.[5,7,8]

Renal status is another important medical consideration in the elderly surgical patient. During surgery, patients older than 65 years undergo more dramatic changes in renal function than younger patients.[9-11] Renal status can be assessed using functions such as the Cockroft-Gault equation ((([140–age] × weight (kg))/ (72 × serum creatinine)) because it corrects for the false elevation of the serum creatinine level, which can occur with a reduction of muscle mass in elderly patients.[12]

Nonsteroidal anti-inflammatory drugs (NSAIDs) are commonly used by elderly patients. These agents have multiple potential negative impacts, especially with respect to kidney function, gastrointestinal bleeding, and bone healing, and must be a source of concern.[13,14] NSAIDs should be avoided in patients undergoing spine fusion, especially during the early inflammatory phase of fusion when the effects of NSAIDs appear to have the greatest impact on bone healing.[15]

Oral bisphosphonates are also commonly used to treat osteoporosis in elderly patients. Although these agents appear to have minimal effect on creatinine clearance,[16] some have been shown to adversely affect bone healing in animal models, depending on the size of the fusion mass and animal model used.[17-20] Discontinuation of oral bisphosphonates before surgery and throughout the perioperative period is prudent until more definitive evidence is available.

Nutritional status is another concern in elderly patients and may be difficult to ascertain through history taking.[21] Assessment of the elderly patient with laboratory data such as total protein, serum albumin, and C-reactive protein levels should be part of the preoperative workup. A well-balanced diet complemented with oral supplements can be used to provide additional calories to correct nutritional deficits preoperatively. Vitamin D (400 to 800 IU/day) and calcium (1,200 mg/day) are also important nutrients for the maintenance of skeletal health in elderly patients[22] (Table 1).

Osteoporosis

Osteoporosis is a major health concern among the elderly population in the United States, with the condition diagnosed in approximately 10 million people and an estimated 44 million people at risk.[22] Although 80% of these patients are women, a significant number of men are also affected.[22,23,24] The financial burden to the medical system because of osteoporotic fractures exceeds $20 billion.[25]

At the biochemical level, bone is composed of an organic and a mineral component. Osteoid, the organic component, is composed of collagen and other proteins, whereas the mineral component is hydroxyapatite (HA). At a cellular level, remodeling depends on the balance between bone formation by osteoblasts and bone resorption by osteoclasts. At a microstructural level, bone is organized into cortical and trabecular bone.

Cortical bone is formed of interconnected cylinders organized around haversian canals, whereas trabecular bone is constructed as a densely interconnected lattice. The greater surface area in trabecular bone results in a higher turnover rate than in cortical bone. Bone loss thus occurs more rapidly in trabecular bone, with replacement of the normal trabecular lattice by thinner and ultimately discontinuous spicules in the disease state referred to as osteoporosis.[26]

Osteoporosis is a metabolic bone disorder that results in decreased bone mineral density. The biochemical composition and microscopic structure of osteoporotic bone are normal, but the volume density of bone is substantially reduced. A reduction of more than 2.5 standard deviations of the bone mineral density of a young adult roughly corresponds to values below 0.8 to 0.9 g/cm^2, depending on gender.[27] This decreased structural density adversely affects the mechanical properties of bone.[28]

Postmenopausal osteoporosis occurs within 10 to 20 years after the onset of menopause and is related to the loss of estrogen, resulting in excess bone resorption, particularly within trabecular bone.[29-31] Senile osteoporosis occurs in men and women and is a result of multisystem, age-related changes in the regulation of overall calcium, vitamin D, and other nutrients.[29] The specific changes in bone resorption and formation are less well defined than for postmenopausal osteoporosis, although both cortical and trabecular bone appear to be affected.[31]

Currently, two methods are used clinically to evaluate bone density. Dual energy x-ray absorptiometry (DEXA) measures bone density by area (g/cm^2). This test is simple, accurate, and carries a low radiation dose. It is also well tolerated, with a procedure duration of 10 to 15 minutes. Quantitative CT scanning is a measurement of volume density (g/cm^3) calculated via cross-sectional images of a vertebral body. The precision of this test is excellent, although it can be compromised by patient positioning and movement. However, the relatively small increase in accuracy of this test over DEXA scanning may not justify the greater expense, greater level of patient discomfort, and exposure of the patient to a greater radiation dose.[32] Osteophyte formation and calcification in the degenerative spine may reduce the accuracy of spinal DEXA scans, a limitation that is usually avoidable by using DEXA scanning of the proximal femur.[33]

Concerns regarding patients with osteoporosis undergoing spinal fusion surgery depend on the underlying pathology and the extent of surgery planned. Specific concerns of hardware failure, adjacent segment fracture, and the possibility of an increased nonunion rate all must be considered in this patient population.

Degenerative Lumbar Spinal Stenosis

Degenerative lumbar spinal stenosis, a common disorder of the elderly population, is an acquired condition resulting from osteoarthritis of the intervertebral disk and the facet joints as well as hypertrophy of the ligamentum flavum.[32,34,35] Most commonly, injury or degenerative changes within the disk initiate a cycle of degeneration of the three-joint complex of the spinal motion segment; however, in some patients, the degenerative process appears to start in the facet joints.[34,36] Progression of the degeneration leads to osteophyte formation at the facet joints, calcification and hypertrophy of the ligamentum flavum, intervertebral disk prolapse, and disk osteophyte formation.[34] All of these features may diminish the room available for the lumbar nerve roots in the central canal, the lateral recess, and the neural foramina.

The classic presentation of patients with lumbar spinal stenosis is neurogenic claudication, which refers to pain in the lower extremities brought on by activity. Although symptoms can be unilateral or bilateral, they are usually asymmetric. Pain is classically described as being exacerbated by activity and by positions of extension of the lumbar spine, with relief occurring following cessation of activity or forward flexion. Reduced pain with activities such as walking uphill or riding a stationary bicycle, which induce flexion of the lumbar spine, may sometimes help distinguish this symptom from vascular claudication.[36] With flexion of the spine, the diameter of the canal is increased and the ligamentum flavum is flat-tened, which is offered as an explanation of the postural relief of symptoms.[37]

The pathogenesis of these symptoms is not completely understood but is likely the result of mechanical compression of the lumbar nerve roots and consequent compromise of the neural blood supply.[36,38] Compression at more than one spinal level has been shown in animal models to produce venous congestion and insufficient arterial inflow, creating a relatively ischemic environment within the neural elements between the areas of congestion.[36,38] Compromised autonomic innervation of the lower limbs may inhibit the appropriate vasodilation response to increased muscle use, which may partially account for similarities in clinical appearance to vascular claudication.[38]

Most patients present with a normal motor examination.[36] Patients with long-standing and severe stenosis may ultimately experience lower extremity weakness or neurogenic bowel and bladder dysfunction.[36] Deep tendon reflexes are often reduced in elderly patients, especially at the Achilles tendon.[39] In addition to a neurologic examination, distal pulses and hip range of motion should also be assessed (Figure 1).

Imaging of the spine in patients suspected of having lumbar spinal stenosis should begin with plain radiographs, including dynamic flexion and extension lateral views. Additional imaging may include MRI and CT with or without myelography.[36,37] Although these studies provide detail regarding the location and extent of stenosis, it is important to remember that the severity of stenosis noted on imaging studies often does not correlate with the severity of symptoms and that stenosis

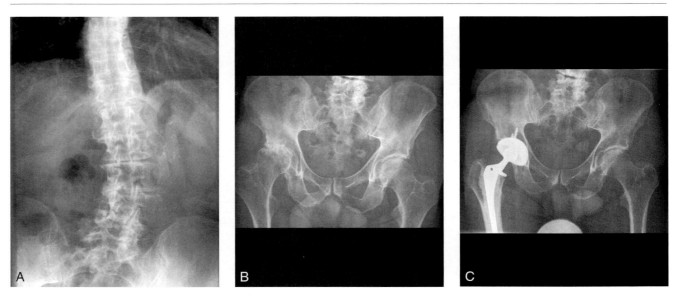

Figure 1 **A,** AP radiograph of the lumbar spine of a 74-year-old man with low back pain and right lower extremity thigh pain. Physical examination revealed stiffness and pain with range of motion of the right hip. **B,** AP pelvis radiograph demonstrating severe degenerative arthritis of the right hip joint. **C,** AP pelvis radiograph obtained 5 years after right total hip replacement. Patient obtained excellent relief of right lower extremity pain, and excellent pain relief was maintained over the duration of follow-up. No procedure to the lumbar spine has been performed to date.

is not a radiographic diagnosis but a clinical diagnosis.[35,40]

Electromyography is most often normal, especially in the early course of the disease, but it can be helpful in ruling out peripheral neuropathy resulting from other causes such as diabetes.[41] Selective nerve root blocks, facet infections, and sacroiliac joint injections may not only be therapeutic, but also are helpful diagnostically in localizing the source of a patient's pain, which can remain unclear even after a thorough clinical and radiographic assessment.[42,43]

Treatment of patients without neurologic deficits should generally begin nonsurgically and progress to surgical options only after more conservative measures have failed. Nonsurgical treatment options include NSAIDs, lumbar flexion and abdominal strengthening exercises, braces, and epidural injections.[44] In general, surgery is indicated for pa-

tients with severe functional compromise and those with persistently troubling symptoms despite efforts at nonsurgical treatment.

Fundamental to the successful surgical treatment of a stenotic segment is decompression, which is accomplished by a thorough removal of all structures contributing to the neurologic compression.[43] Generally, the type of decompression performed will depend on the anatomic site of stenosis and the patient's symptoms. If instability in the form of spondylolisthesis or scoliosis is not demonstrated preoperatively, fusion is generally recommended only when laminectomy is accompanied by greater than 50% resection of both facets or complete facetectomy on one side.[45,46]

Elderly patients often present with central spinal canal stenosis in addition to lateral and foraminal narrowing. Complete laminectomy often provides better neurologic de-

compression than fenestrated laminotomies or limited access procedures, which may fail to address all locations of compression.[47] In at least one clinical study, single-level laminectomies have been associated with diminished outcomes, which suggests that all levels of radiographic stenosis should be decompressed, unless the clinical assessment definitively indicates a specific spinal level.[51,52]

Medicare database studies have shown a correlation between increasing age and the risk of postoperative complications.[48,49] Deyo and associates[48-50] found a complication rate of 14.6% in patients between the ages of 65 and 74 years that increased to 17.7% in patients older than 75 years, with increased complication rates noted for patients undergoing fusion procedures. Such studies, however, do not allow an assessment of specific risk factors, and the age effect noted likely in part reflects the increased rate of associated medical comorbidities in the elderly patient population.

Age alone should not preclude lumbar spinal surgery, although comorbid conditions such as diabetes and heart disease must be discussed with patients because these conditions have been shown to affect surgical outcomes.[51,52] Recently Ragab and associates[53] studied 118 patients older than 70 years, including 21 patients older than 80 years, who were treated for stenosis with decompression alone or decompression and fusion. They described successful outcomes in 109 patients (92%), including 68 of 73 patients (93%) who were treated with decompression alone, which is consistent with the results reported for clinical series that include younger patients.[43,52,53] These authors emphasized the need for close intraoperative monitoring and aggressive fluid management in elderly patients.[53]

To improve the chance of success in patients with medical comorbidities, patients must be optimized medically and educated appropriately before undergoing surgery. One study found that an individual patient's own assessment of personal health and cardiovascular status was the most powerful predictor of success.[54] Other medical comorbidities have also been shown to affect outcomes. For example, Arinzon and associates[55] compared outcomes for 62 diabetic and nondiabetic patients older than 65 years who underwent decompression for spinal stenosis. Although most patients in both groups achieved successful pain relief, nondiabetic patients reported better overall satisfaction, showed more improvement in activities of daily living, required less revision surgery, and experienced fewer perioperative complications. It is impor-

tant to recognize that complications do not always compromise clinical outcomes, as suggested in a retrospective study by Benz and associates,[56] which found that despite a 40% complication rate in laminectomy patients older than 70 years, an overall satisfaction rate of 71% was reported.

Degenerative Lumbar Spondylolisthesis

Degenerative lumbar spondylolisthesis occurs when osteoarthritis of the facet joints leads to anterior displacement of the cranial vertebral body relative to the caudal adjacent vertebrae, which occurs most frequently at the L4-L5 level. Compromise of the vertebral canal results, often worsening preexisting stenosis caused by degenerative disease. More commonly seen in women than men, degenerative spondylolisthesis is a disease of older adults, seldom seen in those younger than 50 years, and perhaps affecting up to 10% of women older than 60 years.[57,58]

Although patients with degenerative lumbar spondylolisthesis report symptoms of lumbar stenosis at higher rates than patients with similar degrees of stenosis but without accompanying spondylolisthesis, many also report back pain.[59,60] Degenerative lumbar spondylolisthesis rarely exceeds 30% of vertebral body width, although slip progression may occur in up to 30% of untreated patients.[59,60] Plain radiography is usually sufficient to determine the nature of the spondylolisthesis and the slip grade.[58,61] MRI or CT with myelography can help evaluate associated compression of the neurologic elements and help screen for other potential causes of back pain in elderly patients, such as vertebral body compression frac-

tures or infectious diskitis.[58,62]

As for patients with stenosis, nonsurgical interventions, including NSAIDs, epidural medications, and lumbar flexibility and strengthening exercises, may be appropriate for patients without neurologic deficit and relatively recent symptom onset.[57] Surgery is an option for patients with severe or persistent symptoms that interfere significantly with quality of life and are refractory to nonsurgical treatment.[59]

Surgical options include decompression alone or decompression combined with a fusion procedure; the fusion procedure may be performed with or without instrumentation. Fusion can be accomplished in several ways, but most commonly is performed via posterior fusion with or without pedicle screw instrumentation. The best available evidence suggests that decompression with arthrodesis results in better clinical outcomes than decompression alone in patients with degenerative spondylolisthesis.[63-67] Despite this evidence, although use of pedicle screw–based instrumentation clearly increases the rate of successful fusion, it is less clearly beneficial in terms of clinical outcome.

Patients with relatively stable spondylolisthesis can be safely treated via laminectomy without fusion.[68] However, the subgroup of patients with degenerative spondylolisthesis that does not benefit from fusion has not been clearly defined. An evidence-based medicine approach, therefore, favors including fusion as a routine part of surgical treatment of these patients.[45,59,69,70] However, current clinical practice does not appear uniform in regard to addition of fusion for these patients.[71] As in patients with lumbar stenosis, the overall risk of compli-

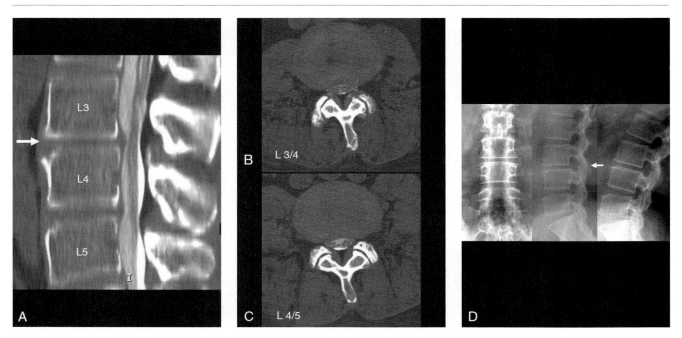

Figure 2   **A,** Sagittal CT myelogram of a 68-year-old woman with neurogenic claudication. A grade I degenerative spondylolisthesis is present the L3-4 disk space (*arrow*). Transverse cuts through the CT myelogram show marked central and lateral recess stenosis at the L3-4 (**B**) and L4-5 disk spaces (**C**). Note relatively coronal orientation of the facet joints at L4-5 with increased sagittal orientation at the L3-4 facet joint. **D,** AP (*left*) and lateral flexion (*center*) and extension (*right*) radiographs obtained 3 years postoperatively following laminectomies of L3, L4, and L5, with posterior facet fusion at L3-4. Note obliteration of the facet joint at L3-4 on the lateral flexion view (*arrow*) and the absence of motion at the L3-4 disk space between the flexion and extension views. The patient had excellent relief of lower extremity pain at 3-year follow-up.

cations, morbidity, and mortality increase with age, and including fusion has been shown to further increase surgical duration and complication rates.[48,49]

When fusion is performed, many authors recommend including instrumentation to improve fusion rates and reduce postoperative activity limitations.[45,59,67] However, avoiding instrumentation is also a reasonable option, particularly when facets are oriented in a relatively coronal plane and segmental instability is limited[45] (Figure 2). It must also be recognized that pedicle screw–based instrumentation is less effective in patients with severe osteoporosis.[72,73] Recently, however, long-term follow-up has suggested that uninstrumented fusion patients with nonunion do ultimately require higher rates of reintervention than patients who gain solid fusion.[65]

Degenerative Scoliosis

Degenerative scoliosis is an acquired disorder of adult patients for which there is no gender preference. It is a distinct diagnosis from that of patients with idiopathic scoliosis who develop secondary spinal degenerative disease because patients with true degenerative scoliosis develop de novo rotational deformity of the spine during the adult years. Patients with degenerative scoliosis typically present with symptoms similar to those of patients with degenerative lumbar stenosis, but often report back pain and may also experience problems with spinal alignment.[74] Patients with symptomatic degenerative scoliosis may have severe functional limitations, especially when sagittal plane imbalance is present.[75,76]

The pathophysiology of degenerative scoliosis is similar to that of lumbar stenosis, but appears to result when there is asymmetric degeneration of the facet joints and disk, resulting in a rotatory effect.[77] The relationship between osteoporosis and degenerative scoliosis is unclear, although the diagnoses often coexist.[78] Vertebral compression fractures can certainly produce sagittal plane and coronal plane deformities, although osteoporosis has not been definitively shown to be a risk factor for development or progression of degenerative scoliosis.[78-80] Severe rotation of the apical vertebrae, a Cobb angle of 30° or more, lateral vertebral translation of 6 mm or more, or a position of L5 above the intercrestal line have all been discussed as features that are predictive of curve progression in patients with degenerative lumbar scoliosis.[81-83]

The choice and success of nonsurgical treatment modalities depends on the type and extent of the deformity, the severity of the stenosis, and the presence of lateral listhesis.[82] In addition to physical therapy and medical treatments, use of spinal orthoses also may be an option. Although bracing generally will not prevent progression of degenerative curves, it may alleviate symptoms of back pain in some patients.[82] Whenever orthotic devices are used in elderly patients, care must be taken to pad bony prominences well to avoid skin breakdown.[81]

Surgical treatment may or may not be appropriate for patients with degenerative scoliosis, depending on the patient's presentation, health status, and expectations from surgery.[77,84] As with degenerative spondylolisthesis, there are conflicting reports regarding the need for spinal stabilization as an adjunct to decompressive surgery in this patient population.[77,84,85] Although the quality of clinical evidence to support the addition of fusion in patients with scoliosis is not as high as in those with degenerative spondylolisthesis, there are several clinical presentations that should generally not be treated by decompression alone, including significant sagittal plane imbalance, lateral listhesis of 5 mm or greater, and patients requiring wide decompression because of associated central canal stenosis.[81-84]

Elderly patients with severe scoliotic curves are not always suitable candidates for the large reconstructive fusion procedures required to treat spinal deformity. It is therefore tempting in patients without severe scoliotic

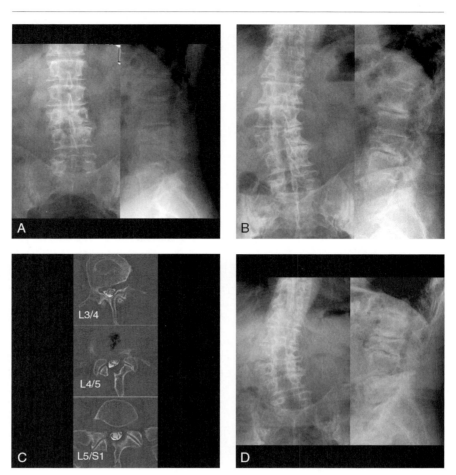

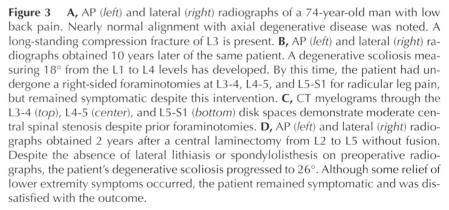

Figure 3 **A,** AP (*left*) and lateral (*right*) radiographs of a 74-year-old man with low back pain. Nearly normal alignment with axial degenerative disease was noted. A long-standing compression fracture of L3 is present. **B,** AP (*left*) and lateral (*right*) radiographs obtained 10 years later of the same patient. A degenerative scoliosis measuring 18° from the L1 to L4 levels has developed. By this time, the patient had undergone a right-sided foraminotomies at L3-4, L4-5, and L5-S1 for radicular leg pain, but remained symptomatic despite this intervention. **C,** CT myelograms through the L3-4 (*top*), L4-5 (*center*), and L5-S1 (*bottom*) disk spaces demonstrate moderate central spinal stenosis despite prior foraminotomies. **D,** AP (*left*) and lateral (*right*) radiographs obtained 2 years after a central laminectomy from L2 to L5 without fusion. Despite the absence of lateral lithiasis or spondylolisthesis on preoperative radiographs, the patient's degenerative scoliosis progressed to 26°. Although some relief of lower extremity symptoms occurred, the patient remained symptomatic and was dissatisfied with the outcome.

curves, significant lateral listhesis, or spinal decompensation to limit surgery to laminectomy or laminotomy alone without fusion.[82] It should be emphasized, however, that there is a lack of specific information regarding the success of decompression without fusion in this patient population, and

the scoliotic curves of some patients will progress following laminectomy despite the absence of these risk factors (Figure 3).

When fusion is elected, the length and location of fusion will vary depending on the patient's presentation. Treatment of mild defor-

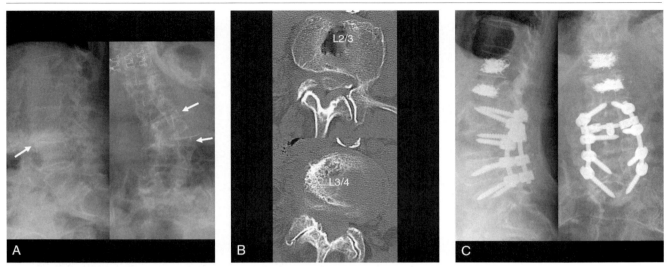

Figure 4 **A,** AP (*left*) and lateral (*right*) radiographs of the lumbar spine of an 86-year-old woman with symptoms of bilateral neurogenic claudication, relatively limited issues of back pain, and severe activity restriction. The patient had no significant medical comorbidities. Note the lateral listhesis at both the L2-3 and L3-4 disk spaces (*arrow*) in the AP view and the anterolisthesis at the L3-4 disk space on the lateral view (*double arrow*). **B,** CT myelograms through the L2-3 (*top*) and L3-4 (*bottom*) disk spaces demonstrate a complete block at the L3-4 level, with a near-complete block at the L2-3 level. **C,** AP (*left*) and lateral (*right*) radiographs after posterior laminectomy and fusion with segmental instrumentation from L2 to L5 using iliac crest bone graft. Prophylactic vertebroplasties of the T12 and L1 vertebrae were performed to prevent adjacent level fractures. At 2-year follow-up, the patient had excellent recovery of functional activities, with near-complete resolution of lower extremity symptoms.

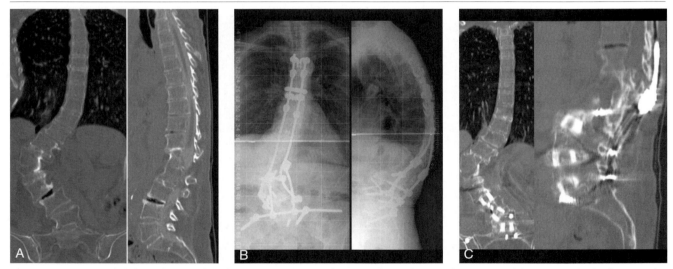

Figure 5 **A,** Sagittal (*left*) and coronal (*right*) reconstructions of postmyelography CT of a 78-year-old woman who had severe degenerative scoliosis of the lumbar spine and was incapacitated by back and leg pain. Although these are not upright images, note the apparent maintenance of both sagittal and coronal balance that was clinically confirmed in this patient. In addition, the CT scan demonstrated that autofusion had occurred from T12 to L3 with severe degenerative disease and lateral lithiasis noted at L3-4 and L4-5; coronal plane deformity and degeneration of the L5-S1 disk space was also noted. **B,** AP (*left*) and lateral (*right*) plain radiographs obtained at 2 years postoperatively demonstrate maintenance of spinal balance with minimal correction through the lumbar curve. Pelvic fixation was used because of the long thoracolumbar fusion and the need to fuse across the L5-S1 disk space. Graft was used in the posterolateral fusion harvested from the left iliac crest during placement of the iliac bolt. On the opposite side, a transiliac bar was placed extending through the right S1 pedicle screw. Vertical cross-extenders were then connected by dominoes to posterior rods extending from T4 to L5. Anterior interbody fusions were performed as a first-stage procedure via a midline retroperoneal approach from L3 to S1, with structural allograft rings filled with autologous bone graft. **C,** Coronal (*left*) and sagittal (*right*) CT reconstructions obtained 2 years postoperatively demonstrate complete consolidation of the anterior interbody grafts at all three levels. The patient had excellent pain relief and recovery of activity after undergoing this procedure.

mities with a coronally and sagittally balanced spine generally can be achieved with decompression and fusion with limited curve correction using instrumentation between the end vertebrae of the Cobb angle. In the senior author's experience, many elderly patients do not require fusion across the lumbosacral junction (Figure 4). Patients with sagittal imbalance, primary lumbar curves larger than 30°, painful lumbosacral fractional curves, or L5-S1 spondylolisthesis may, however, require fusion of the L5-S1 disk space. When fusion to the sacrum is elected, augmentation of sacral pedicle screws with a secondary point of fixation and structural interbody grafting at the L5-S1 disk is important for patients with constructs extending above the thoracolumbar junction. An anterior interbody fusion may be elected in order to better correct sagittal imbalance, for patients requiring fusion over more than three disk spaces, or as a means of increasing fusion rates in patients requiring fusion at the L5-S1 interspace. If anterior lumbar diskectomy and fusion is planned, a midline approach to L3-S1 is better tolerated than the traditional open lateral retroperitoneal (flank) approach with isolated posterior or posterior interbody fusion performed as needed above the L3 level[86] (Figure 5).

When spine surgery is elected in the elderly patient population, efforts to limit the extent of surgery are appropriate, provided the surgical option chosen retains the potential to successfully meet the clinical needs of the patient. Examples of limited surgical approaches include the use of posterior or transforaminal lumbar interbody fusions or transpsoas lateral interbody fusion in favor of anterior approaches[87,88] (Figure 6). In patients with less cen-

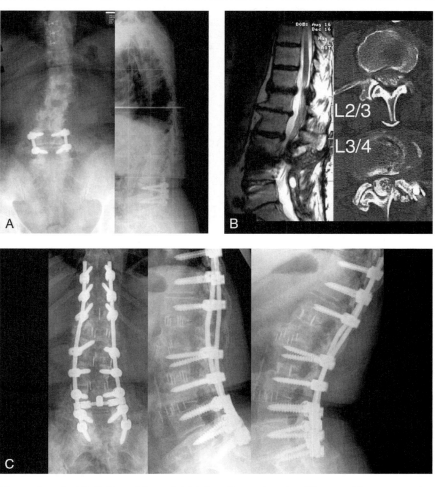

Figure 6   **A,** AP (*left*) and lateral (*right*) radiographs of a 67-year-old woman who had laminectomy and fusion of L4-5 1 year earlier demonstrate severe degenerative disease cranial to the fusion with coronal plane listhesis and lumbar kyphosis. The patient continued to have axial back pain and lumbar radiculopathy, which were likely the result of incomplete treatment of the presenting surgical pathology. **B,** Sagittal plane MRI and CT myelograms at L2-3 (*left*) and L3-4 (*right*) demonstrate persistent lateral recess and foraminal stenosis. **C,** AP (*left*) and lateral flexion (*center*) and extension (*right*) radiographs obtained after T12 to S1 fusion with percutaneous transpsoas approach was performed at the L1-2, L2-3, and L3-4 disk spaces. T12-L1 diskectomy and fusion was performed through a mini-open approach. Bone morphogenetic protein was used for the anterior interbody fusion. By 8-month follow-up, interbody fusions were nearly consolidated and the patient was fully recovered with excellent relief of axial back pain and leg symptoms.

tral canal stenosis, the use of an extended paraspinal (Wiltse) approach may help limit denervation and devascularization of the paraspinal musculature.[89,90]

In patients who require extended constructs for correction and stabilization, attention must be given to spinal balance and load sharing among implants, especially in the presence of osteoporosis. In such patients, significant loads can be placed on mechanically compromised points of fixation and can lead to implant or adjacent segment failure.

Table 2
Methods for Improving Fixation and Reducing Implant Loads in Patients With Osteoporosis*

Method	Citation	Caveat
Increase pedicle screw size	Brantley et al[118] Hirano et al[119]	Larger screws may not increase purchase and may increase risk of pedicle fracture
Conical screws	Ono et al[112] Kwok et al[113]	Loose fixation if backed out
Undertapping or self-tapping screws	Halvorson et al[72]	Possibility of pedicle screw malposition or pedicle fracture
"Up and in" screw orientation	Ruland et al[123] Ono et al[112] McKinley et al[124] Youssef et al[125]	Pullout at end of construct can result in neurologic injury
Pediculolaminar fixation	Hilibrand et al[101] Chiba et al[99] Halvorson et al[72] Hasegawa et al[102] Tan et al[103] Butler et al[107] Hu[93]	Increased volume of instrumentation Requires some soft-tissue disruption at ends of construct
Injectable fillers	Zindrick et al[126] Sarzier et al[127] Lotz et al[129] Wuisman et al[130] Pfeifer et al[134]	Potential for late infection around PMMA Off-label use of cement Potential for cement extravasation
Coated screws	Sanden et al[135, 136] Hasegawa et al[102]	Potential for loosening as coating resorbs
Expandable screws	Cook et al[114, 117] McKoy and An[116]	Potential for screw expansion through end plate or lateral wall May be difficult to remove following ingrowth
Interbody grafting	Polikeit et al[97] Lowe et al[96] Hackenberg et al[98]	Requires additional surgery Vascular risk anteriorly Neurologic risk posteriorly
Adjacent segment augmentation	Hu[93] Kostuik and Shapiro[106]	Off-label cement use Potential to reduce nutrition supply to disk Potential for cement extravasation

*Citations supporting the use of each method and potential concerns are also listed.

Considerations for Instrumentation of the Osteoporotic Spine

Although the mechanical compromise of osteoporotic bone is well known, evidence has demonstrated that spinal instrumentation in patients with osteoporosis can be done with relative safety and effectiveness.[91,92] However, it must be recognized that in the presence of osteoporosis, the mechanical strength of each point of fixation is reduced. For example, the pullout strength, cutout torque, and maximum insertional torque for pedicle screws have all been shown to correlate with bone mineral density and are significantly decreased in osteoporotic vertebrae.[72,73] Therefore, in patients with osteoporosis, careful attention to principles that optimize the strength and minimize loading of individual points of fixation is required[74,93,94] (Table 2).

Minimizing Loads at Individual Fixation Points

Minimizing implant loads at individual points of fixation can be accomplished in several ways. Using multiple points of fixation, obtaining adequate sagittal balance, interbody structural support, accepting lesser degrees of coronal deformity correction, and using accessory means of fixation at individual levels all will reduce pedicle screw or hook loading.[74,93,94] In certain patients, protecting sacral pedicle screws with additional fixation either within the sacrum or at the pelvis should be considered at the end of a long construct.

Using multiple points of fixation, such as segmental pedicle screws, reduces the load applied to individual screws and increases the stiffness of the overall construct. A similar principle applies to hooks or wires, although these implants generally require longer constructs than pedicle screws to provide adequate fixation.[93,95] One disadvantage of using segmental pedicle screw fixation is that the space occupied by the implants can reduce the room available for bone graft.

Sagittal imbalance caused by instrumentation with insufficient lumbar lordosis can result in forward tilt of the head and trunk anterior to the sacrum and pelvis. This can contribute significantly to instrument strains, especially at the cranial and caudal ends of a construct. Efforts to improve sagittal balance are, therefore, important not only to improve patient outcomes, but also from the standpoint of reducing the potential for hardware failure. Shortening of the posterior column may be required to accomplish this, either through aggressive loosening of facet joints and removal of interspinous ligaments or in patients with severe sagittal imbalance, via Smith-Petersen or pedicle subtraction osteotomy techniques. The use of interbody grafting will also help maintain lordosis and reduce loads on posterior instrumentation through load sharing.

Several principles are important in optimizing outcomes of interbody graft placement, specifically in patients with osteoporosis. Careful technique is required to avoid removal of the bony end plate, which provides the greatest mechanical resistance to implant subsidence. Choosing an appropriately sized implant is also important because smaller implants may not engage enough cortical surface and are thus more susceptible to subsidence into the osteoporotic vertebral body.[96,97] Posterior interbody fusion techniques, such as transforaminal lumbar interbody fusion and posterior lumbar interbody fusion, provide surgeons with additional options that may avoid the need for an anterior operation while still providing anterior column support and can be combined with posterior osteotomy techniques to help restore and maintain lordosis.[88,98]

Although sagittal plane balance is important to reduce implant loading, it may be beneficial to accept less correction of coronal deformity in elderly patients with osteoporosis. Whereas maximizing coronal plane balance correction is typically a goal of spinal deformity surgery, in the presence of osteoporosis the strength of bone anchors may not allow strong compression/ distraction or vertebral rotation forces to be applied.[74,93,94] Clinical outcomes in elderly patients are strongly related to achieving sagittal balance and obtaining a solid fusion.

Augmenting pedicle screw fixation at individual segments with offset sublaminar hooks or sublaminar wires also reduces the load at individual screws.[99,100] Sublaminar hooks have been shown to increase pullout strength, construct stiffness, reduce pedicle screw bending moments, and absorb some of the construct strain, especially in significantly osteoporotic bone.[72,99,101-103] Although load sharing can also be considered a means of augmenting fixation at individual vertebrae, the load-sharing effect also reduces loading resulting from the primary fixation devices, which is especially valuable at the cranial and caudal ends of instrumentation constructs.

Supplementary fixation below S1 sacral pedicle screws at the caudal end of long constructs is an important means of reducing pseudarthrosis rates at the L5-S1 disk space.[104,105] Sacral alar screws, S2 pedicle screws, transsacral bars, iliac bolts, and the Galveston iliac rodding technique all can be used effectively.[82] The addition of structural interbody grafting at L5-S1, although it does not necessarily improve the mechanical situation, is an important consideration from the standpoint of increasing the bone surface area available for fusion and thereby increasing fusion rates.

Avoiding Failure of Adjacent Vertebral Segments

Failure of the cranial adjacent segment can occur acutely as a result of vertebral body fracture or loss of implant fixation, or as a longer term complication caused by degeneration of the adjacent motion segment. Avoiding failure of adjacent vertebral segments is also important and may be a particular challenge in longer fusion constructs in elderly patients and those with osteoporosis. Despite this challenge, guidelines for choice of fusion end points remain incompletely defined. In general, ending a fusion of most of the lumbar spine at T12 or L1 should be avoided, particularly in patients with osteoporosis.[106] Most of these constructs should be extended to T9 or T10 to delay or avoid junctional breakdown.

Patients with prior fusion of the thoracic spine or clinically significant deformity in this region should have instrumentation and fusion of remaining unfused segments extending to the upper thoracic spine.[93,107] It is generally not recommended to stop a fusion within a region of kyphosis, such as the midthoracic spine, to avoid excess loading to the cranialmost implants and vertebrae. Augmentation of fixation at the cranial segments with sublaminar wires or the addition of a cranial offset hook is also a potentially useful means of protecting pedicle screws.[74,108]

Consideration should also be given to the prophylactic augmentation of vertebrae adjacent to long fusion constructs through procedures such as vertebroplasty or kyphoplasty, particularly for areas of high mechanical stress such as the thoracolumbar junction. Augmentation of the top instrumented segment and the first cranial adjacent vertebrae is probably most important because these are the most common sites of postoperative vertebral fracture.

Maximizing Strength of Individual Anchor Points

Several studies have demonstrated a direct correlation between bone mineral density and screw pullout forces, with substantially reduced pullout forces noted in osteoporotic bone.[72,73,108-111] Improving the bone-implant interface is fundamental to optimize pedicle screw fixation in osteoporotic bone.[94] Several techniques and devices have been developed that enhance the strength of the interface between bone and pedicle screws, which is generally regarded as the "weakest link" in overall construct stability. These techniques include specific pedicle screw designs, careful pilot hole preparation, optimizing screw orientation, and enhancement with fillers and coatings.

Several unique pedicle screw designs have been described for use in osteoporotic bone. Conical screws, which better approximate pedicle morphometry, have been shown to increase pullout resistance in osteoporotic bone.[112,113] It should be noted, however, that conical screws lose a significant portion of their strength when backed out by even a half turn, which may limit their ability to accommodate rod contour by backing out the screw.[112]

Expandable screws offer additional improvement in pullout strength in severely osteoporotic bone.[114-116] Clinical series using these devices, which include 21 patients with osteoporosis, demonstrated radiographic evidence of fusion in 86% of patients.[114,117] One concern with such implants is that increasing screw diameter could fracture the pedicle, placing the adjacent nerve root at risk.[118] As a guideline, final screw diameters should not exceed 70% of the outer diameter of the pedicle when the bone mineral density is less than 0.7 g/cm^2.[119]

In patients with osteoporosis, undertapping or avoiding tapping of the pilot hole altogether before screw insertion does help improve screw fixation, especially in the lumbar spine.[72,120] Careful evaluation of final screw position in such patients is critical, however, because some tactile feedback during pilot hole preparation is lost, and pedicle fracture can occur during screw placement.[121,122]

Screw orientation also should be optimized in patients with osteoporosis. Screw triangulation via a medial orientation takes advantage of the bone mass between the converging screws for fixation, rather than only that bone lying between threads of a single screw, and has been shown to improve pullout strength in osteoporotic bone.[112,123] Similarly, screws oriented caudal or parallel relative to the vertebral end plate, as opposed to a cranial orientation, avoid increased bending moments at the screw hub in normal vertebrae, and use of this technique is also prudent in osteoporotic bone.[124,125]

Injectable cements of several types have been shown to substantially increase the pullout strength of screw fixation in osteoporotic bone.[74,109,126-133] However, cement extravasation can potentially injure surrounding structures, and permanent cements such as polymethylmethacrylate represent a potential locus for late infection.[74,109] In addition, these techniques currently are considered an off-label use of bone cement. These concerns may be avoided by insertion of cancellous bone chips into the pedicle screw hole before screw insertion, although vertebral body strength is not enhanced by this technique.[110,134]

HA-coated screws have been shown to increase pullout forces, presumably by increasing both the contact surface area as well as the frictional coefficient at the bone-implant interface.[135-137] Hasegawa and associates[137] demonstrated that HA-coated screws had greater pullout force than screws without HA coating specifically in an osteoporotic model. The mechanical behavior of these implants over time as resorption of the HA coating occurs has not been studied, however.

Summary

The elderly patient with lumbar spine degenerative disease presents significant challenges regarding surgical decision making and management. Even the presence of medical comorbidities need not always exclude the elderly patient from elective spine surgery. Both surgeon and patient, however, must be aware of how age and comorbid conditions may affect perioperative management and ultimate clinical outcome.

Osteoporosis is a particularly prevalent comorbidity in the elderly population. The potential presence of osteoporosis, thus, must be a concern in all elderly patients with degenerative disease of the lumbar spine. Several options are available to the spine surgeon that can improve implant fixation and potentially improve outcomes in this patient group. Careful assessment of patients for surgical indications and attention to surgical technique are critical for successful treatment of this challenging patient population.

References

1. Ciol MA, Deyo RA, Howell E, Kreif S: An assessment of surgery for spinal stenosis: Time trends, geographic variations, complications, and reoperations. *J Am Geriatr Soc* 1996;44:285-290.

2. Watters JM, McClaran JC: The elderly surgical patient, in Wilmore DW (ed): *American College of Surgeons: Care of the Surgical Patient, Vol I.* New York, NY, Scientific American, 1991, pp 1-31.

3. Goldman L, Caldera CL, Nussbaum SR, et al: Multifactorial index of cardiac risk in noncardiac surgical procedures. *N Engl J Med* 1977;297:845-850.

4. Tornebrandt K, Fletcher R: Pre-operative chest x-rays in elderly patients. *Anaesthesia* 1982;37:901-902.

5. Smetana GW: Preoperative pulmonary evaluation. *N Engl J Med* 1999;340:937-944.

6. Nunn JF, Milledge JS, Chen D, Dore C: Respiratory criteria of fitness for surgery and anaesthesia. *Anaesthesia* 1988;43:543-551.

7. Joehl RJ: Preoperative evaluation: Pulmonary, cardiac, renal dysfunction and comorbidities. *Surg Clin North Am* 2005;85:1061-1073.

8. Milledge JS, Nunn JF: Criteria of fitness for anaesthesia in patients with chronic obstructive lung disease. *BMJ* 1975;3:670-673.

9. Older P, Smith R: Experience with the preoperative invasive measurement of haemodynamic, respiratory and renal function in 100 elderly patients scheduled for major abdominal surgery. *Anaesth Intensive Care* 1988;16:389-395.

10. Kumle B, Boldt J, Piper S, Schmidt C, Suttner S, Salopek S: The influence of different intravascular volume replacement regimens on renal function in the elderly. *Anesth Analg* 1999;89:1124-1130.

11. Boldt J, Brenner T, Lang J, Kumle B, Isgro F: Kidney-specific proteins in elderly patients undergoing cardiac surgery with cardiopulmonary bypass. *Anesth Analg* 2003;97:1582-1589.

12. Beliveau MM, Multach M: Perioperative care for the elderly patient. *Med Clin North Am* 2003;87:273-289.

13. Niccoli L, Bellino S, Cantini F: Renal tolerability of three commonly employed non-steroidal anti-inflammatory drugs in elderly patients with osteoarthritis. *Clin Exp Rheumatol* 2002;20:201-207.

14. Thaller J, Walker M, Kline AJ, Anderson DG: The effect of non-steroidal anti-inflammatory agents on spinal fusion. *Orthopedics* 2005;28:299-303.

15. Riew KD, Long J, Rhee J, et al: Time dependent inhibitory effects of indomethacin on spinal fusion. *J Bone Joint Surg Am* 2003;85:632-634.

16. Linnebur SA, Milchak JL: Assessment of oral bisphosphonate use in elderly patients with varying degrees of kidney function. *Am J Geriatr Pharmacother* 2004;2:213-218.

17. Huang RC, Khan SN, Sandhu HS, et al: Alendronate inhibits spine fusion in a rat model. *Spine* 2005;30:2516-2522.

18. Xue Q, Li H, Zou X, et al: The influence of alendronate treatment and bone graft volume on posterior lateral spine fusion in a porcine model. *Spine* 2005;30:1116-1121.

19. Xue Q, Li H, Zou X, et al: Healing properties of allograft from alendronate-treated animal in lumbar spine interbody cage fusion. *Eur Spine J* 2005;14:222-226.

20. Lehman RA Jr, Kuklo TR, Freedman BA, Cowart JR, Mense MG, Riew KD: The effect of alendronate sodium on spinal fusion: a rabbit model. *Spine J* 2004;4:36-43.

21. Nourhashemi F, Andrieu S, Rauzy O, et al: Nutrition support and aging in preoperative nutrition. *Curr Opin Clin Nutr Metab Care* 1999;2:87-92.

22. Fast Facts on Osteoporosis. Web site of the National Osteoporosis Foundation. Available at: http://www.NOF.org/statistics. Accessed November 18, 2005.

23. Cummings SR, Melton LJ: Epidemiology and outcomes of osteoporotic fractures. *Lancet* 2002;359:1761-1767.

24. Cauley JA, Fullman RL, Stone KL, et al: Factors associated with the lumbar spine and proximal femur bone mineral density in older men. *Osteoporos Int* 2005;16:1525-1537.

25. Melton LJ: Epidemiology of spinal osteoporosis. *Spine* 1997;22(suppl 24):2S-11S.

26. Lee CA, Einhorn TA: The bone organ system: Form and function, in Feldman MR, Kelsey J (eds): *Osteoporosis*, ed 2. San Diego, CA, Academic Press, 2001, pp 3-30.

27. Wahner HW: Use of densitometry in management of osteoporosis, in Marcus R, Feldman D, Kelsey J (eds): *Ostoeporosis*, San Diego, CA, Academic Press, 1996, pp 1055-1072.

28. Einhorn TA: The structural properties of normal and osteoporotic bone. *Instr Course Lect* 2003;52:533-539.

29. Kahanovitz N: Osteoporosis and fusion. *Instr Course Lect* 1992;41:231-233.

30. Khoska S, Riggs BL, Melton LJ: Clinical spectrum of osteoporosis, in Riggs BL, Melton LJ (eds): *Osteoporosis: Etiology Diagnosis and Management*, ed 2. Philadelphia, PA, Lippincott-Raven, 1995, pp 205-223.

31. Riggs BL, Melton LJ: Involutional osteoporosis. *N Engl J Med* 1986;314:1676-1684.

32. Kirkaldy-Willis WH, Paine KW, Cauchoix J, McIvor G: Lumbar spinal stenosis. *Clin Orthop Relat Res* 1974;99:30-50.

33. Lane JM, Gardner MJ, Lin JT, van der Meulen MC, Myers E: The aging spine: New technologies and therapeutics for the osteoporotic spine. *Eur Spine J* 2003;12(suppl 2):S147-S154.

34. Benoist M: Natural history of the aging spine. *Eur Spine J* 2003;12(suppl 2): S86-S89.

35. Szpalski M, Gunzburg R: Lumbar spinal stenosis in the elderly: An overview. *Eur Spine J* 2003;12(suppl 2):S170-S175.

36. Arbit E, Pannullo S: Lumbar stenosis: A clinical review. *Clin Orthop Relat Res* 2001;384:137-143.

37. Kurz LT, Dvorak J: Clinical radiologic and electrodiagnostic diagnosis of degenerative lumbar stenosis, in Wiesel SW, Weinstein JN, Herkowitz H, Dvorak J, Bell G (eds): *The Lumbar Spine*, ed 2. Philadelphia, PA, WB Saunders, 1996, p 731.

38. Porter RW: Pathophysiology of neurogenic claudication, in Wiesel SW, Weinstein JN, Herkowitz H, Dvorak J, Bell G (eds): *The Lumbar Spine*, ed 2. Philadelphia, PA, WB Saunders, 1996, p 717.

39. Baloh RW, Ying SH, Jacobson KM: A longitudinal study of gait and balance dysfunction in normal older adults. *Arch Neurol* 2003;60:835-839.

40. Boden SD, Davis DO, Dina TS, Patronas NJ, Wiesel SW: Abnormal magnetic resonance scans of the lumbar spine in asymptomatic subjects. *J Bone Joint Surg Am* 1990;72:403-408.

41. Carlson N, Carlson H: Electrodiagnostic studies, in Bernstein J (ed): *Musculoskeletal Medicine*. Rosemont, IL, American Academy of Orthopedic Surgeons, 2003, pp 409-417.

42. Deen HG, Fenton DS, Lamer TJ: Minimally invasive procedures for disorders of the lumbar spine. *Mayo Clin Proc* 2003;78:1249-1256.

43. Sengupta DK, Herkowitz HN: Lumbar spinal stenosis: Treatment strategies and indications for surgery. *Orthop Clin North Am* 2003;34:281-295.

44. Gunzburg R, Szpalski M: The conservative surgical treatment of lumbar spinal stenosis in the elderly. *Eur Spine J* 2003;12(suppl 2):S176-S180.

45. Postacchini F: Surgical management of lumbar spinal stenosis. *Spine* 1999;24:1043-1047.

46. White AA, Panjabi MM (eds): The problem of instability in the human spine: A systematic approach, in *Clinical Biomechanics or the Spine*. Philadelphia, PA, Lippincott, 1990.

47. Epstein NE, Epstein JE: Surgery for spinal stenosis, in Wiesel SW, Weinstein JN, Herkowitz H, Dvorak J, Bell G (eds): *The Lumbar Spine*, ed 2. Philadelphia, PA, WB Saunders, 1996, p 737.

48. Deyo RA, Cherkin DC, Loeser JD, Bigos SJ, Ciol MA: Morbidity and mortality in association with operations on the lumbar spine. *J Bone Joint Surg Am* 1992;74:536-543.

49. Deyo RA, Ciol MA, Cherkin DC, Loeser JD, Bigos SJ: Lumbar spinal fusion: A cohort study of complications, reoperations, and resource use in the Medicare population. *Spine* 1993;18:1463-1470.

50. Malter AD, McNeney B, Loeser JD, Deyo RA: 5-year reoperation rates after different types of lumbar spine surgery. *Spine* 1998;23:814-820.

51. Postacchine F: Classification and treatment, in Weinstein JN, Wiesel SW (eds): *The Lumbar Spine*. Philadelphia. PA, WB Saunders, 1990, p 605.

52. Katz JN, Lipson SJ, Larson MG, McInnes JM, Fossel AH, Liang MH: The outcome of decompressive laminectomy for degenerative lumbar stenosis. *J Bone Joint Surg Am* 1991;73:809-816.

53. Ragab AA, Fye MA, Bohlman HH: Surgery of the lumbar spine for spinal stenosis in 118 patients 70 years of age or older. *Spine* 2003;28:348-353.

54. Katz JN, Stucki G, Lipson SJ, Fossel AH, Grobler LJ, Weinstein JN: Predictors of surgical outcome in degenerative lumbar spinal stenosis. *Spine* 1999;24:2229-2233.

55. Arinzon Z, Adunsky A, Fidelman Z, Gepstein R: Outcomes of decompression surgery for lumbar spinal stenosis in elderly diabetic patients. *Eur Spine J* 2004;13:32-37.

56. Benz RJ, Ibrahim ZG, Afshar P, Garfin SR: Predicting complications in elderly patients undergoing lumbar decompression. *Clin Orthop Relat Res* 2001;384:116-121.

57. Balderston RA, Vaccaro AR: Surgical treatment of adult degenerative spondylolisthesis, in Wiesel SW, Weinstein JN, Herkowitz H, Dvorak J, Bell G (eds): *The Lumbar Spine*, ed 2. Philadelphia, PA, WB Saunders, 1996, p 701.

58. Wiltse LL, Newman PH, Macnab I: Classification of spondylosis and spondylolisthesis. *Clin Orthop Relat Res* 1976;117:23-29.

59. Bassewitz H, Herkowitz H: Lumbar stenosis with spondylolisthesis. *Clin Orthop Relat Res* 2001;384:54-60.

60. Rosenberg NJ: Degenerative spondylolisthesis: Surgical treatment. *Clin Orthop Relat Res* 1976;117:112-120.

61. Meyerding HW: Spondylolisthesis. *Surg Gynecol Obstet* 1932;54:371-379.

62. Phillips FM, Pfeifer BA, Lieberman IH, Kerr EJ, Choi IS, Pazianos AG: Minimally invasive treatments of osteoporotic vertebral compression fractures: Vertebroplasty and kyphoplasty. *Instr Course Lect* 2003;52:559-567.

63. Herkowitz HN, Kurz LT: Degenerative lumbar spondylolisthesis with spinal stenosis. *J Bone Joint Surg Am* 1991;73:802-808.

64. Bjarke Christensen F, Stender Hansen ES, Laursen M, Thomsen K, Bunger CE: Long-term functional outcome of pedicle screw instrumentation as a support for posterolateral spinal fusion: A randomized clinical study with 5-year followup. *Spine* 2002;27:1269-1277.

65. Fischgrund JS, Mackay M, Herkowitz HN, Brower R, Montgomery D, Kurz L: Degenerative lumbar spondylolisthesis with spinal stenosis: A prospective, randomized study comparing decompressive laminectomy and arthrodesis with and without spinal instrumentation. *Spine* 1997;22:2807-2812.

66. Thomsen K, Christiensen FB, Eiskjær SP, Hansen ES, Fruensgaard S, Bunger CE: The effect of pedicle screw instrumentation on functional outcome and fusion rates in posterolateral lumbar spine fusion: A prospective, randomized clinical study. *Spine* 1997;22:2813-2822.

67. Mardjetko SM, Connolly PJ, Shott S: Degenerative lumbar spondylolisthesis: A meta-analysis of literature 1970-1993. *Spine* 1994;19(suppl 20):2256S-2265S.

68. Herron LD, Trippi AC: L4-5 degenerative spondylolisthesis: the results of treatment by decompressive laminectomy without fusion. *Spine* 1989;14:534-538.

69. Guyatt G, Rennie D: *Users' Guide to the Medical Literature*. Chicago, IL, American Medical Association Press, 2004.

70. Sackett DL, Straus SE, Richardson WS, Rosenberg W, Haynes RB: *Evidence Based Medicine*. London, UK, Churchill Livingstone, 2000.

71. Irwin ZN, Hilibrand A, Gustavel M, et al: Variations in surgical decision making for degenerative spinal disorders: Part I. Lumbar spine. *Spine* 2005;30:2208-2213.

72. Halvorson TL, Kelley LA, Thomas KA, Whitecloud TS, Cook SD: Effects of bone mineral density on pedicle screw fixation. *Spine* 1994;19:2415-2420.

73. Okuyama K, Sato K, Abe E, Inaba H, Shimada Y, Murai H: Stability of transpedicle screwing for the osteoporotic spine. *Spine* 1993;18:2240-2245.

74. Glassman SD, Alegre GM: Adult spinal deformity in the osteoporotic spine: Options and pitfalls. *Instr Course Lect* 2003;52:579-588.

75. Schwab F, Dubey A, Pagala M, Gamez L, Farcy JP: Adult scoliosis: A health assessment analysis by SF-36. *Spine* 2003;28:602-606.

76. Jackson RP, Simmons EH, Stripinis D: Incidence and severity of back pain in adult idiopathic scoliosis. *Spine* 1983;8:749-756.

77. Lonstein J: Adult scoliosis, in Bradford D, Lonstein J, Ogilvie T, Winter R (eds): *Moe's Textbook of Scoliosis and Other Spinal Disorders*, ed 2. Philadelphia, PA, WB Saunders, 1987.

78. Healey JH, Lane JM: Structural scoliosis in osteoporotic women. *Clin Orthop Relat Res* 1985;195:216-223.

79. Robin GC, Span Y, Steinberg R, Makin M, Menczel J: Scoliosis in the elderly: A follow-up study. *Spine* 1982;7:355-361.

80. Korovessis P, Piperos G, Sidiropoulos P, Dimas A: Adult idiopathic lumbar scoliosis: A formula for prediction of progression and review of the literature. *Spine* 1994;19:1926-1932.

81. Balderston RA, Albert TJ: Adult Scoliosis: Evaluation and decision making, in Wiesel SW, Weinstein JN, Herkowitz H, Dvorak J, Bell G (eds): *The Lumbar Spine*, ed 2. Philadelphia, PA, WB Saunders, 1996, p 1118.

82. Gupta MC: Degenerative scoliosis: Options for surgical management. *Orthop Clin North Am* 2003;34:269-279.

83. Pritchett JW, Bortel DT: Degenerative symptomatic lumbar scoliosis. *Spine* 1993;18:700-703.

84. Benner B, Ehni G: Degenerative lumbar scoliosis. *Spine* 1979;4:548-552.

85. San Martino A, D'Andria FM, San Martino C: The surgical treatment of nerve root compression caused by scoliosis of the lumbar spine. *Spine* 1983;8:261-265.

86. Esses SI, Botsford DJ: Surgical anatomy and operative approaches to the sacrum, in Frymoyer JW (ed): *The Adult Spine: Principles and Practice*. New York, NY, Raven Press, 1991, pp 2104-2105.

87. Lippman CR, Spence CA, Youssef AS, Cahill DW: Correction of adult scoliosis via a posterior-only approach. *Neurosurg Focus* 2003;14:e5.

88. Potter BK, Freedman BA, Verwiebe EG, Hall JM, Polly DW Jr, Kuklo TR: Transforaminal lumbar interbody fusion: clinical and radiographic results and complications in 100 consecutive patients. *J Spinal Disord Tech* 2005;18:337-346.

89. Wiltse LL: The paraspinal sacrospinal-splitting approach to the lumbar spine. *Clin Orthop Relat Res* 1973;91:48-57.

90. Wiltse LL, Spencer CW: New uses and refinements of the paraspinal approach to the lumbar spine. *Spine* 1988;13:696-706.

91. Kumano K, Hirabayashi S, Ogawa Y, Aota Y: Pedicle screws and bone mineral density. *Spine* 1994;19:1157-1161.

92. McAfee PC, Farey ID, Sutterlin CE, Gurr KR, Warden KE, Cunningham BW: Device related osteoporosis with spinal instrumentation. *Spine* 1989;14:919-926.

93. Hu SS: Internal fixation in the osteoporotic spine. *Spine* 1997;22(suppl 43):43S-48S.

94. Hettwer WH, Hart RA: Principles of instrumentation in the osteoporotic spine: An overview. *Advances in Osteoporotic Fracture Management* 2004;3:1-7.

95. Hart R, Hettwer W, Liu Q, Prem S: Mechanical stiffness of segmental versus nonsegmental pedicle screw constructs: The effect of cross-links. *Spine* 2006;31:E35-E38.

96. Lowe TG, Hashim S, Wilson LA, et al: A biomechanical study of regional endplate strength and cage morphology as it relates to structural interbody support. *Spine* 2004;29:2389-2394.

97. Polikeit A, Ferguson SJ, Nolte LP, Orr TE: Factors influencing stresses in the lumbar spine after the insertion of intervertebral cages: Finite element analysis. *Eur Spine J* 2003;12:413-420.

98. Hackenberg L, Halm H, Bullman V, Volker V, Schneider M, Liljenqvist U: Transforaminal lumbar interbody fusion: A safe technique with satisfactory three to five year results. *Eur Spine J* 2005;14:551-558.

99. Chiba M, McLain RF, Yerby SA, Moseley TA, Smith TS, Benson DR: Short-segment pedicle screw fixation: Biomechanical analysis of supplemental hook fixation. *Spine* 1996;21:288-294.

100. Yerby SA, Ehteshami JR, McLain RF: Offset laminar hooks decrease bending moments of pedicle screws during in situ contouring. *Spine* 1997;22:376-381.

101. Hilibrand AS, Moore DC, Graziano GP: The role of pediculolaminar fixation in compromised pedicle bone. *Spine* 1996;21:445-451.

102. Hasegawa K, Takahashi HE, Uchiyama S, et al: An experimental study of a combination of method using a pedicle screw and laminar hook for the osteoporotic spine. *Spine* 1997;22:958-962.

103. Tan JS, Kwon BK, Dvorak MF, Fisher CG, Oxland TR: Pedicle screw motion in the osteoporotic spine after augmentation with laminar hooks, sublaminar wires, or calcium phosphate cement: A comparative analysis. *Spine* 2004;29:1723-1730.

104. Islam NC, Wood KB, Transfeldt EE, et al: Extension of fusion to the pelvis in idiopathic scoliosis. *Spine* 2001;26:166-173.

105. Alegre GM, Gupta MC, Bay BK, Smith TS, Laubach JE: S1 Screw bending moment with posterior spinal instrumentation across the lumbosacral junction after unilateral iliac crest harvest. *Spine* 2001;26:1950-1955.

106. Kostuik JP, Shapiro MB: Open surgical treatment of osteoporotic fractures and deformity of the spine. *Instr Course Lect* 2003;52:569-578.

107. Butler TE, Asher MA, Jayaraman G, Nunley PD, Robinson RG: The strength and stiffness of thoracic implant anchors in osteoporotic spines. *Spine* 1994;19:1956-1962.

108. Coe JD, Warden KE, Herzig MA, McAfee PC: Influence of bone mineral density on the fixation of thoracolumbar implants: A comparative study of transpedicular screws, laminar hooks, and spinous process wires. *Spine* 1990;15:902-907.

109. Soshi S, Shiba R, Kondo H, Murota K: An experimental study on transpedicular screw fixation in relation to osteoporosis in the lumbar spine. *Spine* 1991;16:1335-1341.

110. Breeze SW, Doherty BJ, Noble PS, LeBlanc A, Heggeness MH: A biomechanical study of anterior thoracolumbar screw fixation. *Spine* 1998;23:1829-1831.

111. Eysel P, Schwitalle M, Oberstein A, Rompe JD, Hopf C, Kullmer K: Preoperative estimation of screw fixation strength in vertebral bodies. *Spine* 1998;23:174-180.

112. Ono A, Brown MD, Latta LL, Milne EL, Holmes DC: Triangulated pedicle screw construct and pullout strength of conical and cylindrical screws. *J Spinal Disord* 2001;14:323-329.

113. Kwok AW, Finkelstein JA, Woodside T, Hearn T, Hu RW: Insertional torque and pullout strengths of conical and cylindrical pedicle screw in cadaveric bone. *Spine* 1996;21:2429-2434.

114. Cook SD, Salkeld SL, Whitecloud TS III, Barbera J: Biomechanical evaluation and preliminary clinical experience with an expansive pedicle screw design. *J Spinal Disord* 2000;13:230-236.

115. Cook SD, Salkeld SL, Stanley T, Faciane A, Miller SD: Biomechanical study of pedicle screw fixation in severely osteoporotic bone. *Spine J* 2004;4:402-408.

116. McKoy BE, An YH: An expandable anchor for fixation in osteoporotic bone. *J Orthop Res* 2001;19:545-547.

117. Cook SD, Barbera J, Rubi M, Salkeld SL, Whitecloud TS III: Lumbosacral fixation using expandable pedicle screws. An alternative in reoperation and osteoporosis. *Spine J* 2001;1:109-114.

118. Brantley AG, Mayfield JK, Koeneman JB, Clark KR: The effects of pedicle screw fit. *Spine* 1994;19:1752-1758.

119. Hirano T, Hasegawa K, Washio T, Hara T, Takahashi H: Fracture risk during pedicle screw insertion in osteoporotic spine. *J Spinal Disord* 1998;11:493-497.

120. Carmouche JJ, Molinari RW, Gerlinger T, Devine J, Patience T: Effects of pilot hole preparation technique on pedicle screw fixation in different regions of the osteoporotic thoracic and lumbar spine. *J Neurosurg Spine* 2005;3:364-370.

121. Ozawa T, Takahashi K, Yamagata M, et al: Insertional torque of the lumbar pedicle screw during surgery. *J Orthop Sci* 2005;10:133-136.

122. Okuyama K, Abe E, Suzuki T, Tamura Y, Chiba M, Sato K: Can insertional torque predict screw loosening and related failures? *Spine* 2000;25:858-864.

123. Ruland CM, McAfee PC, Warden KE, Cunningham BW: Triangulation of pedicular instrumentation: A biomechanical analysis. *Spine* 1991;16(6 Suppl):S270-S276.

124. McKinley TO, McLain RF, Yerby SA, Sharkey NA, Sarigul-Klijin N, Smith TS: Characteristics of pedicle

screw loading: effect of surgical techniques on intravertebral and intrapedicular bending moments. *Spine* 1999;24:18-24.

125. Youssef JA, McKinley TO, Yerby SA, McLain RF: Characteristics of pedicle screw loading: Effect of sagittal insertion angle on intrapedicular bending moments. *Spine* 1999;24:1077-1081.

126. Zindrick MR, Wiltse LL, Widell EH, et al: A biomechanical study of intrapeduncular screw fixation in the lumbosacral spine. *Clin Orthop Relat Res* 1986;203:99-112.

127. Sarzier JS, Evans AJ, Cahill DW: Increased pedicle screw pullout strength with vertebroplasty augmentation in osteoporotic spines. *J Neurosurg* 2002;96:309-312.

128. Hernigou P, Duparc F: Rib graft or cement to enhance screw fixation in anterior vertebral bodies. *J Spinal Disord* 1996;9:322-325.

129. Lotz JC, Hu SS, Chiu DFM, Yu M, Colliou O, Poser RD: Carbonated apatite cement augmentation of pedicle screw fixation in the lumbar spine. *Spine* 1997;22:2716-2723.

130. Wuisman PI, Van Dijk M, Staal H, Van Royen BJ: Augmentation of pedicle screws with calcium apatite cement in patients with severe progression of osteoporotic spinal deformities: An innovative technique. *Eur Spine J* 2000;9:528-533.

131. Bai B, Kummer FJ, Spivak J: Augmentation of anterior vertebral body screw fixation by an injectable, biodegradable calcium phosphate bone substitute. *Spine* 2001;26:2679-2683.

132. Yerby SA, Toh E, McLain RF: Revision of failed pedicles screws using hydroxyapatite cement: A biomechanical analysis. *Spine* 1998;23:1657-1661.

133. Taniwaki Y, Takemasa R, Tani T, Mizobuchi H, Yamamoto H: Enhancement of pedicle screw stability using calcium phosphate cement in osteoporotic vertebrae: In vivo biomechanical study. *J Orthop Sci* 2003;8:408-414.

134. Pfeifer BA, Krag MH, Johnson C: Repair of failed transpedicle screw fixation. *Spine* 1994;19:350-353.

135. Sanden B, Olerud C, Larsson S: Hydroxyapatite coating enhances fixation of loaded pedicle screws: A mechanical in vivo study in sheep. *Eur Spine J* 2001;10:334-339.

136. Sanden B, Olerud C, Johansson C, Larsson S: Improved bone-screw interface with hydroxyapatite coating. *Spine* 2001;26:2673-2678.

137. Hasegawa T, Inufusa A, Imai Y, Mikawa Y, Lim TH, An HS: Hydroxyapatite-coating of pedicle screws improves resistance against pull-out force in the osteoporotic canine lumbar spine model: A pilot study. *Spine J* 2005;5:239-243.

23

Minimally Invasive Techniques for the Treatment of Osteoporotic Vertebral Fractures

Neil A. Manson, MD, FRCSC
Frank M. Phillips, MD

Abstract

Osteoporotic vertebral compression fractures are a leading cause of disability and morbidity in the elderly. The consequences of these fractures include pain, progressive vertebral collapse with resultant spinal kyphosis, and systemic manifestations. Nonsurgical measures have proved unsuccessful in a portion of this population and for this group, minimally invasive vertebral augmentation can be beneficial. Vertebroplasty is designed to address vertebral fracture pain. It involves percutaneous injection of polymethylmethacrylate (PMMA) directly into a fractured vertebral body with the goals of pain relief and prevention of further collapse of the fractured vertebra. Kyphoplasty is designed to address the kyphotic deformity as well as the fracture pain. It involves the percutaneous insertion of an inflatable bone tamp into a fractured vertebral body. Bone tamp inflation works to elevate the end plates and create a cavity to be filled with PMMA with the goals of pain relief, restoration of vertebral body height, and reduced kyphotic deformity. Optimizing surgical technique can improve outcomes and decrease complication rates, and decrease radiation exposure to the patient and surgical team. Obtaining a biopsy prior to cement injection has proved efficacious and may result in the diagnosis of occult pathology underlying a seemingly routine vertebral fracture. As competence and surgical success are acquired, the indications will continue to expand to encompass more challenging pathologies. Recently, vertebral augmentation during spinal decompression and instrumented fusion for burst fracture with neurologic insult has been reported to be successful.

The National Osteoporosis Foundation has estimated that more than 100 million people worldwide are at risk for the development of fragility fractures secondary to osteoporosis. In the United States, the lifetime risk of fractures of the spine, hip, and distal part of the radius is up to 40% for women and 13% for men older than 50 years. This leads to an estimated 700,000 osteoporotic vertebral body compression fractures each year, of which more than one third become chronically painful.[1] Vertebral compression fractures occur in 20% of people older than 70 years and in 16% of postmenopausal women.[2] Not surprisingly, vertebral compression fractures account for a large portion of the more than $17 billion of annual direct costs associated with osteoporotic fractures in the United States.[3]

Osteoporotic Vertebral Fractures

Osteoporotic vertebral compression fractures are a leading cause of disability and morbidity in the elderly.[4-6] The consequences of these fractures include pain, progressive vertebral collapse with resultant spinal kyphosis, and systemic manifestations.

The pain associated with acute vertebral compression fractures may be incapacitating. In several patients, the pain subsides over a period of weeks or months, but it is not uncommon for the pain to become chronic.[7] Chronic pain after vertebral fracture may result from (1) incomplete vertebral healing with progressive osseous collapse, (2) altered spine kinematics as a consequence of spinal deformity, or (3) the development of a pseudarthrosis at the involved vertebra. Chronic pain associated with vertebral compression fractures often leads to impaired quality of life and depression.[7,8]

Kyphotic deformity in the osteoporotic spine may also create a biomechanical environment favoring additional fractures. The kyphotic deformity shifts the patient's center of gravity anteriorly, creating greater flexion bending moments around the apex of the kyphosis, which increase the kyphotic angulation further and promote additional fractures.[9-12] Clinical natural history studies have shown that the risk of a new vertebral fracture in the first year after an incident of vertebral compression fracture increases 5 to 25 times above baseline,[13-15] with the vertebra adjacent to the previously fractured level at particular risk.[16,17] Many patients with fractures and kyphosis become less active because they fear falls and new fractures. This inactivity in turn leads to accelerated osteoporosis and muscle deconditioning.[7] Because of the kyphotic deformity, paraspinal muscles must exert more force to maintain an erect posture. This prolonged exertion can cause backaches and muscle fatigue. Extreme kyphosis places unusual amounts of strain on the ligaments and other soft tissues. Pressure on the lower rib cage near the pelvic rim can produce substantial loin pain and tenderness.[18] Prevention of progressive kyphotic deformity or correction of existing deformity may therefore be important both to reduce the risk of fracture at adjacent levels and to prevent the consequences of spinal kyphosis.

Vertebral compression fractures have been shown to adversely affect quality of life, physical function, mental health, and survival.[7,8,19-22] These effects are related to the severity of the spinal deformity and are partly independent of pain.[7,19] In recent years, researchers have highlighted the impaired pulmonary function that is associated with osteoporotic vertebral compression fractures and spinal deformity.[23,24] Leech and associates[23] reported a 9% decrease in pulmonary vital capacity for each thoracic vertebral fracture. Kyphosis can lead to reduced abdominal space with poor appetite and resultant nutritional problems.[7,25] By shifting the patient's center of gravity forward, kyphotic deformity not only increases the risk of additional fractures,[26] but also may lead to poor balance, which increases the risk of accidental falls.[10,27] In addition to the morbidity associated with vertebral compression fractures, there is an increased mortality rate for older women with vertebral compression fractures compared with that for age-matched controls, as found in a prospective study.[28] The mortality rate was related to pulmonary problems, and it increased with the number of vertebrae fractured.

Nonsurgical Management

Traditionally, acute vertebral compression fractures have been treated nonsurgically except in rare instances in which the fracture is associated with neurologic compromise or advanced spinal instability. In fact, an unknown number of vertebral compression fractures produce no or only slight symptoms and are not seen for acute medical attention. Nonsurgical measures for some symptomatic vertebral compression fractures fail as a result of intolerable pain, deformity, loss of function, or a combination thereof. Open spinal surgery in patients with osteoporosis is fraught with complications because these patients are often of advanced age and frequently have comorbidities and because of the difficulty of securing fixation in osteoporotic bone. Thus, in the past, most patients with painful vertebral compression fractures have been treated with bed rest, analgesic medications, bracing, antiosteoporotic drugs, or some combination thereof.[18,29-31] Although these treatments can be successful, anti-inflammatory and narcotic medications are often poorly tolerated by elderly patients and may predispose them to confusion, an increased risk of falls, and gastrointestinal side effects. Bed rest can lead to an overall physiologic deconditioning and acceleration of bone loss. Bracing is typically poorly tolerated by older patients, is expensive, and may further restrict diaphragmatic excursion. Furthermore, none of these treatments reduces the fracture or corrects the spinal deformity.

Minimally Invasive Interventions

Orthopaedic fracture care emphasizes restoration of anatomy, correction of deformity, and preservation of function. The treatment of osteoporotic vertebral compression fractures ideally should address both the fracture-related pain and the kyphotic deformity. In addition, this should be accomplished without subjecting the elderly patient to inordinate risks or surgical trauma. Vertebroplasty and kyphoplasty are two minimally invasive surgical interventions offering promising results for this patient population.

Definitions

Vertebroplasty Percutaneous injection of a bone filler, typically polymethylmethacrylate (PMMA), directly into a fractured vertebral body with use of fluoroscopic guidance. The goals of vertebroplasty are pain relief and prevention of further collapse of the fractured vertebra. It may be possible to achieve some postural reduction of certain fractures.

Kyphoplasty Percutaneous insertion of an inflatable bone tamp into a fractured vertebral body with use of fluoroscopic guidance. Inflation of the bone tamp elevates the end plates to restore the vertebral body closer to its original height while creating a cavity to be filled with bone void filler, usually PMMA. The goals of kyphoplasty are pain relief, restoration of vertebral body height, and reduction of kyphotic deformity.

Indications

Vertebroplasty and kyphoplasty are indicated for the treatment of painful osteoporotic vertebral fractures, painful vertebrae due to metastasis, multiple myeloma, Kümmell disease, and painful vertebral hemangioma.[32-38] In addition, kyphoplasty may be indicated to correct severe and progressive kyphosis resulting from a vertebral compression fracture.[32,36,39]

The contraindications to both procedures include systemic pathologic conditions such as sepsis, prolonged bleeding times, or cardiopulmonary conditions that preclude the safe completion of the operations. Relative contraindications include vertebral bodies with deficient posterior cortices and neurologic signs or symptoms related to the vertebral fracture. Certain burst or vertebra plana fracture configurations pose technical challenges, and the feasibility of vertebroplasty or kyphoplasty should be cautiously assessed. Treating more than three vertebral levels in one surgical setting is not advocated because of the potential for deleterious cardiopulmonary effects related to PMMA monomer and/or fat or PMMA embolization to the lungs.

The benefits of prophylactic reinforcement of vertebrae "at risk" for fracture remain unproven. Finite element modeling suggested a high potential for complications given the volume of PMMA required for a vertebroplasty to successfully reinforce a vertebra at risk for fracture.[40]

Outcomes and Complications

Vertebroplasty Reports on the outcomes of vertebroplasty have suggested that most patients experience partial or complete pain relief within 72 hours after the procedure.[18,41-49] As reported in the literature, 60% to 100% of patients overall have noted decreased pain after vertebroplasty,[44,48] and improved functional levels and a reduced need for analgesic medication have been reported as well.[46,48,50-53] Zoarski and associates[54] administered the Musculoskeletal Outcomes Data Evaluation and Management Systems (MODEMS) scale before and at 2 weeks after vertebroplasty in 30 patients and found improvement in all four modules of the scale (treatment score, pain and disability, physical function, and mental function). Similarly, improvement in the Nottingham Health Profile scores have been observed after vertebroplasty.[42] Grados and associates,[55] in a longer-term follow-up study in which 25 of 40 patients were evaluated at a mean of 48 months after treatment of osteoporotic vertebral compression fractures with vertebroplasty, reported that the mean score for pain, as measured on a 100-point visual analog scale, decreased from 80 before the vertebroplasty to 37 one month after it. These results remained stable over time, with a pain score of 34 at the time of final follow-up. Published reports have noted a low complication rate after vertebroplasty. Most complications result from extravertebral leakage of PMMA causing spinal cord or nerve root compression or pulmonary embolism.[18,41-49]

Disease-specific questionnaires have further validated the success of vertebroplasty. Using the Roland-Morris Disability Questionnaire, Trout and associates[56] noted decreased pain and disability at 1 week after vertebroplasty, with maintenance of the pain relief at 1 year, in 113 patients who had a total of 164 vertebral fractures. McKiernan and associates[57] thought that the Osteoporosis Quality of Life Questionnaire, with the responses marked on a visual analog scale, was the best tool for evaluating health-related quality-of-life issues in osteoporotic women with back pain caused by vertebral compression fractures. Their prospective evaluation of 46 patients (66 vertebral compression fractures) demonstrated marked improvement in all factors at 1 day after the vertebroplasty with persistence of, although a slight decrease in, the benefit at 6 months. Larger prospective cohort evaluations confirmed these outcomes, demonstrating decreases in pain and analgesic use and improvements in mobility.[58,59] These studies did not show any clinically relevant complications. This suggests an improvement in the understanding and execution of this technique since earlier reports.

The limitations of the vertebroplasty technique are related to the inability of the procedure to correct spinal deformity and the risk of extravertebral PMMA extravasation during injection. During vertebroplasty, low-viscosity PMMA is injected under high pressure directly into cancellous bone. This makes it difficult to control PMMA flow into the vertebral body, creating the risk of extravasation outside of the vertebral body.[60] Extravertebral extravasation of PMMA regularly occurs during vertebroplasty, with reported leak rates of up to 65%.[42] The rate of extravasation has been noted to be higher in patients with metastases or hemangiomas than in patients with osteoporosis.[49,60]

Proponents of vertebroplasty have reported infrequent clinical sequelae of extravertebral leakage of PMMA. Cortet and associates[42] reported extravertebral PMMA in association with 13 of 20 vertebrae that had been treated with vertebroplasty because of an osteoporotic fracture. PMMA leaked into the paravertebral soft tissues in six instances, into the epidural space in three, into the disk space in three, and into the lumbar venous plexus in one. No adverse events were observed. Cyteval and associates[43] noted extravertebral PMMA in 8 of 20 patients treated with vertebroplasty, with leakage into the intervertebral disk in 5 patients, into the neural foramen in 2, and into the lumbar venous plexus in 1. Again, no adverse clinical events were observed. Chiras and associates[41] reported that 4% of patients who had undergone vertebroplasty had radiculopathy that was likely related to intraforaminal PMMA leakage. In a recent study, 3 of 35 patients treated with vertebroplasty had extravasation of PMMA into the epidural space, necessitating open surgical decompression in 2 of the patients.[61] Ryu and associates[62] reported a 26.5% rate of epidural PMMA leakage following 347 vertebroplasties and concluded that the prevalence of epidural leakage depended on the amount of PMMA injected. Use of a PMMA injector tool also increased the prevalence of epidural leakage, whereas the position of the needle tip in the vertebral body did not predict leakage. In summary, despite the substantial prevalence of extravertebral extravasation of PMMA during vertebroplasty, the risk of clinically relevant complications has been reported to be low.

It has been recommended that, to reduce extravertebral leakage of PMMA, studies with intravertebral injections of contrast medium be performed before injection of the PMMA in an attempt to predict potential egress of the PMMA from the vertebral body. Theoretically, extravasation of contrast medium signals the potential for subsequent extravasation of PMMA and thus indicates the need to redirect the needle and repeat the injection of the contrast material until no extravasation is observed. Lower volumes and higher viscosity of PMMA may also be warranted to avoid leakage. McGraw and associates[63] found that intraosseous venography predicted the subsequent flow of PMMA during vertebroplasty in 83% of patients. Gaughen and associates[64] reported that 22 of 42 vertebrae demonstrated PMMA extravasation during vertebroplasty, and venograms had showed correlative extravasation in 14 of the 22 vertebrae. However, the authors concluded that venography did not improve the effectiveness or safety of vertebroplasty performed by experienced physicians. Using intravertebral injections of contrast medium, Phillips and associates[65] showed that rates of transcortical and intravenous leakage of the contrast medium were higher for vertebroplasty than for kyphoplasty. Others have argued that intravertebral injections of contrast medium are not useful and that discontinuing the PMMA injection once the PMMA leaks out of the vertebral body or fills the perivertebral veins remains the best technique for reducing the risk of complications.

The pressurized injection of PMMA during vertebroplasty has also raised concerns about embolization of the PMMA, unreacted PMMA monomer, or bone marrow to the lungs through the venous system.[66] Occasional instances of symptomatic and lethal PMMA pulmonary embolism following vertebroplasty have been reported.[50,67-69]

Groen and associates[70] revisited the vertebral venous system, emphasizing its large volume; numerous valveless connections with cranial, spinal, thoracic, abdominal, and subcutaneous veins; and open connections to the vertebral body and its bone marrow. Because of these characteristics, there is a risk of extrusion of marrow and fat from the vertebral body during a forced external increase of intravertebral pressure. This risk of fat or marrow embolism is present during the PMMA injection in vertebroplasty and also during the balloon inflation in kyphoplasty. Also, PMMA extravasation through this venous system can be expected, particularly with the increased pressures and the more fluid PMMA mixture required during vertebroplasty.[70] Complications including hypotension,[49] pulmonary embolism,[71,72] pulmonary PMMA embolism,[50,68,73,74] adult respiratory distress syndrome,[49] cerebral PMMA embolism,[75] intravascular extension of polymethylmethacrylate,[76] and PMMA toxicity[77] have been reported. An understanding of the pathomechanics, clinical indicators, and optimal technique for vertebroplasty is crucial, despite the low rate of these complications.

Kyphoplasty Early results suggest that kyphoplasty can provide excellent pain relief, improve the height of the collapsed vertebral body, and reduce spinal kyphosis.[29,49,60,78-82] Because kyphoplasty was first reported in 2000, the literature on this procedure is less extensive than that on vertebroplasty. Garfin and Reilley[83] reported the initial multicenter experience with kyphoplasty, in which 2,194 vertebral fractures in 1,439 patients were treated between 1998 and 2000. Ninety percent of the patients reported pain relief within 2 weeks after the procedure. Four neurologic complications were reported in this series; all occurred in the first 50 patients treated, and all were directly attributable to surgeon error and breach of technique. Three instances of postoperative paraparesis were related to insertion of an instrument through the medial pedicle wall, and one epidural hematoma requiring surgical decompression was in a patient who was being treated with anticoagulants. The serious adverse event rate was 0.2% per fracture.

In the study by Wong and associates,[60] 80 of 85 patients reported good to excellent pain relief after kyphoplasty. As experience with kyphoplasty has increased, it has become apparent that the intravertebral cavity created by the inflatable bone tamp allows placement of more viscous, partially cured PMMA. In a prospectively followed cohort of patients treated with kyphoplasty, Lieberman and associates[81] observed improvement in the postoperative scores for physical function, role limitations because of physical health, vitality, mental health, and social function on the Short Form-36 questionnaire. Of 70 vertebral fractures that were treated, five were associated with a clinically irrelevant PMMA leak. The PMMA entered the epidural space in one instance, the disk space in two, and the paraspinal tissues in three. No major

systemic complications or neurologic injuries occurred. In a study of 29 patients treated with kyphoplasty, Phillips and associates[39] reported a decrease in the mean visual analog pain score from 8.6 preoperatively to 2.6 at 1 week postoperatively to 0.6 at 1 year postoperatively. PMMA leaks without apparent clinical consequence occurred at 6 of 61 vertebral levels, with no instances of leakage into the spinal canal.

In addition to pain relief, kyphoplasty affords the opportunity to restore vertebral body height and thereby improve spinal sagittal balance. In an ex vivo study, Belkoff and associates[78] showed a 97% reversal of deformity with kyphoplasty and a 30% reversal with vertebroplasty. Lieberman and associates[81] reported that height was increased (by a mean of 46.8%) in 70% of 70 fractured vertebrae treated with kyphoplasty. Wong and associates[60] similarly noted increased vertebral body height after kyphoplasty. Phillips and associates[84] reported on a series of 40 patients treated with kyphoplasty. In the patients who had reducible fractures, local kyphosis decreased by a mean of 14°. The ability to reduce kyphosis is thought to be a major benefit of kyphoplasty.

The complications of kyphoplasty mirror those discussed regarding vertebroplasty. There are concerns about embolic events initiated by the intravertebral pressure changes caused by inflation of the bone tamp rather than the PMMA injection. Extravasation of PMMA also continues to be a concern, but the rate is lower given the low pressure and increased viscosity during the injection. Complications related to the hardware and balloon rupture have been reported.[32,80] However, subsequent evaluations of larger groups treated with kyphoplasty

support the earlier findings of successful management of both pain and deformity with low complication rates.[85-87] Majd and associates[86] found an 89% rate of clinical success in 360 patients, and Ledlie and Renfro[87] reported radiographic evidence of success in 100 patients.

In an attempt to improve the reliability and extent of fracture reduction, one might consider performing kyphoplasty soon after the fracture. Our experience suggests that, in selected patients, it is easier to elevate the end plates and restore vertebral body height when the kyphoplasty is performed within 1 month after the fracture than when it is performed several months after the fracture. The appropriate duration of nonsurgical treatment of a vertebral fracture before kyphoplasty is considered has not been established. It seems reasonable that patients presenting with an acute vertebral compression fracture and substantial kyphosis might be best managed with earlier intervention in an attempt to maximize improvement in spinal sagittal alignment. This may be particularly important at the thoracolumbar junction, where there is a tendency for the development of kyphosis. However, the efficacy of early intervention has not been elucidated.

Elderly patients with osteoporotic burst fractures and concomitant spinal stenosis can be extremely difficult to treat. Surgical decompression with instrumentation and fusion across the fractured segment is associated with a substantial risk of the instrumentation failing in the osteoporotic bone. Recently, Singh and associates[88] reported the benefits of vertebral augmentation in conjunction with laminectomy to manage this clinical dilemma. Of 25 patients with lumbar spinal stenosis and osteoporotic vertebral fractures (39 fractures) in their series, 9 required concomitant instrumentation for the treatment of spondylolisthesis at the decompressed level. Twenty of the 25 patients demonstrated a good or excellent result. Complications were observed in five patients. Others have reported similar successes with the management of burst fractures that presented without neurologic deterioration.[33,89,90] The ability of kyphoplasty combined with posterior instrumentation to restore vertebral height and spinal alignment following thoracic and lumbar burst fractures was validated in a cadaver model.[91] Unfortunately, the rates of PMMA extravasation secondary to the disruption of the cortical osseous walls of the vertebrae may be a reason for concern, in particular because loss of the integrity of the posterior wall places the neural elements at risk. However, although the use of kyphoplasty for this injury profile is not without risks, the potential to relieve symptoms and provide structural improvement is promising. Presently, there is insufficient information to fully understand the role of PMMA augmentation in the treatment of osteoporotic vertebral burst fractures.

Subsequent Vertebral Fracture After Vertebroplasty and Kyphoplasty

It remains unclear whether subsequent vertebral fractures are related to the natural progression of osteoporosis or are a consequence of augmentation with bone PMMA.[92] A natural history study of 2,725 women with a mean age of 74 years demonstrated a cumulative incidence of new vertebral fractures of 6.6% in the first year.[26] The incidence of second vertebral fractures

in the first year after an initial vertebral fracture was 19%. Only 23% of these second fractures were symptomatic; thus, 5% of women with an untreated compression fracture are expected to sustain a symptomatic subsequent vertebral fracture within 1 year.

The rate of vertebral fracture following vertebroplasty has been reported to be between 12% and 52%, depending on the duration and nature of the follow-up.[55,93] Two thirds of these fractures were identified at levels adjacent to the vertebroplasty and the remainder, at remote levels.[93] Grados and associates[55] reported that the odds ratio of a vertebral fracture occurring in the vicinity of a PMMA-augmented vertebra was 2.27 compared with an odds ratio of 1.44 for a vertebral fracture occurring in the vicinity of a cementless fractured vertebra. This equates to a 57% greater risk of fracture adjacent to a vertebroplasty.

The rate of vertebral fracture following kyphoplasty is 19% to 29%, again depending on the duration and nature of the follow-up. Fribourg and associates[94] documented a subsequent fracture rate of 26%, with 63% of the fractures occurring at adjacent levels. These adjacent-level fractures occurred within 60 days after the kyphoplasty. Thereafter, the fracture incidence mirrored that found in the natural history study previously described,[26] and adjacent-level fractures no longer predominated. Fribourg and associates suggested that patients should be informed of this fracture risk in the early postoperative period.

Harrop and associates[95] found a subsequent vertebral fracture in 23% of 115 patients treated with kyphoplasty. Although no correlation was found between recurrent frac-

tures and age, bone density, T score, gender, or number of augmented levels, stratification by osteoporosis type (primary versus steroid-induced) delineated patients at increased risk. A subsequent fracture was observed in 49% of patients with steroid-induced osteoporosis compared with only 11% of those with primary osteoporosis. Steroid-induced osteoporosis, rather than the kyphoplasty, was thought to be a greater risk factor predicting subsequent fractures. In the only prospective controlled study of kyphoplasty of which we are aware, Kasperk and associates[96] confirmed the nonsignificant differences in the rate of subsequent fractures, at both 6 and 12 months, between patients treated with kyphoplasty and those managed medically.[97] The correction of biomechanical variables following kyphoplasty should work to counteract subsequent fractures.[12] Thus, the concern regarding subsequent vertebral fracture following PMMA augmentation persists but is unconfirmed.

Advantages

Vertebroplasty The advantages of this technique are its simplicity and its ability to relieve pain. The procedure is typically performed with the use of local anesthesia and intravenous sedation. The avoidance of general anesthesia for frail, elderly patients is advantageous. The procedure is straightforward to perform and requires little special equipment. This can equate to faster procedure times and lower costs.

Kyphoplasty The advantages of this technique are deformity correction and relief of pain. Fracture reduction and correction of kyphotic deformity can be achieved with use of specialized instrumentation. It has been hypothesized that restoration of spinal alignment improves the functional capacity of the respiratory, cardiac, gastrointestinal, and musculoskeletal systems. Decreased PMMA extravasation resulting from low-pressure injection of more viscous PMMA reduces complications. Kyphoplasty is more costly than vertebroplasty.

Surgical Technique

Before proceeding with either intervention, the physician must confirm that the back pain is caused by a vertebral compression fracture. This requires careful correlation of the patient's history and findings on clinical examination with radiographic documentation of an acute or unhealed vertebral compression fracture. The possibility of secondary osteoporosis or a malignant tumor producing the back pain must be considered. Degenerative spinal disorders may also present with kyphosis and back pain. A thorough neurologic examination is essential to rule out neurologic compromise. Pain radiating around the trunk in a dermatomal manner may accompany vertebral compression fractures. Pulmonary function should be evaluated in patients in whom advanced kyphosis may have led to respiratory difficulty.

Preoperative planning includes making radiographs to define the fracture geometry and for surgical planning. Lateral radiographs are particularly useful for planning the trajectory for any percutaneous procedure. MRI is typically used to evaluate the acuity of the fracture. When MRI is contraindicated, nuclear bone scans may help the physician to estimate the acuity of the fracture. Osseous edema is readily seen on MRI and can indicate an acute fracture as well as help rule out a tumor or infection. Malignant

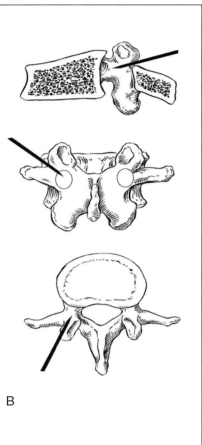

Figure 1   Transpedicular approach for vertebral augmentation. The tip of the injection trocar is started at the lateral aspect of the facet joint corresponding with the upper and outer corner of the pedicle outline as visualized on the posteroanterior image (**A**). The proper sagittal trajectory is confirmed on the lateral image. When the trocar tip is midway along the length of the pedicle on the lateral image, it should be central in the pedicle outline on the posteroanterior image (**B**). When the trocar is through the pedicle and at the posterior vertebral cortical margin on the lateral image, it should be just within the medial border of the pedicle outline on the posteroanterior image.

diseases causing vertebral compression fracture are usually associated with an ill-defined margin, enhancement with gadolinium, and pedicle involvement as well as a paravertebral soft-tissue mass.[98] Sagittal MRI with short tau inversion recovery (STIR) sequences highlight the marrow edema changes associated with acute fractures, and STIR MRI has proved to be useful in determining the acuity of a vertebral compression fracture.

To perform either of the procedures, the patient is positioned prone on the operating room table or in the radiology suite on a spinal frame with cushioned bolsters. Attention to patient positioning and bolster support on the procedure table can provide postural fracture re-

duction, thus improving the chance of correcting kyphosis. Local anesthesia with intravenous conscious sedation (more common for vertebroplasty) or general anesthesia (more common for kyphoplasty) may be used. Local anesthesia may be preferable for patients with medical illness. Fluoroscopy is used throughout the procedure, and we prefer simultaneous biplanar fluoroscopy.

Typically, the transpedicular approach is used in the lumbar spine. The tip of the injection trocar is started at the outer aspect of the pedicle as visualized on the posteroanterior image, and the proper sagittal trajectory is confirmed on the lateral image (Figure 1). When the trocar tip is midway along the length

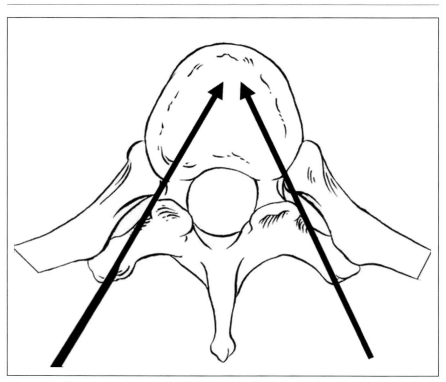

Figure 2 Extrapedicular approach for vertebral augmentation. The starting point is craniolateral toward the costovertebral joint. Contact is made with the neck of the rib or transverse process. The needle is advanced along the neck of the rib, passed under the transverse process, and passed through the ligament complex of the costovertebral joint until the lateral pedicle wall is reached. The needle is then advanced into the vertebral body.

of the pedicle on the lateral image, it should be central in the pedicle outline on the posteroanterior image. When the trocar is through the pedicle and at the posterior vertebral cortical margin on the lateral image, it should be just within the medial border of the pedicle outline on the posteroanterior image. For vertebroplasty, the trocar is advanced until the tip is at the junction of the anterior and middle thirds of the vertebral body. For kyphoplasty, the positioning trocar is exchanged for a working cannula over a guidewire. The cannula is positioned near the posterior margin of the vertebral body while the working instruments are advanced anteriorly until they are 3 mm from the anterior border of the vertebral body.[32]

The extrapedicular approach is commonly used in the thoracic spine because of the smaller pedicle diameter and a less medially angulated pedicle trajectory. The starting point is craniolateral toward the costovertebral joint (Figure 2). Contact is made with the neck of the rib or transverse process. The needle is advanced along the neck of the rib, passed under the transverse process, and passed through the ligament complex of the costovertebral joint until the lateral pedicle wall is reached. The projection of the tip of the needle should be at the upper and outer circumference of the pedicle as seen on the posteroanterior image. On the lateral image, the tip of the needle should be projected between the pedicle margins and an-

terior to the facet joints. Only after the posterior vertebral wall has been passed on the lateral image should the tip of the needle cross the medial pedicle wall on the posteroanterior image. Strict adherence to these landmarks is mandatory to avoid spinal perforation.[32,99] Boszczyk and associates[99] used this technique to perform kyphoplasty at levels from T2 to T8 and noted precise introduction of the tools in all 55 vertebrae, despite the narrow pedicle diameter.

A unipedicular rather than a bipedicular technique has been suggested to decrease risks associated with cannulation, surgical time, radiation exposure, and cost. The unipedicular technique for both vertebroplasty and kyphoplasty has been shown to restore strength, stiffness, and height as well as the bipedicular technique in a cadaver model.[100,101] Lateral wedging was not observed. Using a finite-element model, Liebschner and associates[102] found that, although unipedicular PMMA injection restored stiffness, a medial-lateral bending motion (toggle) toward the untreated side with application of a uniform compressive load was created. This finding has not been confirmed in clinical trials.

Performance of a vertebral body bone biopsy should be considered. When a trephine needle was used before PMMA injection, adequate tissue was obtained for analysis from 67% to 100% of the samples.[36,99] Togawa and associates[103] obtained biopsy specimens from 178 vertebrae and identified possible osteomalacia in 21% of them, with another four confirming an occult or unconfirmed plasma cell dyscrasia. Togawa and associates advocated performance of a biopsy during each first-time vertebral augmentation procedure so as not to miss occult lesions.

Vertebroplasty After proper needle placement and biopsy, PMMA is injected through a cannula into the vertebral body. The PMMA should be of a consistency that minimizes filling pressures and yet prevents leakage. The judicious use of fluoroscopic imaging throughout the procedure is paramount to the success and safety of a vertebroplasty. The procedure is completed when imaging demonstrates adequate vertebral filling or when extravasation of the PMMA is identified.

Kyphoplasty After proper needle placement and biopsy, the inflatable balloon tamp (KyphX Inflatable Bone Tamp; Kyphon, Sunnyvale, California) is inserted through the cannula and expanded under visual (fluoroscopic) and volume and pressure (digital manometer) controls. The bone tamp is inflated until fracture reduction is achieved, the maximal pressure or volume of the balloon is reached, or contact occurs with the cortical wall. The balloon is then deflated and removed. Partially cured PMMA can then be introduced through the cannula under low pressure to fill the void created by the balloon tamp. The volume of the PMMA should approximate that of the intravertebral cavity. Volumes from 3.5 to 8.5 mL have been observed.[36] Again, the judicious use of fluoroscopic imaging throughout the procedure is paramount. To our knowledge, no one has quantified PMMA viscosity to define an optimal injection.

Biomaterials

To date, most vertebroplasty and kyphoplasty procedures have been performed with use of PMMA to augment the fractured vertebral body. The mechanism of pain relief by these procedures is uncertain and may be related to PMMA "stabilization" of the fractured vertebral body or deafferentation related to heating of nerve endings as the PMMA cures. The optimal PMMA volume required to relieve pain and restore strength and stiffness is unknown. In an ex vivo study of experimental osteoporotic compression fractures, injection of 2 mL of PMMA (with barium sulfate) restored vertebral strength (the ability of the vertebral body to bear load) to prefracture levels, whereas 4 to 8 mL of PMMA was required to restore stiffness (resistance to micromotion).[104]

For many years, PMMA has been commonly used around joint prostheses, to fill long bone defects, and to reconstruct the spinal column.[105-107] Potential problems with PMMA include the exothermic reaction during the curing process, when temperatures may reach 100°C and cause thermal damage to adjacent structures; cardiopulmonary toxicity of the unreacted monomer; and the lack of long-term biointegration of the PMMA. A repair process, including primitive mesenchymal cell proliferation, neovascularization, resorption of dead bone, and new bone formation, was found to be absent in a histopathologic assessment following PMMA augmentation of vertebral fractures.[108]

The ideal biomaterial for vertebral augmentation would be radiolucent and nontoxic, would have handling characteristics that allow easy injection, would undergo a gradual transition from a viscous to a solid state with low exothermic temperatures, and would have adequate compressive strength to stabilize the fractured vertebral body. An osteoconductive, biodegradable material, which is replaced by host bone, may be advantageous; however, the ability of osteoporotic bone to remodel and replace a biodegradable material with host bone of adequate quality is uncertain and must be studied before such materials are considered for clinical use. Several alternate biomaterials, including carbonated apatite,[109] bioactive PMMA,[110] and calcium phosphate,[111,112] have been shown to substantially improve compressive strength and load to failure of vertebral bodies. A more extensive understanding of the toxicity profiles and long-term stability of these materials is essential.

Radiation

As the number of minimally invasive techniques to treat spine disorders, and the number of vertebroplasties and kyphoplasty procedures in particular, increases, the use of radiographic guidance in the operating room increases as well. Concerns regarding the radiation exposure to both the patient and the surgeon have been raised.

Boszczyk and associates[113] monitored the radiation exposure to the patients during 60 kyphoplasty procedures guided with biplanar fluoroscopy to treat 104 vertebrae. Exposure times per level during lateral plane imaging were noted to be 2.2 minutes for a single level and 1.7 minutes for a multiple-level session. Exposure times per level during anteroposterior plane imaging were noted to be 1.6 minutes for a single level and 1.1 minutes for a multiple-level session. Imaging times in the lateral plane consistently remained above those in the anteroposterior plane. Entrance skin doses ranged from 0.05 to 1.43 Gy with average values of 0.68 Gy in the lateral plane and 0.32 Gy in the anteroposterior plane. Calculated effective dose values averaged 4.28 mSv with a maximum of 10.14 mSv. In light of a baseline risk of cancer death of 20% to 25%, the postulated increase in lifetime cancer risk after a single kyphoplasty procedure was 0.02% to 0.06%.

Harstall and associates[114] monitored the radiation exposure to the surgeon during 32 vertebroplasty procedures performed with use of a single fluoroscopic unit to image in two planes to treat 136 vertebrae. The average surgical time was 56.2 minutes, and an average of 4.25 vertebrae were augmented. The average exposure time was 2.23 minutes per augmented vertebra. Measurements at the thyroid gland, eye lens equivalent, left and right hands, left arm, and back demonstrated radiation doses per augmented level of 0.052, 0.020, 0.107, 0.049, 0.084, and 0.002 mSv, respectively. Extrapolated radiation doses per year were troubling. Eight percent of the maximum allowed annual dose for the eye lens is expected with this procedure alone. Although the annual morbidity risk for thyroid exposure was calculated to be 0.025%, representing a low to medium 1-year risk, the lifetime risk was considered to be high to very high.

Average whole-body doses are variable and have been calculated to be between 1.44 mSv per level and 96 mSv per patient.[115,116] Theocharopoulos and associates[116] concluded that 90% of the surgeon's effective radiation dose and cancer risk was attributed to kyphoplasty and vertebroplasty procedures, with another 8% attributed to other spine procedures, at their center. Certain intraoperative techniques reduce radiation exposure time. Biplanar fluoroscopy eliminates the unnecessary exposure time required for repositioning of equipment. Surgeon-controlled foot pedals to direct fluoroscopy time streamlined surgical flow. In one study, whenever feasible with regard to fluoroscopic visualization, the PMMA was injected into as many as three adjacent vertebrae simultaneously.[113] Pulsed fluoroscopic operation at 4 pulses/s, positioning of the radiograph tube under the patient table, and use of lead sheets on the patient and a lead apron, lead collar, and goggles by the surgeon further minimize radiation exposure.[114,115] If these measures are followed, exposure levels will be sufficiently low to permit the safe performance of more than 6,700 vertebroplasty procedures by a single surgeon per year.[115]

Summary
Minimally invasive surgical techniques are being used with increasing frequency to manage vertebral compression fractures. Alleviation of fracture pain and optimization of comorbid factors aggravated by these fractures have been demonstrated after use of these techniques. Both vertebroplasty and kyphoplasty demonstrate distinct advantages. Complications do occur during both procedures, but they can be minimized through meticulous surgical technique and surgeon experience. Greater understanding of the histopathologic, biomechanical, and clinical factors involved in these techniques will provide even greater successes in the future.

References
1. Riggs BL, Melton LJ III: The worldwide problem of osteoporosis: Insights afforded by epidemiology. *Bone* 1995;17(5 Suppl):505S-511S.
2. Cohen LD: Fractures of the osteoporotic spine. *Orthop Clin North Am* 1990;21:143-150.
3. National Osteoporosis Foundation: *America's Bone Health: The State of Osteoporosis and Low Bone Mass in Our Nation.* Washington, DC, 2002.
4. Iqbal MM, Sobhan T: Osteoporosis: A review. *Mo Med* 2002;99:19-24.
5. Johnell O: Advances in osteoporosis: Better identification of risk factors can reduce morbidity and mortality. *J Intern Med* 1996;239:299-304.
6. Verbrugge LM, Lepkowski JM, Imanaka Y: Comorbidity and its impact on disability. *Milbank Q* 1989;67:450-484.
7. Silverman SL: The clinical consequences of vertebral compression fracture. *Bone* 1992;13(Suppl 2):S27-S31.
8. Gold DT: The clinical impact of vertebral fractures: Quality of life in women with osteoporosis. *Bone* 1996;18(3 Suppl):185S-189S.
9. Belmont PJ Jr, Polly DW Jr, Cunningham BW, Klemme WR: The effects of hook pattern and kyphotic angulation on mechanical strength and apical rod strain in a long-segment posterior construct using a synthetic model. *Spine* 2001;26:627-635.
10. White AA III, Panjabi MM, Thomas CL: The clinical biomechanics of kyphotic deformities. *Clin Orthop Relat Res* 1977;128:8-17.
11. Gaitanis IN, Carandang G, Phillips FM, et al: Restoring geometric and loading alignment of the thoracic spine with a vertebral compression fracture: Effects of balloon (bone tamp) inflation and spinal extension. *Spine J* 2005;5:45-54.
12. Yuan HA, Brown CW, Phillips FM: Osteoporotic spinal deformity: A biomechanical rationale for the clinical consequences and treatment of vertebral body compression fractures. *J Spinal Disord Tech* 2004;17:236-242.
13. Nevitt MC, Ettinger B, Black DM, et al: The association of radiographically detected vertebral fractures with back pain and function: A prospective study. *Ann Intern Med* 1998;128:793-800.
14. Nevitt MC, Thompson DE, Black DM, et al: Effect of alendronate on limited-activity days and bed-disability days caused by back pain in postmenopausal women with existing vertebral fractures. Fracture Intervention Trial Research Group. *Arch Intern Med* 2000;160:77-85.
15. Wasnich RD: Vertebral fracture epidemiology. *Bone* 1996;18 (3 suppl):179S-183S.

16. Haczynski J, Jakimiuk A: Vertebral fractures: A hidden problem of osteoporosis. *Med Sci Monit* 2001;7:1108-1117.

17. Ross PD, Davis JW, Epstein RS, Wasnich RD: Pre-existing fractures and bone mass predict vertebral fracture incidence in women. *Ann Intern Med* 1991;114:919-923.

18. Rapado A: General management of vertebral fractures. *Bone* 1996;18 (3 suppl):191S-196S.

19. Gold D, Lyles K: Fractures: Effects on quality of life, in Bilezikian JP, Glowacki J, Rosen CJ (eds): *The Aging Skeleton*. San Diego, CA, Academic Press, 1999.

20. Leidig G, Minne HW, Sauer P, et al: A study of complaints and their relation to vertebral destruction in patients with osteoporosis. *Bone Miner* 1990;8:217-229.

21. Lyles KW, Gold DT, Shipp KM, Pieper CF, Martinez S, Mulhausen PL: Association of osteoporotic vertebral compression fractures with impaired functional status. *Am J Med* 1993;94:595-601.

22. Pluijm SM, Tromp AM, Smit JH, Deeg DJ, Lips P: Consequences of vertebral deformities in older men and women. *J Bone Miner Res* 2000;15:1564-1572.

23. Leech JA, Dulberg C, Kellie S, Pattee L, Gay J: Relationship of lung function to severity of osteoporosis in women. *Am Rev Respir Dis* 1990;141:68-71.

24. Schlaich C, Minne HW, Bruckner T, et al: Reduced pulmonary function in patients with spinal osteoporotic fractures. *Osteoporos Int* 1998;8:261-267.

25. Ross PD, Davis JW, Epstein RS, Wasnich RD: Pain and disability associated with new vertebral fractures and other spinal conditions. *J Clin Epidemiol* 1994;47:231-239.

26. Lindsay R, Silverman SL, Cooper C, et al: Risk of new vertebral fracture in the year following a fracture. *JAMA* 2001;285:320-323.

27. Keller TS, Harrison DE, Colloca CJ, Harrison DD, Janik TJ: Prediction of osteoporotic spinal deformity. *Spine* 2003;28:455-462.

28. Kado DM, Browner WS, Palermo L, Nevitt MC, Genant HK, Cummings SR: Vertebral fractures and mortality in older women: A prospective study. Study of Osteoporotic Fractures Research Group. *Arch Intern Med* 1999;159:1215-1220.

29. Eck JC, Hodges SD, Humphreys SC: Vertebroplasty: A new treatment strategy for osteoporotic compression fractures. *Am J Orthop* 2002;31:123-128.

30. Lukert BP: Vertebral compression fractures: How to manage pain, avoid disability. *Geriatrics* 1994;49:22-26.

31. Meunier PJ, Delmas PD, Eastell R, et al: Diagnosis and management of osteoporosis in postmenopausal women: Clinical guidelines. International Committee for Osteoporosis Clinical Guidelines. *Clin Ther* 1999;21:1025-1044.

32. Spivak JM, Johnson MG: Percutaneous treatment of vertebral body pathology. *J Am Acad Orthop Surg* 2005;13:6-17.

33. Boszczyk BM, Bierschneider M, Schmid K, Grillhosl A, Robert B, Jaksche H: Microsurgical interlaminary vertebro- and kyphoplasty for severe osteoporotic fractures. *J Neurosurg* 2004;100:32-37.

34. Cortet B, Cotten A, Deprez X, et al: [Value of vertebroplasty combined with surgical decompression in the treatment of aggressive spinal angioma. Apropos of 3 cases]. *Rev Rhum Ed Fr* 1994;61:16-22.

35. Cotten A, Duquesnoy B: Vertebroplasty: Current data and future potential. *Rev Rhum Engl Ed* 1997;64:645-649.

36. Gaitanis IN, Hadjipavlou AG, Katonis PG, Tzermiadianos MN, Pasku DS, Patwardhan AG: Balloon kyphoplasty for the treatment of pathological vertebral compressive fractures. *Eur Spine J* 2005;14:250-260.

37. Galibert P, Deramond H: [Percutaneous acrylic vertebroplasty as a treatment of vertebral angioma as well as painful and debilitating diseases]. *Chirurgie* 1990;116:326-335.

38. Ide C, Gangi A, Rimmelin A, et al: Vertebral haemangiomas with spinal cord compression: The place of preoperative percutaneous vertebroplasty with methyl methacrylate. *Neuroradiology* 1996;38:585-589.

39. Phillips FM, Ho E, Campbell-Hupp M, McNally T, Todd Wetzel F, Gupta P: Early radiographic and clinical results of balloon kyphoplasty for the treatment of osteoporotic vertebral compression fractures. *Spine* 2003;28:2260-2267.

40. Sun K, Liebschner MA: Biomechanics of prophylactic vertebral reinforcement. *Spine* 2004;29:1428-1435.

41. Chiras J, Depriester C, Weill A, Sola-Martinez MT, Deramond H: [Percutaneous vertebral surgery. Technics and indications]. *J Neuroradiol* 1997;24:45-59.

42. Cortet B, Cotten A, Boutry N, et al: Percutaneous vertebroplasty in the treatment of osteoporotic vertebral compression fractures: An open prospective study. *J Rheumatol* 1999;26:2222-2228.

43. Cyteval C, Sarrabere MP, Roux JO, et al: Acute osteoporotic vertebral collapse: Open study on percutaneous injection of acrylic surgical cement in 20 patients. *AJR Am J Roentgenol* 1999;173:1685-1690.

44. Gangi A, Kastler BA, Dietemann JL: Percutaneous vertebroplasty guided by a combination of CT and fluoroscopy. *AJNR Am J Neuroradiol* 1994;15:83-86.

45. Hardouin P, Grados F, Cotton A, Cortet B: Should percutaneous vertebroplasty be used to treat osteoporotic fractures? An update. *Joint Bone Spine* 2001;68:216-221.

46. Jensen ME, Evans AJ, Mathis JM, Kallmes DF, Cloft HJ, Dion JE: Percutaneous polymethylmethacrylate vertebroplasty in the treatment of osteoporotic vertebral body compression fractures: Technical aspects. *AJNR Am J Neuroradiol* 1997;18:1897-1904.

47. Lapras C, Mottolese C, Deruty R, Lapras C Jr, Remond J, Duquesnel J: [Percutaneous injection of methyl-metacrylate in osteoporosis and severe vertebral osteolysis (Galibert's technic)]. *Ann Chir* 1989;43:371-376.

48. Mathis JM, Petri M, Naff N: Percutaneous vertebroplasty treatment of steroid-induced osteoporotic compression fractures. *Arthritis Rheum* 1998;41:171-175.

49. Watts NB, Harris ST, Genant HK: Treatment of painful osteoporotic vertebral fractures with percutaneous vertebroplasty or kyphoplasty. *Osteoporos Int* 2001;12:429-437.

50. Amar AP, Larsen DW, Esnaashari N, Albuquerque FC, Lavine SD, Teitelbaum GP: Percutaneous transpedicular polymethylmethacrylate vertebroplasty for the treatment of spinal compression fractures. *Neurosurgery* 2001;49:1105-1115.

51. Kim AK, Jensen ME, Dion JE, Schweickert PA, Kaufmann TJ, Kallmes DF: Unilateral transpedicular percutaneous vertebroplasty: Initial experience. *Radiology* 2002;222:737-741.

52. Martin JB, Jean B, Sugiu K, et al: Vertebroplasty: Clinical experience and follow-up results. *Bone* 1999;25 (2 suppl):11S-15S.

53. Tsou IY, Goh PY, Peh WC, Goh LA, Chee TS: Percutaneous vertebroplasty in

the management of osteoporotic vertebral compression fractures: Initial experience. *Ann Acad Med Singapore* 2002;31:15-20.

54. Zoarski GH, Snow P, Olan WJ, et al: Percutaneous vertebroplasty for osteoporotic compression fractures: Quantitative prospective evaluation of long-term outcomes. *J Vasc Interv Radiol* 2002;13:139-148.

55. Grados F, Depriester C, Cayrolle G, Hardy N, Deramond H, Fardellone P: Long-term observations of vertebral osteoporotic fractures treated by percutaneous vertebroplasty. *Rheumatology (Oxford)* 2000;39:1410-1414.

56. Trout AT, Kallmes DF, Gray LA, et al: Evaluation of vertebroplasty with a validated outcome measure: The Roland-Morris Disability Questionnaire. *AJNR Am J Neuroradiol* 2005;26:2652-2657.

57. McKiernan F, Faciszewski T, Jensen R: Quality of life following vertebroplasty. *J Bone Joint Surg Am* 2004;86:2600-2606.

58. Do HM, Kim BS, Marcellus ML, Curtis L, Marks MP: Prospective analysis of clinical outcomes after percutaneous vertebroplasty for painful osteoporotic vertebral body fractures. *AJNR Am J Neuroradiol* 2005;26:1623-1628.

59. Kobayashi K, Shimoyama K, Nakamura K, Murata K: Percutaneous vertebroplasty immediately relieves pain of osteoporotic vertebral compression fractures and prevents prolonged immobilization of patients. *Eur Radiol* 2005;15:360-367.

60. Wong W, Reiley M, Garfin S: Vertebroplasty/ kyphoplasty. *J Wom Imag* 2000;2:117-124.

61. Moreland DB, Landi MK, Grand W: Vertebroplasty: Techniques to avoid complications. *Spine J* 2001;1:66-71.

62. Ryu KS, Park CK, Kim MC, Kang JK: Dose-dependent epidural leakage of polymethylmethacrylate after percutaneous vertebroplasty in patients with osteoporotic vertebral compression fractures. *J Neurosurg* 2002;96 (1 suppl):56-61.

63. McGraw JK, Heatwole EV, Strnad BT, Silber JS, Patzilk SB, Boorstein JM: Predictive value of intraosseous venography before percutaneous vertebroplasty. *J Vasc Interv Radiol* 2002;13:149-153.

64. Gaughen JR Jr, Jensen ME, Schweickert PA, Kaufmann TJ, Marx WF, Kallmes DF: Relevance of antecedent venography in percutaneous vertebroplasty for the treatment of osteoporotic compression fractures. *AJNR Am J Neuroradiol* 2002;23:594-600.

65. Phillips FM, Todd Wetzel F, Lieberman I, Campbell-Hupp M: An in vivo comparison of the potential for extravertebral cement leak after vertebroplasty and kyphoplasty. *Spine* 2002;27:2173-2179.

66. Aebli N, Krebs J, Davis G, Walton M, Williams MJ, Theis JC: Fat embolism and acute hypotension during vertebroplasty: An experimental study in sheep. *Spine* 2002;27:460-466.

67. Levine SA, Perin LA, Hayes D, Hayes WS: An evidence-based evaluation of percutaneous vertebroplasty. *Manag Care* 2000;9:56-60, 63.

68. Padovani B, Kasriel O, Brunner P, Paretti-Viton P: Pulmonary embolism caused by acrylic cement: A rare complication of percutaneous vertebroplasty. *AJNR Am J Neuroradiol* 1999;20:375-377.

69. Perrin C, Jullien V, Padovani B, Blaive B: [Percutaneous vertebroplasty complicated by pulmonary embolus of acrylic cement]. *Rev Mal Respir* 1999;16:215-217.

70. Groen RJ, du Toit DF, Phillips FM, et al: Anatomical and pathological considerations in percutaneous vertebroplasty and kyphoplasty: A reappraisal of the vertebral venous system. *Spine* 2004;29:1465-1471.

71. Chen HL, Wong CS, Ho ST, Chang FL, Hsu CH, Wu CT: A lethal pulmonary embolism during percutaneous vertebroplasty. *Anesth Analg* 2002;95:1060-1062.

72. Tozzi P, Abdelmoumene Y, Corno AF, Gersbach PA, Hoogewoud HM, von Segesser LK: Management of pulmonary embolism during acrylic vertebroplasty. *Ann Thorac Surg* 2002;74:1706-1708.

73. Bernhard J, Heini PF, Villiger PM: Asymptomatic diffuse pulmonary embolism caused by acrylic cement: An unusual complication of percutaneous vertebroplasty. *Ann Rheum Dis* 2003;62:85-86.

74. Jang JS, Lee SH, Jung SK: Pulmonary embolism of polymethylmethacrylate after percutaneous vertebroplasty: A report of three cases. *Spine* 2002;27:E416-E418.

75. Scroop R, Eskridge J, Britz GW: Paradoxical cerebral arterial embolization of cement during intraoperative vertebroplasty: Case report. *AJNR Am J Neuroradiol* 2002;23:868-870.

76. Wenger M, Markwalder TM: Surgically controlled, transpedicular methyl methacrylate vertebroplasty with fluoroscopic guidance. *Acta Neurochir (Wien)* 1999;141:625-631.

77. Lane JM, Johnson CE, Khan SN, Girardi FP, Cammisa FP Jr: Minimally invasive options for the treatment of osteoporotic vertebral compression fractures. *Orthop Clin North Am* 2002;33:431-438.

78. Belkoff SM, Mathis JM, Fenton DC, Scribner RM, Reiley ME, Talmadge K: An ex vivo biomechanical evaluation of an inflatable bone tamp used in the treatment of compression fracture. *Spine* 2001;26:151-156.

79. Garfin S, Reiley M, Wong W: Vertebroplasty and kyphoplasty, in Savitz MH, Chiu JC, Yueng AT (eds): *The Practice of Minimally Invasive Spinal Technique*. Richmond, VA, AAMISMS Education, 2000.

80. Garfin SR, Yuan HA, Reiley MA: New technologies in spine: Kyphoplasty and vertebroplasty for the treatment of painful osteoporotic compression fractures. *Spine* 2001;26:1511-1515.

81. Lieberman IH, Dudeney S, Reinhardt MK, Bell G: Initial outcome and efficacy of "kyphoplasty" in the treatment of painful osteoporotic vertebral compression fractures. *Spine* 2001;26:1631-1638.

82. Theodorou DJ, Theodorou SJ, Duncan TD, Garfin SR, Wong WH: Percutaneous balloon kyphoplasty for the correction of spinal deformity in painful vertebral body compression fractures. *Clin Imaging* 2002;26:1-5.

83. Garfin S, Reilley MA: Minimally invasive treatment of osteoporotic vertebral body compression fracture. *Spine J* 2002;2:76-80.

84. Phillips F, Ho E, Campbell-Hupp M, McNally T, Todd Wetzel F, Gupta P: Early clinical and radiographic results of kyphoplasty for the treatment of osteopenic vertebral compression fractures. *Eur Spine J* 2001;10 (suppl 1):S7.

85. Atalay B, Caner H, Gokce C, Atinors N: Kyphoplasty: 2 years of experience in a neurosurgery department. *Surg Neurol* 2005;64(suppl 2):S72-S76.

86. Majd ME, Farley S, Holt RT: Preliminary outcomes and efficacy of the first 360 consecutive kyphoplasties for the treatment of painful osteoporotic vertebral compression fractures. *Spine J* 2005;5:244-255.

87. Ledlie JT, Renfro MB: Decreases in the number and severity of morphometrically defined vertebral body deformities after kyphoplasty. *Neurosurg Focus* 2005;18:e4.

88. Singh K, Heller JG, Samartzis D, et al: Open vertebral cement augmentation combined with lumbar decompression for the operative management of thoracolumbar stenosis secondary to osteoporotic burst fractures. *J Spinal Disord Tech* 2005;18:413-419.

89. Boszczyk B, Bierschneider M, Potulski M, Robert B, Vastmans J, Jaksche H: [Extended kyphoplasty indications for stabilization of osteoporotic vertebral compression fractures]. *Unfallchirurg* 2002;105:952-957.

90. Chen JF, Lee ST: Percutaneous vertebroplasty for treatment of thoracolumbar spine bursting fracture. *Surg Neurol* 2004;62:494-500.

91. Verlaan JJ, van de Kraats EB, Oner FC, van Walsum T, Niessen WJ, Dhert WJ: The reduction of endplate fractures during balloon vertebroplasty: A detailed radiological analysis of the treatment of burst fractures using pedicle screws, balloon vertebroplasty, and calcium phosphate cement. *Spine* 2005;30:1840-1845.

92. Villarraga ML, Bellezza AJ, Harrigan TP, Cripton PA, Kurtz SM, Edidin AA: The biomechanical effects of kyphoplasty on treated and adjacent nontreated vertebral bodies. *J Spinal Disord Tech* 2005;18:84-91.

93. Uppin AA, Hirsch JA, Centenera LV, Pfiefer BA, Pazianos AG, Choi IS: Occurrence of new vertebral body fracture after percutaneous vertebroplasty in patients with osteoporosis. *Radiology* 2003;226:119-124.

94. Fribourg D, Tang C, Sra P, Delamarter R, Bae H: Incidence of subsequent vertebral fracture after kyphoplasty. *Spine* 2004;29:2270-2277.

95. Harrop JS, Prpa B, Reinhardt MK, Lieberman I: Primary and secondary osteoporosis' incidence of subsequent vertebral compression fractures after kyphoplasty. *Spine* 2004;29:2120-2125.

96. Kasperk C, Hillmeier J, Noldge G, et al: Treatment of painful vertebral fractures by kyphoplasty in patients with primary osteoporosis: A prospective nonrandomized controlled study. *J Bone Miner Res* 2005;20:604-612.

97. Grafe IA, Da Fonseca K, Hillmeier J, et al: Reduction of pain and fracture incidence after kyphoplasty: 1-year outcomes of a prospective controlled trial of patients with primary osteoporosis. *Osteoporos Int* 2005;16:2005-2012.

98. Shih TT, Huang KM, Li YW: Solitary vertebral collapse: Distinction between benign and malignant causes using MR patterns. *J Magn Reson Imaging* 1999;9:635-642.

99. Boszczyk BM, Bierschneider M, Hauck S, Beisse R, Potulski M, Jaksche H: Transcostovertebral kyphoplasty of the mid and high thoracic spine. *Eur Spine J* 2005;14:992-999.

100. Steinmann J, Tingey CT, Cruz G, Dai Q: Biomechanical comparison of unipedicular versus bipedicular kyphoplasty. *Spine* 2005;30:201-205.

101. Tohmeh AG, Mathis JM, Fenton DC, Levine AM, Belkoff SM: Biomechanical efficacy of unipedicular versus bipedicular vertebroplasty for the management of osteoporotic compression fractures. *Spine* 1999;24:1772-1776.

102. Liebschner MA, Rosenberg WS, Keaveny TM: Effects of bone cement volume and distribution on vertebral stiffness after vertebroplasty. *Spine* 2001;26:1547-1554.

103. Togawa D, Lieberman IH, Bauer TW, Reinhardt MK, Kayanja MM: Histological evaluation of biopsies obtained from vertebral compression fractures: Unsuspected myeloma and osteomalacia. *Spine* 2005;30:781-786.

104. Belkoff SM, Mathis JM, Jasper LE, Deramond H: The biomechanics of vertebroplasty: The effect of cement volume on mechanical behavior. *Spine* 2001;26:1537-1541.

105. Bauer TW, Schils J: The pathology of total joint arthroplasty: I. Mechanisms of implant fixation. *Skeletal Radiol* 1999;28:423-432.

106. Jang JS, Lee SH, Rhee CH, Lee SH: Polymethylmethacrylate-augmented screw fixation for stabilization in metastatic spinal tumors: Technical note. *J Neurosurg* 2002;96(1 Suppl):131-134.

107. Wada T, Kaya M, Nagoya S, et al: Complications associated with bone cementing for the treatment of giant cell tumors of bone. *J Orthop Sci* 2002;7:194-198.

108. Huang K-Y, Yan JJ, Lin RM: Histopathologic findings of retrieved specimens of vertebroplasty with polymethylmethacrylate cement: Case control study. *Spine* 2005;30:E585-E588.

109. Schildhauer TA, Bennett AP, Wright TM, Lane JM, O'Leary PF: Intravertebral body reconstruction with an injectable in situ-setting carbonated apatite: Biomechanical evaluation of a minimally invasive technique. *J Orthop Res* 1999;17:67-72.

110. Belkoff SM, Mathis JM, Erbe EM, Fenton DC: Biomechanical evaluation of a new bone cement for use in vertebroplasty. *Spine* 2000;25:1061-1064.

111. Barr JD, Barr MS, Lemley TJ, McCann RM: Percutaneous vertebroplasty for pain relief and spinal stabilization. *Spine* 2000;25:923-928.

112. Lim TH, Brebach GT, Renner SM, et al: Biomechanical evaluation of an injectable calcium phosphate cement for vertebroplasty. *Spine* 2002;27:1297-1302.

113. Boszczyk BM, Bierschneider M, Panzer S, et al: Fluoroscopic radiation exposure of the kyphoplasty patient. *Eur Spine J* 2006;15:347-355.

114. Harstall R, Heini PF, Mini RL, Orler R: Radiation exposure to the surgeon during fluoroscopically assisted percutaneous vertebroplasty: A prospective study. *Spine* 2005;30:1893-1898.

115. Kruger R, Faciszewski T: Radiation dose reduction to medical staff during vertebroplasty: A review of techniques and methods to mitigate occupational dose. *Spine* 2003;28:1608-1613.

116. Theocharopoulos N, Perisinakis K, Damilakis J, Papadokostakis G, Hadjipavlou A, Gourtsoyiannis N: Occupational exposure from common fluoroscopic projections used in orthopaedic surgery. *J Bone Joint Surg Am* 2003;85:1698-1703.

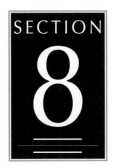

SECTION 8

Advanced Surgical Techniques

Advanced Surgical Techniques

The chapters in this section cover advanced techniques and technologies for spine surgery. In the first chapter, Stock and associates review contemporary methods of occipitocervical fixation and remind the reader of the significant biomechanical demands required for instrumentation in this spinal region, which is the most mobile portion of the cervical spine. A review of the evolution of occipitocervical systems, which includes (in temporal order) halo immobilization, rods and wires, pelvic reconstruction plate-screws, and modern screw-rod constructs, demonstrates the progress that has been made in fixation in this challenging spinal region. The authors describe the occipitocervical anatomy relevant to modern fixation devices, which generally use a plate or plates on the occiput that are connected to rod-screw constructs in the cervical vertebrae. To capture the thickest bone (along the midline at and below the external occipital protuberance) and to provide improved resistance to rotation, most occipital plates now have a combination of midline and lateral screw holes. Stock and associates do a commendable job of thoroughly reviewing the nuances of modern fixation systems and their design features. It is important to keep in mind that fusion is the ultimate goal in most patients requiring occipitocervical fixation. Proper bone grafting techniques, which generally require structural grafts that bridge the occipitocervical junction, are paramount to successful outcomes, although a description of these techniques is beyond the scope of this chapter.

In the second chapter in this section, Sasso provides an excellent technical review of C1 and C2 screw fixation techniques. He also presents a clear anatomic description of the differences between C2 pars interarticularis screws compared with C2 pedicle screws, a topic that remains confusing for many surgeons. All spine surgeons, but particularly those without extensive experience in upper cervical fixation, will benefit from the detailed description of the techniques of screw insertion. C1 lateral mass screws have become increasingly popular not only because of the rigid fixation provided in concert with screw-rod systems, but also because they can be used in circumstances when alternative forms of fixation, such as transarticular screws, may not be appropriate. Such circumstances include anatomic considerations such as C1-C2 malalignment or a high-riding vertebral artery that precludes safe screw passage through the C2 isthmus. C1 screws should be medially angulated to avoid the vertebral artery, internal carotid artery, and the occipitocervical articulation. Another method of C2 fixation, which uses a translaminar screw, is not discussed in this chapter but may be useful in situations in which C2 pars or pedicle screws cannot be inserted because of anatomic constraints from the vertebral artery or revision status.[1]

Daubs and associates review pedicle screw fixation into the upper thoracic pedicles (T1, T2, and T3). The upper thoracic pedicles tend to be larger and thus relatively easier to instrument than those in T4 through T7. T1, in particular, tends to have very large pedicles. Thoracic pedicle screws have gained widespread acceptance in the treatment of thoracic pathology. They generally provide superior fixation compared with hooks and wires, and they also provide greater corrective power in the treatment of spinal deformity. When properly inserted, pedicle screws may actually decrease the risk of neurologic injury because they do not involve placement of implants inside of the spinal canal. Their safety has been established in many studies. Although cortical breaches may occur, mild breaches are rarely of clinical consequence in procedures performed by experienced surgeons. Surgeons who insert thoracic pedicle screws should have a fundamental understanding of structures at potential risk for injury near the upper thoracic spine, including the spinal cord, nerve roots, aorta, esophagus, thoracic duct, and sympathetic ganglia. Lenke's freehand thoracic pedicle screw insertion technique is described in detail. In expert hands, like those of the authors of this chapter, the freehand technique has proven safe and effective; however, for surgeons who do not routinely place thoracic screws, it may be prudent to consider a fluoroscopically assisted approach. The authors also highlight other important concepts in thoracic screw placement, including the ability of pedicles to expand and accept screws that are larger than their original diameters, the biomechanical superiority of the straightforward versus anatomic (15° caudal) insertion technique, the outside-in technique of instrumenting very narrow slit-like pedicles, and the use of the anatomic technique in salvage situations.

In the fourth chapter in this section, Anderson provides a balanced analysis of image guidance in spinal surgery. Major benefits of image-guided surgery include greater accuracy and safety in placing implants, particularly in revision situations where the anatomic landmarks are severely distorted or in minimally invasive applications where access to landmarks is limited. Image-guided surgery may result in less radiation exposure to the patient and the operating team and also can be helpful in making bony cuts in complex procedures such as osteotomies. The disadvantages of image-guided surgery include the so-called fiddle-factor (additional setup and intraoperative time during surgery) and its potential unreliability, leading to paradoxically greater danger amidst a false sense of assurance. As technology evolves, image-guided systems will be of greater benefit and will become easier to use. Currently, the necessity of using image guidance in spine surgery remains unclear; fluoroscopy, even with its disadvantages, remains the modality of choice for most applications.

In the final chapter in this section, Rihn and associates contribute a thorough review of the use of bone morphogenetic proteins (BMPs) in lumbar spine surgery. The rationale for the use of BMPs is that the procurement of autogenous bone is associated with significant morbidity, autografts may be limited in quantity and/or quality, and nonunions still occur despite the use of autograft and rigid fixation. Currently, the only widely available BMP for use in spinal applications is rhBMP-2 (Infuse; Medtronic Sofamor-Danek, Memphis, TN), which is approved by the Food and Drug Administration (FDA) only for spine indications in conjunction with cages for anterior lumbar interbody fusion. BMP-7 (OP-1; Stryker Biotech, Hopkinton, MA), which was initially approved by the FDA under a humanitarian device exemption program for use in fewer than 4,000 patients per year, was not approved for general use by the FDA after a vote in April 2009.

In current clinical practice, most rhBMP-2 is used for off-label indications such as posterolateral or posterior lumbar interbody fusions. The authors review several studies demonstrating that the off-label use of BMPs in the posterolateral lumbar spine generally achieves fusion rates similar to or better than those obtained with iliac crest bone grafts. Safety issues remain a concern, however, more so with posterior interbody applications. Studies suggest a higher rate of postoperative radiculitis with rhBMP-2 in posterior lumbar interbody fusions and transforaminal lumbar interbody fusions than with autograft or allograft alone. Ectopic bone formation may occur when rhBMP-2 is placed into the disk space through a posterior interbody approach, with an unknown but probably small percentage of cases resulting in clinical symptoms. In this era of cost containment, the risk-cost benefit ratio of using BMPs in routine lumbar surgeries needs to be closely examined. Several studies have suggested that the use of BMPs may lower short-term costs by decreasing the complication rate and pain associated with iliac graft harvest, and may reduce long-term costs by lessening the need for pain management and rehabilitation services. The potential to decrease the number of nonunions and revision surgeries also has been suggested. BMPs will continue to play a role in lumbar spine surgery. It is important to remember that proper fusion technique and attention to detail are paramount to achieving successful outcomes even with the introduction and use of new technologies.

John M. Rhee, MD
Assistant Professor
Department of Orthopaedic Surgery
Emory Spine Center
Emory University School of Medicine
Atlanta, Georgia

Reference

1. Wright NM: Posterior C2 fixation using bilateral, crossing C2 laminar screws: Case series and technical note. *J Spinal Disord Tech* 2004;17:158-162.

Dr. Rhee or an immediate family member has received royalties from Biomet; is a member of a speakers' bureau or has made paid presentations on behalf of Biomet and Synthes; is a paid consultant for or is an employee of Synthes; has received research or institutional support from Synthes and Medtronic Sofamor Danek; and owns stock or stock options in Phygen.

Contemporary Posterior Occipital Fixation

Gordon H. Stock, MD

Alexander R. Vaccaro, MD

Andrew K. Brown, MD

Paul A. Anderson, MD

Abstract

Occipitocervical fixation is technically demanding but necessary in many clinical scenarios where junctional occiptocervical instability is present. The surgeon must have a thorough knowledge of the associated anatomy, biomechanics of spinal instrumentation, and familiarity with an ever-growing number of stabilization techniques and implants. The nature of the injury, the patient's anatomy, and the quality of the host bone will ultimately determine which form of fixation is optimal. Although the contemporary modular systems, at first glance, appear to add significant surgical complexity, in truth the designs actually simplify the process by allowing the surgeon to place occipital and spinal anchors in optimal anatomic locations.

Throughout the spine, the vertebral bodies are separated from one another by intervertebral disks. The intervertebral disks provide strength between adjacent segments and limit movement by resisting compressive, rotational, and shear forces placed on the spine. In contrast, the highly mobile occipitocervical (atlanto-occipital and atlantoaxial) joints are synovial joints whose articulations are devoid of an intervertebral disk; instead, they are supported by capsuloligamentous attachments. This region is the most mobile portion of the cervical spine, with nearly one half of cervical flexion-extension and cervical rotation occurring across these cartilagi-nous articulations. However, the anatomic structures that allow this increased mobility also predispose the joints to instability.

The etiology of occipitocervical instability is vast and includes trauma, rheumatoid arthritis, infection, tumor, congenital deformity, and degenerative processes. Instability in this region may be asymptomatic or may manifest as pain, cranial nerve dysfunction, paresis, paralysis, or even sudden death. It is paramount, therefore, that the surgeon fully understand the complex anatomy of the occipitocervical junction, be aware of the presence of instability and its ramifications, and have a practical understanding of the many contemporary methods used to stabilize the occipitocervical articulation.

The goals of surgery at this junction are to decompress the neurologic structures if necessary, normalize alignment, and provide immediate stability to promote osseous fusion. Recent anatomic and biomechanical studies have provided data that have led to more efficient and less morbid strategies of fixation, allowing earlier mobilization and more active participation in rehabilitation.

To better understand current implant systems used to stabilize the occipitocervical junction, it helps to review older instrumentation systems and their advantages and shortcomings.

Evolution of Occipitocervical Fixation

Occipitocervical stabilization was described as early as the 1920s by Foerster, who used a fibular strut-graft construct to span the occipito-cervical articulation.[1] This was followed by in situ onlay bone grafting with wire fixation and attempts to use methylmethacrylate, with and without internal fixation, to stabilize the occipitocervical junction. Although the constructs provided some support, they were associated with a high failure rate as a result of their inability to maintain occipitocervical alignment until osseous fusion could, if ever, occur. In most instances, extended skeletal traction was required for more than 4 weeks.[2-4] In the presence of posttraumatic ligamentous injury, the distraction and translational forces associated with positional changes during immobilization in a halo vest or orthosis at times proved deleterious.[5]

In 1978, Luque[6] introduced contoured steel rods attached to the lamina with wire fixation for thoracic and lumbar spinal fixation. This concept was later adapted to reinforce fusions in the cervical spine and at the occipitocervical junction.[7] Rods could be contoured to achieve a desired alignment, and they also offered improved stability compared with that provided by previous in situ fusion methods. Unfortunately, cumbersome, prolonged postoperative external immobilization was required to improve the otherwise unacceptably low fusion rates. Furthermore, implants were available only in stainless steel, making postoperative imaging impossible. Apostolides and associates[8] introduced a device that could contour titanium rods, which were then fixed to the occiput and the posterior elements of the cervical spine with cables. Thirty-seven of the 39 patients treated with this method had osseous fusion without requiring halo vest immobilization.

For patients with rheumatoid arthritis, Ransford and associates[9] developed a contoured loop that is fixed to the occiput and cervical spine with wires. The loop compresses around C2 with the goal of maintaining the vertical alignment between the occiput and the cervical spine. Ransford and associates did not routinely attempt fusion with bone graft when they used this device. A review of the long-term results in 150 patients suggested that bone grafting in an attempt to obtain a fusion did not improve the results compared with those following fixation alone.[10]

Pelvic plate-and-screw fixation was subsequently adapted for use as segmental internal fixation of the cervical spine.[11-14] This method provided immediate rigidity to the spinal elements and obviated, in many instances, the need for postoperative halo vest immobilization. It was not necessary to pass sublaminar wires, so the most risky part of the Luque technique of fixation was avoided. However, plate-and-screw fixation still had several limitations: plates have a fixed hole-to-hole distance, which at times prevents optimal screw placement; the completed fixation implant leaves very little space for graft material; and plates provide a limited ability to compress or distract across individual interspaces.

Although the screws provided excellent fixation, the plates were less acceptable. Therefore, the longitudinal components of fixation evolved to rods that allowed unlimited superior and inferior screw placement, greater space caudad to the rod for bone grafting, and the ability to compress or distract between spinal segments as desired.

In 1999, Oda and associates[15] performed a cadaveric biomechanical analysis comparing the stability of five different types of occipitoatlantoaxial fixation systems (Figure 1), and drew several important conclusions. First, they showed that C2 transpedicular and C1-C2 transarticular screws significantly increased the stabilizing effect of an occipitocervical implant compared with that provided by rods and sublaminar hooks or wires ($P < 0.05$). Second, the construct with the greatest stability was a combination occipital plate-subaxial rod system with six occipital screws and C2 pedicle screws (Figure 1, E). Their hypothesis that this increased stability would lead to higher fusion rates was supported by an independent clinical study in which all 24 patients treated with rigid internal fixation and bone-grafting obtained an osseous fusion.[16]

An important consideration in the selection of a system is the stiffness of the implants. Anderson and associates[17] recently demonstrated that biomechanical performance correlated with the amount of metallic material and with its distribution as defined by the area moment of inertia. Plates, in general, have a two to three times greater area moment of inertia than do rods. The area moment of inertia correlates directly with biomechanical stiffness. For rods, the area moment of inertia varies to the fourth power of their diameter. Thus, even relatively small increases in rod size can have substantial effects. For example, a change in diameter from 3.2 to 3.5 mm doubles a rod's stiffness. Greater stiffness is believed to be better.

Fixation systems with occipital plates that are not rigidly fixed to the cervical component but can be attached to them with a locking screw mechanism were recently introduced (Figures 2 and 3). This obviates the need for contouring of the longitudinal plate or rod component between the subaxial spine and the occiput and has facilitated implant construction at the time of surgery.

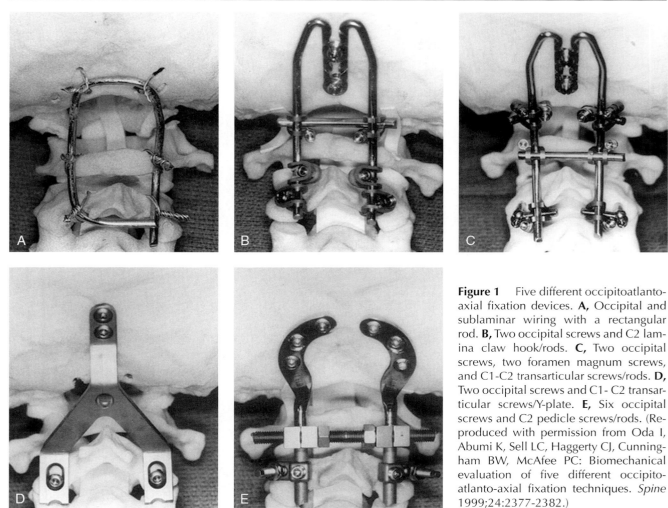

Figure 1 Five different occipitoatlanto-axial fixation devices. **A,** Occipital and sublaminar wiring with a rectangular rod. **B,** Two occipital screws and C2 lamina claw hook/rods. **C,** Two occipital screws, two foramen magnum screws, and C1-C2 transarticular screws/rods. **D,** Two occipital screws and C1- C2 transarticular screws/Y-plate. **E,** Six occipital screws and C2 pedicle screws/rods. (Reproduced with permission from Oda I, Abumi K, Sell LC, Haggerty CJ, Cunningham BW, McAfee PC: Biomechanical evaluation of five different occipito-atlanto-axial fixation techniques. *Spine* 1999;24:2377-2382.)

Currently there remains a variety of fixation methods for stabilization of the occipitocervical junction.[18] There are many factors to consider when choosing which implant to use. The challenge lies in finding a proper balance between the desire for immediate rigid stabilization and the increasing surgical complexity and risk.[19]

In addition to posterior spinal fixation methods, an anterior occipitocervical reconstruction technique with use of screw fixation between the C1 lateral mass and the occipital condyles was recently described by Dvorak and associates.[20,21] Although this method provided stability in axial rotation and lateral bending, it was inferior to contemporary posterior fixation methods with regard to its ability to resist flexion and extension. Although this anterior method of fixation will have only limited application, it may prove helpful in some unique clinical settings where posterior fixation techniques either are not possible or have previously failed.

Contemporary Universal Occipital-Cervical-Thoracic Systems

Some of the device components discussed in this section have not been approved by the US Food and Drug Administration.

At present, there are two popular occipital-cervical-thoracic spinal fixation methods: dual (subaxial) rod-plate (occiput) systems and subaxial rod-independent occipital plate systems (Figures 2 and 3). Most new designs include variations on these themes with components that are all similarly designed to accomplish the same task. In the subaxial and upper cervical spine it is requisite that the skeletal anchors (screws or hooks) form a rigid connection with the longitudinal components (rods) of the implant system. This connection between the spine anchors and the longitudinal components may be direct, or it may be accomplished with

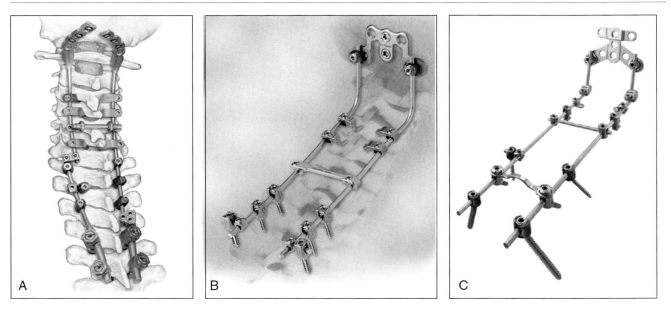

Figure 2 Representative universal posterior fixation systems. **A,** Axon System. (Reproduced with permission from Synthes USA, West Chester, PA.) **B,** Altius M-INI OCT System. (Reproduced with permission from EBI Spine, Parsippany, NJ.) **C,** Mountaineer OCT Spinal System. (Reproduced with permission from DePuy Spine, Raynham, MA.)

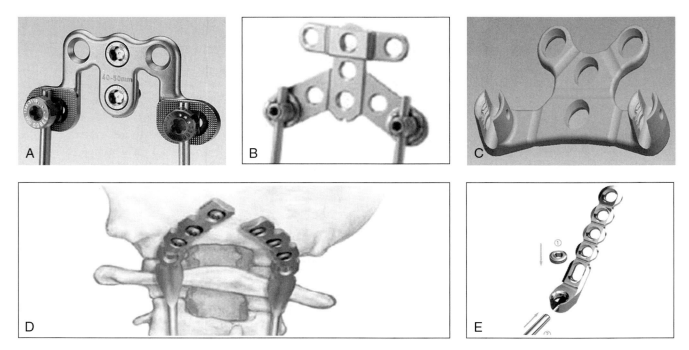

Figure 3 Various independent and bilateral occipitocervical plate designs. **A,** Altius M-INI OCT System. (Reproduced with permission from EBI Spine, Parsippany, NJ.) **B,** Mountaineer OCT Spinal System. The occipital plate is shown with the optional lateral washer. (Reproduced with permission from DePuy Spine, Raynham, MA.) **C,** Vertex Max. (Reproduced with permission from Medtronic Sofamor Danek USA, Memphis, TN.) **D,** Axon System. (Reproduced with permission from Synthes USA, West Chester, PA.) **E,** Oasys. (Reproduced with permission from Stryker, Mahwah, NJ.)

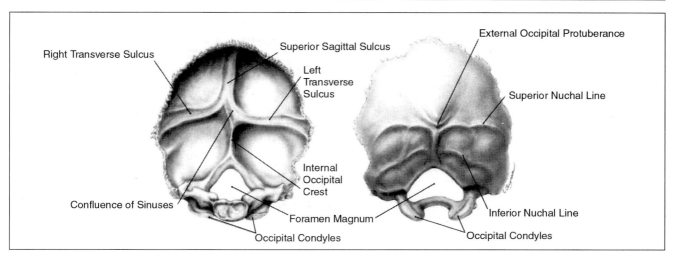

Figure 4 Internal and external osseous anatomy of the posterior aspect of the occiput. (Reproduced with permission from Roberts DA, Doherty BJ, Heggeness MH: Quantitative anatomy of the occiput and the biomechanics of occipital screw fixation. *Spine* 1998;23:1100-1108.)

use of a rod-offset connector or a variable plate-offset connector to allow maximum flexibility in medial-lateral screw or hook location. Additionally, depending on the sagittal contouring of an individual patient's anatomy, the interface between the longitudinal component and the spinal anchors must be able to accommodate substantial screw angulation when needed.

Occipital Fixation

To safely place occipital anchors, it is important to understand the osseous anatomy of the occiput in terms of its thickness in various regions and the location of underlying vascular sinuses[22] (Figure 4). The external occipital protuberance is the most prominent posterior osseous landmark on the occiput. It is located in the midline of the occiput at the confluence of the superior nuchal line and the midoccipital region. From the external occipital protuberance, there are several palpable osseous crests. The superior nuchal line extends laterally from the external occipital protuberance, whereas

the medial nuchal line descends inferiorly along the midline toward the foramen magnum. Finally, the inferior nuchal line extends inferolaterally from the middle of the medial nuchal line bilaterally. On the internal surface of the occiput, there are osseous elevations, or sulci, that contain the large venous sinuses.

In their anatomic study of the occipital bone, Ebraheim and associates[23] projected the course of the large internal venous sinuses onto the external surface of the occiput. The superior nuchal line overlies the transverse sinuses bilaterally whereas the superior sagittal sinus descends from the superior aspect of the cranium inferiorly along the midline to the torcula, or confluence of the sinuses. The torcula lies immediately underneath the external occipital protuberance. These venous structures are at risk for penetrative injury during drilling or screw placement in locations where only the dura mater separates the bone from the lumen of the dural sinuses.

In addition to mapping the large venous sinuses, Ebraheim and asso-

ciates[23] measured the thickness of the occipital bone and used those data to suggest ideal screw-insertion points. They found that the occipital bone is thickest in the midline at the external occipital protuberance. In males it is roughly 11 to 15 mm thick, whereas in females it is 10 to 12 mm thick. Cadaveric sectioning showed that the bone adjacent to the external occipital protuberance was the thickest and densest bone and that the thickness of the bone decreased laterally and inferiorly. Ten- to 12-mm screws can be used close to the external occipital protuberance, and 8-mm screws can be safely inserted lateral and inferior to the external occipital protuberance.

In a separate study on occipital morphology, Zipnick and associates[24] also showed that the occiput was thickest at the external occipital protuberance and that it decreased in thickness in a radial fashion. The outer and middle tables both contributed 45% to the overall bone thickness, whereas the inner table contributed only about 10%. Biomechanical studies have shown that screw pullout strength is related to the thickness of the bone and whether the screw has unicortical or bicortical purchase. Haher and associates[25] found that although unicortical occipital screws had less pullout strength than bicortical screws at the external occipital protuberance, the strength of the unicortical screws was comparable with that of bicortical screws at other locations. Both cortical and cancellous bone-type screws have been tested in occipital bone, but there was no significant biomechanical difference in their pullout strengths.[22]

Fear of venous penetration with bicortical screw fixation limits screw placement to below the superior nuchal line, but the work of Zipnick and associates[24] suggests that unicortical screw purchase both at and above the superior nuchal line is sufficient because the contribution of the inner table to the bone thickness is minimal and that unicortical fixation lowers the risk of intracranial venous penetration.

Because of the thicker bone that descends down the medial nuchal line, midline screws have greater pullout strength than do more laterally placed screws. This finding has been exploited by fixation designs, such as a Y-plate, that involve a single longitudinal series of occipital screw anchors in the midline (Figure 1, D). Although screws placed at the midline had greater pullout strength, this particular design (without lateral support) was found to have much weaker torsional strength than designs that included midline and laterally placed occipital screws.[26] This finding prompted the development of additional designs that either incorporated lateral fixation points in the occiput or even used only lateral fixation, without midline screws.

Anatomic and biomechanical studies have shown that, compared with laterally placed screws, midline screw fixation allows longer screw purchase but decreased torsional resistance.[17] Laterally placed screws theoretically provide better resistance to rotational stresses as a result of the bilateral purchase. In a biomechanical study, Anderson and associates[17] demonstrated that lateral screws had slightly increased stiffness in bending and rotation but not in flexion-extension. This difference was much smaller than that related to changes in rod diameter.[17] A combination of midline and laterally placed screws appears to provide the most optimal screw arrangement to ensure rigid occipital fixation. Most contemporary plates, therefore, have both medial and lateral occipital fixation points incorporated into their design (Figure 3).

To achieve maximum occipital fixation, occipital screws differ from cortical and cancellous bone screws that are used elsewhere; they have a larger diameter and smaller pitch. This design difference is especially important laterally, where the occipital bone is thinner and where shorter screws with a much smaller pitch are necessary for optimal fixation.

An alternative to traditional occipital screw fixation was described by Pait and associates.[27] They described the inside-outside technique, in which a slotted keyhole is first created in the occiput. The head of an occipital screw is then slid down into the created keyhole with the flat head of the screw in the epidural space and with the threads facing out. An occipital bone plate is then secured to the occiput with a nut. Multiple studies[27,28] have shown that this method is also safe and effective for occipital fixation.

A problem with all occipital fixa-

tion devices is implant prominence. Modern occipital plates are designed to be low profile and are precontoured to the approximate shape of the occiput. Bend zones have also been added to some plate designs to facilitate intraoperative manipulation of the plate to achieve an even closer fit between it and the occipital bone. This is shown representatively by the plate in Figure 5, but it can also be seen in Figure 3, C and E. In rod-plate designs, the bilateral occipital plates can be contoured in both the sagittal and the coronal plane for better medial approximation to the occipital bone (Figure 3, D and E).

In designs that use a rod as the longitudinal component connected to an occipital plate, the rod may be a single component that transforms from a rod into a plate in the occipital region (Figure 3, D) or it may be a two-piece design in which the occipital plate and rod are mechanically connected intraoperatively (Figure 3, E). With the latter type of design, the rod is most commonly connected to the plate with use of a slotted connector for flexibility with regard to medial-lateral rod placement. Some of the slotted connections have a fixed orientation (Figure 3, C), whereas others allow one to medialize or lateralize the rod and even rotate the articulation to facilitate plate attachment to the longitudinal rod; this is most clearly seen in Figure 3, A, where up to 5 mm of medial-lateral adjustment and any degree of rotation are possible.

Cervical Spine Fixation

There are multiple techniques for obtaining upper cervical and subaxial spine fixation. A solid upper cervical or subaxial vertebral anchor is the key to a rigid occipitocervical construct. Vertebral anchoring can

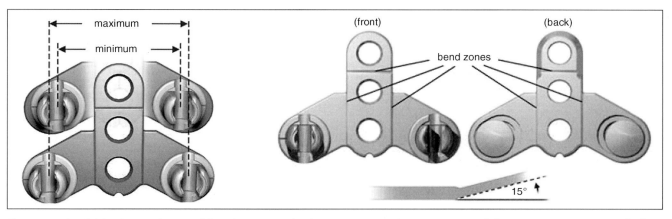

Figure 5 Variable size options and bend zones to facilitate intraoperative contouring of the Mountaineer occipital plate. (Reproduced with permission from DePuy Spine, Raynham, MA.)

be accomplished by using screws (pedicle, lateral mass, or transarticular), laminar hooks, or sublaminar wires. Screws provide the most rigid spinal anchor. Studies have shown that screws can be placed safely in the lateral mass and the cervical pedicles, although the variability in the morphometry and orientation of the pedicles and lateral masses requires very careful preoperative assessment.[29,30] When screws are placed correctly, they avoid the recognized neurologic risks associated with intracanal fixation with laminar hooks, sublaminar wires, or cables.

In addition to the advantage of not violating the canal space, properly placed screws offer several other benefits over laminar hooks that make them preferable for posterior stabilization.

Because hooks engage only the posterior part of the lamina, they can provide only semirigid fixation. On the other hand, a screw in the C1 lateral mass or the C2 pedicle can provide solid three-column fixation. The creation of a stiffer construct often reduces the number of levels that require fusion.

As part of the design versatility of contemporary occipital-cervical-thoracic systems, the bone anchors in the cervical spine—especially those that are most constrained in their anatomic placement, such as C1 and C2 screws—are typically placed first. Once they are placed, these anchors can be used as a guide for choosing a properly sized occipital plate.

In earlier systems, the screw location was limited and mechanically constrained by the implant system. However, with the newer implants, the large variety of screw and connector designs allows the surgeon to place screws where the patient's anatomy dictates and then take advantage of screw and connector design features to facilitate attachment of the anchors to the rods with minimal rod contouring (Figure 6).

Systems currently feature variable axis or polyaxial screws, meaning that there is a certain degree of freedom between the bone screw and screw head or connecting saddle that attaches to the longitudinal rods. Some screws feature a cone of angulation that allows any position within that cone, whereas other screws are more constrained with lesser degrees of freedom, sometimes allowing movement in just

one plane. The screws depicted in Figure 6 have various degrees of freedom between the screw shaft and head. Additional design features, such as biased-angle screws and modular screw designs with multiple connector options, also facilitate rod-anchor attachment.

Longitudinal Components
There are size and shape differences between the rod-plate systems and the independent occipital plate systems. In a rod-plate system, the longitudinal connector options that are available depend on whether the rod and plate are integrated (Figures 2, *A*, and 3, *D*) or are two separate components (Figure 3, *E*). Integrated rod-plate systems avoid the additional mechanical coupling of the rod and plate intraoperatively, but by design they constrain the surgeon more with regard to the location of the cervical or occipital anchors because of the lack of flexibility between a fixed occipital implant location and the attached longitudinal component.

A modular rod-plate system is a design that is intermediate between a pure rod-plate design and an independent occipital plate design. Such a

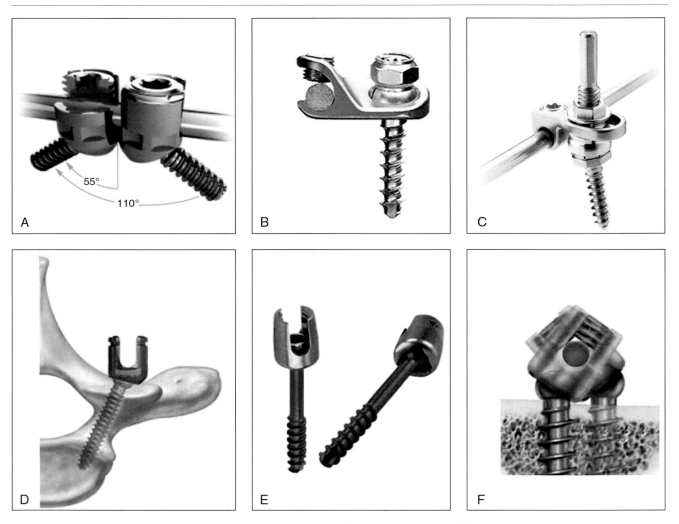

Figure 6 Contemporary screw and connector design features to facilitate attachment of the anchors to the rods with minimal rod contouring. **A,** Oasys biased-angle polyaxial screw. (Reproduced with permission from Stryker, Mahwah, NJ.) **B,** Starlock screw and favored-angle clamp. (Reproduced with permission from Synthes USA, West Chester, PA.) **C,** Altius variable-angle posted screw on lateral connector. (Reproduced with permission from EBI, Parsippany, NJ.) **D,** Mountaineer OCT favored-angle screw. (Reproduced with permission from DePuy Spine, Raynham, MA.) **E,** Vertex multiaxial screw in pivot saddle. (Reproduced with permission from Medtronic Sofamor Danek USA, Memphis, TN.) **F,** Implant detail showing anchor placement versatility. (Reproduced with permission from Medtronic Sofamor Danek USA, Memphis, TN.)

system gives the surgeon the flexibility of changing the rod during surgery without the need to remove the screws from the occipital plate portion of the rod-plate system. However, the fixed-angle interface between the plate and the rod adds an additional constraint to the implant. For example, the connection between the rod and the occipital plate in one system is fixed at 110° (Figure 3, *E*).

Although additional minor contouring of the rod and plate may take place intraoperatively, this fixed-angle design constraint requires that the patient's anatomy be close to this angle for the device to fit well.

Independent occipital plate systems allow ultimate flexibility in plate placement that is independent of the location of the cervical rod. This implant design allows inter-

change or repositioning of the rod without removal of the occipital plate. In the independent occipital plate systems, the rods may come prebent to approximate the anatomy of the occipitocervical junction; minor intraoperative adjustments are then made to further fit the implant to the sagittal plane contouring of the individual patient (Figure 2, *B*).

A recently introduced adjustable

rod (Figure 7) features a joint in the rod at the level of the occipitocervical junction. This innovative design feature allows a full range of angulation to be achieved in a single plane within the rod. This has several advantages. First, surgical time is decreased because rod angulation can be fine-tuned during construct development. In addition, as with other rod-plate systems, the rods can be changed intraoperatively without removing the occipital plate. Finally, depending on the biomechanical strength of the design, long-term fatigue failure may be minimized by the lack of a need for rod-bending or stress transfer, which are traditionally required at this interface.

Several other occipitocervical rod designs are available (Figure 8), including a standard rod, a tapered rod, and a transitional rod. Most systems use rods with a constant cross-sectional area that has been precontoured to fit the occipitocervical angle (Figure 8, A). Although there is some variation in the diameters of the rods, most of the systems use cervical rods that are 3.5 mm in diameter.

The tapered rod is an alternative design with a different diameter at each end separated by a transition zone (Figure 8, B). The increased diameter gives the system added strength, especially at the transition between the occiput and the cervical spine.

A third design is the transitional rod (Figure 8, C). This rod is 3 mm in diameter at each end but 4 mm at the apex of the precontoured bend at the level of the occipitocervical junction. This gives the implant added strength at the apex of the curve, where the mechanical stresses are the greatest, while minimizing the size and weight in other locations along the rod.

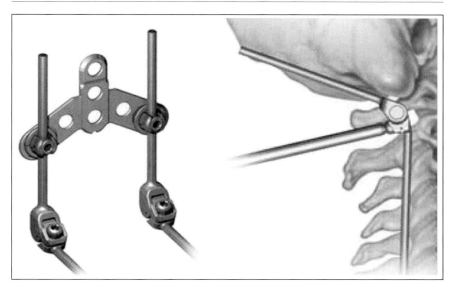

Figure 7 Occipitocervical adjustable rod (Mountaineer OCT Spinal System). The joint allows a full range of angulation in a single plane; angles can be changed intraoperatively without removing the rod. (Reproduced with permission from DePuy Spine, Raynham, MA.)

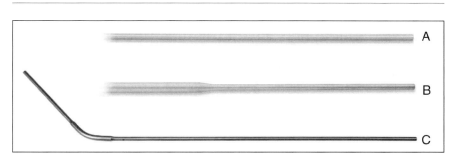

Figure 8 Standard, tapered, and transitional rod designs. **A,** Axon System standard rod. (Reproduced with permission from Synthes USA, West Chester, PA.) **B,** Axon System tapered rod. (Reproduced with permission from Synthes USA, West Chester, PA.) **C,** Summit Spinal System transitional rod. (Reproduced with permission from DePuy Spine, Raynham, MA.)

Other Components of Fixation Systems

To further stabilize the mechanical construct, each system includes cross-connecting bars or transverse connections to stabilize the two rods inferior to the occiput. The cross-connectors attach either directly to the rod or directly onto the heads of the polyaxial screws (head-to-head cross-connectors). The distance between the rods obviously varies with each patient, so each connector has design features that allow it to be easily attached to the rods regardless of the distance between them. Some connectors allow adjustment at the point where the cross-connector connects with the longitudinal rod, whereas others use an adjustable linkage within the connector itself (Figures 1 and 2). The optimal region for attachment of this connector is either right below the occipitocervical bend in the rod or at the cervicothoracic junction for longer constructs to avoid possible contact with the prominent dura in the subaxial spine.

Summary

Occipitocervical fixation is technically very demanding. The surgeon must have a thorough knowledge of the associated anatomy and of the biomechanics of the spinal instrumentation as well as familiarity with an ever-growing number of stabilization techniques and implants. The nature of the injury, the patient's anatomy, and the quality of the host bone ultimately determine which form of fixation is optimal.

Although at first glance the contemporary modular systems appear to add substantial surgical complexity, the designs actually simplify the process by allowing the surgeon to place the spinal anchors in optimal anatomic locations and still easily attach the longitudinal rods with minimal intraoperative contouring of the rods. This flexibility in anchor placement optimizes the chance of obtaining a rigid construct, therefore obviating the need for cumbersome external immobilization. The designs and techniques for obtaining fusion have changed drastically over the past century and will continue to evolve as new design innovations are introduced.

References

1. Foerster O: *Die leitungsbahnen des schmerzgefühls und die chirurgische behandlung der schmerzzustände*. Berlin, Germany, Urban and Schwarzenberg, 1927.

2. Elia M, Mazzara JT, Fielding JW: Onlay technique for occipitocervical fusion. *Clin Orthop Relat Res* 1992;280:170-174.

3. Grantham SA, Dick HM, Thompson RC Jr, Stinchfield FE: Occipitocervical arthrodesis: Indications, technic and results. *Clin Orthop Relat Res* 1969;65:118-129.

4. Hamblen DL: Occipito-cervical fusion: Indications, technique and results. *J Bone Joint Surg Br* 1967;49:33-45.

5. Vaccaro AR, Lim MR, Lee JY: Indications for surgery and stabilization techniques of the occipito-cervical junction. *Injury* 2005;36(suppl 2):B44-B53.

6. Luque ER: The anatomic basis and development of segmental spinal instrumentation. *Spine* 1982;7:256-259.

7. Itoh T, Tsuji H, Katoh Y, Yonezawa T, Kitagawa H: Occipito-cervical fusion reinforced by Luque's segmental spinal instrumentation for rheumatoid diseases. *Spine* 1988;13:1234-1238.

8. Apostolides PJ, Dickman CA, Golfinos JG, Papadopoulos SM, Sonntag VK: Threaded Steinmann pin fusion of the craniovertebral junction. *Spine* 1996;21:1630-1637.

9. Ransford AO, Crockard HA, Pozo JL, Thomas NP, Nelson IW: Craniocervical instability treated by contoured loop fixation. *J Bone Joint Surg Br* 1986;68:173-177.

10. Moskovich R, Crockard HA, Shott S, Ransford AO: Occipitocervical stabilization for myelopathy in patients with rheumatoid arthritis: Implications of not bone-grafting. *J Bone Joint Surg Am* 2000;82:349-365.

11. Grob D, Dvorak J, Panjabi M, Froehlich M, Hayek J: Posterior occipitocervical fusion: A preliminary report of a new technique. *Spine* 1991;16(3 suppl):S17-S24.

12. Lieberman IH, Webb JK: Occipitocervical fusion using posterior titanium plates. *Eur Spine J* 1998;7:308-312.

13. Sasso RC, Jeanneret B, Fischer K, Magerl F: Occipitocervical fusion with posterior plate and screw instrumentation: A long-term follow-up study. *Spine* 1994;19:2364-2368.

14. Smith MD, Anderson P, Grady MS: Occipitocervical arthrodesis using contoured plate fixation: An early report on a versatile fixation technique. *Spine* 1993;18:1984-1990.

15. Oda I, Abumi K, Sell LC, Haggerty CJ, Cunningham BW, McAfee PC: Biomechanical evaluation of five different occipito-atlanto-axial fixation techniques. *Spine* 1999;24:2377-2382.

16. Abumi K, Takada T, Shono Y, Kaneda K, Fujiya M: Posterior occipitocervical reconstruction using cervical pedicle screws and plate-rod systems. *Spine* 1999;24:1425-1434.

17. Anderson PA, Oza AL, Puscak TJ, Sasso R: Biomechanics of occipitocervical fixation. *Spine* 2006;31:755-761.

18. Menezes AH: Complications of surgery at the craniovertebral junction: Avoidance and management. *Pediatr Neurosurg* 1991;17:254-266.

19. Singh SK, Rickards L, Apfelbaum RI, Hurlbert RJ, Maiman D, Fehlings MG: Occipitocervical reconstruction with the Ohio Medical Instruments Loop: Results of a multicenter evaluation in 30 cases. *J Neurosurg* 2003;98(suppl 3):239-246.

20. Dvorak MF, Fisher C, Boyd M, Johnson M, Greenhow R, Oxland TR: Anterior occiput-to-axis screw fixation: Part I. A case report, description of a new technique, and anatomical feasibility analysis. *Spine* 2003;28:E54-E60.

21. Dvorak MF, Sekeramayi F, Zhu Q, et al: Anterior occiput to axis screw fixation: Part II. A biomechanical comparison with posterior fixation techniques. *Spine* 2003;28:239-245.

22. Roberts DA, Doherty BJ, Heggeness MH: Quantitative anatomy of the occiput and the biomechanics of occipital screw fixation. *Spine* 1998;23:1100-1108.

23. Ebraheim NA, Lu J, Biyani A, Brown JA, Yeasting RA: An anatomic study of the thickness of the occipital bone: Implications for occipitocervical instrumentation. *Spine* 1996;21:1725-1730.

24. Zipnick RI, Merola AA, Gorup J, et al: Occipital morphology: An anatomic guide to internal fixation. *Spine* 1996;21:1719-1724.

25. Haher TR, Yeung AW, Caruso SA, et al: Occipital screw pullout strength: A biomechanical investigation of occipital morphology. *Spine* 1999;24:5-9.

26. Sutterlin CE III, Bianchi JR, Kunz DN, Zdeblick TA, Johnson WM, Rapoff AJ: Biomechanical evaluation of occipitocervical fixation devices. *J Spinal Disord* 2001;14:185-192.

27. Pait TG, Al-Mefty O, Boop FA, Arnautovic KI, Rahman S, Ceola W: Inside-outside technique for posterior occipitocervical spine instrumentation and stabilization: Preliminary results. *J Neurosurg* 1999;90(suppl 1):1-7.

28. Sandhu FA, Pait TG, Benzel E, Henderson FC: Occipitocervical fusion for rheumatoid arthritis using the inside-outside stabilization technique. *Spine* 2003;28:414-419.

29. Ebraheim N, Rollins JR Jr, Xu R, Jackson WT: Anatomic consideration of C2 pedicle screw placement. *Spine* 1996;21:691-695.

30. Jones EL, Heller JG, Silcox DH, Hutton WC: Cervical pedicle screws versus lateral mass screws. Anatomic feasibility and biomechanical comparison. *Spine* 1997;22:977-982.

25

C1 Lateral Screws and C2 Pedicle/Pars Screws

Rick C. Sasso, MD

Abstract

A variety of techniques exist for fixation of the upper cervical spine. The development of universal posterior cervical screw-rod instrumentation systems has resulted in recent interest in new and stable segmental fixation into C1 and C2. The C1 lateral mass is a safe and robust anchor point; however, the anatomic corridor to access the screw entry portal is unfamiliar. Understanding the C1 bony landmarks and the course and relationship of the soft-tissue structures (such as the vertebral artery and the C2 nerve root) is critically important. Alternative techniques for achieving segmental screw fixation into C2 are being developed. With polyaxial screw heads and lateral offset connectors, screw anchors can be driven into the most sturdy and safest aspects of C2 without concern for the position of the longitudinal rod.

Historically, anchors into C1 have been limited by the inability to fasten a stable longitudinal structure to connect anchors attached to adjacent vertebrae. Although Magerl originally placed screws into the lateral mass of C1, he was unable to rigidly couple them to a fixation device into C2. Thus, he originated a transarticular screw technique across the C1-C2 facet joint that bears his name.[1] This transarticular screw was a huge advance over the traditional wire/cable techniques of atlantoaxial stabilization.[2] Biomechanically, transarticular

The author or the departments with which he is affiliated has received something of value from a commercial or other party related directly or indirectly to the subject of this chapter.

screws are much more stable under shear and rotational loads compared with wire/cable constructs, and postoperative halo immobilization is not required. Extremely high fusion rates are achieved without the morbidity of halos. Magerl screws, however, do have several disadvantages and carry the distinction of being the most dangerous screw that a spine surgeon can implant. The C1-C2 articulation must be perfectly reduced before attempting transarticular screw insertion, and it is impossible to obtain the steep cranial trajectory in many patients with a fixed cervicothoracic kyphosis. Biplane fluoroscopy is required intraoperatively, and preoperative parasagittal CT reconstructions are mandatory to assess for a high-riding vertebral artery groove in C2, which precludes transarticular screw

implantation in up to 20% of patients. Bilateral vertebral artery injury has proven lethal.

The introduction of universal polyaxial screw/rod instrumentation for the posterior cervical spine has finally allowed surgeons to individually anchor into C1 and C2, provide stability as strong as that of transarticular screws, provide the versatility of incorporating the occiput and the subaxial cervical spine easily into the construct, and allow for safer and less difficult screw insertion. The lateral mass of C1 is a strong and safe anchor point for a screw and may be used to provide additional fixation points in occipitocervical constructs, thus increasing resistance to construct failure in the cervical spine without increasing the number of cervical levels fused. With traditional plate/screw occipitocervical constructs, C1 was entirely bypassed or relatively weak cables were passed under the C1 posterior arch and crimped through the plate holes.

There has been considerable confusion in the literature regarding screws placed into the C2 vertebra from a posterior approach.[3] The distinction between C2 pedicle screws and C2 pars interarticularis screws hinges on the anatomic definitions of the true pedicle and pars interar-

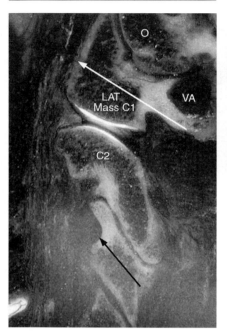

Figure 1 Anatomic specimen of the parasagittal occipitocervical junction through the lateral mass of C1 (Lat Mass C1). The long arrow shows the path of the screw through the C1 lateral mass. O is the occipital condyle, and C2 is the superior articular process of C2. VA is the vertebral artery in the groove along the cephalad aspect of the C1 posterior arch. The short arrow shows the path of the screw through the C3 lateral mass.

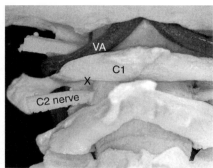

Figure 2 Posterior view photograph of the occipitocervical junction. The entry point for the C1 lateral mass screw is indicated (X). C1 = the posterior arch of C1, VA = the vertebral artery as it runs in the groove of the superior aspect of the C1 posterior arch, C2 nerve = the C2 nerve root. The C1-C2 facet joint lies just anterior to the C2 nerve.

ticularis. C2 screws may be coupled to C1 lateral mass screws to achieve atlantoaxial stabilization.

C1 Lateral Mass Screws

The atlantoaxial joint is challenging to stabilize because of the unique characteristics of the C1 and C2 vertebrae. The anatomic differences between C1 and C2 and the remainder of the subaxial cervical spine require individual strategies for screw insertion. The lateral mass of C1 is not analogous to the lateral mass of the subaxial vertebrae. Therefore, C1 lateral mass screws are distinct from the standard lateral mass screws inserted from C3 to C7 (Figure 1).

The most challenging aspect of implanting C1 lateral mass screws is the exposure of the C1 lateral mass and C1-C2 joint from a cranial to caudal direction. The key to this exposure is mobilization of the C2 nerve root. Although most spine surgeons are comfortable with exposing the C1-C2 joint from a caudal to cranial fashion, as is routinely performed to insert transarticular C1-C2 screws, the dissection of this joint from a cranial to caudal path with mobilization and retraction of the C2 nerve caudally is not common. There has not been a previous reason to expose the C1 lateral mass because there was no advantage or technique to fixate it before the development of universal screw/rod instrumentation.

Dissection of the posterior arch of C1 lateral to 1.5 cm from the midline is performed with caution because the vertebral artery runs in a groove on the superior surface of the posterior arch. It is usually protected by a thin rim of bone from the superior border of this posterior arch,

but it may be exposed; therefore, lateral exposure is focused from the middle aspect to the inferior part of the posterior arch of C1. The venous plexus around the C2 nerve root is cauterized with a bipolar and the C2 root is mobilized caudally. Subperiosteal dissection is performed from the inferior aspect of the posterior arch of C1 and anteriorly down to the lateral mass of C1. The lateral mass of C1 inferior to the C1 arch is exposed. The medial wall of the lateral mass is identified using a forward angle curet to identify the medial limit of screw placement. The medial aspect of the transverse foramen can also be identified and serves as the lateral limit for screw placement. The entry point for screw placement is identified 3 to 5 mm lateral to the medial wall of the lateral mass, at the junction of the lateral mass and inferior aspect of the C1 arch (Figure 2). A high-speed drill with a 3-mm burr is used to remove a small portion of the inferior aspect of the posterior C1 arch overlying the entry point and to create a recess for the screw head. Removing this lip from the inferior aspect of the C1 posterior arch also assists in accessing the vertical wall, which leads to the lateral mass. If this lip is not removed, it is extremely difficult to subperiosteally dissect the venous plexus surrounding the C2 nerve from a cephalad to caudal direction (Figure 3). An assistant retracts the C2 nerve inferiorly and protects it during drilling and screw placement. A cervical probe with a diameter equal to the inner diameter of the polyaxial screw is used to forage a path into the cancellous bone of the C1 lateral mass with 10° to 15° of medial angulation and 10° to 20° of cephalad angulation. The medial angulation is important because it helps surgeons to stay away from the lateral vertebral artery. The spinal canal is not at risk because the starting point for this screw on the lateral mass is near the anterior aspect of the canal. The slight cephalad angulation is necessary to keep the screw out of the C1-C2 facet joint, but the screw should not be steeply angled to prevent the screw head from impinging on the C2 nerve root. Removing the lip of bone from the inferior aspect of the posterior arch assists in allowing a more horizontal trajectory. If this lip remains, it forces a steeper path through the lateral mass. The screw head should sit on the inferior aspect of the posterior arch of C1 that was previously prepared by the drill. Using lateral fluoroscopic imaging, the probe is directed toward the anterior tubercle of C1 midway between the superior and inferior facets of C1. Because this is usually a strong screw with excellent purchase in the lateral mass and the screw is rigidly attached to the rod, bicortical purchase is not routinely obtained through the anterior cortex of C1. If there is concern about the sturdiness of the screw, then a 2.5-mm drill can perforate the anterior cortex. The internal carotid artery is usually just lateral to the entry point of this screw; thus, the importance of medial angulation is strengthened with bicortical purchase. The hole is tapped, and either a 3.5- or 4.0-mm screw is placed. Approximately half of this screw will be within the bone of the C1 lateral mass and half will be exposed under the posterior arch of C1. If preferred, a special C1 partially threaded screw can be used so that no screw threads abut the C2 nerve root (Vertex, Medtronic, Memphis, TN). Anatomic landmarks are used to guide the placement of C1 lateral mass screws; however, a lateral fluo-

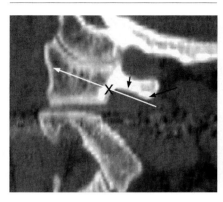

Figure 3   Lateral radiograph of the posterior occipitocervical junction. The entry point for the C1 lateral mass screw is indicated (X). The long arrow shows the trajectory of the screw. The small arrow shows the inferior lip of bone on the posterior arch of C1 that should be removed to allow subperiosteal access to the vertical wall (arrowhead) and provide appropriate trajectory of the screw without excessive cephalad angulation. This also creates a nesting place for the polyaxial screw head on the posterior arch of C1.

roscopic image may be obtained to assure proper sagittal angulation

C2 Pedicle Screws Versus C2 Pars Interarticularis Screws

The pars interarticularis is defined as the portion of the C2 vertebra between the superior and inferior articular surfaces. A screw placed in this portion of C2 has often been called a pedicle screw, but is more appropriately termed a pars interarticularis screw. This screw is placed in a trajectory similar to that of the C1-C2 transarticular screw. The entry point for the C2 pars interarticularis screw is 3 to 4 mm cephalad and 3 to 4 mm lateral to the inferomedial aspect of the inferior articular surface of C2. The screw follows a steep trajectory, paralleling the C2 pars interarticularis. An appropriately steep trajectory ($\geq 40°$) is achieved by aligning the shaft of the drill or screwdriver with the tip of the T1

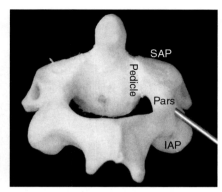

Figure 4   Posterior view photograph of C2. SAP = superior articular process of C2, IAP = inferior articular process of C2.

spinous process. This trajectory may be achieved by using percutaneous stab incisions that are approximately 2 cm lateral to the T1 spinous process. The screws are passed with 10° of medial angulation. Screw length is typically 16 mm, which will stop short of the C1-C2 facet joint. This short screw also usually stops short of the transverse foramen, thereby avoiding injury to the vertebral artery. When possible, a larger (4.0-mm) diameter screw is used to achieve increased pullout resistance because the screw is unicortical.

The C2 pedicle is defined as that portion of the C2 vertebra connecting the dorsal elements with the vertebral body, which is actually a narrow area between the vertebral body and the pars interarticularis (Figure 4). The trajectory of the C2 pedicle screw is different from that of the C2 pars screw, being shallow in relation to the axial plane and more medially angulated.[4] The entry point for C2 pedicle screw fixation is in the pars interarticularis, lateral to the superior margin of the C2 lamina, approximately 2 mm superior and 1 to 2 mm lateral to the entry point for the C2 pars interarticularis screw. The screw is placed with 15°

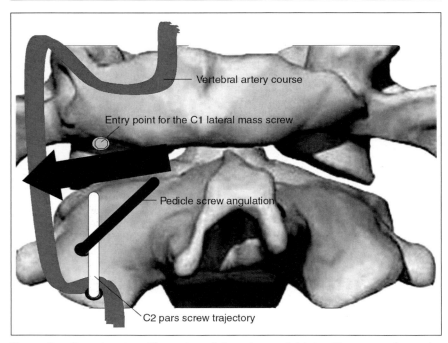

Figure 5 Posterior view illustration of the atlantoaxial joint. The arrow shows the C2 nerve root course.

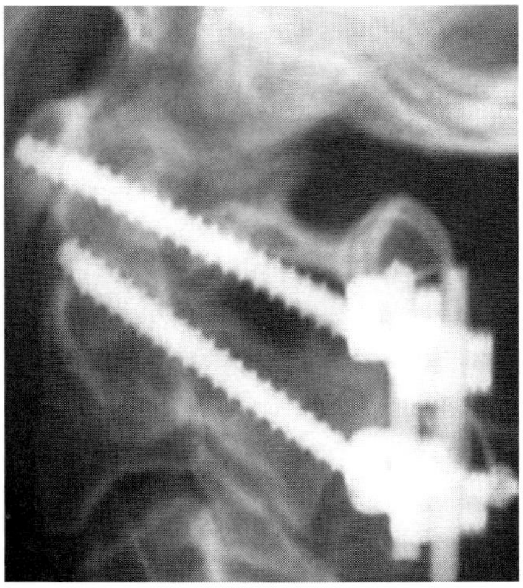

Figure 6 Lateral radiograph of a posterior atlantoaxial fixation construct with C1 lateral mass and C2 pedicle screws. Both screws are 4.0 mm in diameter and 40.0 mm in length.

to 25° of medial angulation, depending on the angulation of the pedicle when palpated by removing a small amount of ligamentum flavum. The thick medial wall of the C2 pedicle will help redirect the screw if necessary and prevent medial wall breakout. The entry point can be adjusted based on the degree of medial angulation of the pedicle as well as the rostrocaudal inclination of the pars interarticularis, which may be determined from the lateral fluoroscopic view. The entry point will generally be 3 to 4 mm lateral to the medial margin of the pars, which may be palpated with a curved spatula. C2 pedicle screws generally should be placed with a slight caudal-to-rostral inclination, which will point toward the ventral C2 body just below the base of the dens. This trajectory (20° up angle) allows safe bicortical purchase if desired and greater resistance to screw pullout. The trajectory of the C2 pedicle screw will be

medial to the C2 transverse foramen (Figure 5).

The fundamental problems with the C2 pars interarticularis screw are that it is short (14 to 18 mm) compared with the C2 pedicle screw (30 to 40 mm) and it carries the same vertebral artery injury risks as the C1-C2 transarticular screw. The C2 pedicle screw, by definition, is positioned into the C2 vertebral body and thus is much longer and biomechanically stronger than the pars interarticularis screw. Also, because it angles medially much more than the pars interarticularis screw, it is less likely to damage the vertebral artery. The pedicle screw also starts more cephalad than the pars interarticularis screw, and this entry point is most often above the vertebral artery as it courses from medial to lateral under the inferior articular process of C2. Because the pars interarticularis screw begins more caudally, its trajectory may take it close to the

underlying vertebral artery in its medial to lateral course. The ability to begin screw placement more cephalad is an advantage because the higher the screw starts, the more likely the vertebral artery has already passed underneath the starting point.

Arthrodesis

Finally, arthrodesis is performed. Posterior arthrodesis with sublaminar cable and interspinous bicortical autograft is preferred if the laminae of C1 and C2 are preserved. Otherwise, lateral arthrodesis is performed by carefully decorticating the exposed surfaces of the C1-C2 joints with a high-speed drill, and then packing cancellous iliac crest autograft into these joints. The rod is then positioned and fixed to the C1 lateral mass and C2 pedicle screws (Figure 6).

Extremely high fusion rates are achieved because of the stability of the segmental C1 and C2 screws, which are rigidly attached to the rods. Postoperative rigid external immobilization is not required. Because pseudarthrosis is rarely needed with this polyaxial screw/rod construct, autogenous iliac crest bone graft harvest is becoming less common. Decortication of the C1-C2 joint surfaces and packing with local bone graft results in a high rate of fusion; the morbidity of the iliac crest bone site is eliminated.

Discussion

This technique can achieve solid fixation of the C1 lateral mass and can be used in a variety of instrumentation constructs for varying indications. The most common indication for the use of C1 lateral mass screws is atlantoaxial instability. Although a variety of techniques exist to treat atlantoaxial instability, certain anatomic factors may preclude their application in specific situations. C1-C2 interspinous fusion techniques using either sublaminar cables or interlaminar clamps in combination with iliac crest autograft require the presence of intact posterior elements.[5,6] These techniques cannot be applied when the C1 arch or C2 laminae have been disrupted by trauma, neoplasm, or other pathologic processes, or when resection of these elements is necessary to achieve neural decompression. Also, rigid postoperative immobilization is required in a halo to achieve satisfactory fusion rates. Even when using the Brooks method of interspinous fusion, which is the most stable of all wire/cable constructs, all patients should be immobilized in a halo vest for 3 months.[7,8]

C1-C2 transarticular screw fixation is likewise precluded by a variety of factors.[2,6,9,10] In up to 20% of patients, a medially located or high-riding vertebral artery will preclude safe passage of C1-C2 transarticular screws unilaterally. In 3% of patients,

vertebral artery anatomy will preclude passage of screws bilaterally.[11,12] Irreducible C1-C2 subluxation will likewise preclude placement of C1-C2 transarticular screws. If C1 is displaced anterior to C2, the resulting trajectory of the transarticular screw is flatter (more horizontal), which jeopardizes the vertebral artery (the steeper the trajectory, the safer the vertebral artery).

Cervicothoracic kyphosis may preclude C1-C2 transarticular screw placement by obstructing the trajectory of the instruments used to insert the screws. Destruction or erosion of the osseous substrate for screw fixation by trauma, neoplasm, or other pathologic processes will similarly preclude transarticular screw placement. In these situations, occipitocervical fusion may be considered as an alternative means to treat atlantoaxial instability. Occipitocervical fusion may be avoided by using C1 lateral mass screws to achieve atlantocervical fixation. By avoiding occipitocervical fixation, range of motion at the atlanto-occipital joint is maintained, and potential morbidity from craniocervical malalignment is reduced. Clinical studies also have suggested that avoidance of occipitocervical fusion may decrease the incidence of delayed subaxial subluxation.[13,14] C1 lateral mass screws can achieve atlantocervical fixation in patients who have demonstrated various anatomic characteristics that precluded traditional methods of atlantoaxial fixation. The rigid internal fixation achieved with this technique allows immediate mobilization with a hard cervical collar, avoiding postoperative halo vest immobilization.

C1 lateral mass screws are extremely useful for occipitocervical fixation. C1 lateral mass screws provide additional fixation points for

occipitocervical constructs, increasing resistance to construct failure. This additional construct integrity is achieved without fusing additional cervical levels, thus preserving cervical motion segments. As the use of polyaxial screw-rod systems for occipitocervical fixation becomes more widespread, C1 lateral mass screws will be used more frequently because the rods and lateral offset connectors used in these systems will allow C1 screws to be easily incorporated into occipitocervical constructs.

All screw techniques in the posterior cervical spine are used "off label" for Food and Drug Administration purposes. Occipital screws and thoracic pedicle screws are considered class II Food and Drug Administration devices. Despite the off-label status of these screw techniques, many types of posterior cervical screws are routinely used by most spine surgeons and are the standard of care in many indications that require cervical stabilization.

In the future, the decision to use a C1 lateral mass screw construct without interspinous fusion or contralateral transarticular screw fixation should be considered on an individual basis in the context of the pathologic process causing instability, bone quality, and other comorbidities that influence bone fusion, as well as the potential morbidity of the alternative treatment, occipitocervical fusion. Larger studies with long-term follow-up will be necessary to determine the safety and efficacy of C1 lateral mass screw constructs.

Lynch and associates[15] evaluated an atlantoaxial construct with C1 lateral mass screws and C2 pedicle screws with and without supplemental interspinous cable and graft and compared this construct with atlantoaxial transarticular screws.

Melcher and associates[16] also performed a human biomechanical cadaveric study of posterior atlantoaxial fixation techniques in an odontoidectomy model. Screw techniques (transarticular and C1 lateral mass/C2 pedicle screw/rod construct) significantly decreased motion compared with all wire/cable techniques. There were no differences between screw techniques; however, the transarticular screw model was tested with a posterior C1-C2 cable, whereas the screw/rod construct was tested without the posterior cable. These findings suggest that C1 lateral mass screw constructs coupled with C2 pedicle screw/rod constructs provide a reasonable alternative to transarticular screws for achieving atlantoaxial stabilization.

Harms and Melcher[17] used a specially modified screw at C1 with an unthreaded proximal shaft to reduce the risk of greater occipital nerve irritation and screw breakage. Fiore and associates[18,19] used standard screws with threads along the entire shaft and did not observe any instances of occipital neuralgia or screw breakage, indicating that standard screws may be used at C1. The risk of greater occipital nerve irritation is low provided there is adequate space caudal to the C1 screw for passage of the nerve.

The risk of vertebral artery injury must always be assessed when placement of lateral mass screws, C2 pars interarticularis screws, C2 pedicle screws, or transarticular screws is planned. Vertebral artery injury has not been reported during placement of C1 screws. The surgeon must note that the trajectory of the C1 lateral mass screw is different from that of lateral mass screws placed in the subaxial cervical spine. Particularly important is that the C1 screw is placed with a slight medial angulation to avoid the vertebral artery laterally.

Summary
The placement of C1 lateral mass screws provides a useful alternative method to achieve atlantoaxial fixation when anatomic factors preclude the placement of atlantoaxial transarticular screws. This method achieves immediate rigid stabilization of the atlantoaxial joint and obviates the need for halo vest immobilization. This technique may be used in certain patients as an alternative to occipitocervical fusion and may also be used to increase construct stability when occipitocervical fixation is used. Placement of C1 lateral mass screws is a technically demanding procedure and should only be performed by surgeons who are highly experienced in the treatment of atlantoaxial instability and have an intimate understanding of the anatomy of the region. The uninitiated surgeon can minimize the possibility of complications during C1 lateral mass screw placement by first performing this procedure in a cadaveric setting. Additional biomechanical analysis of this technique should be performed to quantify the strength of constructs using C1 lateral mass screws compared with other fixation methods. Additional clinical studies should also be performed to determine the safety and efficacy of this technique.

References
1. Sasso RC, Jeanneret B, Fischer K, et al: Occipitocervical fusion with posterior plate and screw instrumentation: A long-term follow-up study. *Spine* 1994;19:2364-2368.
2. Reilly TM, Sasso RC, Hall PV: Atlantoaxial stabilization: Clinical comparison of posterior cervical wiring technique with transarticular screw fixation. *J Spinal Disord Tech* 2003;16:248-253.
3. Benzel EC: Anatomic consideration of C2 pedicle screw placement. *Spine* 1996;21:2301-2302.
4. Borne GM, Bedou GL, Pinaudeau M: Treatment of pedicular fractures of the axis: A clinical study and screw fixation technique. *J Neurosurg* 1984;60:88-93.
5. Dickman CA, Sonntag VK, Papadopoulos SM, et al: The interspinous method of posterior atlantoaxial arthrodesis. *J Neurosurg* 1991;74:190-198.
6. Farey ID, Nadkarni S, Smith N: Modified Gallie technique versus transarticular screw fixation in C1-C2 fusion. *Clin Orthop Relat Res* 1999;359:126-135.
7. Boden SD, Dodge LD, Bohlman HH, et al: Rheumatoid arthritis of the cervical spine: A long-term analysis with predictors of paralysis and recovery. *J Bone Joint Surg Am* 1993;75:1282-1297.
8. McCarron RF, Robertson WW: Brooks fusion for atlantoaxial instability in rheumatoid arthritis. *South Med J* 1988;81:474-476.
9. Dickman CA, Sonntag VK: Posterior C1-C2 Transarticular screw fixation for atlantoaxial arthrodesis. *Neurosurgery* 1998;43:275-281.
10. Haid RW, Subach BR, McLaughlin MR, et al: C1-C2 transarticular screw fixation for atlantoaxial instability: A 6-year experience. *Neurosurgery* 2001;49:65-70.
11. Madawi AA, Casey AT, Solanki GA, et al: Radiological and anatomical evaluation of the atlantoaxial transarticular screw fixation technique. *J Neurosurg* 1997;86:961-968.
12. Paramore CG, Dickman CA, Sonntag VK: The anatomical suitability of the C1-2 complex for transarticular screw fixation. *J Neurosurg* 1996;85:221-224.
13. Clark CR, Goetz DD, Menezes AH: Arthrodesis of the cervical spine in rheumatoid arthritis. *J Bone Joint Surg Am* 1989;71:381-392.
14. Kraus DR, Peppelman WC, Agarwal AK, et al: Incidence of subaxial subluxation in patients with generalized rheumatoid arthritis who had previous occipital cervical fusions. *Spine* 1991;16:S486-489.
15. Lynch JJ, Crawford NR, Chamberlain RH, Bartolomei JC, Sonntag VKH: Biomechanics of lateral mass/pedicle screw fixation at C1-2, in *Proceedings of the 2002 Annual Meeting of the American*

Academy of Neurologic Surgeons. Available at: http://www.aans.org/Library/Article.aspx?ArticleId=12334. Accessed July 17, 2006.

16. Melcher RP, Puttlitz CM, Kleinstueck FS, et al: Biomechanical testing of posterior atlantoaxial fixation techniques.

Spine 2002;27:2435-2440.

17. Harms J, Melcher RP: Posterior C1-C2 fusion with polyaxial screw and rod fixation. *Spine* 2001;26:2467-2471.

18. Fiore AJ, Haid RW, Rodts GE, et al: Atlantal lateral mass screws for posterior

spinal reconstruction: Technical note and case series. *Neurosurg Focus* 2002;12:E5.

19. Fiore AJ, Mummaneni PV, Haid RW, Rodts GE, Sasso RC: C1 lateral mass screws: Surgical nuances. *Tech Orthop* 2002;17:272-277.

Pedicle Screw Fixation (T1, T2, and T3)

Michael D. Daubs, MD

Yongjung J. Kim, MD

Lawrence G. Lenke, MD

Abstract

The indications for thoracic pedicle screw fixation have expanded over the past decade. Thoracic pedicle screws are now being used in the treatment of degenerative, traumatic, neoplastic, congenital, and developmental disorders. The pedicles of T1, T2, and T3 are typically large and ovoid in shape and amenable to pedicle screw fixation in most instances. The placement of thoracic pedicle screws requires knowledge of the topographic and deep bony anatomy of the thoracic spine as well as an appreciation of the surrounding visceral structures at risk. With strict adherence to the surgical techniques of insertion, thoracic pedicle screw fixation is a safe and effective method of stabilization. It offers several advantages over other forms of fixation, especially in the upper thoracic spine where the options are limited.

The use of thoracic pedicle screw fixation in patients requiring spinal surgery has expanded over the past decade. Most spinal surgeons currently consider the placement of pedicle screws into the lumbar spine routine. However, placement of pedicle screws into the thoracic spine is still considered a challenge, and the potential risk of major neurologic and vascular complications, although rare, has caused many surgeons to avoid the technique. Pedicle screws offer distinct advantages over other forms of fixation. Theoretically, pedicle screws provide a form of three-column fixation that allows for greater control in the sagittal, coronal, and rotational planes, resulting in greater stability. They are now commonly used in the treatment of degenerative and traumatic disorders. In the treatment of scoliosis, thoracic pedicle screws have improved the three-dimensional curve correction, decreased the rates of curve progression, and resulted in higher fusion rates.[1-7] Biomechanically, pedicle screws have been shown to provide stronger fixation when compared with hooks,[8] the more traditional form of fixation of the thoracic region.

Several clinical studies have been published evaluating the complications of thoracic screw insertion. The largest study reported a malposition rate of 1.5% and a neurologic complication rate of 0.8%.[5] Kim and associates[7] reported moderate cortical perforation of the pedicle in 6.2% of 3,204 thoracic screws placed, of which 1.7% violated the medial wall. Despite the perforations, there were no reported neurologic complications or need for revisions. At the senior author's institution, more than 10,000 thoracic pedicle screws have now been inserted as an alternative to wire and hook fixation with no neurologic, vascular, or visceral complications. With a thorough knowledge of the thoracic spine anatomy and the surrounding structures, pedicle screw fixation can be safely used.

Relevant Anatomy

In the thoracic spine, three anatomic characteristics of the pedicle affect the size and position of the screw: transverse pedicle diameter, angle of the pedicle trajectory, and length of the pedicle trajectory. These measurements vary throughout the

One or more of the authors or the departments with which they are affiliated have received something of value from a commercial or other party related directly or indirectly to the subject of this chapter.

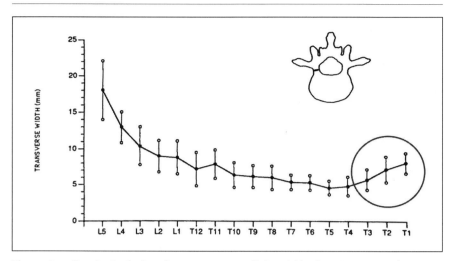

Figure 1 Graph displaying the transverse pedicle widths from T1 to L5. The T1-T3 pedicles are on average significantly wider in diameter than the midthoracic pedicles. (Reproduced with permission from Zindrick MR, Wiltse LL, Doornik A, et al: Analysis of the morphometric characteristics of the thoracic and lumbar pedicles. *Spine* 1987;12:160-166.)

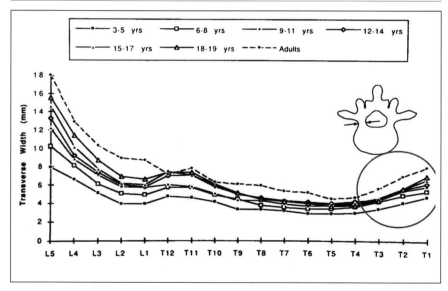

Figure 2 Graph displaying the mean transverse pedicle widths from pediatric age (3 to 5 years) to adulthood (> 20 years). The pedicle width increases with age until adulthood but throughout ages it remains consistently larger at T1, T2, and T3 than the pedicles in the midthoracic spine. (Reproduced with permission from Zindrick MR, Knight GW, Sartori MJ, et al: Pedicle morphology of the immature spine. *Spine* 2000;25:2726-2735.)

racic spine.[11] The average screw diameter used at T1-T3 is 6.0 mm. The pedicle wall is two to three times thicker on the medial side than on the lateral side at all levels.[12] The angle of the trajectory in the transverse plane is approximately 25° convergent for T1 and T2 and decreases to approximately 15° at T3 (Figure 3).[9-11,13] The trajectory in the sagittal angle is approximately 15° caudad.[9-11,13] The length of the pedicle trajectory varies with the age and size of the patient. In 3- to 5-year-old patients, the pedicle trajectory is approximately 22 mm and increases 70% to the adult length of approximately 36 mm.[11] Another important anatomic landmark is the distance from the dorsal lamina to the pedicle isthmus. A cadaver study has demonstrated this average distance to be 12 mm (YJ Kim, MD; LG Lenke, MD; G Cheh, MD; KD Riew, MD; Southampton, Bermuda, unpublished data presented at the 11th International Meeting on Advanced Spine Technologies, 2004).

Thoracic pedicle dimensions vary with each individual. In most patients, the pedicles are large enough for screw fixation, and screws are routinely used in pediatric as well as older adult patients. Even in patients with small pedicles, it has been shown that screws 80% to 115% of the size of the outer pedicle diameter can be safely inserted through gradual plastic deformation with a probe and bone tap[14] (S Suk, MD; JH Lee, MD; Boston MA, unpublished data presented at the 3rd Intermeeting of the Societe Internationale de Recherches Orthopedique et de Traumatologie, 1994). The use of pedicle screws in patients with scoliosis was initially believed to be too dangerous because of the abnormal anatomy. The pedicle morphol-

length of the thoracic spine. From T1 to T3, the pedicle width decreases fairly dramatically[9] (Figure 1). The width is approximately 8.0 mm at T1, 6.5 mm at T2, and 5.0 mm at T3.[9,10] In the immature spine, the pedicle widths are smaller and increase with age.[11] In the 3- to 5-year age group, the mean width is 4.8 mm at T1, 4.0 mm at T2, and 3.4 mm at T3 (Figure 2). The shape is consistently oval in the upper tho-

ogy in patients with scoliotic spines has now been extensively studied. No significant difference has been found when comparing scoliotic vertebrae and normal vertebrae in the thoracic spine in relation to the angle or length of the pedicle trajectory.[13] As the spine becomes more rotated in patients with severe deformity, there is no change in the angle of the pedicle trajectory to the corresponding vertebral body, but there is a change in spatial orientation to the floor. Therefore, although the surgeon has to adjust for the proper angle of insertion, the anatomic landmarks are constant. In adolescent patients with idiopathic scoliosis (average age, 15.5 years) who were evaluated with CT scans, no correlation of pedicle size to age, Risser grade, curve magnitude, or the amount of segmental axial rotation was reported.[15] There is a significant decrease in the width of the concave pedicles compared with the convex side in patients with thoracic scoliosis.[13]

Thoracic pedicles have recently

been morphologically classified. The system of classification is stratified on the basis of ease of pedicle screw insertion (Figure 4). A type A pedicle has a large cancellous channel, a type B pedicle has a small cancellous channel, a type C pedicle has a cortical channel, and a type D

pedicle has an absent channel (slit pedicle). In type C pedicles, intraosseous screw insertion is possible with gradual dilation with the pedicle probe and taps. In type D pedicles, screws are placed juxtapedicular along the lateral pedicle wall into the vertebral body (Fig-

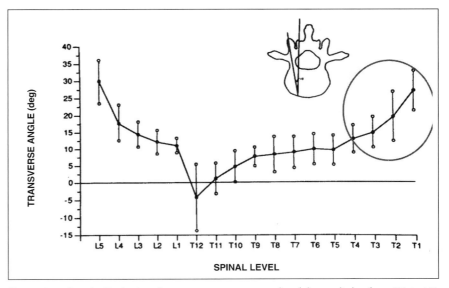

Figure 3   Graph displaying the mean transverse angle of the pedicles from T1 to L5. The angle is extremely convergent at T1 to T3. (Reproduced with permission from Zindrick MR, Wiltse LL, Doornik A, et al: Analysis of the morphometric characteristics of the thoracic and lumbar pedicles. *Spine* 1987;12:160-166.)

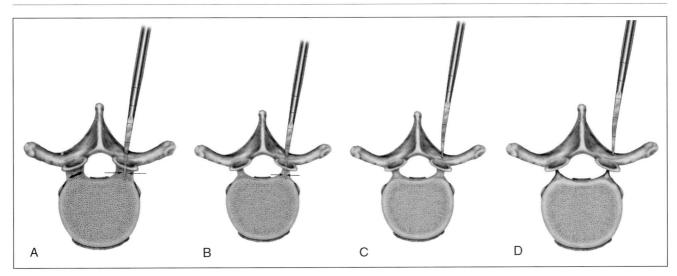

Figure 4   Illustration of the pedicle classification system. **A,** Type A has a large cancellous channel. **B,** Type B has a small cancellous channel. **C,** Type C has a thin cortical channel with absent cancellous bone. **D,** Type D has an absent pedicle channel (slit pedicle). The level of difficulty of pedicle screw insertion increases from type A to D.

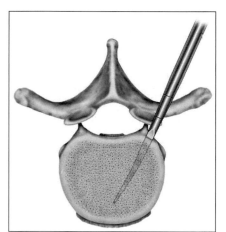

Figure 5 Illustration of a type D pedicle in which the pedicle probe has been inserted along the lateral wall of the pedicle and into the vertebral body in a juxtapedicular fashion.

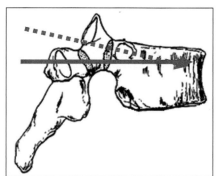

Figure 6 Illustration of the anatomic (*dashed line*) and the straightforward (*solid line*) trajectories for thoracic pedicle insertion.

ure 5). Most upper thoracic pedicles (T1, T2, and T3) will be either type A or B pedicles. However, if scoliosis is present, the concave pedicles may be type C or D.

Structures at Risk

The placement of pedicle screws in the thoracic spine requires a discrete knowledge of the three-dimensional anatomy. Understanding the surface landmarks as well as the deep bony anatomy is essential to correctly identify the pedicle entrance and the proper insertion trajectory. The "safe zone" around the pedicle is extremely small. There is no epidural space between the thoracic pedicle and the dura. The average distance from the pedicle to the nerve root has been determined to be approximately 2.0 mm superiorly and inferiorly at T1 and T2 and 2.8 mm at T3.[16] However, the nerve roots in the thoracic spine exit more horizontally at high angles (120° at T1) compared with the lumbar spine, where they run longitudinally along the medial pedicle wall.[16] Medially, the spinal cord is insulated by the

epidural and subarachnoid spaces, which may explain why breaches in the medial pedicle wall are rarely symptomatic except in instances of gross violation with severe encroachment of the spinal canal. Directly lateral to the pedicle in the upper thoracic spine is the rib. Beyond the rib head is the pleural cavity. Structures anterior to the vertebral body at T1, T2, and T3 include the esophagus, thoracic duct, and sympathetic ganglion. The aorta is present in 30% of patients anteriorly on the left at T3.[17]

Technique

Several pedicle screw insertion techniques have been described: freehand, fluoroscopically-assisted, computer-assisted, and open lamina.[5,6,18-25] The computer-assisted techniques have been developed to improve the accuracy of screw placement, but their ease of use is variable.[19-24] The open-lamina technique has been shown to also improve accuracy. The best technique combines accuracy and ease of use and uses methods and instruments familiar to most spinal surgeons. The freehand technique satisfies these requirements and for this reason is the preferred technique.

Freehand Technique

The freehand technique is based on the insertion techniques used in the lumbar spine. It uses the same instruments (pedicle probe and pedicle sound) used for lumbar pedicle screw insertion and also relies on the knowledge of anatomic landmarks. It is based on three important principles: (1) the correct anatomic starting point, (2) the correct trajectory, and (3) the intraosseous feel while probing the pathway down the pedicle into the vertebral body. It requires a thorough knowledge of the topical landmarks of the pedicle and the underlying bony anatomy to extrapolate the proper three-dimensional pathway. Two approaches have been described: the anatomic approach and the straightforward approach (Figure 6). With the straightforward approach, the sagittal trajectory of the screw parallels the superior end plate of the vertebral body (Figure 6). In the anatomic approach, the screw trajectory follows the anatomic axis of the pedicle, which is 15° caudad in the sagittal plane. The straightforward approach has a 39% increase in maximum insertional technique and a 27% increase in pullout strength compared with the anatomic approach.[26] The increase in fixation strength with the straightforward approach is believed to be a result of improved engagement of the superior cortex of the pedicle and compact cancellous bone along the superior end plate of the vertebral body. The straightforward approach is recommended for most patients, whereas the anatomic approach should be reserved for salvage purposes only.[26]

The technique begins with a meticulous exposure of the posterior elements. The spine is exposed to the tips of the transverse processes bilaterally. The facet joints are then cleared of soft tissue using a combination of cautery and curettage. With an osteotome, the inferior 5 mm of the inferior facet is removed, and the exposed cartilage is scraped from the superior facet surface. The inferior portion of the facet is not removed from the most cephalad level of the construct to avoid disruption of the facet joint.

The starting points for the pedicles at T1, T2, and T3 are shown in Figure 7. At all three levels, the cephalad-caudad starting point is the midpoint of the transverse process. The mediolateral starting point is slightly medial to the lateral border of the superior facet. The more lateral starting point allows for the more convergent transverse trajectory of the pedicles at T1, T2, and T3. Once the starting point is located, a high-speed cortical burr is used to create a posterior cortical breach of approximately 5 mm in depth. A "blush" may be seen that indicates entrance into the cancellous bone at the base of the pedicle; it may not be seen with smaller type B or type C pedicles because of the limited cancellous space. The thoracic gearshift probe (2-mm blunt-tipped, slightly curved) (Figure 8) is placed at the base of the pedicle and gently used to search for the cancellous "soft spot" at the entrance of the pedicle. The gearshift is initially pointed laterally to avoid medial wall perforation. The pressure used for the probe is slightly greater than what is typically used in the lumbar spine. The small 2-mm tip allows the probe to slide down the cancellous channel of the pedicle even if it is extremely small. With extremely small type C pedicles, the ventral surface of the lamina can be gently palpated while sloping down into the pedicle in a funnel-like fashion.

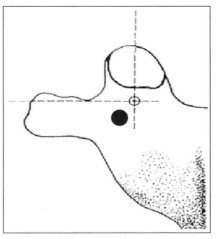

Figure 7 Illustration of the starting point (*black dot*) for insertion of thoracic pedicle screws into T1, T2, and T3. The horizontal dashed line represents the superior edge of the transverse process. The vertical dashed line represents the midpoint of the facet joint. The cephalad-caudad landmark is the midpoint of the transverse process. The mediolateral landmark is just lateral to the midpoint (vertical dashed line) of the facet joint. The lateral starting point allows for the angle of convergence of the pedicles at T1-T3. A starting point medial to the midpoint of the superior facet should be avoided.

This is a helpful step in identifying the pedicle entrance in small pedicles and is frequently used as a confirmatory step for all thoracic pedicles. Once the probe is started, it is inserted 15 to 20 mm just beyond the medially located spinal canal (Figure 9). The gearshift is then removed and the tip is then pointed medially and carefully placed into the base of the hole and advanced 20 to 25 mm. The probe is then rotated 180° to widen the channel for the pedicle screw. It is important to feel bone the entire length of the pedicle and into the body. The probing should be smooth, and consistent pressure should be applied. Any sudden advancement suggests a pedicle wall or vertebral body viola-

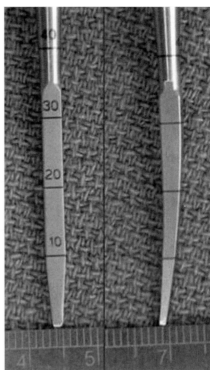
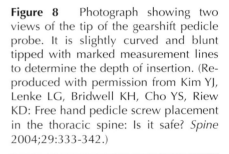

Figure 8 Photograph showing two views of the tip of the gearshift pedicle probe. It is slightly curved and blunt tipped with marked measurement lines to determine the depth of insertion. (Reproduced with permission from Kim YJ, Lenke LG, Bridwell KH, Cho YS, Riew KD: Free hand pedicle screw placement in the thoracic spine: Is it safe? *Spine* 2004;29:333-342.)

tion. The anterior and lateral cortices of the vertebral bodies are weak and can be easily penetrated by the probe. If a sudden advancement does occur, it should be evaluated immediately to avoid complications and possibly salvage the pedicle for fixation.

The gearshift probe is then removed, and the hole is visualized to ensure that only blood and no cerebrospinal fluid is present. Excessive bleeding may indicate a medial wall perforation and secondary epidural bleeding. The flexible ball-tipped sounding probe is then used to palpate the four walls of the pedicle

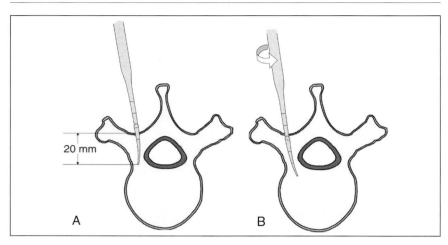

Figure 9 Illustration showing the technique for insertion of the pedicle probe. **A,** The probe is initially started with the curve pointed laterally until it reaches a depth of 20 mm. **B,** It is then reinserted and directed medially into the pedicle and into the vertebral body. (Reproduced with permission from Kim YJ, Lenke LG, Bridwell KH, Cho YS, Riew KD: Free hand pedicle screw placement in the thoracic spine: Is it safe? *Spine* 2004;29:333-342.)

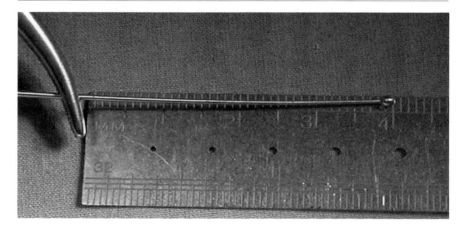

Figure 10 Photograph of the pedicle sounding device. Once the pedicle has been successfully probed, the sounding device is inserted to determine the depth of the pedicle tract and appropriate screw length. (Reproduced with permission from Kim YJ, Lenke LG, Bridwell KH, Cho YS, Riew KD: Free hand pedicle screw placement in the thoracic spine: Is it safe? *Spine* 2004;29:333-342.)

(medial, lateral, superior, and inferior) and the anterior floor. While probing with the sound, the proximal 10 to 15 mm of the channel should be carefully palpated, which is the area of the pedicle isthmus and the location of most pedicle wall perforations. If a perforation is identified, it is possible to carefully redirect the pedicle probe down a new path. If the pedicle is not salvageable, bone wax is placed in the hole to avoid bleeding.

Next, the pedicle tract is tapped with a tap that is 1.0 mm smaller in diameter than the planned screw diameter. If there is resistance to the tap, a tap that is one size smaller should be used to make another attempt. Once tapped, the sounding probe is again

used to palpate the bony ridges of the four walls of the pedicle and the floor. With the sounding probe in position at the proper depth, a hemostat is clamped on the probe at the corresponding entrance of the pedicle tract, marking the appropriate length for the screw (Figure 10). The length of the marked probe is compared with the screw length to ensure accuracy of length. The screw is then inserted slowly by hand using the same trajectory as the pedicle probe that was inserted. The slow insertion allows for the viscoelastic expansion of the pedicle walls. At T1, T2, and T3, the typical screw diameter used is 5.0 to 6.0 mm, although larger screws can be placed depending on the individual pedicle size. The typical length of screw used at these levels is 25 to 35 mm.

There are unique challenges of proximal thoracic pedicle screw insertion. Because the upper level of the thoracic spine is kyphotic, the kyphotic angle can make it difficult to gain the correct sagittal trajectory without interference from the skull and the paraspinal muscles. The lateral wound and muscles can also interfere with the convergent trajectory (25°) needed for screw insertion in the upper thoracic spine. Placing halo skull traction with the patient's neck in a slightly flexed position can reduce the kyphotic angle and ease screw placement.

The transition from cervical to thoracic instrumentation can also be problematic, depending on the system used. Lateral mass screws are typically used at C6 and above, and pedicle screws are typically used at C7 and below. The transition is from the more mediolateral mass fixation points to the laterally placed pedicle screws of the upper thoracic spine. It is best to place the rod medially in the upper thoracic spine. The typical cer-

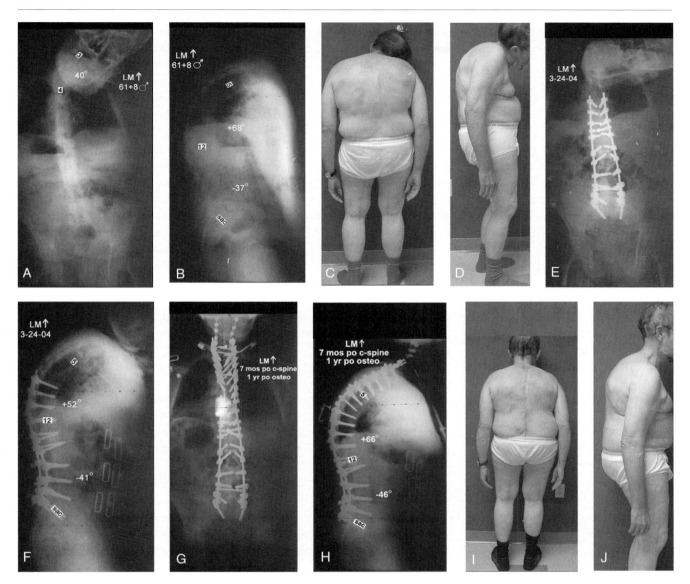

Figure 11 Preoperative AP **(A)** and lateral **(B)** radiographs and photographs **(C** and **D)** of a patient with ankylosing spondylitis with a chronic kyphotic deformity of the thoracolumbar spine secondary to a chronic L1 fracture; the patient also had a severe angular deformity of the cervical spine. Postoperative AP **(E)** and lateral **(F)** radiographs show that the thoracolumbar deformity was initially corrected with a pedicle subtraction osteotomy at L2 followed by a posterior arthrodesis with instrumentation from T9 to the sacrum using a 5.5-mm rod. The patient was placed in cervical traction following the thoracolumbar procedure and 5 months later the cervical deformity was addressed. AP **(G)** and lateral **(H)** radiographs and photographs **(I** and **J)** obtained 1 year postoperatively show that lateral mass fixation was used in the cervical spine with a 3.2-mm rod, which attached to a 4.5-mm rod in the upper thoracic spine and finally into the previously placed 5.5-mm rod.

vical rod construct is 3.5 mm, and the typical upper thoracic rod construct is 4.5 mm to 6.35 mm. The ideal transition is from a 3.5-mm rod in the cervical spine to a 4.5-mm rod in the proximal thoracic spine to a 5.5-mm rod in the lower thoracic spine (Fig-

ure 11). Tapered and screw-in rods are available for this purpose. Dominoes are helpful, but they can be bulky and can impede arthrodesis. If dominoes are used bilaterally, they should be placed at different levels to reduce the chance of pseudarthrosis.

After screw placement, plain radiography or fluoroscopic imaging should be used to assess screw position. Evaluation of thoracic screw position with plain radiography has been extensively studied and has been found to be accurate when compared with CT.[27] Currently, 1% to 2% of pedicle screws are readjusted or removed as a result of intraoperative radiographic findings. It can be difficult to adequately image the upper thoracic spine. Proper preoperative positioning and skull traction both can aid this process.

Pedicle Salvage

If a pedicle breach is found while probing with the sounding device, the pedicle can be salvaged by redirecting the pedicle probe and changing the insertion trajectory. The same degree of caution should be used as the probe is inserted and advanced. Once the new tract is successfully made, the sound is again used to assess the floor and the walls of the new tract. A Kirschner wire can be used to direct a cannulated tap down the new tract if available. If there is any question as to the integrity of the anterior wall of the vertebral body, a Kirschner wire should not be used to avoid advancement of the wire beyond the body wall. After tapping, a screw is carefully directed down the new trajectory. If this technique is unsuccessful, changing to the anatomic trajectory (Figure 6) and repeating the steps of insertion is another option. One study reported that the anatomic trajectory achieved 62% of maximal insertional torque during the salvage of a failed/violated pedicle and provided adequate fixation in the salvage situation.[26]

If the pedicle cannot be salvaged, juxtapedicular screw placement is possible (Figure 5). The starting point is slightly more lateral on the transverse process, and the medial angulation is greater. The pedicle probe is aimed along the lateral wall of the pedicle and aimed medially into the vertebral body at the junction of the pedicle and vertebral body. The purchase is weaker, but

still stronger than hook fixation. If screws cannot be placed and the lamina is intact, hooks or sublaminar wires can be used.

Complications

There are few published reports on complications associated with the use of thoracic pedicle screws. Suk and associates[5] reported their experience with the placement of 4,600 thoracic screws. Using plain AP and lateral radiographic analysis, 1.5% of the thoracic screws were determined to be malpositioned. The malpositioning was lateral in 27% of instances, medial in 6%, superior in 18%, and inferior in 49%. There was one instance of neurologic injury with transient paraparesis resulting from a medial pedicle wall violation. Other reported complications included pedicle fracture (0.24%), screw loosening (0.76%), and infections (1.9%).

Liljenqvist and associates[3] assessed the placement of 120 thoracic pedicle screws using CT. The overall rate of cortical penetration was 25%, with 8.3% of the screws penetrating medially, 14.2% penetrating laterally, and 2.5% penetrating inferiorly. There were no neurologic complications reported. Three screws placed laterally were found to be in close proximity to the aorta.

Kim and associates[6] reported on the safety and reliability of the freehand technique as described previously. More than 3,200 screws were placed by two surgeons and random CT was used to evaluate the placement of 577 screws. Of these, more than 250 were placed at the T1, T2, and T3 level. When evaluating all of the screws placed, 36 (6.9%) were inserted with moderate cortical perforation of which 9 (1.8%) were medial. There were no neurologic, vascular, or visceral complications reported at up to 10-year follow-up.

A few case reports have been published of vascular injuries related to thoracic pedicle screws. Heini and associates[28] reported a case of fatal cardiac tamponade resulting from an injury to the right coronary artery by a Kirschner wire used during screw insertion. Papin and associates[29] reported the unusual clinical symptoms of abdominal pain, mild lower extremity weakness, tremor, thermoalgic discrimination loss, and imbalance related to spinal cord compression from a medially placed thoracic pedicle screw. The symptoms resolved after the screw was removed.

Complication Avoidance

The experience with lumbar pedicle screw placement has shown that most complications occur during the initial learning phase, but dramatically decrease as surgical experience improves.[30] Thoracic screw insertion is no different. The key to avoiding major complications is to use the most familiar and comfortable technique of insertion consistent with the surgeon's personal training. Regardless of the specific method used, there are several key steps to reducing complications. Obtaining intraoperative radiographs on the operating room table is important. AP and lateral radiographs provide an accurate, on-table position of the vertebrae, especially in the sagittal plane. Meticulous exposure of the bony landmarks of the posterior elements and a blood-free surface are also important. By exposing the transverse process, the lamina, the pars interarticularis, and the base of the superior articular process, the entrance point of the pedicle can be accurately identified. Expert knowledge of the topographic anatomic landmarks is essential to understanding the correct three-dimensional trajectory into the pedicle and ensuring accurate placement. Once the screws are inserted, plain radiographs or fluoroscopic images should be obtained to ensure intraosseous placement.

The freehand technique as described previously relies on well-learned methods used in the lumbar spine. The instruments for pedicle probing, tapping, and sounding are the same, as is the reliance on topographic landmarks. With this technique, few major complications have been reported, and the rate of malpositioning is low.

Summary

Pedicle screw fixation in the upper thoracic spine is a safe and effective form of stabilization. It offers advantages over other forms of fixation in the treatment of a variety of spinal disorders. The technique requires expert knowledge of the surface and deep anatomy of the thoracic spine and a thorough awareness of the possible pitfalls. With strict adherence to the surgical methods of insertion, the complication rates are low and similar to those for other forms of fixation.

References

1. Suk SI, Lee CK, Kim WJ, Chung YJ, Park YB: Segmental pedicle screw fixation in the treatment of thoracic idiopathic scoliosis. *Spine* 1995;20:1399-1405.

2. Hamill CL, Lenke LG, Bridwell KH, Chapman MP, Blanke K, Baldus C: The use of pedicle screw fixation to improve correction in the lumbar spine of patients with idiopathic scoliosis: Is it warranted? *Spine* 1996;21:1241-1249.

3. Liljenqvist UR, Halm HF, Link TM: Pedicle screw instrumentation of the thoracic spine in idiopathic scoliosis. *Spine* 1997;22:2239-2245.

4. Halm H, Niemeyer T, Link T, Liljenqvist U: Segmental pedicle screw instrumentation in idiopathic thoracolumbar and lumbar scoliosis. *Eur Spine J* 2000;9:192-197.

5. Suk Si, Kim WJ, Lee SM, Kim JH, Chung ER, Lee JH: Thoracic pedicle screw fixation in spinal deformities: Are they really safe? *Spine* 2001;26:2049-2057.

6. Kim YJ, Lenke LG, Bridwell KH, Cho YS, Riew KD: Free hand pedicle screw placement in the thoracic spine: Is it safe? *Spine* 2004;29:333-342.

7. Kim YJ, Lenke LG, Cho SK, Bridwell KH, Sides B, Blanke K: Comparative analysis of pedicle screw versus hook instrumentation in posterior spinal fusion of adolescent idiopathic scoliosis. *Spine* 2004;29:2040-2048.

8. Hackenberg L, Link T, Liljenqvist U: Axial and tangential fixation strength of pedicle screws versus hooks in the thoracic spine in relation to bone mineral density. *Spine* 2002;27:937-942.

9. Zindrick MR, Wiltse LL, Doornik A, et al: Analysis of the morphometric characteristics of the thoracic and lumbar pedicles. *Spine* 1987;12:160-166.

10. Stanescu S, Ebraheim NA, Yeasting R, et al: Morphometric evaluation of the cervico-thoracic junction. *Spine* 1994;19:2082-2088.

11. Zindrick MR, Knight GW, Sartori MJ, et al: Pedicle morphology of the immature spine. *Spine* 2000;25:2726-2735.

12. Kothe R, O'Holleran JD, Liu W, Panjabi MM: Internal architecture of the thoracic pedicle: An anatomical study. *Spine* 1996;21:264-270.

13. Parent S, Labelle H, Skalli W, de Guise J: Thoracic pedicle morphometry in vertebrae from scoliotic spines. *Spine* 2004;29:239-248.

14. Misenhimer GR, Peek RD, Wiltse LL, Rothman SL, Widell EH Jr: Anatomic analysis of pedicle cortical and cancellous diameter as related to screw size. *Spine* 1989;14:367-372.

15. O'Brien MF, Lenke LG, Mardjetko S, et al: Pedicle morphology, in thoracic adolescent idiopathic scoliosis. *Spine* 2000;25:2285-2293.

16. Ebraheim NA, Jabaly G, Rongming X, Yesting RA: Anatomic relations of the thoracic pedicle to the adjacent neural structures. *Spine* 1997;22:1553-1557.

17. Bailey AS, Stanescu S, Yeasting RA, et al: Anatomic relationships of the cervicothoracic junction. *Spine* 1995;20:1431-1439.

18. Belmont PJ, Klemme WR, Dhawan A, et al: In vivo accuracy of thoracic pedicle screws. *Spine* 2001;26:2340-2346.

19. Kim KD, Johnson PJ, Bloch BS, et al: Computer assisted thoracic pedicle screw placement: An in vitro feasibility study. *Spine* 2001;26:360-364.

20. Amiot LP, Labelle H, De Guise JA, et al: Computer-assisted pedicle screw fixation: A feasibility study. *Spine* 1995;20:1208-1212.

21. Amiot LP, Lang K, Putsier M, et al: Comparative results between conventional and computer assisted pedicle screw installation in the thoracic, lumbar and sacral spine. *Spine* 2000;25:606-614.

22. Choi WW, Breen BA, Levi AD: Computer-assisted fluoroscopic targeting system for pedicle screw insertion. *Neurosurgery* 2000;47:872-878.

23. Kothe R, Matthias Strauss J, Deuretzbacher G, Hemmi T, Lorenzen M, Wiesner L: Computer navigation of parapedicular screw fixation in the thoracic spine: A cadaver study. *Spine* 2001;26:E496-E501.

24. Youkilis AS, Quint DJ, McGillicuddy JE, et al: Stereotactic navigation for placement of pedicle screw in the thoracic spine. *Neurosurgery* 2001;48:771-778.

25. Xu R, Ebraheim NA, Ou Y, Yeasting RA: Anatomic consideration of pedicle screw placement in the thoracic spine: Roy-Camille technique versus open lamina technique. *Spine* 1998;23:1065-1068.

26. Lehman RA, Kuklo TR: Use of the anatomic trajectory for thoracic pedicle screw salvage after failure/violation using the straight-forward technique: A biomechanical analysis. *Spine* 2003;28:2072-2077.

27. Kim YJ, Lenke LG, Cheh G, Riew KD: Evaluation of pedicle screw placement in the deformed spine using intraoperative plain radiographs: A comparison with computerized tomography. *Spine* 2005;30:2084-2088.

28. Heini P, Scholl E, Wyler D, et al: Fatal cardiac tamponade associated with posterior spinal instrumentation: A case report. *Spine* 1998;23:2226-2230.

29. Papin P, Arlet V, Marchesi D, et al: Unusual presentation of spinal cord compression related to misplaced pedicle screws in thoracic scoliosis. *Eur Spine J* 1999;8:156-159.

30. Gertzbein SD, Robbins SE: Accuracy of pedicular screw placement in vivo. *Spine* 1990;15:11-14.

Image Guidance in Spinal Surgery

D. Greg Anderson, MD

Abstract

Image guidance is a rapidly developing surgical technology that allows intraoperative navigation of surgical instruments relative to imaging studies. This technology has the potential to increase the safety, accuracy, and efficiency of certain procedures in spinal surgery. Currently the procedures most applicable to the use of image guidance techniques include the placement of spinal implants, minimal access spinal surgery techniques, and complex osteotomies and spinal arthroplasty. Several types of image guidance systems are currently available, each with certain advantages and disadvantages that must be understood by the operating surgeon. In the future, it is likely that the use of image guidance technology will increase in the field of spinal surgery as image guidance systems become more efficient and less expensive.

Image guidance is a high-tech system of sensors and computers that allows the surgeon to define the location of surgical instruments relative to anatomic landmarks on imaging studies. In its most common form, image guidance registers the positions of fixed markers (fiducials) relative to imaged anatomy and allows real-time tracking of navigated instruments. The navigated instruments are registered in three-dimensional space by a computer and a series of tracking sensors. Because the spine has complex anatomy and because the margin of error is low when performing invasive procedures, image guidance technology is ideal for use in spinal surgery. There are several theoretic benefits to the use of image guidance when performing spinal surgery. The most significant benefit is the potential for increased accuracy and safety when performing invasive procedures.[1-5] However, other benefits include reduction of exposure to ionizing radiation to the patient and surgical team, the potential to perform less invasive procedures, and the ability to follow the position of instruments in multiple planes (images) without the use of intraoperative fluoroscopy.[6] Certain highly technical instrumentation techniques are ideal for image guidance, such as the placement of C1-C2 transarticular screws, because the implant must be placed in a small corridor between critical structures.[7] Image guidance can be invaluable for placement of instrumentation during revision procedures where the normal anatomic landmarks may be absent or obscured.[4,8] Ideally, image guidance should allow a more efficient procedure to be performed, although with the current generation of image guidance systems, this goal is not always achieved.

Although in existence for several years, image guidance systems have not achieved uniform acceptance because of several perceived deficits associated with their use during spinal surgery. First, the equipment is complex, often requiring specially trained personnel to set up and run the equipment. Second, the use of image guidance may in some instances add time and complexity to an already long and tedious spinal procedure. Third, some systems have been perceived as unreliable because imaging data are occasionally erroneous.[6] Finally, image guidance systems are costly and not always economically justifiable in the current health care environment. Despite these perceived limitations, image guidance systems are constantly improving and significant strides have been made in overcoming these potential drawbacks. In many centers, image guidance has become an invaluable aspect of spinal procedures.

Specific Applications of Image Guidance in Spinal Surgery

There are many potential uses of imaging guidance in spinal surgery.

Table 1
Common Sites for the Attachment of the Reference Array During Image-Guided Spinal Surgery

Spinous process

Iliac crest

Pedicle (via a pin, needle, or screw)

Vertebral body (useful in anterior spinal surgery)

Fixed retractor

Skull clamp

Instrumentation construct

One of the most commonly reported indications is for the placement of implants, particularly pedicle screws,[1,3,9,10] facet screws, and trans-articular screws.[7] Using image guidance to define the starting point and trajectory for an implant, the surgeon is provided with useful data that can augment normal anatomic topography. Image guidance is also applicable to percutaneous procedures such as vertebroplasty and kyphoplasty. Image guidance is useful in revision surgery, particularly when a fusion of the posterior elements has been performed, completely obscuring the normal anatomic landmarks with bone.[8,11] Image guidance can be used during decompressive procedures such as a cervical corpectomy where the neural structures must be decompressed without violating the foramen transversarium and the vertebral artery.[4,11] In patients with complex deformity, such as those requiring an osteotomy, image guidance has the potential to assist in the execution of the preoperative plan in terms of the exact angle and starting point for the bony cuts. In the relatively new field of artificial disk replacement, image guidance has the potential to ensure that the implant is placed and aligned correctly, a requirement that is crucial for the device to function correctly.

Components of an Image Guidance System

Image guidance systems include the following components: a computer, a monitor, a tracking system (optical camera or electromagnetic sensor), fiducial references (reference array), and trackable instruments. The system works by attaching the fiducial references to the patient's anatomic landmarks, close to the area of navigation (Table 1). Images are obtained by the computer and displayed on the monitor. Next, the images are calibrated to the position of the fiducial references. Instruments with attached trackers or sensors are then able to be visualized on the monitor relative to the images in the computer system.

The exact form of the tracking can vary because there are competing technologies for instrument tracking.[12] The two most commonly encountered technologies used to study the spine are electro-optical tracking, where a camera optically tracks the position of fiducial references relative to one another geometrically; and electromagnetic tracking, where a sensor creates a surrounding magnetic field that allows the position and alignment of the tracked instrument to be determined. Each technology has certain advantages and disadvantages. For instance, the electro-optical systems are highly accurate but rely on the line of sight between the camera and tracked objects; the line of sight can be blocked by an object such as the surgeon's hand during navigation. Although the electromagnetic systems do not rely on line-of-sight tracking, they are generally confined to a limited navigatable volume around the sensor where tracking can take place because of the decay of the magnetic field strength as the distance from the sensor increases.

These systems are affected by the overall metallic "burden" that distorts the magnetic field and the accuracy of instrument tracking.

Classification of Image Guidance Systems for the Spine

One method for classifying image guidance systems is by the images that are used for tracking during the procedure. Currently, most systems rely on a combination of fluoroscopic or CT images.[3,6] Several navigation systems that rely on MRI are being developed.

Fluoronavigation, perhaps the simplest form of image guidance, uses fluoroscopic images obtained from a C-arm image intensifier at the time of surgery.[1,5] This technique allows the surgeon to track the position of instruments relative to the fluoroscopic images during the procedure. When CT images are used, the images must normally be "loaded" into the image guidance system computer before the procedure. At the time of the procedure, the CT images must be calibrated to the patient's anatomy in the surgical position. One method to calibrate the images is to "touch" points on the patient's anatomy that correspond to points on the imaging study with a calibrated instrument. Another method is to allow the computer to use data obtained from orthogonal fluoroscopic images to define the position and orientation of the patient's anatomy. Some systems use a special C-arm that moves radially around the patient during the operation, taking multiple images that can then be used to create multiplanar reconstructed views of the patient's anatomy, much like a CT scan. Navigation can then be done using the reformatted images in a variety of planes.

Keys to Successful Use of Image Guidance for Spinal Surgery

To successfully use image guidance in spinal surgery, it is first critical to understand the system that is being used. Each system has certain nuances that must be understood to ensure accurate and efficient use of the equipment. Certain tips common to essentially all image guidance systems should be discussed.

The equipment should be set up to allow an ergonomic operation (Figure 1). All systems occupy some space around the operating field and may interfere with the normal positioning of items in the room. Proper positioning of the equipment is important to allow it to function well (line of sight can be limited with some systems) and prevent it from impeding other members of the operating team.

The need to obtain clear images when using a fluoroscopy-based navigation system cannot be over-emphasized. The images must clearly show the anatomic landmarks that the surgeon will be using to allow successful navigation. If fluoroscopic images are to be obtained during surgery, the surgeon must ensure that a radiolucent table is used. Because images are difficult to obtain from certain patients, such as those who are obese or those with severe osteopenia, alternative techniques may be preferable. This limitation should be anticipated when planning an operation. To facilitate accurate intraoperative navigation, the surgeon must take time to align the images well and make sure that the navigated portion of the image is well centered in the field of vision to avoid the parallax phenomenon. Navigation from multiple simultaneous images appears to increase the accuracy of the navigation step.[6]

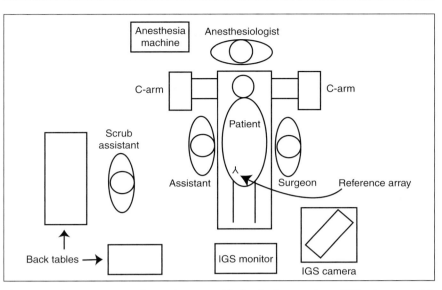

Figure 1 Common setup for an image-guided spinal procedure. IGS = image guidance system.

The fiducial references should be securely attached to the bony anatomy of the spine in a location that is close to the site of navigation and yet unlikely to be displaced or bumped. If the fiducial reference array gets bumped or becomes dislodged, the accuracy of navigation will be severely compromised. There are many potential sites to which a surgeon might attach the fiducial reference array depending on the nature of the surgery. Some common attachment sites include the spinous process, the pedicle,[4] the iliac crest, a skull clamp, or a vertebral body pin.[11,13] Whatever the site chosen, it is important to verify the accuracy of navigation frequently by placing the tip of a reference instrument on a known anatomic landmark.[4]

Summary

Image guidance is a helpful adjuvant to modern spinal procedures. Image guidance techniques have improved substantially since the first generation of image guidance technology. However, because image guidance continues to be highly technical, the surgeon must be prepared to learn the system being used. The amount of preoperative planning must be increased and additional setup time will be required, especially during the early portion of the learning curve. To ensure a smooth-running procedure, the equipment must be well positioned in the room and good quality images must be obtained if using fluoroscopy as an imaging modality for navigation. The fiducial references must be securely attached to the patient's anatomy at a site that is close enough to the navigated site to allow accurate navigation, yet placed at a distance to prevent "bumping" the fiducial reference during the procedure. The accuracy of navigation should be checked frequently during the procedure, by touching the tip of a reference instrument to a known anatomic landmark or by comparing the virtual images to an intraoperative image (such as a fluoroscopy image or radiograph). Image guidance systems can improve the accuracy of spinal surgical procedures and allow increased comfort in performing highly technical procedures including revision surgery.

References

1. Holly LT, Foley KT: Three-dimensional fluoroscopy-guided percutaneous thoracolumbar pedicle screw placement: Technical note. *J Neurosurg* 2003;99(suppl):324-329.

2. Reasoner DK, Warner DS, Todd MM, Hunt SW, Kirchner J: A comparison of anesthetic techniques for awake intubation in neurosurgical patients. *J Neurosurg Anesthesiol* 1995;7:94-99.

3. Resnick DK: Prospective comparison of virtual fluoroscopy to fluoroscopy and plain radiographs for placement of lumbar pedicle screws. *J Spinal Disord Tech* 2003;16:254-260.

4. Holly LT, Bloch O, Obasi C, Johnson JP: Frameless stereotaxy for anterior spinal procedures. *J Neurosurg* 2001;95(suppl): 196-201.

5. Foley KT, Simon DA, Rampersaud YR: Virtual fluoroscopy: computer-assisted fluoroscopic navigation. *Spine* 2001;26:347-351.

6. Mirza SK, Wiggins GC, Kuntz C IV, et al: Accuracy of thoracic vertebral body screw placement using standard fluoroscopy, fluoroscopic image guidance, and computed tomographic image guidance: A cadaver study. *Spine* 2003;28:402-413.

7. Wigfield C, Bolger C: A technique for frameless stereotaxy and placement of transarticular screws for atlanto-axial instability in rheumatoid arthritis. *Eur Spine J* 2001;10:264-269.

8. Austin MS, Vaccaro AR, Brislin B, Nachwalter R, Hilibrand AS, Albert TJ: Image-guided spine surgery: A cadaver study comparing conventional open laminoforaminotomy and two image-guided techniques for pedicle screw placement in posterolateral fusion and nonfusion models. *Spine* 2002;27:2503-2508.

9. Ludwig SC, Kowalski JM, Edwards CC II, Heller JG: Cervical pedicle screws: Comparative accuracy of two insertion techniques. *Spine* 2000;25:2675-2681.

10. Girardi FP, Cammisa FP Jr, Sandhu HS, Alvarez L: The placement of lumbar pedicle screws using computerised stereotactic guidance. *J Bone Joint Surg Br* 1999;81:825-829.

11. Shoda N, Nakajima S, Seichi A, et al: Computer-assisted anterior spinal surgery for a case of recurrent giant cell tumor. *J Orthop Sci* 2002;7:392-396.

12. Sagi HC, Manos R, Park SC, Von Jako R, Ordway NR, Connolly PJ: Electromagnetic field-based image-guided spine surgery part two: Results of a cadaveric study evaluating thoracic pedicle screw placement. *Spine* 2003;28:E351-E354.

13. Vougioukas VI, Hubbe U, Schipper J, Spetzger U: Navigated transoral approach to the cranial base and the craniocervical junction: Technical note. *Neurosurgery* 2003;52:247-251.

28

The Use of Bone Morphogenetic Protein in Lumbar Spine Surgery

Jeffrey A. Rihn, MD
Charley Gates, MD
*Steven D. Glassman, MD
*Frank M. Phillips, MD
*James D. Schwender, MD
*Todd J. Albert, MD

Abstract

Creating a solid lumbar spinal fusion remains a challenge. Despite advances in fixation, a pseudarthrosis still may occur. Recently, attention has focused on creating a more biologically favorable environment to enhance fusion rate. Bone morphogenetic proteins (BMPs) are a group of secreted growth factors that belong to the transforming growth factor-β superfamily. Two recombinant BMP proteins, rhBMP-2 and rhBMP-7 (OP-1), have been used successfully in preclinical and clinical trials and are commercially available for clinical applications.

Lumbar spinal fusion is an integral component of the surgical management of degenerative disease, trauma, deformity, tumor, and infection of the spine. Pseudarthrosis can, in turn, lead to persistent pain, failure of the instrumentation, and the need for revision surgery. It is a challenge to obtain a solid osseous fusion; therefore, both mechanical and biologic variables should be optimized. Mechanical stability is optimized by using pedicle screws and rods for rigid fixation until there is osseous fusion. Internal fixation improves the fusion rates compared with those associated with lumbar fusion without instrumentation, but it does not ensure a 100% fusion rate.

Autogenous bone graft has been used to optimize the biologic environment and is considered the "gold standard" for fusion in lumbar spine surgery; however, pseudarthrosis rates of up to 55% have been reported with use of autogenous bone graft.[1,2] In addition, up to 25% of patients have reported substantial and persistent morbidity associated with the harvesting of autogenous iliac crest bone.[3-8] There is a limited supply of autogenous iliac crest, and it may not be available for a patient requiring revision surgery.

Biologics have been used as alternatives to, or enhancements of, autograft in lumbar fusion surgery over the past decade. One of the most studied and frequently used biologic alternatives to autograft is bone morphogenetic protein (BMP). This chapter reviews the types of BMP used in lumbar spine surgery, the clinical results and complications associated with BMP use, and their economic impact.

What Is BMP?

BMP was discovered by Marshall Urist in 1965.[9] It is a group of

Steven D. Glassman, MD or the department with which he is affiliated has received research or institutional support and royalties from Medtronic and is a consultant for or an employee of Medtronic. Frank M. Phillips, MD or the department with which he is affiliated has received research or institutional support from Medtronic and Stryker. James D. Schwender, MD or the department with which he is affiliated has received royalties from Medtronic and the Orthopedic Development Company and is a consultant for or an employee of Medtronic. Todd J. Albert, MD or the department with which he is affiliated has received royalties from DePuy Spine, holds stock or stock options in K2 Medical and Transi, and is a consultant for or an employee of DePuy Spine.

growth factor proteins within the transforming growth factor-β (TGF-β) superfamily of growth factors.[10] Through molecular cloning techniques and recombinant expression, osteoinductive BMP molecules have been identified and have been produced in mass quantities in their pure form.[11,12] More than 20 types of BMPs have been recognized, but only BMP-2, -4, -6, -7, and -9 have been shown to have significant osteogenic properties.[12-17]

BMP molecules seem to induce bone formation in a stepwise fashion, with individual BMP molecules functioning at different stages of osteoblastic differentiation and osteogenesis. There is probably a synergistic relationship between the different BMP molecules.[15] The BMP molecules combine in vivo to form heterodimers that are much more potent osteoinductive agents than the individual BMP molecules alone.[18] Receptors for these heterodimers have also been discovered.[19] It has been postulated that the signaling pathway of osteoblastic differentiation and osteogenesis is a complex cascade of BMP expression that consists of substantial interaction between the different types of BMPs and other signaling molecules and receptors.[20]

Two commercial forms of recombinant BMP have demonstrated success in preclinical and clinical trials and are available for clinical use. One is rhBMP-2 (Infuse; Medtronic Sofamor Danek, Memphis, TN), and the other is rhBMP-7 (OP-1; Stryker Biotech, Hopkinton, MA). Although both types of BMP have osteogenic properties, only rhBMP-2 has been shown to induce osteoblastic differentiation of mesenchymal stem cells.[17] Currently, the only US Food and Drug Administration (FDA)–approved indication for use of any

BMP in the spine is anterior lumbar interbody fusion with rhBMP-2 within a titanium tapered cage.[21] All other uses in the spine are off label.[22-27]

BMP Carriers

To be effective, the BMP must be maintained at the planned site of fusion until the cascade of osteoblastic differentiation and osteogenesis is underway. Because BMP molecules are relatively soluble, less soluble carriers are used to maintain the BMP at the planned site of fusion. Carriers can either have structural, space-occupying properties (synthetic polymers and calcium phosphate ceramics) or provide little structure or space maintenance (type I collagen sponge). Some of these structural carriers are porous and are composed of calcium compounds, making them osteoconductive (for example, coral). Carriers with structural integrity are more desirable in posterolateral lumbar fusion because they maintain a space around the transverse processes in which the fusion mass can form. Carriers that are deformable, such as the type I collagen sponge, are more suitable for use within interbody cages.

Types of BMP carriers include synthetic polymers, calcium phosphate ceramics, and type I collagen.[28,29] Synthetic polymers are advantageous because they are bioinert and can be manufactured with complete control over their architecture and rate of reabsorption. The most common synthetic polymers are polylactic acid and polyglycolic acid. These polymers are also used to make bioabsorbable implants and suture. When used as a BMP carrier, they are a porous, structural scaffold, which promotes osseous ingrowth and then is absorbed after the fusion mass is established.

Calcium phosphate ceramics are highly crystalline, bioinert materials that, like synthetic polymers, are resorbed over time. The most commonly used are hydroxyapatite and tricalcium phosphate.[29,30] Tricalcium phosphate is resorbed over approximately 6 weeks, which is probably not sufficient time for a bone fusion mass to develop. The resorption rate of hydroxyapatite, on the other hand, is years. Natural coral has an interconnecting porosity that is similar to that of bone. It can either be used in its calcium carbonate form or be processed (that is, the carbonate can be replaced with phosphate) into a form that contains varying amounts of hydroxyapatite. The thickness of the hydroxyapatite determines its rate of dissolution.

Type I collagen, the most abundant protein in bone, binds to noncollagenous protein and has a structure that promotes bone formation. These properties make it an attractive BMP carrier. As a BMP carrier, it is usually manufactured as an absorbable sheet or sponge from either porcine or bovine skin or bone. These type I collagen carriers do not provide structural support or maintain space. They can be combined with calcium phosphate ceramics to form structural scaffolds (for example, Healos [DePuy, Raynham, MA] and Mastergraft Matrix [Medtronic Sofamor Danek]).

The structural support of an interbody fusion is provided by the interbody cage, into which BMP carried on an absorbable type I collagen sponge is inserted directly. A posterolateral lumbar fusion requires a BMP carrier with a structural capacity to withstand collapse under the forces of the surrounding paraspinal muscles and provide a space in which the fusion mass can form. Calcium phosphate ceramic has been shown to be an effective structural carrier in this setting.[30,31] Alternatively, BMP can be carried on an absorbable type I collagen sponge that is combined with a bulking agent (for example, ceramic, allograft cancellous chips, or local autograft bone).[30-34] This combination provides structural integrity and resists compression after placement over the transverse processes.[33]

Preclinical Results of BMP Use in Lumbar Fusion Surgery

Before the use of BMP, a posterior spinal fusion was done by decorticating the osseous surfaces of the posterior vertebral elements and then applying an onlay graft of autogenous or allogenic bone. Most preclinical studies evaluating the safety and efficacy of rhBMP-7 and rhBMP-2 as substitutes for bone graft have shown them to be equal or superior to autogenous iliac crest bone graft in lumbar fusion surgery.

RhBMP-7 and autograft were compared with regard to their effect on the maturation processes of lumbar posterolateral fusions in a canine model.[35] Three treatment groups were compared: autograft alone, autograft plus rhBMP-7, and rhBMP-7 alone. The time to fusion, the resistance of the fusion to motion, and the pathway of bone formation producing the fusion were measured. At 12 weeks, fusion had been achieved at 83% of the posterolateral sites in which autograft plus rhBMP-7 had been implanted and 72% of the sites at which rhBMP-7 alone had been implanted, but fusion was achieved at only 27% of the sites treated with autograft alone. Biomechanical testing indicated that the fusions obtained in both rhBMP-7 treatment groups had substantially less motion in flexion-extension and axial rotation than did those obtained with the autograft bone alone. Plain and polarized light microscopic studies indicated that, in both of the rhBMP-7 treatment groups, bone formation had occurred by means of intramembranous ossification, whereas in the group treated with autograft bone alone, bone had been produced by means of endochondral bone formation. This may partly explain the increased prevalence, speed, and stability of the rhBMP-7–induced fusions.

One potential complication of using BMP is leakage of the BMP resulting in bone formation at remote sites. The effect of rhBMP-7 intentionally placed into the subarachnoid space after thecal sac decompression was studied in a canine model.[36] An opening was created in the dura and arachnoid membranes, and rhBMP-7 was placed into the subarachnoid space in 30 dogs. At 16 weeks, new bone had developed in the subarachnoid space of all animals, with spinal stenosis and compression of the spinal cord. No neurotoxicity was noted. This result suggests that bone growth can occur over exposed dura and that the delivery and containment of rhBMP-7 are important to minimize this potential iatrogenic problem.

RhBMP-2 also has been studied as a bone graft substitute. In a rabbit model, the posterolateral lumbar fusion rate was 100% after using rhBMP-2 on a type I fibrillar collagen sponge, whereas only 42% of the spines fused after using autogenous iliac crest bone graft.[37] In a study of beagle dogs evaluated 12 weeks after L4-L5 intertransverse process fusion with either rhBMP-2 or autograft bone alone, all dogs treated with rhBMP-2 had a fusion, whereas none of the dogs treated with autograft bone alone had a fusion.[38] In that study, several doses of rhBMP-2 were used, with a 40-fold variation between the highest and lowest doses. There were no mechanical, radiographic, or histologic differences in the quality of the fusion masses obtained with the different doses.[38] This finding suggests that, above a threshold dose, the quality of spinal fusion produced with rhBMP-2 does not change with the dose.

Primates are thought to require higher doses of BMP to effect similar outcomes, and in one study concentrations of rhBMP-2 that produced fusions in canines and rabbits failed to do so in rhesus monkeys.[39] One reason for this finding is that primates are believed to have lower concentrations of BMP-responsive cells.[28]

Another problem encountered in nonhuman primates that was not seen in rabbits and dogs was compression of the collagen sponge carrier by the large paraspinal muscles.[39,40] It is possible that this excessive compression squeezed the protein out of the carrier sponge and prevented the development of an adequate fusion mass.[39] A subsequent study showed that a structural ceramic BMP carrier that is able to resist compression may be more suitable for posterolateral fusion in primates: all 15 rhesus monkeys treated with rhBMP-2 in this structural ceramic carrier had a successful posterolateral fusion.[40]

The safety of direct contact of rhBMP-2 with neural tissue was tested in 20 beagles that underwent an L5 laminectomy.[41] Half of the dogs had a puncture wound created in the dura, and either autogenous bone graft or rhBMP-2 was randomly applied to the exposed dura. At 12 weeks, there was no clinical, radiographic, or histologic evidence of neurologic abnormalities. The rhBMP-2 had stimulated bone growth in the laminectomy defect that was in direct contact with the dural membrane, and there was no evidence of abnormal mineralization within the thecal sac or in the spinal cord itself.

Clinical Results of BMP Use in Lumbar Fusion Surgery
Anterior Lumbar Interbody Fusion
The use of rhBMP-2 in spinal surgery was first studied in anterior lumbar interbody fusion, and this is the only FDA-approved indication for its use. In a multicenter, prospective, randomized study, 279 patients with single-level degenerative lumbar disk disease underwent anterior lumbar interbody fusion with two tapered titanium threaded fusion cages.[21] RhBMP-2 on an absorbable collagen sponge was used in the cages in 143 patients, and autograft iliac crest was used in the cages in 136 patients. The dose of rhBMP-2 ranged from 12 to 18 mg (in the form of a 1.5-mg/mL solution), depending on the size of the cage that was used. The mean surgical time and blood loss were less in the rhBMP-2 group. The autograft group had substantial morbidity at the iliac crest donor site, with 5.9% of the patients experiencing an adverse event related to graft harvest and 32% of the patients reporting discomfort at the graft site after 2 years. Two years after the surgery, plain radiographs and CT scans were used to evaluate the osseous fusion. The rhBMP-2 group was reported to have a 94.5% fusion rate compared with an 88.7% fusion rate in the autograft group. Both groups had similar improvements in clinical outcome measures through the duration of the study.

Two different prospective multicenter studies were performed to compare rhBMP-2 and autogenous iliac crest used in threaded allograft cortical dowels for single-level anterior lumbar interbody fusion.[22,23] Plain radiographs and CT scans were used to evaluate the fusion. In the first study, all 24 patients in the rhBMP-2 group and only 68% of the 22 in the autograft group had a solid osseous fusion at 2 years after the surgery.[22] At the time of final follow-up, the patients in the rhBMP-2 group had a better neurologic status and less back and lower limb pain than the patients in the autograft group. No adverse events were associated with the use of rhBMP-2. In the second study, 131 patients had a single-level anterior lumbar interbody fusion with threaded allograft dowels; 79 received rhBMP-2, and 52 received autograft.[23] The authors reported a 100% fusion rate in the rhBMP-2 group at 1 and 2 years and an 89% fusion rate at 1 year and an 81.5% fusion rate at 2 years in the autograft group. Eighteen percent of the patients in the rhBMP-2 group had transient vertebral osteolysis; all of these cases resolved by 2 years and had no effect on the clinical outcome.

Posterolateral Lumbar Fusion
The use of rhBMP-2 was compared with the use of autograft iliac crest bone in posterolateral lumbar fusion in two prospective, randomized, multicenter, FDA-regulated investigational device exemption clinical studies. Part of the first FDA-regulated study was a prospective, randomized clinical pilot study comparing posterolateral lumbar spine fusion in three groups of patients.[32] Five patients were treated with autograft with pedicle screw fixation;

11 patients with rhBMP-2 with pedicle screw fixation; and 9 patients with rhBMP-2 without pedicle screw fixation. All patients had single-level degenerative disk disease with no greater than grade I spondylolisthesis. The dose of rhBMP-2 was 20 mg per side of the spine (in a 2 mg/mL solution), which was larger than the dose used in the anterior lumbar interbody fusion procedures,[21-23] carried on calcium phosphate ceramic granules. At an average of 17 months postoperatively, only 40% of the spines in the autograft group were fused, whereas 100% of those in the groups that had received rhBMP-2 (both with and without pedicle screw fixation) were fused; also, clinical improvement was seen earlier in the rhBMP-2 groups. The patients treated with rhBMP-2 without pedicle screws had the greatest improvement in the Oswestry Disability Index at the time of final follow-up.

In the second ongoing prospective, randomized, FDA-regulated study, rhBMP-2 at a dose of 20 mg per side (in a 2 mg/mL solution) on a compression-resistant matrix (hydroxyapatite and tricalcium phosphate/collagen) carrier was compared with autograft iliac crest for use in a single-level posterolateral lumbar fusion.[42] The patients in the study had degenerative lumbar disk disease with no greater than grade I spondylolisthesis and a failure of at least 6 months of conservative treatment. The rhBMP-2 group had a significantly higher mean fusion grade than the autograft group at both 6 months ($P < 0.0001$) and 12 months ($P < 0.0023$; Figure 1). In a later report of the 2-year results of this study,[43] which included 45 patients in the autograft group and 53 in the rhBMP-2 group, there was a shorter surgical time and less blood loss in

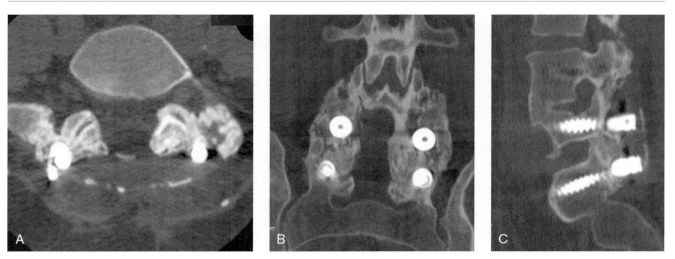

Figure 1 Axial (**A**), coronal (**B**), and sagittal (**C**) CT images acquired 12 months after an L4-L5 posterolateral fusion with the use of rhBMP-2. RhBMP-2 was delivered at a dosage of 20 mg per side on a compression-resistant matrix consisting of hydroxyapatite and tricalcium phosphate/collagen. These CT images demonstrate a solid bilateral fusion.

the rhBMP-2 group. There were no differences in clinical outcomes. The fusion rates were 73% in the autograft group and 91% in the rhBMP-2 group ($P = 0.051$). Complication rates were similar, and most complications were secondary to gastrointestinal, traumatic, or cardiac events.

A separate publication involving the same data presented a comparison of patients who smoked and those who did not.[44] At 2 years after the surgery, solid lumbar fusion was obtained in 100% of the 55 nonsmokers and 95% of the 21 smokers in the rhBMP-2 group. In the autograft group, solid fusion was achieved in 94% of the 55 nonsmokers and 76% of the 21 smokers. Despite the improved rate of solid fusion in the smokers who had received rhBMP-2, the values for the clinical outcome measures for the smokers were decreased compared with the values for the nonsmokers. The authors concluded that rhBMP-2 can enhance the fusion rate in smokers who undergo single-level posterolateral lumbar fusion.

In another study, a group of 41 patients who had a posterolateral lumbar fusion with rhBMP-2 (12 mg in the form of a 1.5 mg/mL solution) on a collagen sponge placed along with autograft iliac crest was compared with a group of 11 age- and sex-matched patients who had been treated with autograft iliac crest alone.[45] The rhBMP-2/autograft group had an increased rate of fusion of 97% (68 of 70 surgically treated levels) compared with the autograft group, which had a fusion rate of 77% (17 of 22 surgically treated levels; $P < 0.05$). Although the combination of rhBMP-2 and autograft iliac crest provided the highest reported fusion rate following posterolateral lumbar arthrodesis, to our knowledge it does not eliminate the substantial potential for morbidity at the iliac crest harvest site.

In a retrospective study, 91 patients who had been treated, at a single institution, with a posterolateral lumbar spine fusion with rhBMP-2 (12 mg in the form of a 1.5 mg/mL solution) on a collagen sponge that

was wrapped around local bone and bone graft extender were compared with a group of 35 patients who had undergone single-level posterolateral lumbar fusion with the use of autogenous iliac bone graft.[27] In the rhBMP-2 group, 48 patients had a primary single-level fusion, 27 had a primary multilevel fusion, and 16 patients had revision fusion surgery because of nonunion. At the time of follow-up, at a minimum of 2 years, the nonunion rates in these three groups were 4.2%, 0%, and 25%, respectively. The autograft group had a nonunion rate of 11.4%. Within the rhBMP-2 group, a subgroup of patients who were identified as smokers had no nonunions. The men in the rhBMP-2 group had a significantly higher nonunion rate than the women (11.1% and 3.4%, respectively; $P = 0.036$). The authors of the study concluded that a lower dose of rhBMP-2 (compared with that used in prior studies), applied with local bone and bone graft extender, results in a fusion rate similar to that following use of autograft iliac crest in posterolateral

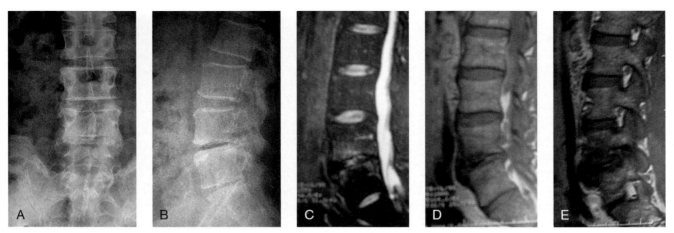

Figure 2   Images demonstrating the transforaminal lumbar interbody fusion procedure with the use of rhBMP-2 in a 40-year-old man who presented with low back pain and right lower limb pain that were equal in severity. An extensive course of nonsurgical treatment had failed. **A** and **B,** Anteroposterior and lateral radiographs demonstrating substantial disk degeneration at the L4-L5 level. **C,** T2-weighted midsagittal MRI showing substantial L4-L5 disk degeneration with vertebral end plate changes. **D** and **E,** Parasagittal T1-weighted MRIs showing evidence of a right-sided foraminal disk herniation that is causing substantial compression of the L4 nerve root. An L4-L5 transforaminal lumbar interbody fusion was performed from the right side with the use of rhBMP-2 and local autograft bone.

lumbar fusion. It also appeared that rhBMP-2 may increase fusion rates in smokers.

Several investigators have evaluated the clinical efficacy of rhBMP-7 (OP-1), particularly in posterolateral lumbar fusion.[46-50] These early studies did not show the fusion rate following the use of OP-1 combined with autograft to be superior to that achieved with autograft alone, but there were no documented complications related to the use of OP-1. A larger multicenter, prospective, randomized, FDA-approved investigational device exemption clinical study was performed to evaluate the use of OP-1 putty as a replacement for iliac crest autograft in single-level posterolateral lumbar fusion in patients with symptomatic lumbar stenosis and grade I or II degenerative spondylolisthesis.[48-51] Twenty-four patients were randomized to receive OP-1 putty and 12 to receive iliac crest autograft. The OP-1 putty (3.5 mg per side of the spine) was placed between the transverse pro-

cesses at the level of interest. No local autograft bone or instrumentation was used. At 1 year,[48] 2 years,[49] and 4 years[50] postoperatively, the OP-1 and iliac crest autograft groups had similar fusion rates (approximately 50%) and clinical outcomes. No adverse effects had resulted from the use of OP-1.[51]

In a prospective randomized study, OP-1 putty (3.5 mg per side, in 9 patients) was compared with a mixture of local autograft and calcium phosphate ceramic granules (in 10 patients) for a single-level posterolateral lumbar fusion with internal fixation in patients with spinal stenosis and degenerative spondylolisthesis. At 1 year postoperatively, radiographic evidence of fusion was present in 7 of the 9 patients who had received OP-1 and 9 of the 10 patients who had received the autograft-ceramic mixture.[51] In 16 patients, the hardware was removed, and the fusion mass was explored. In that group of 16 patients, only 4 of the 7 patients treated with

OP-1 and 7 of the 9 treated with the autograft-ceramic mixture had a solid fusion. The authors concluded that although OP-1 does stimulate new bone formation at the site of a posterolateral fusion, the rate of solid fusion is low.

Transforaminal Lumbar Interbody Fusion

This procedure, first described by Harms and Rolinger[52] in 1982, allows an anterior interbody fusion and a posterolateral fusion to be achieved through a single posterior approach. An interbody cage with bone graft is placed into a distracted disk space through a posterolateral transforaminal approach, and a standard posterolateral fusion with pedicle screw stabilization is done. To eliminate the need for iliac crest autograft and the morbidity associated with its harvest, off-label use of rhBMP-2 in transforaminal lumbar interbody fusion has become increasingly popular (Figures 2 through 4).

In a preliminary study of transforaminal lumbar interbody fusions, with an average duration of follow-up of 9 months, the fusion rate associated with the use of rhBMP-2 and autograft (in 21 patients) was compared with the fusion rate associated with the use of iliac crest autograft alone (in 19 patients).[24] Of the 21 patients who were treated with rhBMP-2 and autograft, 12 received iliac crest autograft and 9 received autograft obtained locally from the laminectomy. In this group, the autograft was packed posterior to the rhBMP-2-filled cage. The mean time to fusion was 6 months in the autograft group, 4 months in the rhBMP-2/iliac crest autograft group, and 3 months in the rhBMP-2/local bone group. One patient in the autograft group and one patient in the rhBMP-2/local bone group had a pseudarthrosis. No patient in the rhBMP-2/iliac crest autograft group had a pseudarthrosis or symptomatic foraminal bone formation. The authors concluded that rhBMP-2 is a safe and effective alternative to iliac crest autograft for use in transforaminal lumbar interbody fusion and leads to more rapid fusion while eliminating harvest-site morbidity.

The use of rhBMP-2 in both minimally invasive and open transforaminal lumbar interbody fusion procedures was reported in 74 patients followed for an average of 20 months.[26] The study included single-level and multilevel transforaminal lumbar interbody fusions, many of which were performed in the setting of previous lumbar surgery. The BMP-2 was applied on an absorbable collagen sponge and was combined with autogenous local bone and/or allograft bone. All patients in the study had a solid fusion within 10 months after the surgery, with a mean time to fusion of 4.1 months. There were no complications or allergic reactions that the authors attributed specifically to the use of rhBMP-2. Two patients, however, were noted to have persistent, postoperative radiculitis. No ectopic bone formation was observed.

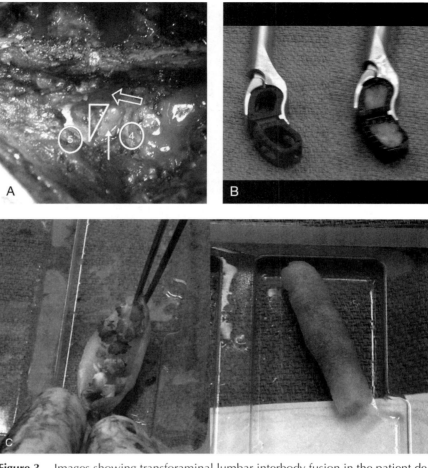

Figure 3 Images showing transforaminal lumbar interbody fusion in the patient described in Figure 2. **A,** Intraoperative photograph demonstrating the approach for the transforaminal lumbar interbody fusion. The inferior articulating facet, the pars interarticularis, and a portion of the lamina of the L4 vertebral body were removed with an osteotome and a Kerrison rongeur. The locations of the L4 and L5 pedicles are defined by the white circles. The solid white arrow points to the exiting L4 nerve root, and the open arrow points to the thecal sac. The triangle highlights the area through which the transforaminal lumbar interbody fusion is performed. Its borders are formed by the exiting nerve root, the thecal sac, and the inferior aspect of the disk space of interest. The anulus fibrosus is incised, and the disk space is prepared through this triangle. **B,** After the disk space is prepared, the BMP-soaked collagen sponge is packed into the interbody cage, and the cage is inserted into the anterior two thirds of the disk space to maximize lordosis and minimize the risk of exposing the nerve root to BMP. **C,** A BMP-soaked collagen sponge is rolled around local autograft bone and placed posterolaterally, bridging the transverse processes. Some surgeons avoid placing BMP posterolaterally on the side of the transforaminal lumbar interbody fusion to avoid nerve root irritation and postoperative radiculitis.

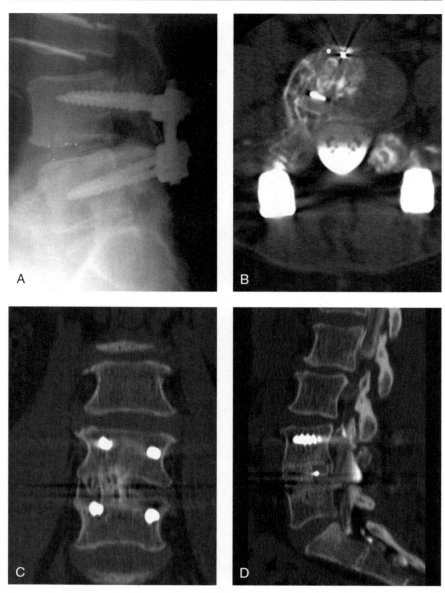

Figure 4 **A,** Lateral radiograph made following a transforaminal lumbar interbody fusion procedure in the patient described in Figure 2. Note that the interbody cage (marked by metallic beads) is located in the anterior two thirds of the disk space. Axial (**B**), coronal (**C**), and sagittal (**D**) CT scans demonstrating a solid interbody fusion 12 months after the transforaminal lumbar interbody fusion was performed with rhBMP-2.

Safety of BMP in Lumbar Spine Surgery

Few documented adverse events can be attributed to BMP. Nonetheless, certain complications and safety issues related to the use of BMP in the lumbar spine are concerns. Adverse reactions with repeat BMP exposure include postoperative radiculitis, vertebral osteolysis and edema, and neurocompressive ectopic bone formation (that is, bone formation in the central canal or intervertebral foramen).

As a foreign protein, BMP has the potential to stimulate the formation of antibodies. Antibodies to BMP can, on reexposure, lead to a hyperinflammatory response with local (for example, wound) problems and systemic consequences (for example, anaphylaxis), but there is no clinical evidence to suggest that reexposure to BMP can have detrimental effects (L. Carreon and associates, unpublished data presented at the 22nd Annual Meeting of the North American Spine Society, 2007). The use of BMP, particularly in transforaminal lumbar interbody fusion and posterior lumbar interbody fusion, has been associated with severe postoperative radiculitis, which can start days after the surgery without neural compression. The cause is thought to be a BMP-related proinflammatory reaction and/or ectopic bone formation in the vicinity of the nerve root sleeve and the intervertebral foramen. Postoperative nerve injury (that is, a new or increased neurologic deficit) was reported in 20.7% and 14.3% of patients who had undergone one- and two-level minimally invasive transforaminal lumbar interbody fusion with rhBMP-2, respectively.[26] The authors stated that none of the complications were specifically attributed to rhBMP-2. Two of the patients in their study had persistent postoperative radiculitis that was still present at the time of the latest follow-up. In another study, with a retrospective design, radiculitis that lasted more than 6 months developed in 9 of 39 patients who had a transforaminal lumbar interbody fusion with the use of rhBMP-2 and only 1 of 29 patients who had the fusion with the use of iliac crest autograft (JA Sanfilippo and associates, unpublished data presented at the 22nd Annual

Meeting of the North American Spine Society, 2007). The average duration of the postoperative radiculitis in the rhBMP-2 group was 13.4 months. There is anecdotal evidence that the use of a sealant, such as DuraSeal Xact Sealant System (Confluent Surgical, Waltham, MA), to minimize the amount of rhBMP-2 in the vicinity of the nerve root may decrease the prevalence of postoperative radiculitis. Clinical studies are needed to further explore this issue.

Ectopic bone formation can potentially occur in the anterior epidural space and near the nerve root, along the track of insertion of BMP, when an interbody fusion is performed from a posterolateral or transforaminal approach[53] (Figure 5). Although the risks of ectopic bone formation developing with BMP use remain unknown, hematoma seems to be a carrier, and excessive bleeding can disperse the BMP. Hemostatic agents, such as Gelfoam (Pfizer, New York, NY), have also been implicated as carriers. An early study of the use of BMP in posterior lumbar interbody fusion demonstrated a high rate of substantial ectopic bone formation in the spinal canal.[53] No clinical symptoms, however, developed secondary to this ectopic bone formation.[55] Clinical studies of the use of BMP in transforaminal lumbar interbody fusion have not revealed problems with ectopic bone formation.[24-26] Placement of the rhBMP-2 anterior to and within the interbody cage in the anterior column, but not in the middle column near the anulotomy, is thought to minimize the risk of ectopic bone formation in the spinal canal and/or intervertebral foramen following a transforaminal lumbar interbody fusion.

Vertebral osteolysis and vertebral

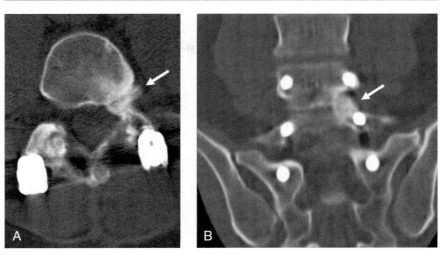

Figure 5 Axial (**A**) and coronal (**B**) CT scans demonstrating ectopic bone formation in the intervertebral foramen (white arrows) following a transforaminal lumbar interbody fusion performed with rhBMP-2.

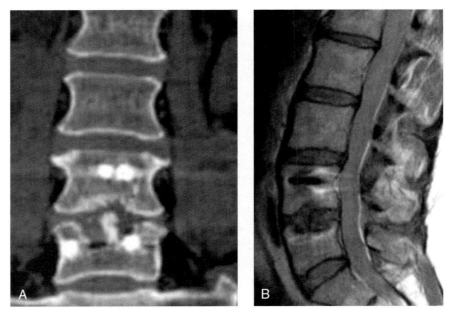

Figure 6 Coronal CT scan (**A**) and sagittal T1-weighted MRI (**B**) demonstrating vertebral osteolysis 6 months after a transforaminal lumbar interbody fusion performed with the use of rhBMP-2. Although this finding is often associated with increased back pain and radiculitis, it seems as though the vertebral body reaction to BMP is a self-limiting process that does not affect the clinical outcome or the rate of fusion.

edema have been observed after using BMP in an interbody fusion.[23,54] The pathophysiology and relevance of the vertebral osteolysis are unknown. It has been reported to occur in 8% to 18% of cases.[23,54] It

seems to resolve spontaneously, but patients may have pain while it is present (Figure 6). It may be due, at least in part, to a violation of the vertebral body end plate during preparation of the disk space.

Economics of BMP Use in Spine Surgery

There have been several economic evaluations comparing the cost of BMP use with the cost of traditional autogenous iliac crest bone grafting.[55-57] Most investigators have concluded that BMPs will prove to be cost neutral. The costs associated with the use of BMPs are largely offset by the prevention of the pain and complications associated with the harvest of autogenous iliac crest bone graft. Ultimately, the largest long-term cost offset may be associated with a reduced number of fusion failures and the reduced need for revision.[55] An economic model based on clinical trial data, peer-reviewed literature, and clinical expert opinion suggested that, over a 2-year period after surgery, the upfront cost of BMP is likely to be offset to a substantial extent by more efficient use of other medical resources, including a decreased length of hospital stay and decreased use of pain clinics and rehabilitation services.[56]

In an economic prospective, randomized, controlled trial of 102 patients older than 60 years, 50 patients were treated with lumbar spine surgery with rhBMP-2 and 52 patients were treated with lumbar spine surgery with iliac crest bone graft, with or without graft extender.[57] All costs during the first 3 months after surgery (the perioperative Medicare global billing period) were recorded. A research nurse followed all patients throughout their hospital stay and posthospitalization recovery to identify any adverse events or additional outpatient medical care. The total payer expenditure for the 3 months averaged $33,860 in the rhBMP-2 group and $37,227 in the iliac crest bone-graft group. In the rhBMP-2 group, the mean surgical time was 22 minutes shorter, the mean length of stay in the hospital was almost 1 day shorter, and inpatient rehabilitation was used less frequently.

Summary

The use of BMPs in lumbar fusion surgery has increased over the past several years. Both rhBMP-2 and rhBMP-7 are members of the TGF-β superfamily and have been used with success in both preclinical and clinical trials. The only FDA-approved indication for BMP in the spine is anterior lumbar interbody fusion with the use of rhBMP-2 in a titanium tapered cage. Off-label uses of BMPs are becoming increasingly popular as enthusiasm for them grows and indications for their clinical application expand. Several randomized trials are currently being performed to study the use of BMPs in both posterolateral lumbar fusion and transforaminal lumbar interbody fusion. These studies have produced promising early results. Important concerns regarding the clinical application of BMP include safety and cost. Finally, the large upfront cost of BMPs appears to be offset by the prevention of complications associated with iliac crest harvest, including a longer surgical time, more blood loss, and longer inpatient and rehabilitation stays. Ultimately, if BMPs are able to reduce the number of fusion failures, then they will prove to be cost sparing in the long run.

References

1. Fischgrund JS, Mackay M, Herkowitz HN, Brower R, Montgomery DM, Kurz LT: Degenerative lumbar spondylolisthesis with spinal stenosis: A prospective, randomized study comparing decompressive laminectomy and arthrodesis with and without spinal instrumentation. *Spine* 1997;22:2807-2812.

2. France JC, Yaszemski MJ, Lauerman WC, et al: A randomized prospective study of posterolateral lumbar fusion: Outcomes with and without pedicle screw instrumentation. *Spine* 1999;24:553-560.

3. Younger EM, Chapman MW: Morbidity at bone graft donor sites. *J Orthop Trauma* 1989;3:192-195.

4. Kurz LT, Garfin SR, Booth RE Jr: Harvesting autogenous iliac bone grafts: A review of complications and techniques. *Spine* 1989;14:1324-1331.

5. Banwart JC, Asher MA, Hassanein RS: Iliac crest bone graft harvest donor site morbidity: A statistical evaluation. *Spine* 1995;20:1055-1060.

6. Arrington ED, Smith WJ, Chambers HG, Bucknell AL, Davino NA: Complications of iliac crest bone graft harvesting. *Clin Orthop Relat Res* 1996;329:300-309.

7. Silber JS, Anderson DG, Daffner SD, et al: Donor site morbidity after anterior iliac crest bone harvest for single-level anterior cervical discectomy and fusion. *Spine* 2003;28:134-139.

8. Ahlmann E, Patzakis M, Roidis N, Shepherd L, Holtom P: Comparison of anterior and posterior iliac crest bone grafts in terms of harvest-site morbidity and functional outcomes. *J Bone Joint Surg Am* 2002;84:716-720.

9. Urist MR: Bone: Formation by auto-induction. *Science* 1965;150:893-899.

10. Kingsley DM: The TGF-beta superfamily: New members, new receptors, and new genetic tests of function in different organisms. *Genes Dev* 1994;8:133-146.

11. Wang EA, Rosen V, Cordes P, et al: Purification and characterization of other distinct bone-inducing factors. *Proc Natl Acad Sci USA* 1988;85:9484-9488.

12. Wozney JM, Rosen V, Celeste AJ, et al: Novel regulators of bone formation: Molecular clones and activities. *Science* 1988;242:1528-1534.

13. Israel DI, Nove J, Kerns KM, Moutsatsos IK, Kaufman RJ: Expression and characterization of bone morphogenetic protein-2 in Chinese hamster ovary cells. *Growth Factors* 1992;7:139-150.

14. Wozney JM, Rosen V, Byrne M, Celeste AJ, Moutsatsos I, Wang EA: Growth factors influencing bone development. *J Cell Sci Suppl* 1990;13: 149-156.

15. Celeste AJ, Iannazzi JA, Taylor RC, et al: Identification of transforming growth factor beta family members present in bone-inductive protein purified from bovine bone. *Proc Natl Acad Sci USA* 1990;87:9843-9847.

16. Wozney JM, Rosen V: Bone morphogenetic protein and bone morphogenetic protein gene family in bone formation and repair. *Clin Orthop Relat Res* 1998;346:26-37.

17. Cheng H, Jiang W, Phillips FM, et al: Osteogenic activity of the fourteen types of human bone morphogenetic proteins (BMPs). *J Bone Joint Surg Am* 2003;85:1544-1552. Erratum in *J Bone Joint Surg Am* 2004;86:141.

18. Israel DI, Nove J, Kerns KM, et al: Heterodimeric bone morphogenetic proteins show enhanced activity in vitro and in vivo. *Growth Factors* 1996; 13:291-300.

19. Mayer H, Scutt AM, Ankenbauer T: Subtle differences in the mitogenic effects of recombinant human bone morphogenetic proteins -2 to -7 on DNA synthesis on primary bone-forming cells and identification of BMP-2/4 receptor. *Calcif Tissue Int* 1996;58:249-255.

20. Zlotolow DA, Vaccaro AR, Salamon ML, Albert TJ: The role of human bone morphogenetic proteins in spinal fusion. *J Am Acad Orthop Surg* 2000;8:3-9.

21. Burkus JK, Gornet MF, Dickman CA, Zdeblick TA: Anterior lumbar interbody fusion using rhBMP-2 with tapered interbody cages. *J Spinal Disord Tech* 2002;15:337-349.

22. Burkus JK, Transfeldt EE, Kitchel SH, Watkins RG, Balderston RA: Clinical and radiographic outcomes of anterior lumbar interbody fusion using recombinant human bone morphogenetic protein-2. *Spine* 2002;27: 2396-2408.

23. Burkus JK, Sandhu HS, Gornet MF: Influence of rhBMP-2 on the healing patterns associated with allograft interbody constructs in comparison with autograft. *Spine* 2006;31:775-781.

24. Mummaneni PV, Pan J, Haid RW, Rodts GE: Contribution of recombinant human bone morphogenetic protein-2 to the rapid creation of interbody fusion when used in transforaminal lumbar interbody fusion: A preliminary report. Invited submission from the Joint Section Meeting on Disorders of the Spine and Peripheral Nerves, March 2004. *J Neurosurg Spine* 2004;1:19-23.

25. Schwender JD, Holly LT, Rouben DP, Foley KT: Minimally invasive transforaminal lumbar interbody fusion (TLIF): Technical feasibility and initial results. *J Spinal Disord Tech* 2005;18(suppl):S1-S6.

26. Villavicencio AT, Burneikiene S, Nelson EL, Bulsara KR, Favors M, Thramann J: Safety of transforaminal lumbar interbody fusion and intervertebral recombinant human bone morphogenetic protein-2. *J Neurosurg Spine* 2005;3:436-443.

27. Glassman SD, Carreon L, Djurasovic M, et al: Posterolateral lumbar spine fusion with INFUSE bone graft. *Spine J* 2007;7:44-49.

28. Sandhu HS: Bone morphogenetic proteins and spinal surgery. *Spine* 2003;28(suppl 15):S64-S73.

29. Boden SD, Martin GJ Jr, Morone M, Ugbo JL, Titus L, Hutton WC: The use of coralline hydroxyapatite with bone marrow, autogenous bone graft, or osteoinductive bone protein extract for posterolateral lumbar spine fusion. *Spine* 1999;24:320-327.

30. Khan SN, Fraser JF, Sandhu HS, Cammisa FP Jr, Girardi FP, Lane JM: Use of osteopromotive growth factors, demineralized bone matrix, and ceramics to enhance spinal fusion. *J Am Acad Orthop Surg* 2005;13: 129-137.

31. Minamide A, Kawakami M, Hashizume H, Sakata R, Tamaki T: Evaluation of carriers of bone morphogenetic protein for spinal fusion. *Spine* 2001;26:933-939.

32. Boden SD, Kang J, Sandhu H, Heller JG: Use of recombinant human bone morphogenetic protein-2 to achieve posterolateral lumbar spine fusion in humans: A prospective, randomized clinical pilot trial. *Spine* 2002;27:2662-2673.

33. Suh DY, Boden SD, Louis-Ugbo J, et al: Delivery of recombinant human bone morphogenetic protein-2 using a compression-resistant matrix in posterolateral spine fusion in the rabbit and in the non-human primate. *Spine* 2002;27:353-360.

34. Kraiwattanapong C, Boden SD, Louis-Ugbo J, Attallah E, Barnes B, Hutton WC: Comparison of Healos/bone marrow to INFUSE (rhBMP-2/ACS) with a collagen-ceramic sponge bulking agent as graft substitutes for lumbar spine fusion. *Spine* 2005;30: 1001-1007.

35. Cunningham BW, Shimamoto N, Sefter JC, et al: Osseointegration of autograft versus osteogenic protein-1 in posterolateral spinal arthrodesis: Emphasis on the comparative mechanisms of bone induction. *Spine J* 2002;2:11-24.

36. Paramore CG, Lauryssen C, Rauzzino MJ, et al: The safety of OP-1 for lumbar fusion with decompression: A canine study. *Neurosurgery* 1999;44:1151-1156.

37. Schimandle JH, Boden SD, Hutton WC: Experimental spinal fusion with recombinant human bone morphogenetic protein-2. *Spine* 1995;20: 1326-1337.

38. Sandhu HS, Kanim LE, Kabo JM, et al: Effective doses of recombinant human bone morphogenetic protein-2 in experimental spinal fusion. *Spine* 1996;21:2115-2122.

39. Martin GJ Jr, Boden SD, Marone MA, Moskovitz PA: Posterolateral inter-

transverse process spinal arthrodesis with rhBMP-2 in a nonhuman primate: Important lessons learned regarding dose, carrier, and safety. *J Spinal Disord* 1999;12:179-186.

40. Boden SD, Martin GJ Jr, Morone MA, Ugbo JL, Moskovitz PA: Posterolateral lumbar intertransverse process spine arthrodesis with recombinant human bone morphogenetic protein 2/hydroxyapatite-tricalcium phosphate after laminectomy in the nonhuman primate. *Spine* 1999;24: 1179-1185.

41. Meyer RA Jr, Gruber HE, Howard BA, et al: Safety of recombinant human bone morphogenetic protein-2 after spinal laminectomy in the dog. *Spine* 1999;24:747-754.

42. Glassman SD, Dimar JR, Carreon LY, Campbell MJ, Puno RM, Johnson JR: Initial fusion rates with recombinant human bone morphogenetic protein-2/compression resistant matrix and a hydroxyapatite and tricalcium phosphate/collagen carrier in posterolateral spinal fusion. *Spine* 2005;30:1694-1698.

43. Dimar JR, Glassman SD, Burkus KJ, Carreon LY: Clinical outcomes and fusion success at 2 years of single-level instrumented posterolateral fusions with recombinant human bone morphogenetic protein-2/compression resistant matrix versus iliac crest bone graft. *Spine* 2006;31:2534-2540.

44. Glassman SD, Dimar JR III, Burkus K, et al: The efficacy of rhBMP-2 for posterolateral lumbar fusion in smokers. *Spine* 2007;32:1693-1698.

45. Singh K, Smucker JD, Gill S, Boden SD: Use of recombinant human bone morphogenetic protein-2 as an adjunct in posterolateral lumbar spine fusion: A prospective CT-scan analysis at one and two years. *J Spinal Disord Tech* 2006;19:416-423. Erratum in *J Spinal Disord Tech* 2007;20:185.

46. Vaccaro AR, Patel T, Fischgrund J, et al: A pilot safety and efficacy study of OP-1 putty (rhBMP-7) as an adjunct to iliac crest autograft in posterolateral lumbar fusions. *Eur Spine J* 2003;12:495-500.

47. Vaccaro AR, Patel T, Fischgrund J, et al: A 2-year follow-up pilot study evaluating the safety and efficacy of op-1 putty (rhbmp-7) as an adjunct to iliac crest autograft in posterolateral lumbar fusions. *Eur Spine J* 2005;14: 623-629.

48. Vaccaro AR, Patel T, Fischgrund J, et al: A pilot study evaluating the safety and efficacy of OP-1 putty (rhBMP-7) as a replacement for iliac crest autograft in posterolateral lumbar arthrodesis for degenerative spondylolisthesis. *Spine* 2004;29:1885-1892.

49. Vaccaro AR, Anderson DG, Patel T, et al: Comparison of OP-1 putty (rhBMP-7) to iliac crest autograft for posterolateral lumbar arthrodesis: A minimum 2-year follow-up pilot study. *Spine* 2005;30:2709-2716.

50. Vaccaro AR, Whang PG, Patel T, et al: The safety and efficacy of OP-1 (rhBMP-7) as a replacement for iliac crest autograft for posterolateral lumbar arthrodesis: Minimum 4-year follow-up of a pilot study. *Spine J* 2008;8:457-465.

51. Kanayama M, Hashimoto T, Shigenobu K, Yamane S, Bauer TW, Togawa D: A prospective randomized study of posterolateral lumbar fusion using osteogenic protein-1 (OP-1) versus local autograft with ceramic bone substitute: Emphasis of surgical exploration and histologic assessment. *Spine* 2006;31:1067-1074.

52. Harms J, Rolinger H: [A one-stager procedure in operative treatment of spondylolistheses: Dorsal traction-reposition and anterior fusion (author's transl)] . *Z Orthop Ihre Grenzgeb* 1982;120:343-347.

53. Haid RW Jr, Branch CL Jr, Alexander JT, Burkus JK: Posterior lumbar interbody fusion using recombinant human bone morphogenetic protein type 2 with cylindrical interbody cages. *Spine J* 2004;4:527-539.

54. Lewandrowski KU, Nanson C, Calderon R: Vertebral osteolysis after posterior interbody lumbar fusion with recombinant human bone morphogenetic protein 2: A report of five cases. *Spine J* 2007;7:609-614.

55. Ackerman SJ, Mafilios MS, Polly DW Jr: Economic evaluation of bone morphogenetic protein versus autogenous iliac crest bone graft in single-level anterior lumbar fusion: an evidence-based modeling approach. *Spine* 2002;27(16, suppl 1): S94-S99.

56. Polly DW Jr, Ackerman SJ, Shaffrey CI, et al: A cost analysis of bone morphogenetic protein versus autogenous iliac crest bone graft in single-level anterior lumbar fusion. *Orthopedics* 2003;26:1027-1037.

57. Glassman SD, Carreon LY, Campbell MJ, et al: The perioperative cost of Infuse bone graft in posterolateral lumbar spine fusion. *Spine J* 2008;8: 443-448.

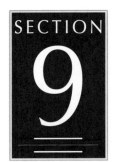

SECTION 9

Degenerative Cervical Disorders

Degenerative Cervical Disorders

In this section, the authors discuss a spectrum of degenerative cervical disorders of the spine along with treatment options and techniques for avoiding potential pitfalls and managing those that occur. Together, the chapters in this section review the current management algorithms of common clinical scenarios related to this group of cervical disorders.

The first chapter by Rao and associates begins with an overview of degenerative cervical spondylosis. Degenerative changes in the cervical spine occur often but usually do not result in significant clinical sequelae. A practical approach to organizing initial patient evaluations based on symptoms and degenerative findings is developed. Patients are categorized into three general groups—those with axial neck pain, cervical radiculopathy, and cervical myelopathy.

The findings from the patient history, physical examination, and diagnostic studies allow characterization of a clinical entity. Although nonsurgical options are the initial mainstay of treatment for most cervical conditions, surgical options may be considered if limiting axial or radicular symptoms persist, if a progressive neurologic deficit develops, or if significant myelopathy is observed. Anterior and posterior surgical procedures are reviewed. Specific procedures may be appropriate based on the location of the pathology, levels of the disease, extent of the disease, and other patient- and surgeon-related factors.

Data from reviews of the surgical outcomes of different degenerative cervical conditions are critically presented by Rao and associates. Common complications, including neurologic disorders, neck pain, neck stiffness, instability,

kyphosis, dysphagia, adjacent segment deterioration, and implant-related problems, are reviewed.

The second chapter by Anderson and associates specifically considers a new technology in the armamentarium of cervical spine surgery—cervical artificial disk replacement. This is a timely topic because motion-sparing technologies are currently receiving increased consideration.

With both arthrodesis and arthroplasty, the primary goal of the surgery is decompression of the neural elements and relief of neurologic symptoms and/or avoidance of progressive neurologic deficit. The driving force behind disk arthroplasty is the potential for avoiding adjacent level degeneration, which has been associated with fusion procedures. The authors also discuss the difficulty of differentiating adjacent segment degeneration from the effects of the natural history of cervical spondylosis.

The mechanical considerations of disk replacements are reviewed. Theoretic advantages to motion-preserving surgery are reported to be retained motion, avoidance of adjacent segment degeneration, and earlier return to activities. These advantages are balanced by the strong track record of fusions, the potential resorption of osteophytes that may occur in accordance with the Wolfe law, and the potential beneficial effects of limiting continued motion around compromised neural elements.

The chapter references seven cervical disk prostheses undergoing clinical investigation by the US Food and Drug Administration. (Since the publication of the chapter by Anderson and associates, three of the devices [the Bryan Cervical

Disc, Medtronic Sofamor Danek, Memphis, TN; the Prestige Artificial Cervical Disc System, Medtronic Sofamor Danek; and the ProDisc-C, Synthes Spine, Paoli, PA] have been approved for general use.)[1] Design considerations and testing paradigms of disk prostheses are reviewed. Clinical outcomes from early studies with short-term follow-up are then presented. In general, these studies showed results similar to those of arthrodesis. Some studies suggested that disk replacement can result in improved outcomes and earlier return to activities. Few complications were reported and there were no reports of catastrophic neural injury; however, the authors noted that longer term follow-up data are needed. A more recent 2009 study reported encouraging short-term outcomes for cervical disk arthroplasty,[2] although intermediate- and long-term study results are still needed.

In the chapter by Devin and associates, techniques for the prevention, identification, and treatment of inadequate decompressions of the cervical spine are presented. The authors also offer insights into considerations for avoiding pitfalls and discuss their management if encountered. Certainly, the primary approach to surgical complications is prevention. The preoperative evaluation of a patient with a cervical spine disorder is reviewed with reference to identifying the pathology and defining the optimal surgical approach. Other considerations to best achieve surgical objectives are then reviewed. For example, the assessment of cervical alignment is stressed, management options for ossification of the posterior longitudinal ligament are presented, the relative role of anterior cervical diskectomy versus corpectomy is introduced, and a careful review of the cervical levels needing attention is highlighted. Specific surgical pearls also are presented.

Patients in whom prior surgery has failed are discussed. Surgical indications, initial diagnoses, procedural or technical errors, and a review of all preoperative and postoperative imaging studies are necessary to understand the reasons that the initial surgery failed. Revision surgery can be successful if general treatment principles are followed.

Overall, the three chapters in this section present a comprehensive overview of current management strategies for patients with degenerative conditions of the cervical spine. Practical approaches are defined for patients with neck pain, radiculopathy, and myelopathy. Although most patients respond favorably to conservative treatments, surgical options may be clearly indicated based on certain clinical scenarios. From decompression alone to fusion or disk replacement, the key to successful surgical management of patients with degenerative disorders of the cervical spine is achieving adequate decompression and stabilization.

Jonathan N. Grauer, MD
Associate Professor
Department of Orthopaedics
    and Rehabilitation
Yale University School of Medicine
New Haven, Connecticut

Shawn Hermenau, MD
Spine Fellow
Department of Orthopaedics
    and Rehabilitation
Yale University School of Medicine
New Haven, Connecticut

References

1. US Food and Drug Administration Website. Devices. http://www.accessdata.fda.gov/scripts/cdrh/devicesatfda/index.cfm. Accessed September 10, 2009.

2. Anderson PA, Puschak TJ, Sasso RC: Comparison of short-term SF-36 results between total joint arthroplasty and cervical spine decompression and fusion or arthroplasty. *Spine* (Phila Pa 1976) 2009;34:176-183.

Dr. Grauer or an immediate family member is a member of a speakers' bureau or has made paid presentations on behalf of Stryker; is a paid consultant for or is an employee of Stryker, Smith & Nephew, and DePuy; and has received research or institutional support from Medtronic Sofamor Danek, Stryker, and Regeneration Technologies. Dr. Hermenau or an immediate family member has received research or institutional support from DePuy.

29

Degenerative Cervical Spondylosis: Clinical Syndromes, Pathogenesis, and Management

Raj D. Rao, MD
*Bradford L. Currier, MD
*Todd J. Albert, MD
Christopher M. Bono, MD
Satyajit V. Marawar, MD
Kornelis A. Poelstra, MD, PhD
Jason C. Eck, DO, MS

Abstract

Degenerative changes in the cervical spinal column are ubiquitous in the adult population, but infrequently symptomatic. The evaluation of patients with symptoms is facilitated by classifying the resulting clinical syndromes into axial neck pain, cervical radiculopathy, cervical myelopathy, or a combination of these conditions. Although most patients with axial neck pain, cervical radiculopathy, or mild cervical myelopathy respond well to initial nonsurgical treatment, those who continue to have symptoms or patients with clinically evident myelopathy are candidates for surgical intervention.

Spondylosis refers to age-related degenerative changes within the spinal column. Radiographic evidence of cervical spondylosis is frequent in asymptomatic adults.[1,2] Approximately 25% of individuals younger than 40 years of age, 50% of individuals older than 40 years of age, and 85% of individuals older than 60 years of age have some degree of disk degeneration.[2,3] Occupations that place increased loads on the head predispose individuals to the development of cervical spondylosis. Activities such as rugby, soccer, and horseback riding and occupations such as flying fighter jets may also predispose individuals to the development of cervical spondylosis.[4-8]

Symptoms caused by cervical spondylosis can be categorized broadly into three clinical syndromes: axial neck pain, cervical radiculopathy, and cervical myelopathy. Patients can have a combination of these syndromes. Axial posterior neck pain occasionally radiates to the shoulder or periscapular region in a nondermatomal distribution. Axial neck pain is more common in women, has a lifetime prevalence of 66% in North American adults, and 5% of the population has disabling pain at any given time.[9-11] Cervical radiculopathy refers to pain, sensory findings, or a neurologic deficit in a dermatomal distribution in the upper extremity, with or without neck pain. The annual incidence of cervical radiculopathy was reported to be 83 per 100,000 population, whereas the prevalence was found to be 3.5 per 1,000 population with a peak incidence in the sixth decade of life.[12,13] Cervical myelopathy refers to the syndrome of long-tract clinical findings in the upper and lower extremities arising from involvement of the spinal cord by the spondylotic changes in the cervical

*Bradford L. Currier, MD or the department with which he is affiliated has received research or institutional support from Synthes Spine and royalties from DePuy Spine and Stryker Spine. Todd J. Albert, MD is a consultant or employee for DePuy Spine.

spinal column. The true incidence is difficult to ascertain because of the subtle findings in its early stages.

Pathogenesis of Symptoms

Neck Pain

Subaxial neck pain is most often caused by muscular and ligamentous factors related to improper posture, poor ergonomics, and muscle fatigue. Numerous potential causes have been reported, but their contribution is unclear. Low levels of high-energy phosphates such as adenosine triphosphate (ATP), adenosine diphosphate, and phosphoryl creatine have been found in the trapezius muscles of patients with fibromyalgic neck pain.[14] Patients with chronic trapezius myalgia have shown lower muscle blood flow and higher intramuscular tension on the symptomatic side when compared with the contralateral, asymptomatic side of the same patient and with healthy controls.[15] Prior neck injury has been found to be an independent risk factor.[16] Degenerative changes at the cervical disk and facet joints can be a source of symptoms. Nerve fibers and nociceptive nerve endings are present in the peripheral portions of the disk and in the capsule and synovium of the facet joints.[17-20] Findings of diskography and provocative injections of the facet joint have supported the role of these structures in the causation of neck pain.[21,22]

Cervical Radiculopathy

Biochemical and biomechanical changes that occur with age result in a degenerative cascade. The intervertebral disk gradually loses height, posterior portions of the disk bulge into the spinal canal and the neuroforamina, the ligamentum flavum and facet joint capsule infold, and osteophytes form. All of this leads to decreases in canal and foraminal size. Subluxation and hypermobility between vertebral bodies may occur.

It is not clear why compression of a nerve causes pain. It is generally believed that only an inflamed or irritated nerve root can result in radicular pain on compression. Neurogenic chemical mediators of pain released from the cell bodies of the sensory neurons and non-neurogenic mediators released from disk tissue may play a role in initiating and perpetuating an inflammatory response.[23,24] Chronic edema and fibrosis within the nerve root caused by compression can also potentially alter the response threshold and increase the sensitivity of the nerve root to pain.[25] It may be that the dorsal root ganglion is the source of pain, as it is exquisitely sensitive to deformation.[26] In addition to mechanical compression of the dorsal root ganglion, the prolapsed nucleus pulposus elutes inflammatory mediators, initiating a local inflammatory response that leads to increased permeability at the dorsal root ganglion and pain.[27]

Cervical Myelopathy

Mechanical compression of the spinal cord is widely held to be the primary pathophysiologic mechanism of cervical myelopathy. Animal studies have shown that at least 40% cord compression was necessary to produce reversible neurologic deficits.[28] Patients with less than 40% compression and myelopathy are likely to have additional factors such as a developmentally reduced anteroposterior diameter of the spinal canal, dynamic cord compression, dynamic changes in the intrinsic morphology of the spinal cord, or an impaired vascular supply of the spinal cord. The anteroposterior diameter of the subaxial spine in normal adults measures 17 to 18 mm. Individuals with an anteroposterior diameter of the canal of less than 13 mm are considered to have developmental stenosis and may be predisposed to the development of cervical myelopathy.[29] The shape and cross-sectional area of the spinal canal are important predictors of the development of cervical myelopathy. A cross-sectional area of the spinal cord of less than 60 mm² and a banana-shaped cord both have been found to be associated with the development of clinical signs or symptoms of myelopathy.[30,31] An anteroposterior cord compression ratio (the ratio of the anteroposterior to the transverse cord diameter) of less than 40% suggested substantial flattening of the cord and also was found to be associated with worse neurologic dysfunction.[32] Changes in the dimensions of the spinal canal during normal neck movement or as a result of abnormal segmental mobility may play a role in the development of cervical myelopathy by causing dynamic cord compression. The segmental anteroposterior diameter as well as the volume of the cervical spinal canal have been found to be reduced in extension.[33,34] Retrolisthesis of C3 on C4 could accentuate cord compression in elderly individuals with myelopathy.[35] Instability at a segment cephalad to a motion segment with severe disk degeneration may lead to dynamic cord compression.[36]

Morphologic changes also occur within the spinal cord with flexion and extension. Breig and associates[37] previously showed that the spinal cord stretches with flexion of the cervical spine and shortens and thickens with extension of the cervical spine. Thickening of the cord in extension makes it more susceptible to pressure from the infolded ligamentum flavum or the lamina. In flexion, the stretched cord may be prone to higher intrinsic pressure if it abuts against a disk or a vertebral body anteriorly.

Experimental studies have shown that ischemia of the cord has an additive effect on the clinical manifestations of myelopathy resulting from compression.[38,39] Tenting of the anterior spinal arteries as well as reduced flow in the anterior radicular arteries and especially the transverse intramedullary arterioles arising from the anterior sulcal artery can lead to ischemia of the anterior horn and the adjacent lateral columns.[37,40] Abnormal movement of a motion segment can trigger a vasospastic response that can also compromise the cord's intrinsic blood supply.[41]

Clinical Evaluation
Neck Pain
Localized pain and tenderness in the posterior muscles of the neck suggest a muscle sprain or a soft-tissue injury. Deep palpation of "trigger points" produces referred patterns of pain along the course of the myofascial structures. Determining a position of maximal discomfort may also provide a clue to the underlying pathologic entity. Pain in the posterior neck muscles that is worsened by flexion of the head suggests a myofascial etiology. Pain in the posterior aspect of the neck that is aggravated by extension, and especially by rotation of the head to one side, suggests a discogenic component. Predominant suboccipital pain radiating to the back of the ear, occiput, or neck raises the possibility of pathologic involvement of the upper cervical spine. Restricted rotation of the head to one side suggests involvement of the ipsilateral atlantoaxial articulation.

Pain in the neck and shoulder girdle can be referred from the heart, lungs, and abdominal viscera. Morning stiffness, polyarticular involvement, rigidity, or cutaneous manifestations accompanying the neck pain suggest a systemic inflammatory arthritic process. Fever, weight loss, or nonmechanical neck pain may point to an infectious or neoplastic lesion in the cervical spine, causing neck pain.

Cervical Radiculopathy
Henderson and associates[42] reviewed the clinical presentations in 736 patients with cervical radiculopathy and reported that 99% had arm pain, 85% had sensory deficits, 80% had neck pain, 71% had reflex deficits, 68% had motor deficits, 52% had scapular pain, 18% had anterior chest pain, 10% had headaches, and 1% presented with left-sided chest and arm pain ("cervical angina"). The symptoms are usually aggravated by extension or lateral rotation of the head to the side of the pain (the Spurling maneuver). Patients with radicular pain may obtain some relief by elevating the arm overhead (the shoulder abduction sign) and sometimes by flexing and tilting the neck to the contralateral side.[43]

Upper cervical radiculopathies occasionally present as suboccipital pain with referral to the back of the ear. C4 radiculopathy can present as neck and shoulder pain with accompanying ipsilateral diaphragmatic palsy.[44] Paresthesias along the superior border of the trapezius are a clue to a radicular etiology. Nonspondylotic pathologic conditions can occasionally simulate cervical radiculopathy (Figure 1, Table 1).

Cervical Myelopathy
Patients with cervical myelopathy generally present with clumsiness or a loss of fine motor skills in the hands. An increasingly awkward gait or difficulty with maintaining balance may have been noted by the patient or family members. Patients may report urinary urgency, hesitation, or frequency but rarely incontinence or retention of urine. Concomitant axial neck pain and/or radiculopathy are frequent. Motor weakness and wasting may be present in the upper or lower extremities. Pain, temperature, proprioception and vibratory sensations, and touch all may be diminished in the extremities and the trunk, depending on the location of the spinal cord compromise. Abnormal reflex findings include hyperreflexia or clonus of normal deep tendon reflexes, absence of superficial reflexes, or the presence of pathologic reflexes (the inverted radial reflex, the Hoffmann reflex, and the extensor plantar response) (Figure 1). Myelopathy hand is a term used to refer to a constellation of findings, including loss of dexterity, diffuse numbness, wasting of the intrinsic hand muscles, inability to rapidly grasp and release the fist, and ulnar and flexor drift of the ulnar two digits while attempting to keep the fingers adducted and extended (finger escape sign).[32,45] Myelopathy resulting from a cord level cephalad to C3 may result in a hyperactive scapulohumeral reflex—that is, tapping of the spine of the scapula or acromion results in scapular elevation and/or abduction of the humerus.

Investigations
Patients with warning signs and symptoms of serious pathologic involvement of the cervical spine, such as tumor, infection, fracture, or neurologic injury, should undergo appropriate imaging studies without delay (Table 2). For all other

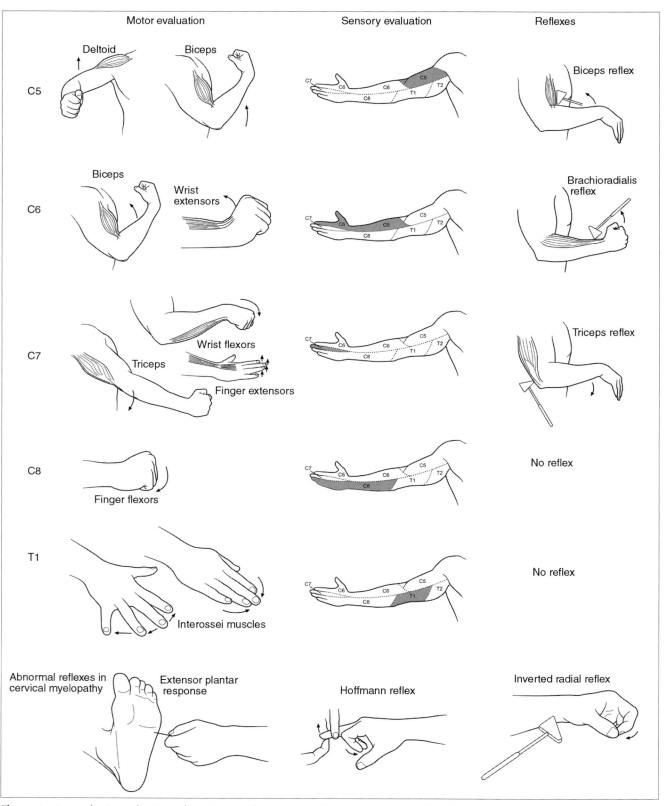

Figure 1 Neurologic evaluation of a patient with cervical radiculopathy and myelopathy.

Table 1
Differential Diagnosis of Cervical Radiculopathy

Peripheral entrapment syndromes

Rotator cuff/shoulder abnormalities

Brachial plexitis

Herpes zoster

Thoracic outlet syndrome

Sympathetic mediated pain syndrome

Intraspinal or extraspinal tumor

Epidural abscess

Cardiac ischemia

Table 2
Warning Signs of Serious Cervical Spine Disorders Necessitating Immediate Imaging Studies

Potential Cause	Clinical Characteristics
Fracture	Clinically relevant trauma in adolescent or adult; minor trauma in elderly patient; ankylosing spondylitis
Neoplasm	Pain worse at night; unexplained weight loss; history of neoplasm; age older than 50 years or younger than 20 years
Infection	Fever, chills, night sweats; unexplained weight loss; history of recent systemic infection; recent invasive procedure; immunosuppression; intravenous drug use
Neurologic injury	Progressive neurologic deficit; upper and lower extremity symptoms; bowel or bladder dysfunction

patients, imaging studies are delayed for 4 to 6 weeks to allow time for spontaneous recovery.

Plain Radiographs

Plain radiographs should be made with the patient in an upright position when possible. Degenerative changes such as intervertebral disk space narrowing, osteoarthrosis of the facet and uncovertebral joints, osteophytes, and end-plate sclerosis are ubiquitous in the adult population and are not diagnostic.[46] The Pavlov ratio is calculated by dividing the anteroposterior diameter of the spinal canal by the anteroposterior diameter of the vertebral body. A normal value is 1.0. A value of less than 0.8 suggests developmental canal stenosis but does not correlate with the space available for the spinal cord.[47,48] Lateral flexion-extension radiographs are used to measure the cervical range of motion and to identify ankylosed segments and cervical instability (translation of > 3.5 mm and relative sagittal plane angulation of > 11°).[49]

Computed Tomography With Myelography

Compressive osteophytes, foraminal stenosis, and ossification of the posterior longitudinal ligament are best identified with use of CT scans. CT myelography, an invasive procedure, is reportedly better than MRI in distinguishing osseous from soft-tissue impingement of neural structures and in detecting foraminal stenosis.[50,51] Shafaie and associates[52] found that concordance between CT and MRI findings was only moderately good in the interpretation of degenerative cervical spine changes that led to radiculopathy or myelopathy. CT myelography tended to upgrade the degree of spinal canal compromise, neural foraminal encroachment, and cord diameter reduction. They concluded that, while CT myelography and MRI should be considered complementary studies, CT myelography may be preferable to MRI because of its superior differentiation of bone and soft tissues.[52] CT myelography also provides better imaging detail in patients with postoperative metal artifacts or scoliotic deformity.

Magnetic Resonance Imaging

MRI is the diagnostic standard for evaluation of the soft tissues of the cervical spine, including the neural elements, disk, joint capsule, and ligaments. Abnormalities are frequently seen on the MRIs of adults, and it is important to correlate imaging and clinical findings. Teresi and associates[53] found disk degeneration on the MRIs of 5 of 25 asymptomatic individuals between 45 and 54 years of age and those of 24 of 42 asymptomatic individuals who were older than 64 years. Spinal cord compression was found on the images of 9 of 58 individuals who were younger than 64 years and on those of 11 of 42 individuals who were older than 64 years.[53] Boden and associates[1] detected foraminal stenosis on the images of 1 of 40 asymptomatic patients who were younger than 40 years and on those of 5 of 23 patients who were older than 40 years.

MRI also allows direct visualization of intramedullary cord changes. Ohshio and associates[54] reported a direct correlation between histopathologic features and intramedullary signal changes on MRI. Isolated areas of high signal intensity on T2-weighted images indicate edema, which may resolve. A combination of low signal intensity on T1-weighted images and high signal intensity on T2-weighted images indicates severe lesions in gray matter with necrosis, myelomalacia, or spongiform changes.

Intramedullary signal changes in the cord have been detected in more than 60% of patients with symptomatic cervical myelopathy.[55-57] It is, however, not clear if the presence and the type of intramedullary signal changes in patients with symptomatic cervical myelopathy can be

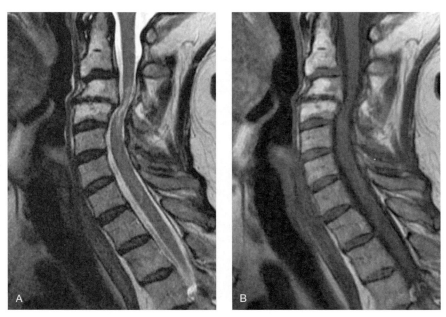

Figure 2 Sagittal MRIs of the cervical spine of a patient with cervical myelopathy. **A,** T2-weighted image showing a well-circumscribed and extensive high signal intensity lesion at the site of compression in the cephalad part of the cervical spinal cord. **B,** T1-weighted image showing low signal intensity change at the site of compression.

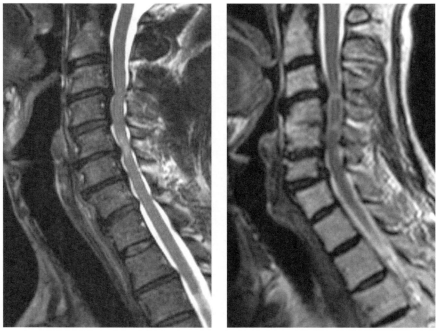

Figure 3 Sagittal T2-weighted MRI of a patient with cervical myelopathy. A high signal intensity lesion with a faint and ill-defined border is seen at the site of spinal cord compression at the level of the C5-C6 disk space.

Figure 4 Sagittal T2-weighted MRI of the cervical spine showing compression over several levels and multisegmental areas of high signal intensity.

used to predict either the prognosis or the outcome of treatment with any accuracy. High-intensity signal changes on T2-weighted images are found frequently and can be diffuse or well demarcated, focal or multisegmental; however, their clinical relevance is unclear (Figures 2 through 4). Well-demarcated high-intensity signal changes on T2-weighted images combined with low-intensity signal changes on T1-weighted images are rare; they usually are found in late stages of cervical myelopathy and indicate a more severe, irreversible pathologic condition such as late-stage myelomalacia and cystic necrosis.[58,59] Bednarik and associates[58] found high-intensity intramedullary signal changes on T2-weighted images of 23 of 66 asymptomatic patients with cervical stenosis, but they identified no patients with a combination of high-intensity intramedullary signal changes on T2-weighted images and low-intensity intramedullary signal changes on T1-weighted images. The presence of intramedullary signal changes does not predict a poor outcome after nonsurgical treatment in patients with mild myelopathy.[56]

Morio and associates[55] identified intramedullary signal changes in 71 of 73 patients who underwent surgery for clinically evident myelopathy. They concluded that, while low-intensity signal changes on T1-weighted images may indicate a poor prognosis, high-intensity signal changes on T2-weighted images can be caused by a broad spectrum of compressive myelomalacic pathologic conditions and reflect a broad spectrum of spinal cord recuperative potentials. In another surgical series, Suri and associates[57] identified intramedullary signal changes in 121 of 146 symptomatic patients. Of these 121 patients, 33% had changes only on the T2-weighted images and 67% had changes on both the T1- and the T2-weighted images. Patients without intramedullary signal changes or with changes only on T2-weighted images had significantly better postoperative motor strength than did patients with changes on both T1- and T2-weighted images ($P < 0.05$). There have also been reports that patients with focal high-intensity intramedullary signal changes on T2-weighted images have better clinical outcomes following surgery than do patients with multisegmental high-intensity intramedullary signal changes on T2-weighted images.[60,61]

The transverse area and shape of the spinal cord at the compressed segment may predict outcomes, with a preoperative transverse spinal cord area of less than 0.45 cm² correlating with poor surgical results.[62] With progressive compression, the cross section of the spinal cord changes from a boomerang shape to a teardrop shape to a triangular shape.[63] The boomerang and teardrop shapes have a better potential for recovery than do the triangular shape.

Metabolic neuroimaging technology recently has been applied to the spinal cord. Uchida and associates[64] compared findings on preoperative high-resolution[18] F-fluorodeoxyglucose-positron emission tomography (FDG-PET) with Japanese Orthopaedic Association (JOA) scores and findings on MRI in 23 patients undergoing surgery for myelopathy. FDG-PET findings correlated with preoperative JOA scores, postoperative JOA scores, and the rate of postoperative improvement, but they had no correlation with high-intensity intramedullary signal changes on T2-weighted images. Currently, the major limitation of

this technology is the poor resolution of PET scans. (Accurate measurements of glucose utilization are difficult to obtain.) Future technologic advancements in PET scanning may facilitate evaluation of early spinal cord damage and provide indications for surgical intervention.

Electrodiagnostic Studies

Electrodiagnostic studies may help to differentiate between various causes of symptoms, including myelopathy, radiculopathy, peripheral entrapment syndromes, peripheral neuropathy, shoulder dysfunction, and brachial plexopathy. Recommended investigations for neurophysiologic examination of patients with cervical myelopathy include testing of somatosensory-evoked potentials by stimulation of the tibial nerve and motor-evoked potentials from the upper and lower extremities.[65] Both motor-evoked potentials and somatosensory-evoked potentials can be abnormal in patients with spinal cord compression who have no clinical features of myelopathy.[66,67] Bednarik and associates[67] prospectively followed 30 patients with evidence of spinal cord compression on MRI, but no clinical evidence of cervical myelopathy, by testing motor- and somatosensory-evoked potentials for a period of 2 years. The authors detected electrophysiologic abnormalities in 15 of the 30 patients at the beginning of the study. Clinical signs of cervical myelopathy were detected in 5 of these 15 patients over the next 2 years, with at least one test of evoked potentials showing deterioration at the time of the appearance of the signs of cervical myelopathy. Myelopathy did not develop in any of the patients with normal motor- and somatosensory-evoked potentials at the beginning

of the study. Bednarik and associates concluded that there was a significant association between abnormal findings on evoked-potential studies and the development of cervical myelopathy in patients with spinal cord compression ($p = 0.02$).

Studies of motor- and somatosensory-evoked potentials might be useful in detecting subclinical myelopathy. In patients with evidence of spinal cord compression on MRI and symptoms but no definitive signs of myelopathy, motor-evoked potentials are more commonly abnormal than are somatosensory-evoked potentials.[66] Clinical features of cervical myelopathy can be masked in patients with peripheral neuropathy, and studies of evoked potentials can detect clinically silent myelopathy in these patients.[68] In patients with diagnosed cervical spondylotic myelopathy, upper extremity motor-evoked potentials are most commonly abnormal. Patients who have normal preoperative median somatosensory-evoked potentials may have better recovery rates after surgery for myelopathy than patients who have abnormal somatosensory-evoked potentials.[69] A decrease in motor-evoked potentials of 50% or more correlates well with a postoperative motor deficit.[70]

Electromyography can show increased insertional activity, fibrillations, and fasciculations and diminished motor unit recruitment, which are signs of denervation caused by pathologic changes at the nerve root or anterior horn cells. Electromyography in combination with nerve conduction velocity studies can help to distinguish cervical radiculopathy from peripheral neuropathy or peripheral root entrapment syndromes in some patients. The value of electromyography as a primary diagnostic modality for patients with clinical signs of radiculopathy is offset by its low sensitivity.[71,72] Its concordance with MRI findings in patients is low. Nardin and associates[73] reported that, in 19 of 47 patients with cervical radiculopathy, electromyographic results did not correlate with findings on MRI. Additionally, electromyography is less likely to show abnormal findings in patients with predominantly sensory radiculopathy.[73,74] It may be possible to improve the sensitivity of electromyography for detecting cervical radiculopathy by the addition of paraspinal muscles to the electromyography screen.[75]

Nonsurgical Management

Narcotic analgesics, nonsteroidal anti-inflammatory agents, corticosteroids, muscle relaxants, and antidepressants are commonly used to relieve neck pain and radiculopathy. A short period of rest or cessation of pain-provoking activities and the use of a soft collar with the neck in mild flexion may sometimes alleviate acute pain and spasm. In a meta-analysis of the literature, physical modalities such as heat, cold, therapeutic ultrasound, massage, use of transcutaneous electrical nerve stimulation (TENS), and cervical traction were not found to have any reproducible benefit in the treatment of acute or chronic neck pain.[76] A 4- to 6-week program of physical therapy, including isometric exercises, active range-of-motion exercises, aerobic conditioning, and resistive exercises has been found to be helpful for patients with chronic neck pain.[77,78] There have been a few reports of substantial relief of radicular pain and improved functional outcome after the use of cervical traction for the treatment of cervical radiculopathy.[79,80] Long-

term success has been reported in 40% to 70% of patients who received translaminar or transforaminal epidural corticosteroid injections for treatment of cervical radiculopathy.[81-83] Rare but potentially catastrophic complications can be associated with these injection techniques.[84] In a cohort of patients with neck pain or radicular symptoms in the upper extremities followed for 10 to 25 years, Gore and associates[85] found that nonsurgical management resulted in complete resolution of symptoms in 43% of the patients and partial resolution in 25%, whereas 32% had continued moderate or severe pain.

Patients with mild myelopathy are occasionally offered a trial of observation or nonsurgical management, but nonsurgical management is generally not successful in reversing or permanently halting the progress of myelopathy. Conservative treatment includes intermittent cervical immobilization in a soft collar; anti-inflammatory medications and bed rest; and active discouragement of high-risk activities, manipulation therapies, and vigorous or prolonged flexion of the head.[86] A greater anteroposterior diameter of the spinal canal, a transverse area of the spinal cord greater than 70 mm², and age older than 56 years are factors that seem to be associated with a better response to conservative treatment by patients with mild myelopathy.[87]

Indications for Surgical Intervention

Success rates for nonsurgical management of neck pain and cervical radiculopathy may vary depending on the patient population studied. Even in a referral practice, 70% to 80% of patients with neck pain respond favorably to nonsurgical treatment.[88,89]

Surgical intervention is considered for the following patients with predominantly axial neck pain.

1. Those with severely limiting pain caused by cervical degenerative disease that is not relieved by nonsurgical treatment of more than 12 months. It is difficult to identify the symptomatic level in these patients with MRI alone,[90,91] and objective confirmation of the disk as the "pain generator" with use of both MRI and provocative diskography should be considered to improve the clinical success rates. A nonorganic component to the pain should be absent. Anterior diskectomy and fusion is the surgical intervention of choice for these patients with discogenic neck pain.

2. Patients with C3 or C4 nerve root impingement can present with features simulating axial neck pain. Patients with such "pseudoaxial" neck pain who do not respond to nonsurgical measures for 6 to 12 weeks may be candidates for surgical intervention.

3. Patients with pseudarthrosis of the cervical spine with graft collapse or hardware migration and disabling axial neck pain are candidates for revision anterior surgery. Patients without implant failure may have higher fusion rates and superior clinical outcomes after posterior cervical fusion with instrumentation than after anterior revision.[92,93]

Surgery is an option for patients with persistent cervical radiculopathy following failure of a 3-month trial of nonsurgical measures to relieve disabling radicular pain. These patients must have neuroimaging studies that show a pathologic condition that corresponds to the clinical features. Surgery is also an option for patients with a progressive motor deficit or a disabling motor deficit from the radiculopathy.[94]

Studies of the natural history of cervical myelopathy suggest that most patients with clinically established disease will have progression of symptoms, possibly in a stepwise fashion with time.[95-98] Bednarik and associates[58] found that clinical signs or symptoms of myelopathy developed in 13 of 66 patients with asymptomatic spinal cord compression seen on MRI in a study with a minimum 2-year follow-up. Patients with mild myelopathy probably do not benefit from surgery. In a prospective randomized study with a duration of follow-up of 3 years, patients with mild to moderate nonprogressive or slowly progressive myelopathy were found to have similar outcomes after either nonsurgical or surgical treatment.[86] A trial of nonsurgical treatment did not decrease the potential for ultimate recovery of patients with mild myelopathy.[99] Patients with severe or progressive myelopathy are candidates for surgical intervention. Several factors are considered in the decision regarding when to proceed with surgery in patients with myelopathy; these include the degree of neurologic dysfunction, patient disability, findings on radiographs and MRI, duration of symptoms, and presence of comorbidity.

Surgical Options and Techniques

The two options typically considered for the surgical management of cervical radiculopathy are (1) anterior cervical diskectomy and fusion and (2) posterior laminotomy-foraminotomy. An anterior approach is preferred for patients with a central or bilateral disk lesion, whereas a lateral cervical disk herniation can be approached either anteriorly or posteriorly. The long-term results of the two procedures are comparable, but anterior cervical diskectomy and fusion is preferred for patients who have substantial neck pain associated with radicular symptoms.[100-102] Patients with myelopathy should be treated with anterior cervical diskectomy or corpectomy when there is pathologic compression at up to three levels or when cervical lordosis is reversed.[103] A laminectomy or laminoplasty is used in patients requiring decompression at four or more segments, those with a developmentally narrow canal, and those in whom the anterior column is already fused. Cervical lordosis is critical for a posterior approach because it allows the cord to migrate dorsally after the decompression.

Anterior Cervical Diskectomy and Corpectomy

A subtotal diskectomy with removal of cartilaginous end plates and anterior osteophytes is done through a Smith-Robinson approach[104] (Figure 5). We prefer to use a left-sided approach because the course of the recurrent laryngeal nerve is more sheltered within the tracheoesophageal groove on this side.

After removal of disk material within the interspace, posterior osteophytes may need to be removed to adequately decompress the spinal cord and nerve root. Removal of posterior osteophytes increases the risk of injury to the spinal cord, and large osteophytes may be removed more safely with a partial corpectomy.[105] Osteophytes may resorb after a successful anterior fusion, but this theory is controversial.[106,107] Removal of the posterior longitudinal ligament similarly increases the risk of cord contusion and postoperative epidural hematoma,[108] but it should be done if a rent in the posterior longitudinal ligament is detected or if there is clinical or imaging-based suspicion of an extruded fragment posterior to the ligament.

During the corpectomy, a 15- to 19-mm central trough is removed from the anterior aspect of the vertebral body with a rongeur or a high-speed burr. A thin residue of posterior wall and the posterior longitudinal ligament are resected with use of a diamond-tipped burr, small curets, and a 1-mm Kerrison rongeur as required. The adequacy of the decompression is assessed by visual inspection of the decompressed posterior longitudinal ligament or dura.

Anterior cervical diskectomy without fusion results in a higher prevalence of postoperative neck pain, can lead to a reduction in the neuroforaminal area, and is rarely advised.[109,110]

Anterior Fusion

All cartilaginous material is removed, but the integrity of the osseous end plate is preserved to provide mechanical stability to the inserted graft. Four or five tiny perforations are created within the cephalad and caudad osseous end plates with use of a small curet or burr to facilitate fusion across the interspace. Some surgeons remove the osseous end plates and seat the inserted graft within the exposed cancellous bone, with the aim of improving fusion rates.[111] The graft should be 2 mm taller than the measured height of the disk space to maintain sagittal alignment. The graft is recessed 2 mm posterior to the anterior cortical margin of the adjacent vertebral bodies.

Following anterior diskectomy, the placement of a tricortical horseshoe-shaped autograft harvested from the anterior iliac crest has led to excellent fusion rates.[112-114]

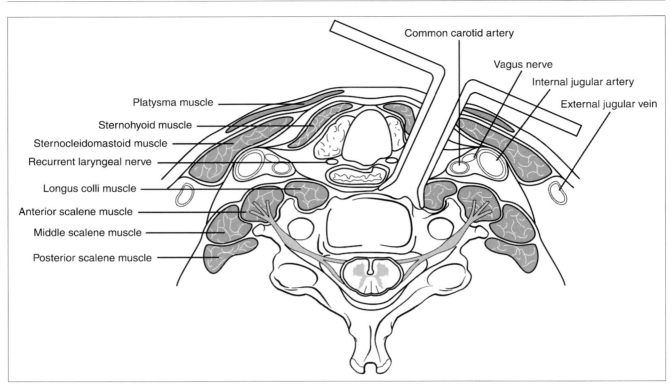

Figure 5 Cross-sectional anatomy through the midcervical spine, illustrating the fascial planes used in the anterior cervical approach. The strap muscles, the trachea, and the esophagus are retracted medially while the carotid sheath is retracted laterally. (Reproduced from Rao RD, Bagario V: Anterior approaches to the cervical and cervicothoracic spine, in *Orthopaedic Knowledge Online*. Rosemont, IL, American Academy of Orthopaedic Surgeons, 2005.)

Equivalent fusion rates have been reported after allografting and autografting, combined with use of anterior plates and segmental screw fixation, for intervertebral fusions of up to three levels.[115,116] Longer-term results are required before definite recommendations can be made regarding the use of titanium cages, carbon-fiber cages, and polyetheretherketone (PEEK) cages.[117-119]

Tricortical iliac crest autograft struts are the best option for anterior column reconstruction after a one- or two-level anterior cervical corpectomy, but they are associated with donor site morbidity. A fibular strut is preferred when the iliac crest is mechanically insufficient or for corpectomy defects that are longer than two levels. The use of longer strut grafts after multilevel corpectomies is associated with complications. Settling of the graft with kyphotic change in the angulation and fracture of the fibular strut graft has been reported after the use of long fibular grafts.[120,121] Wang and associates[122] found the risk of graft displacement and migration to be higher as the number of removed vertebral bodies increased and when the fusion extended down to C7. Use of metallic cages and synthetic spacers in conjunction with local autograft or allograft after single- or multiple-level corpectomies (Figure 6) has resulted in comparable fusion rates, but the long-term results are still unclear.[123,124] High rates of early failure of the reconstruction, cage subsidence, and plate loosening have been reported following the use of titanium mesh cages in multilevel corpectomies.[125,126]

Anterior Cervical Plates

After either diskectomy or corpectomy, anterior osteophytes are removed from the margins of the adjacent vertebrae to prepare a flat bed for the plate. The length of the plate is selected so that a minimum distance of 5 mm is maintained between the ends of the plate and the adjacent disks (Figure 7). This helps to decrease adjacent-level disk ossification.[127] The use of screws locked to the plate obviates the need for bicortical purchase in the vertebral body. When multisegmental fixation is performed, an attempt should be made to fix the plate to all vertebral levels.

The use of an anterior cervical plate in an anterior cervical diskectomy and fusion involving two or more levels improves fusion rates, reduces the need for postoperative stabilization, reduces graft-related complications, and is associated with less postoperative kyphosis.[128,129] Use of an anterior cervical plate after a single-level anterior cervical diskectomy and fusion with autograft bone does not improve clinical results or fusion rates but reduces graft collapse.[130,131] An anterior plate may be beneficial when allograft bone is used for a single-level anterior cervical diskectomy and fusion.[132] Fusion occurs in approximately 90% of patients who have a single-level anterior cervical diskectomy.[133,134] The prevalence of pseudarthrosis increases with the number of levels that are operated on.[112]

The use of an anterior plate has been found to reduce pseudarthrosis rates following single-level corpectomy.[135] Failure rates ranging from 6 of 12 to 5 of 7 have been reported following corpectomy involving three or more levels, even with use of an anterior plate, and supplemental posterior instrumentation should be considered for such patients.[136,137]

Cervical Disk Replacement

Artificial disk replacement has not yet been approved by the US Food and Drug Administration for clinical use. Cervical disk replacement has been proposed as an alternative to anterior cervical diskectomy and fusion in patients with pathologic involvement of a cervical disk. Although the causes of deterioration of motion segments adjacent to a "stiff" fusion are unclear, a theoretic benefit of disk replacement is a reduction in

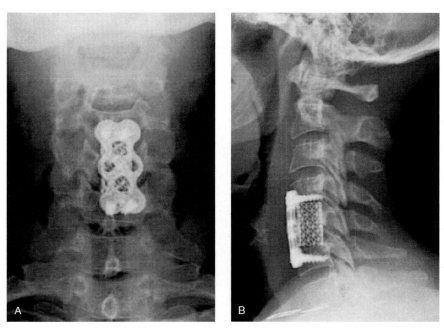

Figure 6   AP (**A**) and lateral (**B**) radiographs of the cervical spin of a patient with cervical spondylotic myelopathy treated with C5 corpectomy, insertion of a titanium mesh cage packed with local autogenous bone in the trough, and application of an anterior cervical plate from C4 to C6.

this risk of adjacent segment deterioration.[138-140] Cadaver and clinical studies with a 2-year follow-up have demonstrated maintenance of motion at a surgical segment following disk replacement.[141,142] Selection of patients for cervical disk replacement currently is not standardized. Common exclusion criteria mentioned in the current literature are substantial cervical deformity, radiographic findings of segmental instability, isolated axial neck pain, a lack of motion at the segment preoperatively, and severe facet arthrosis.[143-145] In a series of 49 patients with a one-level disk replacement, 32 had an excellent result; 2, a good result; 10, a fair result; and 5, a poor result.[142] Comparable clinical outcomes were reported 2 years following Bryan artificial disk replacement and 2 years following anterior cervical diskectomy and fusion. Other early results have been similar.[146,147] In one study, the

prevalence of symptomatic adjacent-level degenerative disk disease in patients treated with fusion was reported to be significantly higher than that in patients treated with disk replacement ($P = 0.009$).[148] Heterotopic ossification, persistent pain, prosthetic migration, segmental kyphosis, and device failure have been reported following cervical disk replacement.[142,145,149,150]

Posterior Laminotomy-Foraminotomy

The keyhole foraminotomy technique was originally described by Scoville[151] and is used for patients with unilateral radicular findings caused by a lateral or foraminal soft cervical disk herniation or foraminal stenosis. The procedure involves removal of the lateral one third of the superior and inferior hemilaminae with removal of the medial one third of the facet joint. In the case of a soft cervical disk, the foraminot-

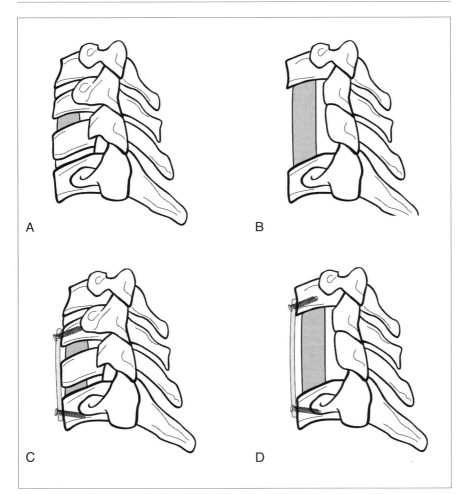

Figure 7 Common anterior surgical interventions used for cervical spondylosis. **A,** Anterior cervical diskectomy and insertion of a spacer for fusion. **B,** Anterior cervical corpectomy and insertion of a strut bone graft. **C,** Anterior cervical diskectomy followed by insertion of a bone spacer for fusion and application of an anterior plate. **D,** Anterior cervical corpectomy, insertion of a strut graft, and application of an anterior plate. (Reproduced with permission from Rao RD, Gourab K, David KS: Surgical treatment of cervical spondylotic myelopathy. *J Bone Joint Surg Am* 2006;88:1624.)

the risk of kyphosis, limits constriction of the dura from extradural scar formation, and obviates the need for fusion.[154,155]

Intraoperatively, visible expansion of the dural sac and pulsation of the dura after opening of the laminoplasty doors or following laminectomy suggest good canal expansion.[156] A laminoplasty opening gap of 8 to 10 mm and an average increase in the canal diameter of approximately 5 mm usually result in adequate decompression.[157,158] Foraminotomy is considered following a laminoplasty or laminectomy in patients who show foraminal stenosis from a disk protrusion or foraminal osteophytes and concordant radicular symptoms. A prophylactic C5 foraminotomy can be performed to reduce the prevalence of C5 palsy from posterior translation of the cord, although there is no clear evidence that it reduces the prevalence of C5 palsy.

The laminoplasty door is held open by anchoring the spinous process to the facet joint on the hinge side with use of suture or wire, or by insertion of autograft, allograft, or ceramic spacers on the open side. Stabilization of the open door with use of mini-plates fixed to the lamina and the lateral mass without major complications has been reported by multiple authors[159,160] (Figure 8).

omy is followed by excision of the extruded disk fragment with use of a small, blunt-tipped nerve hook. Foraminotomy alone is adequate in patients with foraminal stenosis because of an osteophytic ridge.[152] Microendoscopic posterior cervical foraminotomy techniques may further reduce the postoperative pain and disability associated with muscle stripping during an open foraminotomy.[153]

Laminoplasty

Laminoplasty increases the effective diameter of the spinal canal from C3 to C7 by shifting the laminae dorsally with use of either a so-called single door with a single lateral hinge or a double door with lateral hinges on both sides. In contrast to laminectomy, laminoplasty retains a covering of posterior laminar bone and ligamentum flavum over the spinal cord, minimizes the instability and

Laminectomy

Laminectomy can be considered when decompression is required at more than three levels, particularly in elderly patients, in whom comorbidities increase surgical risk. All levels with radiographic evidence of stenosis should be included in the decompression. Limiting the number of segments that are decompressed does not influence the development of postlaminectomy

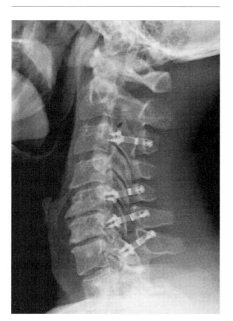

Figure 8 Lateral radiograph of the cervical spine of a patient with cervical spondylotic myelopathy managed with C3-C7 laminoplasty and mini plate fixation.

kyphosis or instability, but inclusion of C2 and T1 in the laminectomy increases the likelihood of kyphosis and instability developing.[161,162] Concern about postlaminectomy kyphosis and instability has led to the development of the laminectomy with fusion and posterior instrumentation.

Laminectomy without instrumentation should be restricted to patients with preserved cervical lordosis. In patients with a flexible cervical kyphosis, laminectomy may be combined with application of posterior instrumentation with the neck extended to restore cervical lordosis and maximize posterior shift of the spinal cord.

Posterior Cervical Instrumentation

Instrumentation options for posterior cervical fixation after laminectomy include sublaminar and facet wires connected to a longitudinal rod or a rectangular construct, and interspinous wires.[163,164] Lateral mass and cervical pedicle-based screw fixation systems are alternative options for patients with deficient posterior elements, but they have not yet been approved by the Food and Drug Administration for clinical use in the United States.[165-167] To reduce the risk of spinal cord injury during the use of lateral mass or pedicle screws, the screw holes should be drilled before the laminectomy. Pedicle screws may be preferable at C2 and C7 because the lateral masses are poorly developed at these levels. The reported prevalence of fusion in patients treated with instrumentation is better than that in patients treated with bone grafting alone.[166,168,169]

Outcomes Following Cervical Surgery

Neck Pain

Most patients with axial neck pain respond favorably to nonsurgical management.[85,88,89,96] Clinical outcomes in patients with predominantly axial neck pain may be influenced by psychologic factors.[114,170] The benign natural history of neck pain, difficulty in identifying an accurate pain generator, and the lack of randomized controlled studies comparing surgical and nonsurgical management have led many surgeons to recommend nonsurgical management for patients with axial neck pain, but some studies have demonstrated a substantial decrease in pain and improved function following anterior cervical diskectomy and fusion for axial neck pain.[91,171] Use of both MRI and provocative diskography to determine whether fusion should be performed in patients with axial neck pain has been found to reduce the number of levels that need to be fused, and sometimes painful levels are revealed to be morphologically normal on the MRI.[91]

Cervical Radiculopathy

Anterior cervical diskectomy and fusion is an excellent surgical option for the treatment of cervical radiculopathy, with good to excellent clinical results in 70% to 90% of patients.[112,172,173] The age of the patient, the duration of symptoms, and the type of disk (soft or hard) have not been found to affect the clinical outcome.[174,175] Nonsmokers tend to have significantly more relief of arm pain and a better clinical outcome than smokers ($P < 0.01$).[133] Additionally, male gender, greater segmental kyphosis, a greater preoperative range of motion of the neck, greater right and left hand grip strength, an organic type of pain drawing, and a low disability score on the Neck Disability Index (NDI) have been significantly correlated with better postoperative pain relief in patients with radiculopathy ($P < 0.1$).[176]

Wirth and associates[101] found no significant difference between the clinical outcomes following anterior cervical diskectomy and fusion and those following posterior foraminotomy for the treatment of cervical radiculopathy. Recurrence of radiculopathy at the same level was more common after foraminotomy, whereas recurrence at other levels was more common after anterior cervical diskectomy and fusion. Patients treated with posterior foraminotomy more frequently have persistent neck pain postoperatively.[100] Herkowitz and associates[102] concluded that there was not a significant difference between the results of anterior cervical diskectomy and fusion and those of posterior foraminotomy, although there was a trend for better clinical outcomes after anterior cervical diskectomy and fusion.

Cervical Myelopathy

Good restoration of spinal canal dimensions, earlier decompression, lack of comorbidity, and either a complete lack of intramedullary cord changes or only isolated changes on T2-weighted MRIs predict better outcomes following anterior decompression for the treatment of cervical myelopathy.[57,177,178] Emery and associates[179] reported on 106 patients with cervical myelopathy who had undergone either anterior diskectomy or corpectomy and fusion without instrumentation. Eighty-two of these patients had preoperative gait abnormalities; 38 of them recovered normal gait, and an additional 33 had an improvement in gait. Substantial improvements in hand function and sensory deficits also have been reported after anterior decompression for the treatment of myelopathy.[177,179,180]

A meta-analysis revealed that 55% of more than 2,000 patients showed some neurologic recovery following laminoplasty.[181] The neurologic outcome was not influenced by the laminoplasty technique and was similar after laminoplasty and laminectomy.

In a study comparing 23 patients treated with cervical corpectomy and 24 patients treated with cervical laminoplasty for multilevel spondylotic myelopathy, no significant difference in neurologic recovery was found between the groups at 1 year, at 5 years, or at the time of final follow-up, which ranged from 10 to 14 years.[182] Longer surgical times and more blood loss were reported with the anterior cervical surgery, whereas frequent axial neck pain and more postoperative stiffness were reported after the laminoplasties.

Common Complications of Surgical Intervention
Neurologic Complications

Flynn[183] reported 311 neurologic complications following more than 36,000 anterior cervical diskectomy and fusion procedures done by 704 neurosurgeons. Radiculopathy accounted for 40% of the complications; substantial permanent myelopathy, 25%; and recurrent laryngeal nerve palsy, 17%. Recurrent laryngeal nerve palsy has been reported in 2% to 11% of patients following an anterior cervical approach.[184,185] A prospective study in which preoperative and postoperative laryngoscopy was performed in 123 patients who underwent single- or multiple-level anterior cervical diskectomy or corpectomy with fusion demonstrated a 24% initial prevalence of recurrent laryngeal nerve palsy with persistence of the palsy at 3 months in 13%.[186] Comparative studies have not shown any significant correlation between the side of the approach and the prevalence of recurrent laryngeal nerve palsy.[187] Avoidance of prolonged retraction, knowledge of the anatomy, careful dissection, and deflation of the endotracheal tube cuff after placement of the retractor may all help to diminish the prevalence of this complication.

Postoperative C5 radiculopathy can occur after laminoplasty or laminectomy, presumably as a result of traction on the short C5 nerve root due to posterior migration of the cord after posterior decompression or as a result of closure of the laminoplasty door causing nerve impingement. The complication is equally frequent following anterior surgery, possibly because of impingement of the ventral aspect of the spinal cord against the edges of a corpectomy trough. C5 radiculopa-

thy occurred in approximately 4% of patients after anterior surgery or laminoplasty and in 1% of patients after laminectomy.[188] Patients with a postoperative C5 palsy were found to have more severe cord compression at the C3-C4 and C4-C5 levels than did patients without palsy.[189] Spontaneous recovery is expected in most patients, but it may be delayed for up to 12 months.[105,189] Concurrent foraminotomy and intraoperative electromyographic monitoring of the C5 nerve root may help to diminish the prevalence of this condition.[190,191] Injury to the superior laryngeal nerve leading to easy voice fatigue and difficulty with high-pitched tones, and Horner syndrome from injury to the sympathetic nerves, occur infrequently after anterior surgery.

Neck Pain

More than half of patients experience posterior neck and shoulder girdle pain after laminoplasty, and the pain may be severe.[192] The prevalence of axial pain and stiffness following multilevel posterior decompression has been reportedly lowered by preservation of the extensor muscle and ligament attachments by performing partial or complete laminectomies or interlaminar decompression at a few levels or by reattaching osteotomized spinous processes after laminoplasty, and by early postoperative mobilization.[182,193-196] In addition, restricting the laminoplasty to the C3-C6 level and avoiding the inclusion of C7 in the procedure reduce the prevalence of early postoperative axial neck pain.[197]

Neck Stiffness

Neck stiffness is common after laminoplasty or laminectomy with fusion and instrumentation. In a meta-analysis of laminoplasty, approximately half of the range of motion of the neck was found to be lost postoperatively.[181] Postoperative interlaminar osseous fusion, which occurs most frequently at C2-C3, may be one of the major causes of restriction of the range of motion following laminoplasty.[198] Substantial postoperative stiffness is not common following anterior cervical diskectomy and fusion. Stiffness following corpectomy and fusion is more pronounced in patients who have undergone a three- or four-level procedure.[199]

Instability and Kyphosis

Laminectomy alone, especially in children and young adults or in patients with preexisting kyphosis or segmental mobility, can result in postoperative instability, kyphosis, and worsening of the neurologic deficit.[200] Laminectomy with fusion and instrumentation maintains lordosis that is close to its preoperative value.[165] Kyphosis can also result following laminoplasty, especially when C2 is included, when preoperative lordosis is less than 10°, and when the range of preoperative flexion is greater than the range of preoperative extension.[181,201,202]

Dysphagia

Hematoma, local edema, denervation of the pharyngeal plexus, adhesions between the esophagus, trachea, and prevertebral fascia, and a displaced graft or instrumentation are potential causes of dysphagia after anterior surgery. A prevalence of dysphagia of as high as 50% at 1 month, but with gradual improvement over time, has been reported.[203,204] The risk of dysphagia is higher after multilevel procedures and in patients with long-standing neck pain, but the type of procedure

(diskectomy or corpectomy) and the use of an anterior plate do not influence the prevalence of postoperative dysphagia.[203,204]

Adjacent Segment Deterioration

The prevalence of adjacent segment degeneration increases each year following anterior cervical fusion, with about 25% of patients having symptomatic adjacent segment disease at 10 years.[205] The facts that segments most prone to adjacent-segment deterioration are C5-C6 and C6-C7, which are also most likely to naturally show degenerative changes, and that this prevalence is similar to that found following foraminotomy without fusion, suggest that adjacent segment disease may be a consequence of the natural evolution of spondylotic disease and not necessarily related to the adjacent fusion.

Complications With Instrumentation

Breakage or loosening of a plate or screws has been reported in 35% of patients after anterior surgery.[206] Hardware failure was more common when the screws were not locked to the plate.[206] Migration of the loosened screws into the esophagus is a potential complication.[207,208]

Nerve root injury is the most common complication after posterior instrumentation, but it occurs in fewer than 1% of patients. In one study, cortical penetration was reported in association with 10 of 190 pedicle screws inserted (5%), with no resulting neurovascular complications in these patients.[167]

Summary

Degenerative cervical spondylosis can present clinically as axial neck pain, cervical radiculopathy, or cer-

vical myelopathy. Pathoanatomic changes are generally well visualized on imaging studies and must be correlated with the clinical findings. Most patients with axial neck pain, cervical radiculopathy, or mild cervical myelopathy respond well to an initial trial of nonsurgical management.

Anterior cervical diskectomy and fusion and laminotomy-foraminotomy are options for the surgical management of cervical radiculopathy. The clinical outcome after the performance of either of these procedures to treat cervical radiculopathy is excellent. Surgical considerations in patients with cervical myelopathy include the number of levels involved, the alignment of the cervical spine, and the dimensions of the spinal canal. The clinical outcome following surgery for cervical myelopathy depends primarily on the duration since the onset of symptoms, the presence and pattern of intramedullary signal changes on MRI, and the adequacy of decompression. Both anterior and posterior decompressions of the cervical spinal cord result in satisfactory outcomes. Approach-related complications such as dysphagia and injury to the laryngeal nerves are concerns with the anterior neck approach, whereas persistent neck pain, stiffness, and the development of instability are concerns with the posterior approach.

Instrumentation is frequently used in conjunction with anterior or posterior fusion to increase the rigidity of the construct and to enhance the success of the fusion. The use of a plate following anterior fusion improves fusion rates after multilevel anterior cervical diskectomy or single-level corpectomy and can reduce the prevalence of postoperative dislodgment of the graft and the development of kyphosis even following single-level diskectomy. The prevalence of complications remains high after multilevel anterior cervical corpectomies, despite the addition of an anterior cervical plate, and supplemental posterior stabilization ought to be considered for these patients. Artificial disk replacement in the cervical spine is still in its infancy, and long-term outcomes are required before it can be recommended.

References

1. Boden SD, McCowin PR, Davis DO, Dina TS, Mark AS, Wiesel S: Abnormal magnetic-resonance scans of the cervical spine in asymptomatic subjects: A prospective investigation. *J Bone Joint Surg Am* 1990;72:1178-1184.

2. Lehto IJ, Tertti MO, Komu ME, Paajanen HE, Tuominen J, Kormano MJ: Age-related MRI changes at 0.1 T in cervical discs in asymptomatic subjects. *Neuroradiology* 1994;36:49-53.

3. Matsumoto M, Fujimura Y, Suzuki N, et al: MRI of cervical intervertebral discs in asymptomatic subjects. *J Bone Joint Surg Br* 1998;80:19-24.

4. Mahbub MH, Laskar MS, Seikh FA, et al: Prevalence of cervical spondylosis and musculoskeletal symptoms among coolies in a city of Bangladesh. *J Occup Health* 2006;48:69-73.

5. Berge J, Marque B, Vital JM, Senegas J, Caille JM: Age-related changes in the cervical spines of front-line rugby players. *Am J Sports Med* 1999;27:422-429.

6. Kartal A, Yildiran I, Senkoylu A, Korkusuz F: Soccer causes degenerative changes in the cervical spine. *Eur Spine J* 2004;13:76-82.

7. Tsirikos A, Papagelopoulos PJ, Giannakopoulos PN, et al: Degenerative spondyloarthropathy of the cervical and lumbar spine in jockeys. *Orthopedics* 2001;24:561-564.

8. Hendriksen IJ, Holewijn M: Degenerative changes of the spine of fighter pilots of the Royal Netherlands Air Force (RNLAF). *Aviat Space Environ Med* 1999;70:1057-1063.

9. Cote P, Cassidy JD, Carroll LJ, Kristman V: The annual incidence and course of neck pain in the general population: A population-based cohort study. *Pain* 2004;112:267-273.

10. Cote P, Cassidy JD, Carroll L: The Saskatchewan Health and Back Pain Survey: The prevalence of neck pain and related disability in Saskatchewan adults. *Spine* 1998;23:1689-1698.

11. Cote P, Cassidy JD, Carroll L: The factors associated with neck pain and its related disability in the Saskatchewan population. *Spine* 2000;25:1109-1117.

12. Radhakrishnan K, Litchy WJ, O'Fallon WM, Kurland LT: Epidemiology of cervical radiculopathy: A population-based study from Rochester, Minnesota, 1976 through 1990. *Brain* 1994;117:325-335.

13. Salemi G, Savettieri G, Meneghini F, et al: Prevalence of cervical spondylotic radiculopathy: A door-to-door survey in a Sicilian municipality. *Acta Neurol Scand* 1996;93:184-188.

14. Bengtsson A, Henriksson KG, Larsson J: Reduced high-energy phosphate levels in the painful muscles of patients with primary fibromyalgia. *Arthritis Rheum* 1986;29:817-821.

15. Larsson R, Oberg PA, Larsson SE: Changes of trapezius muscle blood flow and electromyography in chronic neck pain due to trapezius myalgia. *Pain* 1999;79:45-50.

16. Croft PR, Lewis M, Papageorgiou AC, et al: Risk factors for neck pain: A longitudinal study in the general population. *Pain* 2001;93:317-325.

17. Ferlic DC: The nerve supply of the cervical intervertebral disc in man. *Bull Johns Hopkins Hosp* 1963;113:347-351.

18. McLain RF: Mechanoreceptor endings in human cervical facet joints. *Spine* 1994;19:495-501.

19. Chen C, Lu Y, Kallakuri S, Patwardhan A, Cavanaugh JM: Distribution of A-delta and C-fiber receptors in the cervical facet joint capsule and their response to stretch. *J Bone Joint Surg Am* 2006;88:1807-1816.

20. Inami S, Shiga T, Tsujino A, Yabuki T, Okado N, Ochiai N: Immunohistochemical demonstration of nerve fibers in the synovial fold of the human cervical facet joint. *J Orthop Res* 2001;19:593-596.

21. Grubb SA, Kelly CK: Cervical discography: Clinical implications from 12 years of experience. *Spine* 2000;25:1382-1389.

22. Dwyer A, Aprill C, Bogduk N: Cervical zygapophyseal joint pain patterns: I. A study in normal volunteers. *Spine* 1990;15:453-457.

23. Chabot MC, Montgomery DM: The pathophysiology of axial and radicular neck pain. *Semin Spine Surg* 1995;7:2-8.

24. Cornefjord M, Olmarker K, Farley DB, Weinstein JN, Rydevik B: Neuropeptide changes in compressed spinal nerve roots. *Spine* 1995;20:670-673.

25. Cooper RG, Freemont AJ, Hoyland JA, et al: Herniated intervertebral disc-associated periradicular fibrosis and vascular abnormalities occur without inflammatory cell infiltration. *Spine* 1995;20:591-598.

26. Rydevik BL, Myers RR, Powell HC: Pressure increase in the dorsal root ganglion following mechanical compression. Closed compartment syndrome in nerve roots. *Spine* 1989;14:574-576.

27. Murata Y, Onda A, Rydevik B, Takahashi I, Takahashi K, Olmarker K: Changes in pain behavior and histologic changes caused by application of tumor necrosis factor-alpha to the dorsal root ganglion in rats. *Spine* 2006;31:530-535.

28. Hukuda S, Mochizuki T, Ogata M, Shichikawa K, Shimomura Y: Operations for cervical spondylotic myelopathy: A comparison of the results of

anterior and posterior procedures. *J Bone Joint Surg Br* 1985;67:609-615.

29. Bohlman HH: Cervical spondylosis and myelopathy. *Instr Course Lect* 1995;44:81-97.

30. Penning L, Wilmink JT, van Woerden HH, Knol E: CT myelographic findings in degenerative disorders of the cervical spine: Clinical significance. *AJR Am J Roentgenol* 1986;146: 793-801.

31. Houser OW, Onofrio BM, Miller GM, Folger WN, Smith PL: Cervical spondylotic stenosis and myelopathy: Evaluation with computed tomographic myelography. *Mayo Clin Proc* 1994;69:557-563.

32. Ono K, Ebara S, Fuji T, Yonenobu K, Fujiwara K, Yamashita K: Myelopathy hand: New clinical signs of cervical cord damage. *J Bone Joint Surg Br* 1987;69:215-219.

33. Gu R, Zhu Q, Lin Y, Yang X, Gao Z, Tanaka Y: Dynamic canal encroachment of ligamentum flavum: An in vitro study of cadaveric specimens. *J Spinal Disord Tech* 2006;19:187-190.

34. Holmes A, Han ZH, Dang GT, Chen ZQ, Wang ZG, Fang J: Changes in cervical canal spinal volume during in vitro flexion-extension. *Spine* 1996; 21:1313-1319.

35. Mihara H, Ohnari K, Hachiya M, Kondo S, Yamada K: Cervical myelopathy caused by C3-C4 spondylosis in elderly patients: A radiographic analysis of pathogenesis. *Spine* 2000; 25:796-800.

36. Wang B, Liu H, Wang H, Zhou D: Segmental instability in cervical spondylotic myelopathy with severe disc degeneration. *Spine* 2006;31: 1327-1331.

37. Breig A, Turnbull I, Hassler O: Effects of mechanical stresses on the spinal cord in cervical spondylosis: A study on fresh cadaver material. *J Neurosurg* 1966;25:45-56.

38. Gooding MR, Wilson CB, Hoff JT: Experimental cervical myelopathy: Effects of ischemia and compression of the canine cervical spinal cord. *J Neurosurg* 1975;43:9-17.

39. Hukuda S, Wilson CB: Experimental cervical myelopathy: Effects of compression and ischemia on the canine cervical cord. *J Neurosurg* 1972;37: 631-652.

40. Doppman JL: The mechanism of ischemia in anteroposterior compression of the spinal cord 1975. *Invest Radiol* 1990;25:444-452.

41. Gooding MR: Pathogenesis of myelopathy in cervical spondylosis. *Lancet* 1974;2:1180-1181.

42. Henderson CM, Hennessy RG, Shuey HM Jr, Shackelford EG: Posterior-lateral foraminotomy as an exclusive operative technique for cervical radiculopathy: A review of 846 consecutively operated cases. *Neurosurgery* 1983;13:504-512.

43. Davidson RI, Dunn EJ, Metzmaker JN: The shoulder abduction test in the diagnosis of radicular pain in cervical extradural compressive monoradiculopathies. *Spine* 1981;6:441-446.

44. Cloward RB: Diaphragm paralysis from cervical disc lesions. *Br J Neurosurg* 1988;2:395-399.

45. Ebara S, Yonenobu K, Fujiwara K, Yamashita K, Ono K: Myelopathy hand characterized by muscle wasting: A different type of myelopathy hand in patients with cervical spondylosis. *Spine* 1988;13:785-791.

46. Gore DR, Sepic SB, Gardner GM: Roentgenographic findings of the cervical spine in asymptomatic people. *Spine* 1986;11:521-524.

47. Pavlov H, Torg JS, Robie B, Jahre C: Cervical spinal stenosis: Determination with vertebral body ratio method. *Radiology* 1987;164:771-775.

48. Prasad SS, O'Malley M, Caplan M, Shackleford IM, Pydisetty RK: MRI measurements of the cervical spine and their correlation to Pavlov's ratio. *Spine* 2003;28:1263-1268.

49. White AA III, Panjabi MM: Update on the evaluation of instability of the lower cervical spine. *Instr Course Lect* 1987;36:513-520.

50. Modic MT, Masaryk TJ, Mulopulos GP, Bundschuh C, Han JS, Bohlman H: Cervical radiculopathy: Prospective evaluation with surface coil MR imaging, CT with metrizamide, and metrizamide myelography. *Radiology* 1986;161:753-759.

51. Jahnke RW, Hart BL: Cervical stenosis, spondylosis, and herniated disc disease. *Radiol Clin North Am* 1991;29: 777-791.

52. Shafaie FF, Wippold FJ II, Gado M, Pilgram TK, Riew KD: Comparison of computed tomography myelography and magnetic resonance imaging in the evaluation of cervical spondylotic myelopathy and radiculopathy. *Spine* 1999;24:1781-1785.

53. Teresi LM, Lufkin RB, Reicher MA, et al: Asymptomatic degenerative disk disease and spondylosis of the cervical spine: MR imaging. *Radiology* 1987; 164:83-88.

54. Ohshio I, Hatayama A, Kaneda K, Takahara M, Nagashima K: Correlation between histopathologic features and magnetic resonance images of spinal cord lesions. *Spine* 1993;18:1140-1149.

55. Morio Y, Teshima R, Nagashima H, Nawata K, Yamasaki D, Nanjo Y: Correlation between operative outcomes of cervical compression myelopathy and MRI of the spinal cord. *Spine* 2001;26:1238-1245.

56. Matsumoto M, Toyama Y, Ishikawa M, Chiba K, Suzuki N, Fujimura Y: Increased signal intensity of the spinal cord on magnetic resonance images in cervical compressive myelopathy: Does it predict the outcome of conservative treatment? *Spine* 2000;25: 677-682.

57. Suri A, Chabbra RP, Mehta VS, Gaikwad S, Pandey RM: Effect of intramedullary signal changes on the surgical outcome of patients with cervical spondylotic myelopathy. *Spine J* 2003;3:33-45.

58. Bednarik J, Kadanka Z, Dusek L, et al: Presymptomatic spondylotic cervical cord compression. *Spine* 2004;29: 2260-2269.

59. Wada E, Ohmura M, Yonenobu K: Intramedullary changes of the spinal

cord in cervical spondylotic myelopathy. *Spine* 1995;20:2226-2232.

60. Wada E, Yonenobu K, Suzuki S, Kanazawa A, Ochi T: Can intramedullary signal change on magnetic resonance imaging predict surgical outcome in cervical spondylotic myelopathy? *Spine* 1999;24:455-462.

61. Papadopoulos CA, Katonis P, Papagelopoulos PJ, Karampekios S, Hadjipavlou AG: Surgical decompression for cervical spondylotic myelopathy: Correlation between operative outcomes and MRI of the spinal cord. *Orthopedics* 2004;27: 1087-1091.

62. Fukushima T, Ikata T, Taoka Y, Takata S: Magnetic resonance imaging study on spinal cord plasticity in patients with cervical compression myelopathy. *Spine* 1991;16 (10 suppl): S534-S538.

63. Matsuyama Y, Kawakami N, Yanase M, et al: Cervical myelopathy due to OPLL: Clinical evaluation by MRI and intraoperative spinal sonography. *J Spinal Disord Tech* 2004;17:401-404.

64. Uchida K, Kobayashi S, Yayama T, et al: Metabolic neuroimaging of the cervical spinal cord in patients with compressive myelopathy: A high-resolution positron emission tomography study. *J Neurosurg Spine* 2004;1: 72-79.

65. Dvorak J, Sutter M, Herdmann J: Cervical myelopathy: Clinical and neurophysiological evaluation. *Eur Spine J* 2003;12(suppl 2):S181-S187.

66. Simo M, Szirmai I, Aranyi Z: Superior sensitivity of motor over somatosensory evoked potentials in the diagnosis of cervical spondylotic myelopathy. *Eur J Neurol* 2004;11: 621-626.

67. Bednarik J, Kadanka Z, Vohanka S, et al: The value of somatosensory and motor evoked potentials in preclinical spondylotic cervical cord compression. *Eur Spine J* 1998;7: 493-500.

68. Chistyakov AV, Soustiel JF, Hafner H, Kaplan B, Feinsod M: The value of motor and somatosensory evoked potentials in evaluation of cervical myelopathy in the presence of peripheral neuropathy. *Spine* 2004;29: E239-E247.

69. Lyu RK, Tang LM, Chen CJ, Chen CM, Chang HS, Wu YR: The use of evoked potentials for clinical correlation and surgical outcome in cervical spondylotic myelopathy with intramedullary high signal intensity on MRI. *J Neurol Neurosurg Psychiatry* 2004;75:256-261.

70. Nakagawa Y, Tamaki T, Yamada H, Nishiura H: Discrepancy between decreases in the amplitude of compound muscle action potential and loss of motor function caused by ischemic and compressive insults to the spinal cord. *J Orthop Sci* 2002;7: 102-110.

71. Ashkan K, Johnston P, Moore AJ: A comparison of magnetic resonance imaging and neurophysiological studies in the assessment of cervical radiculopathy. *Br J Neurosurg* 2002;16: 146-148.

72. Berger AR, Busis NA, Logigian EL, Wierzbicka M, Shahani BT: Cervical root stimulation in the diagnosis of radiculopathy. *Neurology* 1987;37: 329-332.

73. Nardin RA, Patel MR, Gudas TF, Rutkove SB, Raynor EM: Electromyography and magnetic resonance imaging in the evaluation of radiculopathy. *Muscle Nerve* 1999;22: 151-155.

74. Wilbourn AJ, Aminoff MJ: AAEE minimonograph #32: The electrophysiologic examination in patients with radiculopathies. *Muscle Nerve* 1988;11:1099-1114.

75. Dillingham TR, Lauder TD, Andary M, et al: Identification of cervical radiculopathies: Optimizing the electromyographic screen. *Am J Phys Med Rehabil* 2001;80:84-91.

76. Philadelphia Panel: Philadelphia Panel evidence-based clinical practice guidelines on selected rehabilitation interventions for neck pain. *Phys Ther* 2001;81:1701-1717.

77. Wang WT, Olson SL, Campbell AH, Hanten WP, Gleeson PB: Effectiveness of physical therapy for patients with neck pain: An individualized approach using a clinical decision-making algorithm. *Am J Phys Med Rehabil* 2003;82:203-221.

78. Chiu TT, Lam TH, Hedley AJ: A randomized controlled trial on the efficacy of exercise for patients with chronic neck pain. *Spine* 2005;30: E1-E7.

79. Olivero WC, Dulebohn SC: Results of halter cervical traction for the treatment of cervical radiculopathy: Retrospective review of 81 patients. *Neurosurg Focus* 2002;12:ECP1.

80. Joghataei MT, Arab AM, Khaksar H: The effect of cervical traction combined with conventional therapy on grip strength on patients with cervical radiculopathy. *Clin Rehabil* 2004;18: 879-887.

81. Bush K, Hillier S: Outcome of cervical radiculopathy treated with periradicular/epidural corticosteroid injections: A prospective study with independent clinical review. *Eur Spine J* 1996;5:319-325.

82. Cicala RS, Thoni K, Angel JJ: Long-term results of cervical epidural steroid injections. *Clin J Pain* 1989;5: 143-145.

83. Vallee JN, Feydy A, Carlier RY, Mutschler C, Mompoint D, Vallee CA: Chronic cervical radiculopathy: Lateral-approach periradicular corticosteroid injection. *Radiology* 2001; 218:886-892.

84. Rathmell JP, Aprill C, Bogduk N: Cervical transforaminal injection of steroids. *Anesthesiology* 2004;100: 1595-1600.

85. Gore DR, Sepic SB, Gardner GM, Murray MP: Neck pain: A long-term follow-up of 205 patients. *Spine* 1987; 12:1-5.

86. Kadanka Z, Mares M, Bednanik J, et al: Approaches to spondylotic cervical myelopathy: Conservative versus surgical results in a 3-year follow-up study. *Spine* 2002;27:2205-2211.

87. Kadanka Z, Mares M, Bednarik J, et al: Predictive factors for spondylotic cervical myelopathy treated conservatively or surgically. *Eur J Neurol* 2005;12:55-63.

88. DePalma AF, Subin DK: Study of the cervical syndrome. *Clin Orthop Relat Res* 1965;38:135-142.

89. Rothman RH, Rashbaum RF: Pathogenesis of signs and symptoms of cervical disc degeneration. *Instr Course Lect* 1978;27:203-215.

90. Schellhas KP, Smith MD, Gundry CR, Pollei SR: Cervical discogenic pain: Prospective correlation of magnetic resonance imaging and discography in asymptomatic subjects and pain sufferers. *Spine* 1996;21:300-312.

91. Zheng Y, Liew SM, Simmons ED: Value of magnetic resonance imaging and discography in determining the level of cervical discectomy and fusion. *Spine* 2004;29:2140-2146.

92. Carreon L, Glassman SD, Campbell MJ: Treatment of anterior cervical pseudoarthrosis: Posterior fusion versus anterior revision. *Spine J* 2006;6: 154-156.

93. Kuhns CA, Geck MJ, Wang JC, Delamarter RB: An outcomes analysis of the treatment of cervical pseudarthrosis with posterior fusion. *Spine* 2005;30:2424-2429.

94. Albert TJ, Murrell SE: Surgical management of cervical radiculopathy. *J Am Acad Orthop Surg* 1999;7: 368-376.

95. Clarke E, Robinson PK: Cervical myelopathy: A complication of cervical spondylosis. *Brain* 1956;79:483-510.

96. Lees F, Turner JW: Natural history and prognosis of cervical spondylosis. *BMJ* 1963;2:1607-1610.

97. Nurick S: The natural history and the results of surgical treatment of the spinal cord disorder associated with cervical spondylosis. *Brain* 1972;95: 101-108.

98. Symon L, Lavender P: The surgical treatment of cervical spondylotic myelopathy. *Neurology* 1967;17:117-127.

99. Matsumoto M, Chiba K, Ishikawa M, Maruiwa H, Fujimura Y, Toyama Y: Relationships between outcomes of conservative treatment and magnetic resonance imaging findings in patients with mild cervical myelopathy caused by soft disc herniations. *Spine* 2001;26:1592-1598.

100. Onimus M, Destrumelle N, Gangloff S: Surgical treatment of cervical disk displacement: Anterior or posterior approach?. *Rev Chir Orthop Reparatrice Appar Mot* 1995;81:296-301.

101. Wirth FP, Dowd GC, Sanders HF, Wirth C: Cervical discectomy: A prospective analysis of three operative techniques. *Surg Neurol* 2000;53:340-348.

102. Herkowitz HN, Kurz LT, Overholt DP: Surgical management of cervical soft disc herniation: A comparison between the anterior and posterior approach. *Spine* 1990;15:1026-1030.

103. Rao RD, Gourab K, David KS: Operative treatment of cervical spondylotic myelopathy. *J Bone Joint Surg Am* 2006;88:1619-1640.

104. Robinson RA, Smith GW: Anterolateral cervical disc removal and interbody fusion for cervical disc syndrome. *Bull Johns Hopkins Hosp* 1955; 96:223-224.

105. Yonenobu K, Okada K, Fuji T, Fujiwara K, Yamashita K, Ono K: Causes of neurologic deterioration following surgical treatment of cervical myelopathy. *Spine* 1986;11:818-823.

106. Connolly ES, Seymour RJ, Adams JE: Clinical evaluation of anterior cervical fusion for degenerative cervical disc disease. *J Neurosurg* 1965;23:431-437.

107. Stevens JM, Clifton AG, Whitear P: Appearances of posterior osteophytes after sound anterior interbody fusion in the cervical spine: A high-definition computed myelographic study. *Neuroradiology* 1993;35:227-228.

108. Bertalanffy H, Eggert HR: Complications of anterior cervical discectomy without fusion in 450 consecutive patients. *Acta Neurochir (Wien)* 1989;99: 41-50.

109. Yamamoto I, Ikeda A, Shibuya N, Tsugane R, Sato O: Clinical long-term results of anterior discectomy without interbody fusion for cervical disc disease. *Spine* 1991;16:272-279.

110. Lieu AS, Howng SL: Clinical results of anterior cervical discectomy without interbody fusion. *Kaohsiung J Med Sci* 1998;14:212-216.

111. Emery SE, Bolesta MJ, Banks MA, Jones PK: Robinson anterior cervical fusion comparison of the standard and modified techniques. *Spine* 1994; 19:660-663.

112. Bohlman HH, Emery SE, Goodfellow DB, Jones PK: Robinson anterior cervical discectomy and arthrodesis for cervical radiculopathy: Long-term follow-up of one hundred and twenty-two patients. *J Bone Joint Surg Am* 1993;75:1298-1307.

113. Clements DH, O'Leary PF: Anterior cervical discectomy and fusion. *Spine* 1990;15:1023-1025.

114. Riley LH Jr, Robinson RA, Johnson KA, Walker AE: The results of anterior interbody fusion of the cervical spine: Review of ninety-three consecutive cases. *J Neurosurg* 1969;30: 127-133.

115. Papadopoulos EC, Huang RC, Girardi FP, Synnott K, Cammisa FP Jr: Three-level anterior cervical discectomy and fusion with plate fixation: Radiographic and clinical results. *Spine* 2006;31:897-902.

116. Samartzis D, Shen FH, Matthews DK, Yoon ST, Goldberg EJ, An HS: Comparison of allograft to autograft in multilevel anterior cervical discectomy and fusion with rigid plate fixation. *Spine J* 2003;3:451-459.

117. Moreland DB, Asch HL, Clabeaux DE, et al: Anterior cervical discectomy and fusion with implantable titanium cage: Initial impressions, patient outcomes and comparison to fusion with allograft. *Spine J* 2004;4: 184-191.

118. Frederic S, Benedict R, Payer M: Implantation of an empty carbon fiber cage or a tricortical iliac crest autograft after cervical discectomy for single-

level disc herniation: A prospective comparative study. *J Neurosurg Spine* 2006;4:292-299.

119. Sekerci Z, Ugur A, Ergun R, Sanli M: Early changes in the cervical foraminal area after anterior interbody fusion with polyetheretherketone (PEEK) cage containing synthetic bone particulate: A prospective study of 20 cases. *Neurol Res* 2006;28:568-571.

120. Hughes SS, Pringle T, Phillips F, Emery S: Settling of fibula strut grafts following multilevel anterior cervical corpectomy: A radiographic evaluation. *Spine* 2006;31:1911-1915.

121. Jones J, Yoo J, Hart R: Delayed fracture of fibular strut allograft following multilevel anterior cervical spine corpectomy and fusion. *Spine* 2006;31: E595-E599.

122. Wang JC, Hart RA, Emery SE, Bohlman HH: Graft migration or displacement after multilevel cervical corpectomy and strut grafting. *Spine* 2003;28:1016-1022.

123. Woiciechowsky C: Distractable vertebral cages for reconstruction after cervical corpectomy. *Spine* 2005;30: 1736-1741.

124. Sevki K, Mehmet T, Ufuk T, Azmi H, Mercan S, Erkal B: Results of surgical treatment for degenerative cervical myelopathy: Anterior cervical corpectomy and stabilization. *Spine* 2004; 29:2493-2500.

125. Daubs MD: Early failures following cervical corpectomy reconstruction with titanium mesh cages and anterior plating. *Spine* 2005;30:1402-1406.

126. Hee HT, Majd ME, Holt RT, Whitecloud TS III, Pienkowski D: Complications of multilevel cervical corpectomies and reconstruction with titanium cages and anterior plating. *J Spinal Disord Tech* 2003;16:1-8.

127. Park JB, Cho YS, Riew KD: Development of adjacent-level ossification in patients with an anterior cervical plate. *J Bone Joint Surg Am* 2005;87: 558-563.

128. Wang JC, McDonough PW, Endow KK, Delamarter RB: Increased fusion rates with cervical plating for two-level anterior cervical discectomy and fusion. *Spine* 2000;25:41-45.

129. Connolly PJ, Esses SI, Kostuik JP: Anterior cervical fusion: Outcome analysis of patients fused with and without anterior cervical plates. *J Spinal Disord* 1996;9:202-206.

130. Wang JC, McDonough PW, Endow K, Kanim LE, Delamarter RB: The effect of cervical plating on single-level anterior cervical discectomy and fusion. *J Spinal Disord* 1999;12: 467-471.

131. Samartzis D, Shen FH, Lyon C, Phillips M, Goldberg EJ, An HS: Does rigid instrumentation increase the fusion rate in one-level anterior cervical discectomy and fusion? *Spine J* 2004; 4:636-643.

132. Kaiser MG, Haid RW Jr, Subach BR, Barnes B, Rodts GE Jr: Anterior cervical plating enhances arthrodesis after discectomy and fusion with cortical allograft. *Neurosurgery* 2002;50: 229-238.

133. Cauthen JC, Kinard RE, Vogler JB, et al: Outcome analysis of noninstrumented anterior cervical discectomy and interbody fusion in 348 patients. *Spine* 1998;23:188-192.

134. Martin GJ Jr, Haid RW Jr, MacMillan M, Rodts GE Jr, Berkman R: Anterior cervical discectomy with freeze-dried fibula allograft: Overview of 317 cases and literature review. *Spine* 1999;24:852-859.

135. Epstein NE: The management of one-level anterior cervical corpectomy with fusion using Atlantis hybrid plates: Preliminary experience. *J Spinal Disord* 2000;13:324-328.

136. Vaccaro AR, Falatyn SP, Scuderi GJ, et al: Early failure of long segment anterior cervical plate fixation. *J Spinal Disord* 1998;11:410-415.

137. Sasso RC, Ruggiero RA Jr, Reilly TM, Hall PV: Early reconstruction failures after multilevel cervical corpectomy. *Spine* 2003;28:140-142.

138. Hilibrand A, Berta S, Daffner S: The impact of anterior cervical fusion upon overall range of motion and neck flexibility. *Proceedings of the Annual Meeting of the North American Spine Society.* Burr Ridge, IL, North American Spine Society, 2005.

139. Rao RD, Wang M, McGrady LM, Perlewitz TJ, David KS: Does anterior plating of the cervical spine predispose to adjacent segment changes? *Spine* 2005;30:2788-2793.

140. Dmitriev AE, Cunningham BW, Hu N, Sell G, Vigna F, McAfee PC: Adjacent level intradiscal pressure and segmental kinematics following a cervical total disc arthroplasty: An in vitro human cadaveric model. *Spine* 2005;30:1165-1172.

141. Puttlitz CM, Rousseau MA, Xu Z, Hu S, Tay BK, Lotz JC: Intervertebral disc replacement maintains cervical spine kinetics. *Spine* 2004;29:2809-2814.

142. Goffin J, Van Calenbergh F, van Loon J, et al: Intermediate follow-up after treatment of degenerative disc disease with the Bryan Cervical Disc Prosthesis: Single-level and bi-level. *Spine* 2003;28:2673-2678.

143. Pracyk JB, Traynelis VC: Treatment of the painful motion segment: Cervical arthroplasty. *Spine* 2005;30 (16 suppl):S23-S32.

144. Anderson PA, Sasso RC, Rouleau JP, Carlson CS, Goffin J: The Bryan Cervical Disc: Wear properties and early clinical results. *Spine J* 2004;4 (6 suppl):303S-309S.

145. Pickett GE, Sekhon LH, Sears WR, Duggal N: Complications with cervical arthroplasty. *J Neurosurg Spine* 2006;4:98-105.

146. Coric D, Finger F, Boltes P: Prospective randomized controlled study of the Bryan Cervical Disc: Early clinical results from a single investigational site. *J Neurosurg Spine* 2006;4:31-35.

147. Sasso RC, Hacker R, Heller JG: Artificial disc versus fusion: Abstract: A prospective, randomized study with 2-year follow-up on 99 patients. *Final Program: The 34th Annual Meeting of the Cervical Spine Research Society.* Rosemont, IL, Cervical Spine Research Society, 2006, p 66.

148. Robertson JT, Papadopoulos SM, Traynelis VC: Assessment of adjacent-segment disease in patients treated with cervical fusion or arthroplasty: A prospective 2-year study. *J Neurosurg Spine* 2005;3:417-423.

149. Leung C, Casey AT, Goffin J, et al: Clinical significance of heterotopic ossification in cervical disc replacement: A prospective multicenter clinical trial. *Neurosurgery* 2005;57:759-763.

150. Shim CS, Lee SH, Park HJ, Kang HS, Hwang JH: Early clinical and radiologic outcomes of cervical arthroplasty with Bryan Cervical Disc prosthesis. *J Spinal Disord Tech* 2006;19:465-470.

151. Scoville WB: Types of cervical disk lesions and their surgical approaches. *JAMA* 1966;196:479-481.

152. Russell SM, Benjamin V: Posterior surgical approach to the cervical neural foramen for intervertebral disc disease. *Neurosurgery* 2004;54:662-666.

153. Adamson TE: Microendoscopic posterior cervical laminoforaminotomy for unilateral radiculopathy: Results of a new technique in 100 cases. *J Neurosurg* 2001;95(1 suppl): 51-57.

154. Mikawa Y, Shikata J, Yamamuro T: Spinal deformity and instability after multilevel cervical laminectomy. *Spine* 1987;12:6-11.

155. Ishida Y, Suzuki K, Ohmori K, Kikata Y, Hattori Y: Critical analysis of extensive cervical laminectomy. *Neurosurgery* 1989;24:215-222.

156. Naito M, Ogata K, Kurose S, Oyama M: Canal-expansive laminoplasty in 83 patients with cervical myelopathy: A comparative study of three different procedures. *Int Orthop* 1994;18:347-351.

157. Itoh T, Tsuji H: Technical improvements and results of laminoplasty for compressive myelopathy in the cervical spine. *Spine* 1985;10:729-736.

158. Hirabayashi K, Toyama Y, Chiba K: Expansive laminoplasty for myelopathy in ossification of the longitudinal ligament. *Clin Orthop Relat Res* 1999; 359:35-48.

159. Deutsch H, Mummaneni PV, Rodts GE, Haid RW: Posterior cervical laminoplasty using a new plating system: Technical note. *J Spinal Disord Tech* 2004;17:317-320.

160. O'Brien MF, Peterson D, Casey AT, Crockard HA: A novel technique for laminoplasty augmentation of spinal canal area using titanium miniplate stabilization: A computerized morphometric analysis. *Spine* 1996;21:474-484.

161. Guigui P, Benoist M, Deburge A: Spinal deformity and instability after multilevel cervical laminectomy for spondylotic myelopathy. *Spine* 1998;23:440-447.

162. Kaptain GJ, Simmons NE, Replogle RE, Pobereskin L: Incidence and outcome of kyphotic deformity following laminectomy for cervical spondylotic myelopathy. *J Neurosurg* 2000;93(2 suppl):199-204.

163. Kumar VG, Rea GL, Mervis LJ, McGregor JM: Cervical spondylotic myelopathy: Functional and radiographic long-term outcome after laminectomy and posterior fusion. *Neurosurgery* 1999;44:771-778.

164. Epstein NE: Laminectomy with posterior wiring and fusion for cervical ossification of the posterior longitudinal ligament, spondylosis, ossification of the yellow ligament, stenosis, and instability: A study of 5 patients. *J Spinal Disord* 1999;12:461-466.

165. Houten JK, Cooper PR: Laminectomy and posterior cervical plating for multilevel cervical spondylotic myelopathy and ossification of the posterior longitudinal ligament: Effects on cervical alignment, spinal cord compression, and neurological outcome. *Neurosurgery* 2003;52:1081-1088.

166. Heller JG, Edwards CC II, Murakami H, Rodts GE: Laminoplasty versus laminectomy and fusion for multilevel cervical myelopathy: An independent matched cohort analysis. *Spine* 2001;26:1330-1336.

167. Abumi K, Kaneda K, Shono Y, Fujiya M: One-stage posterior decompression and reconstruction of the cervical spine by using pedicle screw fixation systems. *J Neurosurg* 1999;90 (1 suppl):19-26.

168. Callahan RA, Johnson RM, Margolis RN, Keggi KJ, Albright JA, Southwick WO: Cervical facet fusion for control of instability following laminectomy. *J Bone Joint Surg Am* 1977; 59:991-1002.

169. Hamanishi C, Tanaka S: Bilateral multilevel laminectomy with or without posterolateral fusion for cervical spondylotic myelopathy: Relationship to type of onset and time until operation. *J Neurosurg* 1996;85:447-451.

170. Peolsson A, Vavruch L, Oberg B: Predictive factors for arm pain, neck pain, neck specific disability and health after anterior cervical decompression and fusion. *Acta Neurochir (Wien)* 2006;148:167-173.

171. Palit M, Schofferman J, Goldthwaite N, et al: Anterior discectomy and fusion for the management of neck pain. *Spine* 1999;24:2224-2228.

172. Gore DR, Sepic SB: Anterior cervical fusion for degenerated or protruded discs. A review of one hundred forty-six patients. *Spine* 1984;9:667-671.

173. Goldberg EJ, Singh K, Van U, Garretson R, An HS: Comparing outcomes of anterior cervical discectomy and fusion in workman's versus non-workman's compensation population. *Spine J* 2002;2:408-414.

174. Arnasson O, Carlsson CA, Pellettieri L: Surgical and conservative treatment of cervical spondylotic radiculopathy and myelopathy. *Acta Neurochir (Wien)* 1987;84:48-53.

175. Lunsford LD, Bissonette DJ, Jannetta PJ, Sheptak PE, Zorub DS: Anterior surgery for cervical disc disease: Part 1. Treatment of lateral cervical disc herniation in 253 cases. *J Neurosurg* 1980;53:1-11.

176. Peolsson A, Hedlund R, Vavruch L, Oberg B: Predictive factors for the outcome of anterior cervical decom-

pression and fusion. *Eur Spine J* 2003; 12:274-280.

177. Fujiwara K, Yonenobu K, Ebara S, Yamashita K, Ono K: The prognosis of surgery for cervical compression myelopathy: An analysis of the factors involved. *J Bone Joint Surg Br* 1989;71: 393-398.

178. Kawaguchi Y, Kanamori M, Ishihara H, Ohmori K, Abe Y, Kimura T: Pathomechanism of myelopathy and surgical results of laminoplasty in elderly patients with cervical spondylosis. *Spine* 2003;28:2209-2214.

179. Emery SE, Bohlman HH, Bolesta MJ, Jones PK: Anterior cervical decompression and arthrodesis for the treatment of cervical spondylotic myelopathy: Two to seventeen-year follow-up. *J Bone Joint Surg Am* 1998; 80:941-951.

180. Prabhu K, Babu KS, Samuel S, Chacko AG: Rapid opening and closing of the hand as a measure of early neurologic recovery in the upper extremity after surgery for cervical spondylotic myelopathy. *Arch Phys Med Rehabil* 2005;86:105-108.

181. Ratliff JK, Cooper PR: Cervical laminoplasty: A critical review. *J Neurosurg* 2003;98(3 suppl):230-238.

182. Wada E, Suzuki S, Kanazawa A, Matsuoka T, Miyamoto S, Yonenobu K: Subtotal corpectomy versus laminoplasty for multilevel cervical spondylotic myelopathy: A long-term follow-up study over 10 years. *Spine* 2001;26:1443-1448.

183. Flynn TB: Neurologic complications of anterior cervical interbody fusion. *Spine* 1982;7:536-539.

184. Apfelbaum RI, Kriskovich MD, Haller JR: On the incidence, cause, and prevention of recurrent laryngeal nerve palsies during anterior cervical spine surgery. *Spine* 2000;25:2906-2912.

185. Heeneman H: Vocal cord paralysis following approaches to the anterior cervical spine. *Laryngoscope* 1973;83: 17-21.

186. Jung A, Schramm J, Lehnerdt K, Herberhold C: Recurrent laryngeal nerve palsy during anterior cervical spine surgery: A prospective study. *J Neurosurg Spine* 2005;2:123-127.

187. Kilburg C, Sullivan HG, Mathiason MA: Effect of approach side during anterior cervical discectomy and fusion on the incidence of recurrent laryngeal nerve injury. *J Neurosurg Spine* 2006;4:273-277.

188. Yonenobu K, Hosono N, Iwasaki M, Asano M, Ono K: Neurologic complications of surgery for cervical compression myelopathy. *Spine* 1991;16: 1277-1282.

189. Ikenaga M, Shikata J, Tanaka C: Radiculopathy of C-5 after anterior decompression for cervical myelopathy. *J Neurosurg Spine* 2005;3:210-217.

190. Komagata M, Nishiyama M, Endo K, Ikegami H, Tanaka S, Imakiire A: Prophylaxis of C5 palsy after cervical expansive laminoplasty by bilateral partial foraminotomy. *Spine J* 2004;4: 650-655.

191. Jimenez JC, Sani S, Braverman B, Deutsch H, Ratliff JK: Palsies of the fifth cervical nerve root after cervical decompression: Prevention using continuous intraoperative electromyography monitoring. *J Neurosurg Spine* 2005;3:92-97.

192. Hosono N, Yonenobu K, Ono K: Neck and shoulder pain after laminoplasty: A noticeable complication. *Spine* 1996;21:1969-1973.

193. Yoshida M, Otani K, Shibasaki K, Ueda S: Expansive laminoplasty with reattachment of spinous process and extensor musculature for cervical myelopathy. *Spine* 1992;17:491-497.

194. Shiraishi T, Fukuda K, Yato Y, Nakamura M, Ikegami T: Results of skip laminectomy-minimum 2-year follow-up study compared with open-door laminoplasty. *Spine* 2003; 28:2667-2672.

195. Kawaguchi Y, Kanamori M, Ishiara H, Nobukiyo M, Seki S, Kimura T: Preventive measures for axial symp-

toms following cervical laminoplasty. *J Spinal Disord Tech* 2003;16:497-501.

196. Takeuchi K, Yokoyama T, Aburakawa S, et al: Axial symptoms after cervical laminoplasty with C3 laminectomy compared with conventional C3-C7 laminoplasty: A modified laminoplasty preserving the semispinalis cervicis inserted into axis. *Spine* 2005;30: 2544-2549.

197. Hosono N, Sakaura H, Mukai Y, Yoshikawa H: Abstract: The source of axial pain after cervical laminoplasty-C7 is more crucial than deep extensor muscles. *Final Program: The 34th Annual Meeting of the Cervical Spine Research Society*. Rosemont, IL, Cervical Spine Research Society, 2006, p 112.

198. Iizuka H, Iizuka Y, Nakagawa Y, et al: Interlaminar bony fusion after cervical laminoplasty: Its characteristics and relationship with clinical results. *Spine* 2006;31:644-647.

199. Hanai K, Fujiyoshi F, Kamei K: Subtotal vertebrectomy and spinal fusion for cervical spondylotic myelopathy. *Spine* 1986;11:310-315.

200. Kaptain GJ, Simmons NE, Replogle RE, Pobereskin L: Incidence and outcome of kyphotic deformity following laminectomy for cervical spondylotic myelopathy. *J Neurosurg* 2000;93(2 suppl):199-204.

201. Takeshita K, Seichi A, Akune T, Kawamura N, Kawaguchi H, Nakamura K: Can laminoplasty maintain the cervical alignment even when the C2 lamina is contained? *Spine* 2005; 30:1294-1298.

202. Suk K-S, Kim K-T, Lee J-H, Lee S-H: Sagittal alignment of the cervical spine after laminoplasty. *Proceedings of the North American Spine Society 21st Annual Meeting*. Burr Ridge, IL, North American Spine Society, 2006.

203. Bazaz R, Lee MJ, Yoo JU: Incidence of dysphagia after anterior cervical spine surgery: A prospective study. *Spine* 2002;27:2453-2458.

204. Riley LH III, Skolasky RL, Albert TJ, Vaccaro AR, Heller JG: Dysphagia after anterior cervical decompression and fusion: Prevalence and risk factors from a longitudinal cohort study. *Spine* 2005;30:2564-2569.

205. Hilibrand AS, Carlson GD, Palumbo MA, Jones PK, Bohlman HH: Radiculopathy and myelopathy at segments adjacent to the site of a previous anterior cervical arthrodesis. *J Bone Joint Surg Am* 1999;81:519-528.

206. Lowery GL, McDonough RF: The significance of hardware failure in anterior cervical plate fixation: Patients with 2- to 7-year follow-up. *Spine* 1998;23:181-186.

207. Geyer TE, Foy MA: Oral extrusion of a screw after anterior cervical spine plating. *Spine* 2001;26:1814-1816.

208. Pompili A, Canitano S, Caroli F, et al: Asymptomatic esophageal perforation caused by late screw migration after anterior cervical plating: Report of a case and review of relevant literature. *Spine* 2002;27:E499-E502.

Update on Cervical Artificial Disk Replacement

Paul A. Anderson, MD
Rick C. Sasso, MD
K. Daniel Riew, MD

Abstract

Cervical disk arthroplasty, one of the emerging motion-sparing technologies, is currently undergoing evaluation in the United States as an alternative to arthrodesis for the treatment of cervical radiculopathy and myelopathy. With both arthrodesis and arthroplasty, the primary surgical goal is thorough decompression of neurocompressive pathology—directly by removal of osteophyte and disk and indirectly by disk distraction. There is, however, one principal difference between arthrodesis and arthroplasty. With a solid fusion, resorption of osteophytes (in accordance with Wolff's law) further enhances decompression. In contrast, osteophyte resorption will not occur with motion-preserving arthroplasty. There are many challenges when deciding between arthrodesis and arthroplasty. Prosthetic performance demands exacting implantation techniques to ensure correct placement, thus placing increasing demands on special instrumentation and surgical skills. It is also important to understand the tribology (the study of prosthetic lubrication, wear, and biologic effects) of disk arthroplasty and to be familiar with currently available information regarding kinematics, basic science, testing, and early clinical results.

The primary rationale for disk arthroplasty is motion preservation, with the theoretic advantage of avoiding adjacent segment degeneration. It is believed that motion preservation allows fewer activity restrictions and earlier return to activities, including work and driving.

Rationale for Disk Arthroplasty

Adjacent-Level Degeneration

There is general consensus that degeneration occurs in segments adjacent to fusion. However, no study has definitively established that this adjacent-level degeneration is primarily caused by the adverse mechanical effect of fusion versus the natural history of degenerative disk disease.

Numerous studies have demonstrated the incidence of adjacent level degeneration following arthro-

deses. Baba and associates[1] examined 106 patients following anterior fusion for myeloradiculopathy over an average of 8.6 years. Overall, 25% of patients had progressive neurologic changes at adjacent levels; 17 of these patients required additional surgery. As expected, patients who underwent multilevel arthrodesis had a greater chance of adjacent-level degeneration. Gore and Sepic[2,3] similarly reported short- and long-term follow-up of anterior cervical diskectomy and arthrodesis. At 5-year follow-up, 18 of 37 patients had symptoms at adjacent levels. The authors compared these patients with a cohort of asymptomatic patients who were followed over the same period and found no differences in radiographic evidence of deterioration, except for increased osteophyte formation.[4] Gore and Sepic did not comment on whether there were any changes in symptoms. In reporting their 21-year results, Gore and Sepic noted that 16 of 50 patients at 10-year follow-up had new onset of symptoms related to adjacent-level disease, half of whom required further surgery.[3] Based on these long-term data, they recommended that this patient population be informed of the significant chance of revision surgery at long-term follow-up.

The most often cited article on adjacent-level disease is by Hilibrand and associates,[5] who analyzed the results of Bohlman's surgical cases. They reported long-term follow-up in 374 patients at 2 to 21 years after anterior cervical diskectomy and arthrodesis. The annual incidence of symptomatic, adjacent-level degenerative disease was 2.9%, and the prevalence at 10-year follow-up was 25.9%. In contrast to the findings of Baba and associates,[1] single-level fusions, especially at C5-6 or C6-7, were associated with a greater risk of symptomatic degeneration than multilevel fusions. Patients who had a three-level arthrodesis from C4 to C7 had the lowest risk of requiring additional surgery. The authors, therefore, concluded that the risk for adjacent-level disease is not increased in patients who undergo longer fusions. As expected, patients with preoperative disease at adjacent levels were more likely to have symptomatic adjacent-level disease postoperatively. Consequently, the authors suggested that adjacent-level degeneration more likely resulted from the natural history of spondylosis as opposed to the increased stresses of multilevel fusions.

To determine whether the indication for the procedure had an effect on adjacent-level degeneration, Goffin and associates[6] compared the 5-year follow-up results of cohorts who underwent arthrodeses for degeneration and trauma. They found that 85% of both groups had postoperative evidence of progressive radiographic deterioration and that there was no difference between the groups based on the index indication. These findings imply that the etiology of the adjacent-level degen-

eration may have been mechanically related to the fusion rather than the natural history of spondylosis. Thus, there appears to be an 85% incidence of radiographic degenerative changes and a 25% incidence of new symptomatic radiculopathy in patients who undergo anterior fusion.

In an effort to determine the natural history of spondylosis, Gore and associates[7] determined the incidence of cervical degeneration in 200 asymptomatic patients. They found that significant degenerative changes were common in patients older than 50 years. By age 60 years, 95% of men and 65% of women had degenerative changes. In a follow-up study, significant degenerative changes were found in most patients, but surprisingly 15% had now developed pain.[8] This finding suggests that degenerative disk disease is common and symptomatic disease occurs in the absence of fusion. With the limitations of these studies, conflicting data, and the lack of adequate controlled studies, no conclusions can be drawn regarding the mechanical versus biologic etiology of degenerative disk disease. Nevertheless, the high incidence of adjacent-level degeneration has provided a justifiable reason to develop new technologies to limit disk deterioration.

Viscoelasticity

The intervertebral disk functions as a shock absorber based on the viscoelastic properties of its collagen and proteoglycan molecular structure. Proteoglycans, in particular, absorb water molecules, creating a large matrix of negative charges that repel under load. Loss of this viscoelastic property by fusion is therefore believed to be a major factor leading to adjacent-level degeneration. However, none of the cur-

rently available prostheses allow viscoelasticity comparable to that provided by the normal disk. Furthermore, LeHuec and associates[9] compared the ability of a metal-polymer and metal-on-metal lumbar prosthesis to absorb impulse and vibrational load. Despite an order of magnitude difference in elastic properties between the two implants, no difference in the shock-absorbing effect was noted. Similarly, Dahl and associates[10] compared a simulated fusion with cervical artificial disks having different elastic properties. They found significant difference between all arthroplasties and fusion. However, no differences were found among arthroplasties with different elasticities. Thus, any motion-sparing device appeared to be protective of adjacent segments compared with fusion under impulse and vibrational stresses.

Maintenance of Motion

Loss of overall range of motion following fusion is poorly documented and, in fact, is rarely reported by patients with successful pain relief. Although 7° to 10° of motion at the surgical level has been reported following cervical arthroplasty, no evidence of functional impairment has been reported.[11,12] Most patients having arthroplasty do not require immobilization and therefore regain overall motion faster than patients treated with fusion.

The pattern of motion in normal individuals and patients who underwent fusion or arthroplasty was studied by Goffin and associates.[13] Using video fluoroscopy and digital processing, the patients who underwent fusion were noted to have asynchronous (jerky) motion at adjacent segments, whereas motion in patients who underwent arthroplasty was similar to that of normal asymptomatic individuals.

Perioperative Morbidity

Because arthroplasty generally does not require postoperative immobilization, return to function, including work and driving, can theoretically occur much earlier than in patients who undergo arthrodesis. Furthermore, complications related to fusion, such as hardware failure and pseudarthrosis, are avoided. Anderson and associates[14] compared revision rates in 1,229 patients who underwent cervical arthroplasty or arthrodesis and found that in the 580 patients who underwent arthrodesis, 4.8% had revisions by 2 years postoperatively, whereas only 2.9% of the 649 patients who underwent arthroplasty had revisions. These data suggest that symptomatic adjacent-level degeneration may be decreased by arthroplasty because significantly fewer patients who undergo arthroplasty require revisions to treat adjacent-level degeneration.

Mitigation of Fusion Effects by Arthroplasty

Dmitriev and associates[15] compared the biomechanical effects on adjacent segments for cervical disk arthroplasty and fusion and found that significant increases in intradiskal pressures occurred at both the cranial and caudal levels. Puttlitz and associates[16] performed a similar analysis and found that motion at adjacent levels after arthroplasty mimicked that of the normal functional unit, including coupled motion. DiAngelo and associates[17,18] also found that motion normalized to the intact segment after arthroplasty and that increased range of motion was seen after fusion. These results are similar to those reported for lumbar arthroplasty and indicate that cervical arthroplasty normalizes

the adverse biomechanical consequences of fusion. The findings of these basic investigations have been confirmed by postoperative human kinematic studies.

Sasso and Rouleau[19] studied cervical motion in 22 patients enrolled in a prospective, randomized clinical trial. Radiographic data, including flexion, extension, and neutral lateral radiographs, were obtained preoperatively and at regular postoperative intervals for up to 24 months. Cervical vertebral bodies were tracked on digital radiographs using quantitative motion analysis software to calculate the functional spinal unit motion parameters. The anterior-posterior translation during flexion-extension activities remained unchanged for the disk replacement group (8.3% preoperatively, 8.4% at 6 months, and 8.2% at 12 months) for the level above the disk. In contrast, the anterior-posterior translation increased for the level above the fusion (8.5% preoperatively, 12.4% at 6 months, and 11.0% at 12 months). This increase was dramatic for some patients who underwent fusion, but was not uniformly noted. At 6-month follow-up, the increase in translation was significantly greater for patients who underwent fusion ($P < 0.02$) than for those who received a disk replacement. Pickett and associates[20] performed a similar analysis and found that the center of rotation following arthroplasty was similar to the center of rotation that was present preoperatively. The importance of these clinical and biomechanical findings in reducing the risk of adjacent-level degeneration is unknown at this time.

Design Considerations
Kinematics

One of the primary goals of cervical disk replacement is to reproduce

normal kinematics. Normal range of motion in the subaxial cervical spine is 10° to 20° of flexion-extension, 5° to 15° of lateral bending, and 5° to 10° of rotation. Additionally, coupled motions are present, including anterior-posterior translation during flexion and extension and axial rotation during lateral bending. Also, the instantaneous axis of rotation in flexion-extension is located inferior to the caudal end plate and is relatively posterior in the vertebral body. This position changes during motion as a result of combined angulation and translation. In flexion-extension, there is 1 to 2 mm of anterior translation. Current implant designs differ in how well these normal mechanics are reproduced.

Cervical disk replacements can be classified as unconstrained, semiconstrained, and constrained, depending on how they mimic normal kinematics. Unconstrained devices allow coupled translation with angulation. Two types of unconstrained designs are available: a three-piece device in which the center or nuclear core can translate forward or backward and a device with saddle joints. A semiconstrained prosthesis allows coupled motion in some directions (flexion-extension), but has a fixed center of rotation in other directions (lateral bending). The Prestige ST Artificial Cervical Disc and the Prestige LP Cervical Disc (Medtronic, Minneapolis, MN), both with a ball and trough design, are examples of semiconstrained prostheses. A constrained device has a constant center of rotation and a ball and socket design that does not allow anterior-posterior translation. The clinical effects of the differences in prostheses designs are unknown. Theoretically, an important distinction between constrained and unconstrained designs is a change in balance of loads between the disk and facets, especially in extension. When the spine is in flexion, the facets "unshingle" and are less active in constraining the motion of the functional spine unit. However, when the spine is in extension, the facets "shingle" and become more involved in constraining the motion. Thus, with a constrained facet joint and a constrained disk joint, binding or limited motion (also known as "kinematic conflict") would be expected because one joint works against the other. This conflict would give rise to decreased motion or increased stress on the system and would potentially reduce motion.

DiAngelo and associates[17] investigated constrained and unconstrained designs in human cadaver spines to compare the motion of the harvested spine and the implanted spine. The results demonstrated that the unconstrained device mimicked normal mechanics, whereas the semiconstrained device failed to reproduce normal motion in extension. Both devices should achieve greater than normal segmental motion, which occurs in ± 15° in flexion/extension.

Materials

The most likely mode of failure is wear of the bearing surface, which is largely determined by the materials used. Current cervical disk replacements are made from materials similar to those used for joint arthroplasty, including cobalt-chromium-molybdenum alloy, stainless steel, and ultra high-density molecular weight polyethylene. Additionally, because lower load occurs in the spine than in joints such as the knee, other materials have been used for cervical disk replacements, including titanium, polyurethane, and titanium carbide, the latter of which has the advantage of much better imaging quality.

Bone Fixation

Biologic fixation to bone is important for the long-term function of the prosthesis. A variety of stabilization and surface treatments are used. Cervical prostheses are initially stabilized to prevent expulsion or displacement into the spinal canal with screws, keels, ridges, and specially machined cavities. Surface treatments include titanium plasma spray with calcium phosphate and cinctured beads. Bone ingrowth into the Porous Coated Motion (PCM) Artificial Cervical Disc (Cervitech, Rockaway, NJ) and the Bryan Cervical Disc System (Medtronic) appears to be satisfactory. McAfee and associates[21] evaluated bone ingrowth in the PCM device and found a 40% to 50% rate of incorporation in a nonhuman primate model. In human explants, Jensen and associates[22] reported a 32% rate of bone ingrowth with Bryan Cervical Disc System explants.

Testing of Cervical Devices

Seven cervical disk prostheses are currently undergoing clinical testing in the United States (Figure 1). The basic design parameters of each of these prostheses are provided in Table 1. Extensive preclinical and clinical testing of new motion-sparing devices such as cervical disk prostheses are required to ensure safety and efficacy. Cervical disk prostheses are intended for use in patients who are younger than those who undergo arthroplasties for appendicular joints; therefore, long-term wear characteristics are a major concern. In total hip and knee arthroplasty implantations, younger, more active patients experience a much higher failure rate. During testing, the response of the implant to the host as well as the response of the host to the implant should be measured. Clinical testing of efficacy should also be conducted via rigorous randomized controlled trials that measure the primary outcome variables of pain, neurologic function, and functional outcomes.

Mechanical Testing

All components initially should be tested for fatigue. Because of the large number of cycles required (a minimum of 10 million) for fatigue testing, this is done on a simulator. Unlike hip and knee implants for which protocols are well established and have a track record of predicting long-term function, spine simulators are undergoing evolution. Simulator wear results for the Bryan and Prestige cervical prostheses have been reported.[23,24] At 10 million cycles, a mean volume loss for the Bryan disk was 0.76%. Failure occurred when end plates contacted each other at 39 million cycles. The wear debris consisted of large elliptical particles with a mean ferret diameter of 3.89 μm and aspect ratio of 1.38. The Prestige metal-on-metal disk had less wear than the Bryan disk (0.19% at 20 million cycles); a linear wear rate of 0.18 mm^3 per 1 million cycles was reported.

Inflammatory Reaction

Wear particles are bioactive and under certain conditions can induce a significant inflammatory response, resulting in failure and loosening of the device. In the spine, additional concerns arise because of the location of the devices adjacent to vascular, visceral, and neurologic structures. Devices are tested for their

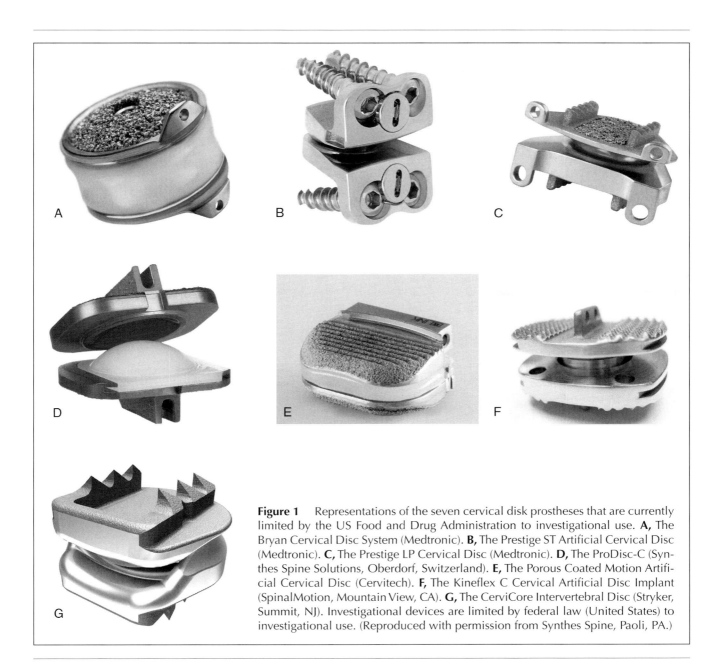

Figure 1   Representations of the seven cervical disk prostheses that are currently limited by the US Food and Drug Administration to investigational use. **A,** The Bryan Cervical Disc System (Medtronic). **B,** The Prestige ST Artificial Cervical Disc (Medtronic). **C,** The Prestige LP Cervical Disc (Medtronic). **D,** The ProDisc-C (Synthes Spine Solutions, Oberdorf, Switzerland). **E,** The Porous Coated Motion Artificial Cervical Disc (Cervitech). **F,** The Kineflex C Cervical Artificial Disc Implant (SpinalMotion, Mountain View, CA). **G,** The CerviCore Intervertebral Disc (Stryker, Summit, NJ). Investigational devices are limited by federal law (United States) to investigational use. (Reproduced with permission from Synthes Spine, Paoli, PA.)

inflammatory properties in two manners: in a rabbit laminectomy defect model in which large amounts of wear debris are installed directly into the epidural space, and by implantation in a suitable animal. McAfee and associates[21] reported minimal change in the dura mater and no effect on the neuronal elements of polyethylene particles for the PCM prosthesis.

Placement of the device in the cervical spine in animals allows for analysis of responses of the implant to the host and the host to the implant. This type of analysis is limited, however, by time and cost considerations as well as by an unequal biomechanical environment in humans. Anderson and associates[23] assessed the Bryan disk in goats and reported that debris was observed in 8 of 11 specimens, but only

a minimal inflammatory response was observed in the periprosthetic tissue. No toxic effects were noted in the neural elements, draining lymph nodes, or distant sites such as liver and spleen.

Retrieval Studies

Retrieval analysis of implants from humans is important to understand the in vivo biologic reaction of the

Table 1
Cervical Disk Prostheses in US Food and Drug Administration Investigations (2005)

Prosthesis	Material	Bearing Surface	Articulation(s) No.	Articulation(s) Type	US Food and Drug Administration (FDA) Status	Bone Ingrowth	Fixation
Bryan Cervical Disc System (Medtronic)	Titanium alloy Polyurethane	Metal-on-polymer	2	Three piece Nuclear core	Completed enrollment	Titanium shards	Mortise
Prestige ST Artificial Cervical Disc (Medtronic)	Stainless steel	Metal-on-metal	1	Ball and trough	Completed enrollment	Grit blast	Screws
Prestige LP Cervical Disc (Medtronic)	Titanium ceramic composite	Metal-on-metal	1	Ball and trough	Completed enrollment	Titanium plasma spray	Rails
ProDisc-C (Synthes Spine Solutions)	Cobalt-chromium-molybdenum-polyethylene	Metal-on-polymer	1	Ball and socket	Completed enrollment	Titanium plasma spray	Keel
Porous Coated Motion (PCM) Artificial Cervical Disc (Cervitech)	Cobalt-chromium-molybdenum-polyethylene	Metal-on-polymer	1	Ball and socket	In FDA trial	Titanium plasma spray using calcium phosphates	Surface ridges or screws
Kineflex C Cervical Artificial Disc Implant (SpinalMotion)	Cobalt-chromium-molybdenum	Metal-on-metal	2	Three piece Nuclear core	In FDA trial	Unconstrained	Keel
CerviCore Intervertebral Disc (Stryker)	Cobalt-chromium-molybdenum	Metal-on-metal	1	Saddle	In FDA trial	Unconstrained	Rails

implant and the potential implications of wear. These results can help validate preclinical testing in simulators and animal models. Anderson and associates[24] reported retrievals of 11 Bryan disks and 3 Prestige disks because of infection, failure to relieve initial symptoms, and adjacent segment degeneration. None of the devices had mechanical failure. The prosthetic wear patterns of the Prestige disk were similar to those observed in simulators. However, the amount of wear was less than one tenth of that predicted, based on 1 million cycles per year. In both brands/types of prostheses, revision was achieved relatively easily without corpectomy. The polyurethane nucleus of the Bryan disk was assessed chemically with spectroscopy and chromatography. After implan-

tation of up to 11 months, no oxidation was observed, and the molecular weight of the polymer was similar to that of a control implant. No observable changes in the surface were present and all nuclei were dimensionally normal, without evidence of loss from wear. These results were reassuring, indicating that the prosthesis, at least in the short term, was durable and had wear rates much less than those predicted by design and reported in testing protocols.

Indications

In the United States, the indications for surgery in Investigational Device Exemption studies are radiculopathy or myelopathy at a single level between C3 and C7; the contraindications are osteoporosis, instability of

more than 3 mm, moderate or severe facet arthritis, or a history of infection. The intent is to use an arthroplasty as an alternative to an arthrodesis. The results of using the Bryan disk at two levels was reported in Europe, with slightly better outcomes than when used at a single level, but this device has not been tested in a randomized controlled study in which it is compared with fusion.[11] Another study reported the successful treatment of levels adjacent to a prior fusion.[25] Concerns regarding the treatment of myelopathy using arthroplasty have been raised because maintaining motion may be a disadvantage to neural recovery. In one report, satisfactory outcomes have been reported in a small number of patients treated with the Bryan disk.[26]

Clinical Outcomes

Reports of early clinical experience with disk arthroplasty devices have been uniformly favorable. Studies have shown that the outcomes of cervical arthroplasty are at least as good, if not better, than arthrodesis. Although it is certainly possible that long-term clinical results will also be favorable, good short-term outcomes do not necessarily predict good long-term outcomes. For example, the early results of lumbar cage fusions showed excellent clinical results and led to an increase in the use of lumbar cages; however, the popularity of such procedures has significantly diminished over the past several years. It is entirely possible that the use of cervical disk arthroplasty may undergo a similar evolution.

Goffin and associates[11,27] reported the results of a multicenter European study. For both single-level and bilevel arthroplasty, 90% of patients had excellent, good, or fair results at 2 years postoperatively. Lafuente and associates[28] evaluated 46 consecutive patients who underwent disk arthroplasty using the Bryan device and reported a highly statistically significant difference between preoperative and 12-month postoperative scores for the Visual Analog Scale (VAS), the Medical Outcomes Study Short Form 36-Item Health Survey (SF-36), and the Neck Disability Index (NDI). Two patients (4.3%) were found to have a bony ankylosis of the disk arthroplasty.

Duggal and associates[29] reported on the results of 26 patients undergoing one- and two-level Bryan disk replacement for radiculopathy and/or myelopathy. They found that motion was preserved (mean range of motion, 7.8°) at up to 24 months postoperatively. Postoperative NDI scores were significantly improved and there was a trend toward improvement of the SF-36 physical component score.

Bertagnoli and associates[30] reported on 16 patients with cervical spondylosis who prospectively underwent cervical arthroplasty using the ProDisc-C (Synthes Spine Solutions). There were 12 single-level and 4 two-level procedures; a total of 20 artificial disks were implanted. At a maximum follow-up of 12 months, Oswestry Disability Index and VAS scores were significantly improved. The arthroplasty levels had motion from 4° to 12° postoperatively and no complications were noted.

The Prestige disk has undergone several modifications. The Prestige I disk, which was used for the treatment of adjacent-level degeneration, demonstrated excellent outcomes and a satisfactory range of motion in 14 of the original 14 patients.[31] The Prestige II added bone ingrowth surfaces, a lower profile, and a trough to allow coupled motions. Porchet and Metcalf[32] reported the results of a prospective randomized controlled multicenter study in which NDI and SF-36 scores were measured preoperatively and for up to 24 months postoperatively. In comparison to patients who underwent fusion, all of the outcome measures showed equivalency at up to 24 months postoperatively. Radiographic analysis revealed preservation of motion for all prostheses.

Pimenta and associates[33] reported the results of an uncontrolled study of the PCM Artificial Cervical Disc. Fifty-three patients underwent 83 arthroplasties, and outcomes were measured using the VAS, NDI, and the Treatment Intensity Gradient Test. Scores for all of these measures improved postoperatively. The authors noted one complication in which a device migrated 4 mm. This complication was kept under observation without any further treatment. At up to 3-month follow-up, 90% of the patients had good to excellent results using Odom's criteria.

Myelopathy

Thus far, results for the treatment of myelopathy appear satisfactory, but data are limited because the results of randomized controlled studies have not been reported. Concerns when using arthroplasty for this condition have been raised because preservation of motion may have an adverse effect on spinal cord recovery. Sekhon[26] reported a case series of nine patients with cervical spondylotic myelopathy who were treated with anterior decompression and reconstruction with the Bryan disk. Follow-up ranged from 1 to 17 months. On average, the Nurick grade improved by 0.72 and Oswestry NDI scores improved by 51.4 points. Improvement in cervical lordosis was noted in 29% of the patients. No complications were reported.

Summary and Critique of Clinical Data

When examining these cervical arthroplasty studies, it is important to be aware that there may be significant placebo effects associated with the clinical outcome measures. Any patient who received the disk in a nonrandomized or randomized study knew that they had been treated with the new study device. Virtually all of these patients were pleased that they received this new device. On the other hand, in the randomized trials, most of the patients who underwent arthrodesis were disappointed that they were not in the arthroplasty group. This realization has the potential for setting different expectations for the surgical procedure, which might ultimately affect the postoperative clinical outcome measures. Whether this theoretic critique is actually valid remains to be determined and would require a study in which patients are blinded to their treatment, even postoperatively.

It should be noted that most of these studies only reported short-term results, some with only a 3-month follow-up. It remains to be determined whether the early enthusiasm for artificial cervical disks will be borne out by long-term studies. Despite these concerns, the data from prospective, randomized clinical trials of cervical prostheses in the United States suggest that artificial cervical disk replacements, in general, produce outcomes similar to those of anterior fusions, but maintain motion across the disk space.

Complications

Few complications of cervical disk arthroplasty have been reported. Perioperative complications included a possibly higher rate of hematoma (epidural and retropharyngeal) and infections.[24] Technical complications that have been anecdotally reported have included reports of vertebral body fracture during implantation and early dislodgement requiring reoperation.

Adverse inflammatory reactions with osteolysis have not been observed. Paravertebral ossification of unknown etiology has been reported to occur in up to 5% of patients.[11,34] It has been demonstrated, however, that treatment with anti-inflammatory agents may decrease this tendency.[34] Failure of clinical improvement is the most common cause for reoperation,[24] and often

results from incomplete removal of compressive pathology posterior to the uncinate process. Arthroplasty requires more aggressive decompression because maintenance of motion will not result in bony remolding such as occurs following fusion. Neurologic complications have been rarely reported.

Summary

Cervical disk arthroplasty was developed to maintain motion hypothetically to reduce the risk of future adjacent-level degeneration. Other advantages are believed to be earlier return to activity and reduced surgical morbidity. Seven devices are currently undergoing US Food and Drug Administration investigation. The differences in materials, design, and implantation techniques on device performance are unknown. Preclinical testing for durability, stability, bony ingrowth, and inflammatory reactions shows that current designs are meeting established criteria for success.

Early follow-up of human studies are encouraging, demonstrating outcomes comparable to those of fusion, with the added advantage of motion preservation. Reported complications are few and manageable and have not resulted in catastrophic neural injury. The rate of revision has also been low. Longer follow-up is needed to determine whether these devices can function well over time and to determine long-term implant to host and host to implant reactions.

References

1. Baba H, Furusawa N, Imura S, Kawahara N, Tsuchiya H, Tomita K: Late radiographic findings after anterior cervical fusion for spondylotic myeloradiculopathy. *Spine* 1993;18:2167-2173.

2. Gore DR, Sepic SB: Anterior cervical fusion for degenerated or protruded discs: A review of one hundred forty-six patients. *Spine* 1984;9:667-671.

3. Gore DR, Sepic SB: Anterior discectomy and fusion for painful cervical disc disease: A report of 50 patients with an average follow-up of 21 years. *Spine* 1998;23:2047-2051.

4. Gore DR, Gardner GM, Sepic SB, Murray MP: Roentgenographic findings following anterior cervical fusion. *Skeletal Radiol* 1986;15:556-559.

5. Hilibrand AS, Carlson GD, Palumbo MA, Jones PK, Bohlman HH: Radiculopathy and myelopathy at segments adjacent to the site of a previous anterior cervical arthrodesis. *J Bone Joint Surg Am* 1999;81:519-528.

6. Goffin J, Geusens E, Vantomme N, et al: Long-term follow-up after interbody fusion of the cervical spine. *J Spinal Disord Tech* 2004;17:79-85.

7. Gore DR, Sepic SB, Gardner GM: Roentgenographic findings of the cervical spine in asymptomatic people. *Spine* 1986;11:521-524.

8. Gore DR: Roentgenographic findings in the cervical spine in asymptomatic persons: A ten-year follow-up. *Spine* 2001;26:2463-2466.

9. LeHuec JC, Kiaer T, Friesem T, Mathews H, Liu M, Eisermann L: Shock absorption in lumbar disc prosthesis: A preliminary mechanical study. *J Spinal Disord Tech* 2003;16:346-351.

10. Dahl MC, Rouleau JP, Papadopoulos SM, Nuckley RP, Ching RP: A dynamic characteristic comparison of the intact, fused, and prosthetic replaced cervical disc, in *Proceedings of the 5th Combined Meeting of the Orthopaedic Research Societies*, Banff, Alberta, Canada, July 1, 2004.

11. Goffin J, Van Calenbergh F, van Loon J, et al: Intermediate follow-up after treatment of degenerative disc disease with the Bryan cervical disc prosthesis: Single-level and bi-level. *Spine* 2003;28:2673-2678.

12. Bertagnoli R, Duggal N, Pickett GE, et al: Cervical total disc replacement: Part II. Clinical results. *Orthop Clin North Am* 2005;36:355-362.

13. Goffin J, Komistek R, Mahfouz H, Wong D, Macht D: In vivo kinematics of normal, degenerative, fused and disk-replaced cervical spines, in *Proceedings of the 2003 Annual Meeting*. Rosemont, IL, American Academy

of Orthopaedic Surgeons, 2003, pp 473-474.

14. Anderson PA, Sasso R, Riew KD, Metcalf NH: Reoperation rates of cervical arthroplasty versus arthrodesis. *Spine J* 2005;5:S76-S77.

15. Dmitriev AE, Cunningham BW, Hu N, Sell G, Vigna F, McAfee PC: Adjacent level intradiscal pressure and segmental kinematics following a cervical total disc arthroplasty: An in vitro human cadaveric model. *Spine* 2005;30:1165-1172.

16. Puttlitz CM, Rousseau MA, Xu Z, Hu S, Tay BK, Lotz JC: Intervertebral disc replacement maintains cervical spine kinetics. *Spine* 2004;29:2809-2814.

17. DiAngelo DJ, Roberston JT, Metcalf NH, McVay BJ, Davis RC: Biomechanical testing of an artificial cervical joint and an anterior cervical plate. *J Spinal Disord Tech* 2003;16:314-323.

18. DiAngelo DJ, Foley KT, Morrow BR, et al: In vitro biomechanics of cervical disc arthroplasty with the ProDisc-C total disc implant. *Neurosurg Focus* 2004;17:E7.

19. Sasso R, Rouleau JP: Kinematics of a cervical disc prosthesis. *Spine J* 2005;5:S87.

20. Pickett GE, Rouleau JP, Duggal N: Kinematic analysis of the cervical spine following implantation of an artificial cervical disc. *Spine* 2005;30:1949-1954.

21. McAfee PC, Cunningham BW, Orbegoso CM, Sefter JC, Dmitriev AE, Fedder IL: Analysis of porous ingrowth in intervertebral disc prostheses: A nonhuman primate model. *Spine* 2003;28:332-340.

22. Jensen WK, Anderson PA, Rouleau JP: Bone ingrowth in retrieved Bryan Cervical Disc prostheses. *Spine* 2005;30:2497-2502.

23. Anderson PA, Rouleau JP, Bryan VE, Carlson CS: Wear analysis of the Bryan Cervical Disc prosthesis. *Spine* 2003;28:S186-S194.

24. Anderson PA, Rouleau JP, Toth JM, Riew KD: A comparison of simulator-tested and retrieved cervical disc prostheses: Invited submission from the Joint Section Meeting on Disorders of the Spine and Peripheral Nerves, March 2004. *J Neurosurg Spine* 2004;1:202-210.

25. Sekhon LH: Reversal of anterior cervical fusion with a cervical arthroplasty prosthesis. *J Spinal Disord Tech* 2005;18:S125-S128.

26. Sekhon LH: Cervical arthroplasty in the management of spondylotic myelopathy. *J Spinal Disord Tech* 2003;16:307-313.

27. Goffin J, Casey A, Kehr P, et al: Preliminary clinical experience with the Bryan cervical disc prosthesis. *Neurosurgery* 2002;51:840-845.

28. Lafuente J, Casey AT, Petzold A, Brew S: The Bryan cervical disc prosthesis as an alternative to arthrodesis in the treatment of cervical spondylosis. *J Bone Joint Surg Br* 2005;87:508-512.

29. Duggal N, Pickett GE, Mitsis DK, Keller JL: Early clinical and biomechanical results following cervical arthroplasty. *Neurosurg Focus* 2004;17:E9.

30. Bertagnoli R, Yue JJ, Pfeiffer F, et al: Early results after ProDisc-C cervical disc replacement. *J Neurosurg Spine* 2005;2:403-410.

31. Wigfield CC, Gill SS, Nelson RJ, Metcalf NH, Robertson JT: The new Frenchay artificial cervical joint: Results from a two-year pilot study. *Spine* 2002;27:2446-2452.

32. Porchet F, Metcalf NH: Clinical outcomes with the Prestige II cervical disc: Preliminary results from a prospective randomized clinical trial. *Neurosurg Focus* 2004;17:E6.

33. Pimenta L, McAfee PC, Cappuccino A, Bellera FP, Link HD: Clinical experience with the new artificial cervical PCM (Cervitech) disc. *Spine J* 2004;4:315S-321S.

34. Heller J, Goffin J: Classification of paravertebral ossification after insertion of the Bryan cervical disc prosthesis, in *Proceedings of the 31st Annual Meeting of the Cervical Spine Research Society*. Cervical Spine Research Society, 2003.

Prevention, Identification, and Treatment of Inadequate Decompression of the Cervical Spine

Clinton J. Devin, MD

Michael T. Espiritu, MD

James D. Kang, MD

Abstract

Inadequate decompression is one of the most common reasons for failed spinal surgery. Understanding the common areas where neural impingement occurs in the cervical spine, recognizing these changes on imaging studies, and recognizing the clinical manifestations help provide an intraoperative template for thorough decompression. A thorough preoperative workup assesses sagittal alignment of the cervical spine, determines if instability exists, identifies the location of the compression, and determines the etiology of the compressive lesion. This information guides the surgeon in deciding whether an anterior, a posterior, or a combined anterior and posterior approach will provide the most adequate decompression. It also will help determine whether arthrodesis is needed to provide optimal neurologic recovery. Patients who have had surgery and present with persistent neurologic symptoms, or who do not recover as expected, pose a unique challenge. The surgeon must determine if persistent compression exists, look for evidence of instability, and evaluate for irreversible spinal cord changes. Alternatively, other causes of neurologic changes, unrelated to neurologic impingement, must be ruled out. The initial step in achieving the goal of complete neurologic decompression is a thorough preoperative evaluation for static and dynamic causes of compression. The most important concept regarding inadequate decompression is to avoid it with careful preoperative planning of the index procedure.

Inadequate decompression is one of the most common reasons for unsuccessful surgery of the cervical spine. To provide an intraoperative template for thorough decompression, it is important to understand the common areas where neural impingement occurs in the cervical spine, to recognize these changes on imaging studies, and to be aware of the clinical manifestations of such changes.

Preoperative Considerations
Static and Dynamic Compression

Cervical spondylosis typically follows a stepwise cascade of degeneration. The disk degenerates and begins to collapse and bulge posteriorly into the spinal canal, altering motion and increasing stress on the uncovertebral and facet joints, with the resultant development of arthrosis. With disk collapse, the ligamentum develops re-dundancy and folds inward, further compressing the spinal canal. Certain anatomic characteristics predispose patients to spinal cord impingement. The space available for the spinal cord in the subaxial spine is determined by measuring the distance between the posterior vertebral line and the spinolaminar line. In normal adults, it measures 17 to 18 mm. Congenital stenosis is defined as a space of less than 13 mm.[1] The normal cervical spinal cord diameter is 9 to 10 mm ± 1.5 mm.[2] Because of the limited reserve space, symptoms develop earlier in the spondylotic process in patients with congenital narrowing than in those with a normal cervical canal diameter. These patients most frequently present with myelopathic symptoms, including deterioration of hand use (75%), upper extremity numbness and paresthesias (82.9%), and gait difficulties (80.3%).[3] Radicular symptoms, can develop in combination with myelopathy or as an isolated entity. Isolated nerve root impingement occurs when there is a decrease in the area of the neuroforamen. This can be caused by a spondylotic process with spurring of the uncovertebral and facet joints altering the anteroposterior diameter, as well as collapse of the disk space, thus decreasing the cranial-caudal diameter. Nerve root impingement

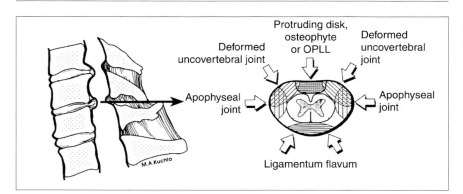

Figure 1 Schematic demonstrating various structures that can cause compression in spondylotic myelopathy. OPLL = ossification of the posterior longitudinal ligament. (Reproduced with permission from Law MD Jr, Bernhardt M, White AA: Evaluation and management of cervical spondylotic myelopathy. *J Bone Joint Surg Am* 1994;76:1420-1433.)

also can occur because of extrusion of nucleus pulposus material. The mechanical compression and chemical factors in the nucleus pulposus material act in combination to potentiate the inflammatory cascade. The dorsal root ganglion is particularly sensitive to pressure and inflammation, resulting in prolonged and abnormal discharges into its respective distribution[4] (Figure 1). Neural impingement from static causes usually is detectable with modern MRI and CT myelography; however, dynamic causes can be subtle and often are overlooked in the preoperative workup.

A dynamic component to spinal cord and nerve root impingement may be in the form of positional stenosis or instability. Chen and associates[5] evaluated changes in the spinal canal diameter in five human cadavers when tension/compression and flexion/extension were applied. The most dramatic decrease in diameter was with extension, whereby infolding of the ligamentum flavum and shingling of the lamina resulted in a reduction of canal diameter by 24.3%.[5] Other studies reported similar findings with MRI performed in flexion and extension.[6,7] Conventional MRI and CT myelography studies are performed with the body in a static position within the gantry and may miss truly symptomatic forms of stenosis. The idea of dynamic neural impingement is further supported by outcome studies. Morio and associates[8] evaluated patients who were treated with French-door laminaplasty with posterolateral bone grafting. Patients who lost more than 30% of preoperative intervertebral motion had higher Japanese Orthopaedic Association (JOA) scores and neurologic recovery than those who retained their preoperative motion.[8]

Instability also may contribute to dynamic stenosis. This instability may be part of the degenerative process or may be iatrogenic from previous surgery. Instability on static radiographs is defined as subluxation of more than 3.5 mm or 11° of angulation between adjacent levels. On dynamic views, instability is defined as 4 mm of subluxation.[9] Retrolisthesis is aggravated in extension and reduced in flexion. In contrast, spondylolisthesis is more symptomatic in flexion and reduced in ex-

tension. Areas above stiffened segments are particularly prone to the development of degenerative instability. This often is seen at the C3-C4 level in elderly patients.[10] Iatrogenic instability occurs from destabilizing the spine by a wide decompression in the absence of arthrodesis. Iatrogenic instability has been described when more than 50% of the facet complex is resected during a posterior decompression.[11] These patients may not recover as expected or may have a period of recovery followed by recurrence of myelopathy or radiculopathy. Guigui and associates[12] obtained dynamic radiographs of 58 patients who had a laminectomy and found that those with evidence of instability had inferior neurologic recovery. In the setting of instability or wide resection, supplemental arthrodesis should be considered to prevent recurrent neurologic compromise and provide an environment for optimal neurologic recovery.

Sagittal Alignment, Location of Compressive Pathology, and Number of Levels Involved

Currently, there is no level I evidence to guide the surgeon in determining whether an anterior or posterior approach provides the optimal outcome, and there is poor agreement among spine surgeons.[13] Despite differences in opinion, surgeons agree that carefully assessing the sagittal alignment of the cervical spine on an upright lateral plain radiograph, identifying the location of the pathology, and determining the number of levels involved can help guide the choice of surgical approach. A full, plain radiographic series, including flexion and extension views, provides the best evaluation of sagittal alignment. Laminectomies and laminaplasties directly decompress posterior pathology; however, in the setting of anterior pathology, they rely on posterior drift of the spinal cord. To achieve this, some amount of lordosis is required. The definition of adequate lordosis has been debated. Komotar and associates[9] have described effective lordosis as a line drawn from the posterior inferior aspect of the spinous process of C2 to a similar spot on C7. No portion of C3-C6 spinous process may be dorsal to this line.[9] Hamanishi and Tanaka[14] stated that a minimal lordosis of 10° must exist to provide adequate drift and decompression. Anatomically, the nerve roots that exit the spinal cord anteriorly at their respective foramina limit dorsal spinal cord shift. Neuroforaminal stenosis may further tether the nerve root and limit spinal cord drift. The maximal amount of spinal cord shift is 6.0 to 6.6 mm, and this occurs at the midcervical level.[15,16] This should be taken into consideration if an osteophyte or ossification of the posterior longitudinal ligament (OPLL) exists anteriorly with a size greater than 6.0 mm. Even with maximal posterior drift, the spinal cord will still be draped over the anterior pathology. Lee and associates[15] demonstrated the importance of the amount of stenosis at the level directly cephalad to the level of decompression. The cephalad space available for the cord should be twice the diameter of the cord itself to provide adequate posterior drift. If this ratio is less than 2, the decompression should be extended cephalad until this requirement is met. The level caudad to the decompression was not determined to be statistically significant in allowing posterior drift.[15] If retrovertebral pathology exists in a straight or kyphotic spine, and a posterior approach is performed, the spinal cord and nerve roots will not be able to drift away from the ventral pathology and neurologic function can remain static or even decline.[17]

A rigid kyphosis is an absolute contraindication to an isolated posterior approach. Decompression is more appropriately achieved with an anterior cervical diskectomy and fusion (ACDF), an anterior cervical corpectomy and fusion (ACCF), or a combination of the procedures. Multilevel ACDF provides more biomechanical stability than a corpectomy, and segmental interbody grafts are a powerful means of re-creating lordosis.[18] Unfortunately, the risk of pseudarthrosis increases in a linear fashion with the increasing number of levels fused. In three- to four-level ACDF procedures, the reported fusion rate has been as low as 47% to 56%.[19,20] A multilevel diskectomy also will not adequately treat retrovertebral disease, and an ACCF should be considered. A corpectomy provides retrovertebral decompression and corrects kyphosis.[21] In addition, a corpectomy has only two bony interfaces that require healing, with reported fusion rates of 86% to 99%.[22,23] The disadvantage of a multilevel corpectomy is the risk of graft-related complications, with statistical significance demonstrated in isolated three-level ACCF. Because graft failure has been reported in 50% to 71% of patients with isolated three-level ACCF, augmentation with a posterior arthrodesis is recommended.[24,25] An alternative method of anterior decompression that does not compromise stability is combining a corpectomy at one level and a diskectomy at another level. This method demonstrated a 96% neurologic recovery and fusion rate in a group of patients with multilevel cervical spondylotic myelopathy[26] (Figure 2).

The number of levels involved, patient comorbidities, and the fusion environment also should be considered when determining the approach. A three-level compressive pathology is best approached posteriorly in the absence of an excessively large anterior lesion or focal kyphosis. A posterior approach also may provide a more optimal outcome in elderly patients with multilevel disease and medical comorbidities. Posterior procedures typically can be done more expediently, have less blood loss, and carry a lower risk of airway compromise.[27,28] Osteoporosis provides a unique challenge, with an increased risk of subsidence and hardware failure with an anterior approach.[29] A combined anterior and posterior approach to multilevel disease should be considered if there are risk factors indicating a poor fusion environment, such as a patient who smokes or has renal failure.[29]

Determining the number of levels to decompress can be as challenging as deciding on the optimal approach. In multilevel cervical disease, there often is a level of maximal compression; however, additional levels may demonstrate evidence of mild stenosis that, if not treated, may lead to a less than ideal outcome. MRI findings may help guide the surgeon to decompress a level or leave it alone. The presence of either increased signal within the spinal cord on a T2-weighted sequence alone, or in combination with a low signal on a T1-weighted sequence, correlates with a spectrum of histologic changes. If the patient is symptomatic and surgery is planned, these MRI findings should cause inclusion of that level in the decompression. The transverse area of the cord as determined on axial MRI or CT myelography

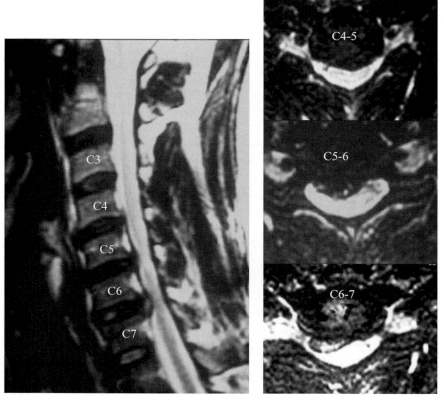

Figure 2 MRI scan showing multilevel spondylotic myelopathy (left) and magnified images (right).

should also be used in determining the extent of the decompression. A transverse area of the spinal cord measuring less than 60 mm² is associated with the development of myelopathy.[30,31] It has been suggested that any level demonstrating a transverse area of less than 60 mm² should be decompressed.

The issue of disk degeneration and the later development of adjacent level disease (ALD) is less well defined. ALD is defined as the development of radicular or myelopathic signs and symptoms referable to a motion segment adjacent to a prior cervical arthrodesis. There is some debate about whether ALD is the natural progression of the spondylotic process or is hastened by, or is a direct result of, the biomechanical changes created by the arthrodesis.[32-37] Not all MRI findings of disk degeneration are significant, given that these changes are seen in a large percentage of elderly asymptomatic individuals.[38,39] If a decompression and arthrodesis are being considered, evidence of disk degeneration adjacent to the level of interest also should be considered. Yonenobu and associates[40] compared early and late onset of neurologic deterioration in 110 patients undergoing decompression for myelopathy. In the early onset group, four patients deteriorated within 6 months because of ALD. Retrospective analysis of these early failures demonstrated degenerative changes on preoperative myelograms. The authors concluded that a fusion should not stop adjacent to a degenerated level; rather, it should include the degenerated level.[40] Ishihara and associates[41] retrospectively evaluated 112 patients clinically and radiologically to determine predictors for the development of ALD following ACDF. Symptomatic ALD developed in 17% of those followed, with an average of 6.5 years (range, 1 to 17 years) from the first operation to the development of ALD. The age, sex, and number of levels fused were clinically analyzed. Radiographic parameters evaluated included preoperative cervical spine alignment, preoperative range of motion from C2 to C7, AP spinal canal diameter at C5 only, the presence of adjacent segment degeneration on preoperative plain radiographs, and evidence of indentation of the dura on MRI or myelography on preoperative imaging. The only statistically significant factor for the development of symptomatic ALD was the presence of indentation of the dura mater on preoperative myelography or MRI. This suggests the need to fuse asymptomatic levels that demonstrate disk degeneration with associated dura mater indentation.[41] Hilibrand and associates[33] provided some insight into the significance of degeneration at various levels and later development of ALD. They demonstrated symptomatic ALD in 25% of all patients within 10 years of anterior cervical arthrodesis. This equates to an average annual incidence of 2.9%. The levels at greatest risk for ALD were the C5-6 and C6-7 interspaces. The intermediate risk levels were the C3-4 and C4-5 levels. Those at lowest risk of being involved in ALD were the C2-3 and C7-T1 levels. Interestingly, ALD was less likely to develop in multilevel fusions, probably because the fusion included those levels at highest risk for the later development of ALD. The amount of preexisting disk degeneration at the adjacent level correlated with the time to the development of symptoms. Adjacent-level disks that demonstrated significant degeneration at the time of the initial surgery showed symptomatic disease within 2 years, whereas adjacent disks without evidence of degeneration at the index procedure were disease free for more than 7 years. Of 46 patients in whom symptomatic ALD developed, only 13 responded to nonsurgical treatment. A single-level arthrodesis involving C5 or C6 and preexisting radiographic evidence of degeneration at adjacent levels are the greatest risk factors for the development of ALD. This indicates that if there is severe degeneration at an asymptomatic level and it involves one of the high-risk levels, consideration should be given for including it in the index fusion.[33] This recommendation is further supported by the fact that revision surgery provides a lower rate of fusion and worse neurologic recovery than the index procedure.[42,43] Evidence of disk degeneration with indentation of the dura or degeneration at a high-risk level should be carefully discussed with the patient. Even though the level may be causing minimal compression, these factors may lead to early development of ALD and the recurrence of symptoms. Some patients desire a less extensive procedure and are willing to accept the risk of revision surgery, whereas others prefer treatment at the index procedure. Given the lack of strong evidence guiding treatment, the patient should be afforded the opportunity to make a well-informed decision.

Intraoperative Considerations
Anterior Procedures
A balance exists in anterior cervical surgery between providing adequate decompression and not unnecessarily destabilizing the spine or placing neurovascular structures at risk. There is some debate as to whether resection of the posterior longitudinal ligament (PLL) or the uncovertebral joints during ACDF improves neurologic outcome. Proponents for resecting the PLL believe that it is necessary to adequately search for and remove sequestered disk fragments that are posterior to the PLL. These disk fragments can be small in size; however, there is no direct correlation to the size of disk fragment and the patient's neurologic deficit.[44] This finding suggests that the pain and symptoms from herniated nucleus pulposus may be primarily caused by inflammatory chemical mediators rather than mechanical compression.[45] Some surgeons determine the need to resect the PLL based on preoperative MRI findings, whereas others intraoperatively examine the PLL for a rent. MRI has demonstrated poor sensitivity for detecting sequestered cervical disk fragments. In one study, the preoperative MRI scans of some patients were reviewed by multiple examiners and compared with intraoperative evidence of a disk fragment after PLL resection.[46] MRI demonstrated a sensitivity of 46.2%; however, if a fragment was observed on MRI, it had a 92.2% specificity. In this same study, appreciation of a rent in the PLL before resection showed a sensitivity of 88.5%.[46] Therefore, visual inspection or palpation is more accurate in determining the need to resect the PLL. An awareness of the potential for an extruded fragment should be heightened with a soft-disk herniation. Other surgeons believe that resection of the PLL creates unnecessary risks of a dural tear, neurologic injury, bleeding, and increased surgical

time. Some believe that distraction alone from the interbody graft provides adequate space for the spinal cord and nerve root, rendering the effect of sequestered fragments negligible.

Another debate about ACDF is whether the uncovertebral joint requires resection to adequately decompress the exiting nerve root. Because the exiting nerve root passes just posterior to the uncovertebral joint, many physicians argue that resection of uncovertebral spurs is required to provide adequate decompression.[47] Others believe that indirect widening of the foramen with an interbody graft and reabsorption of these spurs after achieving a solid arthrodesis are adequate.[48] Resecting the uncovertebral joint can cause morbidity. Biomechanical studies have shown that the posterior portion of the uncovertebral joint is the most stabilizing portion of the joint.[49,50] The vertebral artery is very close to the uncovertebral joint, especially at the more cephalad levels.[51] In a retrospective review of 109 patients who had ACDF with plate fixation, Shen and associates[52] compared 71 patients who had direct uncovertebral decompression (group 1) with 38 patients who did not (group 2). Flexion and extension views were used to determine fusion, and Odom criteria were used to determine clinical outcome. There was a 95.8% union rate in group 1 and a 100% union rate in group 2. All of those with nonunions reported good outcomes. The overall outcomes were not statistically different between groups.[52] Albert and associates[53] further confirmed the indirect increase in area of the neural foramen by measuring the area on sagittal CT scans before and after placement of an anterior cervical interbody graft,

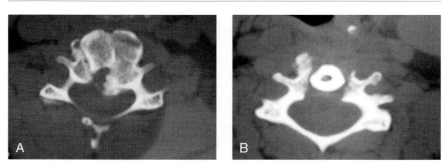

Figure 3 **A,** Axial CT scan demonstrating an inadequately performed anterior decompression with angled decompression and residual compression of the neural elements. **B,** Postoperative axial CT scan demonstrating decompression and strut grafting after revision anterior surgery on the same patient.

reporting a 33% increase in foraminal area after ACDF.[53] Resection should likely be reserved for patients with a large osteophyte and associated symptoms in a distribution that correlates, but even this has not been proven to be necessary.

ACCF poses its own unique intraoperative challenges. Performing a corpectomy requires a thorough understanding of the relative anatomic locations of the vertebral arteries, exiting nerve roots, and spinal cord. The general course of the vertebral artery and its respective foramen from C3 to C6 is from medial and posterior to anterior and lateral.[51] The distance between the neural foramina provides a maximal allowable width of resection, but this is much wider than is required to adequately decompress the spinal cord and exiting nerve root. Performing a too narrow decompression leads to poor outcomes in myelopathic patients.[40,54] The width of the spinal canal is relatively constant in the subaxial spine, measuring approximately 13 to 14.5 mm.[55,56] Before corpectomy, the longus colli should be elevated so that both uncovertebral joints are visible. This provides definition of the true midline and avoids an asymmetric resec-

tion that could result in a vertebral artery injury or inadequate decompression. Many anatomic landmarks have been evaluated as intraoperative reference points for maintaining a safe distance from the vertebral artery while providing adequate lateral decompression. Most surgeons use the uncovertebral joint as a reference for adequate lateral decompression. The distance between the medial margins of the uncovertebral joints at C3 is approximately 15 mm; at C6, it is 19 mm. When completed, a multilevel corpectomy should have a trapezoidal shape, being narrower at the cephalad portion and wider at the caudad portion. It is important to assess the width of the resection with something of known length, such as the surgeon's index fingertip. Decompressing up to the medial margin of the uncovertebral joint leaves approximately 5 mm of bone protecting the vertebral artery.[55] For a thorough foraminotomy, the osteophytes should be resected with a curet or Kerrison punch off the uncus and in line with the exiting nerve root up to the medial edge of the pedicle. Extra care should be taken at C3 and C4 because the vertebral artery has a more posterior location. Adequate lateral

decompression is further confirmed by the presence of epidural fat and veins surrounding the exiting nerve root[55] (Figure 3).

Using these anatomic landmarks generally will avoid a vertebral artery injury between C3 and C6, but a careful review of preoperative axial images is necessary to ensure that an anomalous vertebral artery does not exist. In the presence of a tortuous vertebral artery, a posterior decompressive procedure should be considered. If an anterior procedure is required because of focal kyphosis or significant retrovertebral disease, a hybrid anterior decompression should be performed in which a diskectomy is done above the vertebra with a tortuous artery and a corpectomy below. Theoretically, this technique leaves the tortuous vertebral artery alone because the abnormality occurs in the midbody of the respective vertebrae.[57-59]

Freidberg and associates[60] used intraoperative CT scans to assess the adequacy of resection after diskectomy or corpectomy in 31 consecutive patients. In 17 patients, the CT scans showed inadequate resection, and further surgery was performed. Albert and associates[61] evaluated the proximity of the lateral extent of the decompression to the foramen transversarium, using image-guided frameless stereotaxy compared with anatomic landmarks. The image-guided stereotaxy resulted in an average distance from the lateral edge of the trough to the vertebral artery of 4.34 mm compared with 5.10 mm when using anatomic landmarks. This finding indicates that a potentially wider decompression can be safely performed with image-guided stereotaxy; however, the clinical significance of this difference is unknown. More importantly, there was less variability in the width of the remaining bone in the stereotaxy group (range, 3.3 to 5.48 mm) compared with the anatomic group (range, 1.72 to 7.71 mm).[61] Ultrasound confirmation of adequate trough width also has been described.[62]

One theoretic risk of an excessively wide corpectomy is anterior drift of the spinal cord and development of a C5 palsy. Almost all C5 palsies are unilateral and occur within 1 week after surgery. The overall average frequency of C5 palsy is 4.6% regardless of the approach.[63] In a three-level or more ACCF, the senior author (JDK) leaves the PLL intact, believing that it prevents excessive anterior drift and traction on the C5 nerve root. When a C5 palsy occurs, imaging studies are obtained to ensure that no residual compressive lesion is present. If none are found, treatment includes conservative care with physical therapy, with most patients having return of deltoid and biceps function.

Posterior Procedures

Options for posterior treatment of cervical spondylotic myelopathy and radiculopathy include laminectomy, laminaplasty, and laminoforaminotomy or "keyhole" foraminotomy. With the correct indication, adequate training, and attention to detail, these procedures can provide excellent results with minimal complications.

The primary indication for laminectomy is multilevel (usually three or more levels) spondylotic myelopathy with or without radiculopathy.[64] Historically, laminectomy was the only procedure available for treating cervical spondylotic myelopathy, but complications with postlaminectomy kyphosis, increases in instability, progression of

OPLL, and neurologic deterioration limited its use after anterior procedures were developed.[65,66] As with all posterior procedures, the requirement for preoperative cervical lordosis cannot be overemphasized because these procedures require posterior drift for decompression. Posterior fusion with instrumentation after multilevel laminectomy should be considered because of the high rates of complications related to instability. Comparing ACDF with laminectomy for the treatment of multilevel spondylotic radiculopathy, Herkowitz[67] found that postlaminectomy kyphosis (25%) and anterior subluxation (40%) compromised the results of laminectomy alone (66% good to excellent results with laminectomy compared with 92% for ACDF). Subsequent reports have suggested that fusion should be strongly considered when hypermobility is found on preoperative flexion-extension radiographs or when complete unilateral or bilateral facetectomy compromises more than 50% of the total facet complex.[11,12,68] The laminectomy technique involves the use of a burr, after initial posterior midline cervical exposure, to thin the cortices at the junction of the laminae and lateral masses. If fusion is not planned, the exposure should not violate the capsule over the facet joints. A small Kerrison rongeur can be used to complete the cut, or a Cobb elevator can be used to lever up on the bony segments to break the thin shell of remaining bone. Meticulous hemostasis must be maintained to prevent postoperative hematoma. Foraminotomies should be considered if a radicular component exists.

Laminaplasty was developed in Japan to provide expansion of the spinal canal posteriorly without the need for fusion.[68,69] It is similar to

laminectomy in that both are midline posterior procedures requiring a lordotic or neutral spine to accomplish spinal decompression. Indications for its use are myelopathy and radiculopathy caused by multilevel cervical spinal stenosis.[70] In addition to a kyphotic spine, other contraindications for laminaplasty are situations in which adhesions or scar may tether the dura or nerve roots and prevent drift, such as prior decompressive surgery, ossification of the ligamentum flavum, idiopathic epidural fibrosis, or dorsal epidural abscess. Laminaplasty (like laminectomies) also can be combined with foraminotomies to accomplish nerve root decompression. The foraminotomies on the hinge side need to be done before the "door" is opened. Multiple methods of laminaplasty have been described, including the open door, the French door, and Z-plasty, but the literature does not provide any conclusive proof that one method is superior to another.[71,72] Keeping the hinge open also has led to multiple methods of fixation, including plates, simple bony suture techniques, suture anchors, and bone grafts on the door side. The results of laminaplasty generally have been good, with some reports of an 86% rate of successful outcomes, similar to anterior procedures but superior to laminectomy.[67] Combined foraminotomies with laminaplasty also have fared well, with 91% improvement in radiculopathy reported by Lee and associates.[73] Laminaplasties result in a 30% to 50% loss of cervical motion, but this is better than the loss of motion that occurs with multilevel arthrodesis.[74,75] The most common complications are C5 root palsy and persistent axial neck pain.[70] Other less common complications are postoperative kyphosis and closure

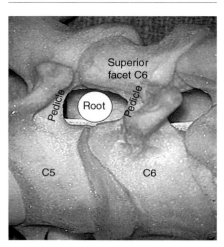

Figure 4 The boundaries of the neural foramen. (Reproduced from Lehman RA, Riew KD: Thorough decompression of the posterior cervical foramen. *Instr Course Lect* 2007;56:301-309.)

or fracture of the lamina with recurrent myelopathy.[67,76] It has been reported, however, that with advances in laminaplasty, these sources of mechanical failure are now rare, even with minimal bracing and activity as tolerated.[77] Adherence to the indications, contraindications, and surgical fixation technique should allow adequate decompression.

Foraminotomies can be done alone or combined with a laminaplasty, as described above, to decompress the cervical nerve roots. Adequate decompression relies on knowing the relevant anatomy of the neural foramen. The neural foramen is bordered anteriorly by the uncovertebral joint and lateral disk, posteriorly by the superior articular facet of the caudal vertebral segment, and cranially and caudally by the pedicles of the superior and inferior respective vertebrae (Figure 4). Lehman and Riew[78] advised that to thoroughly decompress the foramen, the dorsal aspect must be unroofed from the medial border of the pedicle laterally until the lateral border of the pedicle can be felt.

The decompression needs to be done in an anteroposterior direction only, by resecting approximately 50% of the superior articular facet. The uncovertebral joint also can be burred down; however, the nerve root must be mobile enough to retract out of the way with minimal force. One other caveat to keep in mind is that, as the decompression progresses ventrally, the location of the vertebral artery lies laterally, anterior to the root. This procedure can be performed through a standard midline posterior cervical incision or more percutaneous approaches, using a paramedian incision 1.5 to 2.0 cm off the midline.[79] Regardless of the approach, a common mistake leading to inadequate decompression is not seeing the cranial border of the superior facet.[78] Without seeing or palpating the entire cranial border, bone can be left behind, which can continue to impinge on the root. Inadequate decompression also is caused by not going laterally enough. Because the foramen is bordered superiorly and inferiorly by the pedicles, if an adequate decompression has been done, the lateral edge of the pedicle should be palpable. In general, results have been good, with Henderson and associates[80] reporting a 96% rate of arm pain relief in a study of 736 patients. Zeidman and Ducker[81] reported similar results, with 167 of 172 patients (97%) who were treated with laminoforaminotomies showing improvement in radicular pain.

Cervical Arthroplasty

Successful fusion after ACDF allows for resorption of the osteophytes posteriorly through stress shielding;[48] however, this cannot occur in a motion-preserving procedure such as total disk replacement in the cervical spine. Exacting removal of all osteophytes and compressing structures must be done with disk arthroplasty.[82] Although the short-term results appear to be favorable for cervical disk replacement, long-term follow-up is lacking.[83] The frequency of lumbar total disk replacement has increased, but, because of the relatively young age of those receiving these disks, it would seem prudent to use these devices with caution until more long-term data are available.[84,85]

Use of the Operating Microscope

The commercial surgical microscope was introduced in 1953 and was first used in spinal surgery in 1978. Since then, several advantages have been cited for the operating microscope for both anterior and posterior cervical surgery. Usually in cervical surgery, the area of the surgical site is small. With loupe magnification, a maximum of two people can see into the incision; however, with a modern microscope, multiple eyepieces are available. There also is the option to show the image on a display so other operating room personnel can see the surgery and anticipate the next step. With the correct instruments, the microscope allows the hand to be out of the wound, allowing the use of multiple instruments at the same time. In addition to these advantages, the light in the microscope is perfectly collinear with the lens and can be turned up or down along with the magnification to provide the optimal view. This higher magnification allows the surgeon to better see all pathologic structures, such as osteophytes or small disk fragments, so they are properly treated. Riew and associates,[86] suggested that using the operating microscope allows more rapid decompressions and improved safety because of improved visualization.

One pitfall in the use of the microscope is that the microscope must be perfectly perpendicular to the area of resection or the surgeon may become disoriented and believe that the decompression is being taken straight down when in reality the decompression is being done asymmetrically, potentially destabilizing the spine or endangering the vertebral artery.

Ossification of the Posterior Longitudinal Ligament

OPLL should be thought of differently than cervical spondylotic myelopathy when determining a surgical plan. The four types of OPLL include segmental, which is posterior to the vertebral body (39%); continuous, which is retrovertebral and crosses the disk space (27%); mixed, with both continuous and segmental characteristics (29%); and other (5%).[87] Nonsurgical treatment of OPLL has a limited role and is appropriate for patients with minimal neurologic deficits and those with significant medical comorbidities that preclude surgery. Katoh and associates,[88] reported that of 27 patients treated for OPLL who sustained minor trauma, myelopathy developed in 13 (48%), deterioration of preexisting myelopathy occurred in 7 (26%), and 7 (26%) had no neurologic change. These findings were similar to those of Matsunaga and associates[89] who followed 450 patients with OPLL for a mean of 17.6 years; 304 were treated nonsurgically and 146 surgically. During the follow-up period, myelopathy developed in 55 of the 323 patients (17%) who did not have myelopathy at the initial visit. Risk factors for the development of myelopathy were

OPLL stenosis of more than 60% and increased cervical range of motion. Kaplan-Meier analysis demonstrated a myelopathy-free rate of 71% at 30 years. No difference in final function was seen in those with a Nurick grade of 1 or 2 managed surgically or nonsurgically. In patients with a Nurick grade of 3 or 4 managed surgically, only 12% were wheelchair bound or bedridden compared with 89% of those treated nonsurgically.[89]

Certain characteristics of OPLL help guide the choice of an anterior or posterior approach. OPLL can erode through the dura and if directly resected, may result in the formation of a cerebrospinal fluid fistula. Predictions about the formation of a cerebrospinal fluid leak can be made based on CT myelogram findings. The single-layer sign is ossification of the PLL from the inside out, and the double-layer sign is ossification of the PLL on the periphery with a central hypodense layer. At the time of surgery, Hida and associates[90] found that 11% of those with a single-layer sign demonstrated a dural defect, whereas 83% of those with a double-layer sign demonstrated a dural defect. Min and associates[91] retrospectively evaluated 197 patients who had anterior decompression and fusion for OPLL. They found dural defects in 52.6% of patients with a double-layer sign compared with 13.6% of patients with a single-layer sign. In addition, they found continuous-type OPLL more likely to be associated with a dural defect.[91] A dural defect carries a fairly significant morbidity and may require lumbar drain placement, prolonged bed rest, and even placement of a myocutaneous flap.[92] To avoid exposing the dural defect, the "floating method" has been proposed. The floating method allows the ossi-

fied ligament to float anteriorly without resecting the PLL and decreases the risk of exposing a dural defect and the subsequent formation of a cerebrospinal fluid fistula. This is accomplished by providing a wide enough decompression in the lateral and cephalad-caudad directions to allow the bone to float anteriorly. The transverse decompression often must extend between the pedicles, up to 20 to 25 mm, to ensure sufficient decompression.[93,94] The ossification should migrate 4 to 5 mm. Inadequate anterior flotation may be caused by a strut graft that was placed too far posterior, inadequate peripheral release of the bone or ligament, or the ossification itself may be more mature with less buoyancy.[94] Uncinatectomies often are required because the OPLL can cause foraminal stenosis. The width of resection and the need for foraminotomies should be determined based on the patient's history, physical examination, and preoperative images. The inherent risks with this approach include inadequate decompression, recurrence if the OPLL island reossifies with its periphery, and vertebral artery injury caused by wide decompression.[87] Advantages include a decreased risk of hemorrhage from epidural veins and a decreased risk of epidural hematoma. In addition, it allows a gradual anterior migration with less risk of iatrogenic nerve root deficits.

Matsuoka and associates[93] reported on the results of the anterior floating method in 63 patients with 13-year follow-up. The JOA score improved from a mean of 8.3 preoperatively to 14.0 at 10-year follow-up, and declined slightly to 13.5 at 13-year follow-up. Delayed deterioration was attributed to inadequate decompression and progression of the ossification outside the original surgical field. There was no recurrent ossification within the margins of the prior decompression.[93]

A posterior procedure avoids the risk of vertebral artery injury and formation of a cerebrospinal fluid leak; however, certain patient characteristics are necessary to use this procedure. As previously discussed, posterior approaches require lordosis to allow the spinal cord to drift. Multiple structures anchor the spinal cord anteriorly, including the dentate ligament, nerve root, and root sleeves. OPLL can form adhesions between the ossified ligament and dura preventing posterior drift.[94] The maximal amount of spinal cord shift is 6.0 to 6.6 mm, which occurs at the midcervical level.[15,95] This shift should be considered if OPLL exists anteriorly with a size greater than 6.0 mm. Even with maximal posterior drift, the spinal cord will still be draped over the anterior pathology. In general, OPLL requires a much larger postoperative canal diameter than does spondylotic myelopathy to provide adequate decompression and neurologic recovery.[96] The configuration of the ossified lesion and its overall occupation of the canal also are important in predicting outcomes based on the approach. Iwasaki and associates[97,98] compared anterior decompression and fusion ($n = 27$) to laminaplasty ($n = 66$) for the treatment of OPLL. The anterior decompression consisted of the floating method if the OPLL could not be easily removed or if complete resection of the OPLL was followed by placement of allograft or autograft and halo immobilization. Patients were evaluated at a mean follow-up of 6 years for anterior decompression and 10.2 years for laminaplasty using the JOA score. Anterior decompression and fusion yielded better results when the occupying ratio of the OPLL was more than or equal to 60% or the OPLL lesion had a hill-type configuration. The anterior surgery group had a much higher complication rate, requiring additional surgery in 26% of patients compared with only 1.5% of the laminaplasty group. Anterior surgery carries increased risk but may provide better decompression in those with hill-type lesions or a compression-occupying ratio of more than 60%.[97,98]

Another consideration is that an ossification lesion is more likely to progress after posterior surgery. Progression of OPLL following laminaplasty has been reported in 70% to 73% of patients, with an increased risk in those younger than age 59 years.[97] In contrast, the risk of progression after anterior surgery is 36% to 64%.[97] This progression may not correlate with neurologic outcome. Hori and associates[99] reported on 55 patients who had laminaplasty for OPLL (follow-up > 5 years). Outcome measures included JOA scores and serial radiographs. In 12 patients (21.8%), ossification progressed; there was a higher risk in younger patients, those with C3 involvement, and mixed-type or continuous-type OPLL. Progression did not correlate with the JOA score.[99]

Revision Surgery

Patients who present with persistent symptoms or who are not expected to recover after a cervical decompression pose a unique set of challenges and should be thoroughly evaluated. The causes of unsuccessful surgery are often multifactorial and may include an improper diagnosis, inadequate decompression, iatrogenic neurologic injury, irreversible changes at the index procedure, the development of postoperative instability, or the presence of a pseudarthrosis. It must be confirmed that the appropriate diagnosis was made at the index procedure. Other neurologic disorders can cause clinical manifestations similar to cervical myelopathy. Patients with multiple sclerosis often have paresthesias involving the extremities, with associated weakness and hand clumsiness. Clinical characteristics of multiple sclerosis are facial numbness and visual changes. MRI of the brain and spinal cord show demyelinating lesions, and the cerebrospinal fluid often has oligoclonal bands. Amyotrophic lateral sclerosis is an isolated disease of the anterior horn cells. Patients initially present with muscle cramps, which is followed by rapid deterioration of strength. Guillain-Barré syndrome is a demyelinating polyneuropathy with symmetric ascending paralysis, areflexia, paresthesias, and diffuse pain. Cerebrospinal fluid shows increased protein. Pernicious anemia is secondary to insufficient vitamin B_{12} absorption caused by inadequate dietary intake or decreased absorption and can result in peripheral paresthesias and weakness, later progressing to an unsteady gait. The complete blood cell count demonstrates macrocytic anemia; B_{12} levels are abnormal. Peripheral nerve entrapment, such as cubital tunnel or carpal tunnel syndromes, can occur as an isolated entity or in combination with cervical radiculopathy or myelopathy and is termed double-crush syndrome. Patients with a peripheral nerve entrapment have a delay of nerve conduction velocities at the site of the entrapment. Patients with a spinal cord tumor or infection have persistent nonmechanical neck pain and possible nerve pain and often have constitutional symptoms. Each of these conditions demonstrates unique findings on MRI and often is associated with elevated laboratory indices. The spinal cord should be carefully evaluated for evidence of a syrinx, which causes weakness and sensory deficits depending on the level of involvement.[100] Imaging studies and the results of the physical examination should be used to determine the diagnosis. If the diagnosis remains in question, electrodiagnostic studies and a neurologic consultation are indicated.

Inadequate decompression at the level of interest often can be seen with MRI or CT myelography; however, dynamic stenosis can go undetected on these static studies. Standard MRI or CT may not adequately detect persistent foraminal stenosis, which is better seen on oblique MRIs.[101] Inadequate decompression also can be secondary to unrecognized stenosis at a level not imaged at the initial procedure. Upper motor neuron symptoms and findings caused by spinal cord compression can occur in the cervical or thoracic spine. Patients with both a cervical and thoracic disk herniation have been decribed.[102] OPLL has been reported to occur in both the cervical and thoracic spine. Seventy percent of OPLL involves the cervical spine, and the remaining 30% is evenly divided between the proximal thoracic (T1 through T4) and proximal lumbar (L1 through L3) levels.[87] If a patient does not improve after cervical decompression, imaging of the thoracic spine should be considered.

Iatrogenic intraoperative neurologic injury is caused by direct trauma or hypoperfusion of the spinal cord resulting from intraoperative hypotension. This injury often is detected intraoperatively by changes seen with somatosensory or motor-evoked potentials.[103] The patient awakens with the neurologic deficit, and, over time, histologic changes can occur, which can be seen on MRI. Patients who do not clinically improve after surgical decompression may have had preexisting chronic and irreversible spinal cord dysfunction caused by prolonged cord compression. When counseling patients at the index or revision procedure, it is important that surgeons recognize irreversible changes on MRI scans along with other factors that predict outcome. Compression of the spinal cord leads to a stepwise progression of spinal cord involvement, beginning with the anterior horn and intermediate zone of the gray matter, followed by the lateral and posterior funiculi, and eventually throughout the entire gray matter and lateral funiculus.[104] These histologic changes take time, and MRI findings can represent a spectrum of pathology.[105] Increased signal seen on T2-weighted sequences can represent reversible histologic changes, such as edema, or irreversible changes such as necrosis, myelomalacia, or spongiform necrosis.[106] The quality of this signal can indicate the reversibility on a histologic level, with faint T2 hyperintensities indicating reversible changes; and distinct, well-defined hyperintensities indicating irreversible changes and a worse prognosis with decompression.[107,108] A more ominous MRI finding is the combination of a high signal on T2-weighted sequences and a low signal on T1-weighted sequences, indicating irreversible changes.[106] The presence of a high-signal–intensity lesion in the central gray matter on both the left and right side, the so called snake-eye appearance, on axial T2-weighted sequences indicates irreversible cystic necrosis of the anterior horn cells.[109] Other factors that negatively affect outcome include chronicity of symptoms of more than 18 months, increased neurologic involvement on presentation, a patient age of older than 60 years, a transverse area of the spinal cord less than 50 mm^2, and multilevel compression.[110-113]

Instability can occur at the level of decompression or adjacent to a successful arthrodesis. Instability and postoperative kyphosis can develop in laminectomies without fusion if an excessively wide decompression is performed.[11] Over time, neurologic function deteriorates in patients with instability.[114] Instability can develop in those previously treated with decompression and successful arthrodesis. This hypermobility and dynamic stenosis is most common at the upper adjacent level.[115] Evidence of instability is best diagnosed with flexion-extension radiographs. Microinstability and persistent symptoms also can occur when there is a pseudarthrosis. Persistent motion at a pseudarthrosis can result in axial neck pain or recurrent myelopathy or radiculopathy. A pseudarthrosis can be identified by a 2-mm difference in the interspace between adjacent spinous processes on flexion and extension radiographs.[116] A CT scan with reconstructions also can be used to look for traversing bony trabeculae.[117] Intraoperative assessment remains the gold standard. Phillips and associates[118] reported that 33% of those with a failed arthrodesis who were treated nonsurgically were asymptomatic at 5 years, indicating that few patients are pain-free in the long term. Successful treatment has been reported using revision anterior arthrodesis and posterior arthrodesis.[21,119]

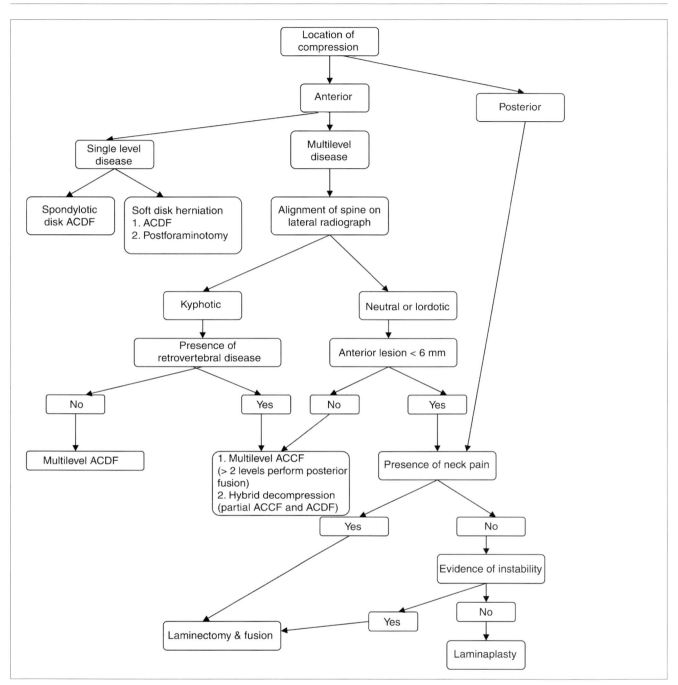

Figure 5 Decision-making flowchart for subaxial cervical spine spondylotic myelopathy.

Summary

Inadequate decompression of the cervical spine usually can be avoided by carefully assessing all the pertinent preoperative factors (Figure 5). After careful preoperative planning has been completed, understanding and identifying all of the intraoperative technical issues for a complete decompression are vitally important to achieve a well-decompressed spinal canal. In patients who present with an inadequately decompressed spinal canal, a thorough reevaluation is necessary. Revision surgery can be successful if the general principles of spinal decompression are followed.

References

1. Rao R: Neck pain, cervical radiculopathy, and cervical myelopathy: Pathophysiology, natural history, and clinical evaluation. *Instr Course Lect* 2003;52:479-488.

2. Murone I: The importance of the sagittal diameters of the cervical spinal canal in relation to spondylosis and myelopathy. *J Bone Joint Surg Br* 1974;56:30-36.

3. Chiles BW III, Leonard MA, Choudhri HF, Cooper PR: Cervical spondylotic myelopathy: Patterns of neurological deficit and recovery after anterior cervical decompression. *Neurosurgery* 1999;44:762-770.

4. Chabot MC: The pathophysiology of axial and radicular neck pain. *Semin Spine Surg* 1995;7:2-8.

5. Chen IH, Vasavada A, Panjabi MM: Kinematics of the cervical spine canal: Changes with sagittal plane loads. *J Spinal Disord* 1994;7:93-101.

6. Chen CJ, Hsu HL, Niu CC, et al: Cervical degenerative disease at flexion-extension MR imaging: Prediction criteria. *Radiology* 2003;227:136-142.

7. Muhle C, Metzner J, Weinert D, et al: Classification system based on kinematic MR imaging in cervical spondylitic myelopathy. *AJNR Am J Neuroradiol* 1998;19:1763-1771.

8. Morio Y, Yamamoto K, Teshima R, Nagashima H, Hagino H: Clinicoradiologic study of cervical laminoplasty with posterolateral fusion bone graft. *Spine* 2000;25:190-196.

9. Komotar RJ, Mocco J, Kaiser MG: Surgical management of cervical myelopathy: Indications and techniques for laminectomy and fusion. *Spine J* 2006;6:252S-267S.

10. Mihara H, Ohnari K, Hachiya M, Kondo S, Yamada K: Cervical myelopathy caused by C3-C4 spondylosis in elderly patients: A radiographic analysis of pathogenesis. *Spine* 2000;25:796-800.

11. Zdeblick TA, Zou D, Warden KE, McCabe R, Kunz D, Vanderby R: Cervical stability after foraminotomy: A biomechanical in vitro analysis. *J Bone Joint Surg Am* 1992;74:22-27.

12. Guigui P, Benoist M, Deburge A: Spinal deformity and instability after multilevel cervical laminectomy for spondylotic myelopathy. *Spine* 1998;23:440-447.

13. Irwin ZN, Hilibrand A, Gustavel M, et al: Variations in surgical decision making for degenerative spinal disorders: Part II. Cervical spine. *Spine* 2005;30:2214-2219.

14. Hamanishi C, Tanaka S: Bilateral multilevel laminectomy with or without posterolateral fusion for cervical spondylotic myelopathy: Relationship to type of onset and time until operation. *J Neurosurg* 1996;85:447-451.

15. Lee JY, Sharan A, Baron EM, et al: Quantitative prediction of spinal cord drift after cervical laminectomy and arthrodesis. *Spine* 2006;31:1795-1798.

16. Waltz TA: Physical factors in the production of myelopathy of cervical spondylosis. *Brain* 1967;90:395-404.

17. Epstein N: Posterior approaches in the management of cervical spondylosis and ossification of the posterior longitudinal ligament. *Surg Neurol* 2002;58:194-207.

18. Papadopoulos EC, Huang RC, Girardi FP, Synnott K, Cammisa FP Jr: Three-level anterior cervical discectomy and fusion with plate fixation. *Spine* 2006;31:897-902.

19. Bolesta MJ, Rechtine GR II, Chrin AM: Three- and four-level anterior cervical discectomy and fusion with plate fixation: A prospective study. *Spine* 2000;25:2040-2044.

20. Emery SE, Bohlman HH, Bolesta MJ, Jones PK: Anterior cervical decompression and arthrodesis for the treatment of cervical spondylotic myelopathy: Two to seventeen-year follow-up. *J Bone Joint Surg* 1998;80:941-951.

21. Zdeblick TA, Hughes SS, Riew KD, Bohlman HH: Failed anterior cervical discectomy and arthrodesis: Analysis and treatment of thirty-five patients. *J Bone Joint Surg Am* 1997;79:523-532.

22. Eleraky MA, Llanos C, Sonntag VK: Cervical corpectomy: Report of 185 cases and review of the literature. *J Neurosurg* 1999;90:35-41.

23. Mayr MT, Subach BR, Comey CH, Rodts GE, Haid RW Jr: Cervical spinal stenosis: Outcome after anterior corpectomy, allograft reconstruction, and instrumentation. *J Neurosurg* 2002;96:10-16.

24. Sasso RC, Ruggiero RA Jr, Reilly TM, Hall PV: Early reconstruction failures after multilevel cervical corpectomy. *Spine* 2003;28:140-142.

25. Vaccaro AR, Falatyn SP, Scuderi GJ, et al: Early failure of long segment anterior cervical plate fixation. *J Spinal Disord* 1998;11:410-415.

26. Ashkenazi E, Smorgick Y, Rand N, Millgram MA, Mirovsky Y, Floman Y: Anterior decompression combined with corpectomies and discectomies in the management of multilevel cervical myelopathy: A hybrid decompression and fixation technique. *J Neurosurg Spine* 2005;3:205-209.

27. Wada E, Suzuki S, Kanazawa A, Matsuoka T, Miyamoto S, Yonenobu K: Subtotal corpectomy versus laminoplasty for multilevel cervical spondylotic myelopathy: A long-term follow-up study over 10 years. *Spine* 2001;26:1443-1447.

28. Emery SE, Smith MD, Bohlman HH: Upper-airway obstruction after multilevel cervical corpectomy for myelopathy. *J Bone Joint Surg Am* 1991;73:544-551.

29. Kim PK, Alexander JT: Indications for circumferential surgery for cervical spondylotic myelopathy. *Spine J* 2006;6:299S-307S.

30. Kadanka Z, Kerkovsky M, Bednarik J, Jarkovsky J: Cross-sectional transverse area and hyperintensities on magnetic resonance imaging in relation to the clinical picture in cervical spondylotic myelopathy. *Spine* 2007;32:2573-2577.

31. Penning L, Wilmink JT, van Woerden HH, Knol E: CT myelographic findings in degenerative disorders of the cervical spine: Clinical significance. *AJR Am J Roentgenol* 1986;146: 793-801.

32. Goffin J, van Loon J, Van Calenbergh F, Plets C: Long-term results after anterior cervical fusion and osteosynthetic stabilization for fractures and/or dislocations of the cervical spine. *J Spinal Disord* 1995;8:500-508.

33. Hilibrand AS, Carlson GD, Palumbo MA, Jones PK, Bohlman HH: Radiculopathy and myelopathy at segments adjacent to the site of a previous anterior cervical arthrodesis. *J Bone Joint Surg Am* 1999;81:519-528.

34. Kolstad F, Nygaard ØP, Leivseth G: Segmental motion adjacent to anterior cervical arthrodesis. *Spine* 2007; 32:512-517.

35. Reitman CA, Hipp JA, Nguyen L, Esses SI: Changes in segmental intervertebral motion adjacent to cervical arthrodesis: Prospective study. *Spine* 2004;29:E221-E226.

36. Eck JC, Humphreys SC, Lim TH, et al: Biomechanical study on the effect of cervical spine fusion on adjacent-level intradiscal pressure and segmental motion. *Spine* 2002;27: 2431-2434.

37. Park DH, Ramakrishnan P, Cho TH, et al: Effect of lower two-level anterior cervical fusion on the superior adjacent level. *J Neurosurg Spine* 2007; 7:336-340.

38. Boden SD, McCowin PR, Davis DO, Dina TS, Mark AS, Wiesel S: Abnormal magnetic-resonance scans of the cervical spin in asymptomatic subjects: A prospective investigation. *J Bone Joint Surg* 1990;72:1178-1184.

39. Matsumoto M, Fujimura Y, Suzuki N, et al: MRI of cervical intervertebral discs in asymptomatic subjects. *J Bone Joint Surg Br* 1998;80: 19-24.

40. Yonenobu K, Okada K, Fuji T, Fujiwara K, Yamashita K, Ono K: Causes of neurologic deterioration following surgical treatment of cervical myelopathy. *Spine* 1986;11:818-823.

41. Ishihara H, Kanamori M, Kawaguchi Y, Nakamura H, Kimura T: Adjacent segment disease after anterior cervical interbody fusion. *Spine J* 2004;4:624-628.

42. Hilibrand AS, Yoo JU, Carlson GD, Bohlman HH: The success of anterior cervical arthrodesis adjacent to a previous fusion. *Spine* 1997;22:1574-1579.

43. Matsumoto M, Nojiri K, Chiba K, Toyama Y, Fukui Y, Kamata M: Open-door laminoplasty for cervical myelopathy resulting from adjacent-segment disease in patients with previous anterior cervical decompression and fusion. *Spine* 2006;31:1332-1337.

44. Saal JA: Natural history and nonoperative treatment of lumbar disc herniation. *Spine* 1996;21:2S-9S.

45. Saal JS: The role of inflammation in lumbar pain. *Spine* 1995;20:1821-1827.

46. Humphreys SC, Hodges SD, Fisher DL, Eck JC, Covington LA: Reliability of magnetic resonance imaging in predicting disc material posterior to the posterior longitudinal ligament in the cervical spine: A prospective study. *Spine* 1998;23:2468-2471.

47. Bohlman HH, Emery SE, Goodfellow DB, Jones PK: Robinson anterior cervical discectomy and arthrodesis for cervical radiculopathy: Long-term follow-up of one hundred and twenty-two patients. *J Bone Joint Surg Am* 1993;75:1298-1307.

48. An HS, Evanich CJ, Nowicki BH, Haughton VM: Ideal thickness of Smith-Robinson graft for anterior cervical fusion: A cadaveric study with computed tomographic correlation. *Spine* 1993;18:2043-2047.

49. Kotani Y, McNulty PS, Abumi K, Cunningham B, Kaneda K, McAfee P: The role of anteromedial foraminotomy and the uncovertebral joints in the stability of the cervical spine: A biomechanical study. *Spine* 1998;23:1559-1565.

50. Chen TY, Crawford NR, Sonntag VK, Dickman CA: Biomechanical

effects of progressive anterior cervical decompression. *Spine* 2001;26:6-13.

51. Vaccaro AR, Ring D, Scuderi G, Garfin SR: Vertebral artery location in relation to the vertebral body as determined by two-dimensional computed tomography evaluation. *Spine* 1994;19:2637-2641.

52. Shen FH, Samartzis D, Khanna N, Goldberg EJ, An HS: Comparison of clinical and radiographic outcome in instrumented anterior cervical discectomy and fusion with or without direct uncovertebral joint decompression. *Spine J* 2004;4:629-635.

53. Albert TJ, Smith MD, Bressler E, Johnson LJ: An in vivo analysis of the dimensional changes of the neuroforamen after anterior cervical diskectomy and fusion: A radiologic investigation. *J Spinal Disord* 1997;10: 229-233.

54. Ou Y, Lu J, Mi J, et al: Extensive anterior decompression for mixed cervical spondylosis: Resection of uncovertebral joints, neural transverse foraminotomy, subtotal corpectomy, and fusion with strut graft. *Spine* 1994;19:2651-2657.

55. Oh SH, Perin NI, Cooper PR: Quantitative three-dimensional anatomy of the subaxial cervical spine: Implication for anterior spinal surgery. *Neurosurgery* 1996;38:1139-1144.

56. Smith MD, Emery SE, Dudley A, Murray KJ, Leventhal M: Vertebral artery injury during anterior decompression of the cervical spine. *J Bone Joint Surg Br* 1993;75:410-415.

57. Oga M, Terada K, Shimizu A, Sugioka Y: Tortuosity of the vertebral artery in patients with cervical spondylotic myelopathy: Risk factor for the vertebral artery injury during anterior cervical decompression. *Spine* 1996; 21:1085-1089.

58. Curylo LJ, Mason HC, Bohlman HH, Yoo JU: Tortuous course of the vertebral artery and anterior cervical decompression. *Spine* 2000; 25:2860-2864.

59. Tumialan LM, Wippold FJ II, Morgan RA: Tortuous vertebral artery injury

complicating anterior cervical spinal fusion in a symptomatic rheumatoid cervical spine. *Spine* 2004;29:E343-E348.

60. Freidberg SR, Pfeifer BA, Dempsey PK, et al: Intraoperative computerized tomography scanning to assess the adequacy of decompression in anterior cervical spine surgery. *J Neurosurg* 2001;94:8-11.

61. Albert TJ, Klein GR, Vaccaro AR: Image-guided anterior cervical corpectomy: A feasibility study. *Spine* 1999;24:826-830.

62. Goto S, Mochizuki M, Kita T, et al: Anterior surgery in four consecutive technical phases for cervical spondylotic myelopathy. *Spine* 1993;18:1968-1973.

63. Sakaura H, Hosono N, Mukai Y, Ishii T, Yoshikawa H: C5 palsy after decompression surgery for cervical myelopathy: A review of the literature. *Spine* 2003;28:2447-2451.

64. An HS, Ahn NU: Posterior decompressive procedures for the cervical spine. *Instr Course Lect* 2003;52:471-477.

65. Albert TJ, Vacarro A: Postlaminectomy kyphosis. *Spine* 1998;23:2738-2745.

66. Yonenobu K, Fuji T, Ono K, Okada K, Yamamoto T, Harada N: Choice of surgical treatment for multisegmental cervical spondylotic myelopathy. *Spine* 1985;10:710-716.

67. Herkowitz HN: A comparison of anterior cervical fusion, cervical laminectomy, and cervical laminoplasty for the surgical management of multiple level spondylotic radiculopathy. *Spine* 1988;13:774-780.

68. Mikawa Y, Shikata J, Yamamuro T: Spinal deformity and instability after multilevel cervical laminectomy. *Spine* 1987;12:6-11.

69. Snow RB, Weiner H: Cervical laminectomy and foraminotomy as surgical treatment of cervical spondylosis: A follow-up study with analysis of failures. *J Spinal Disord* 1993;6:245-250.

70. Herkowitz HN, Garfin SR, Eismont FJ, Bell GR, Balderston RA (eds): *Rothman-Simeone The Spine*, ed 5. Philadelphia, PA, Saunders Elsevier, vol 2, 2006.

71. Hirabayashi K, Watanabe K, Wakano K, Suzuki N, Satomi K, Ishii Y: Expansive open-door laminoplasty for cervical spinal stenotic myelopathy. *Spine* 1983;8:693-699.

72. Kawai S, Sunago K, Doi K, Saika M, Taguchi T: Cervical laminoplasty (Hattori's method): Procedure and follow-up results. *Spine* 1988;13:1245-1250.

73. Lee TT, Green BA, Gromelski EB: Safety and stability of open-door cervical expansive laminoplasty. *J Spinal Disord* 1998;11:12-15.

74. Seichi A, Takeshita K, Ohishi I, et al: Long-term results of double-door laminoplasty for cervical stenotic myelopathy. *Spine* 2001;26:479-487.

75. Inoue H, Ohmori K, Ishida Y, Suzuki K, Takatsu T: Long-term follow-up review of suspension laminotomy for cervical compression myelopathy. *J Neurosurg* 1996;85:817-823.

76. Hirabayashi K, Toyama Y, Chiba K: Expansive laminoplasty for myelopathy in ossification of the longitudinal ligament. *Clin Orthop Relat Res* 1999;359:35-48.

77. Morimoto T, Uranishi R, Nakase H, Kawaguchi S, Hoshido T, Sakaki T: Extensive cervical laminoplasty for patients with long segment OPLL in the cervical spine: An alternative to the anterior approach. *J Clin Neurosci* 2000;7:217-222.

78. Lehman RA Jr, Riew KD: Thorough decompression of the posterior cervical foramen. *Instr Course Lect* 2007;56:301-309.

79. Adamson TE: Microendoscopic posterior cervical laminoforaminotomy for unilateral radiculopathy: Results of a new technique in 100 cases. *J Neurosurg* 2001;95(suppl 1):51-57.

80. Henderson CM, Hennessy RG, Shuey HM Jr, Shackelford EG: Posterior-lateral foraminotomy as an exclusive operative technique for cervical radiculopathy: A review of 846 consecutively operated cases. *Neurosurgery* 1983;13:504-512.

81. Zeidman SM, Ducker TB: Posterior cervical laminoforaminotomy for radiculopathy: Review of 172 cases. *Neurosurgery* 1993;33:356-362.

82. Anderson PA, Sasso RC, Riew KD: Update on cervical artificial disk replacement. *Instr Course Lect* 2007;56:237-245.

83. Mummaneni PV, Burkus JK, Haid RW, Traynelis VC, Zdeblick TA: Clinical and radiographic analysis of cervical disc arthroplasty compared with allograft fusion: A randomized controlled trial. *J Neurosurg Spine* 2007;6:198-209.

84. Ross R, Mirza AH, Norris HE, Khatri M: Survival and clinical outcome of SB Charite III disc replacement for back pain. *J Bone Joint Surg Br* 2007;89:785-789.

85. Putzier M, Funk JF, Schnieder SV, et al: Charit total disc replacement: Clinical and radiographical results after an average follow-up of 17 years. *Eur Spine J* 2006;15:183-195.

86. Riew KD, McCulloch JA, Delamarter RB, An HS, Ahn NU: Microsurgery for degenerative conditions of the cervical spine. *Instr Course Lect* 2003;52:497-508.

87. Epstein N: Diagnosis and surgical management of cervical ossification of the posterior longitudinal ligament. *Spine J* 2002;2:436-449.

88. Katoh S, Ikata T, Hirai N, Okada Y, Nakauchi K: Influence of minor trauma to the neck on the neurological outcome in patients with ossification of the posterior longitudinal ligament (OPLL) of the cervical spine. *Paraplegia* 1995;33:330-333.

89. Matsunaga S, Sakou T, Taketomi E, Komiya S: Clinical course of patients with ossification of the posterior longitudinal ligament: A minimum 10-year cohort study. *J Neurosurg* 2004;100:245-248.

90. Hida K, Iwasaki Y, Kohanagi I, Abe H: Bone window computed

tomography for detection of dural defect associated with cervical ossified posterior longitudinal ligament. *Neurol Med Chir (Tokyo)* 1997;37:173-175.

91. Min JH, Jang JS, Lee SH: Significance of the double-layer and single-layer signs in ossification of the posterior longitudinal ligament of the cervical spine. *J Neurosurg Spine* 2007;6:309-312.

92. Belanger TA, Roh JS, Hanks SE, Kang JD, Emery SE, Bohlman HH: Ossification of the posterior longitudinal ligament: Results of anterior cervical decompression and arthrodesis in sixty-one North American patients. *J Bone Joint Surg Am* 2005;87:610-615.

93. Matsuoka T, Yamaura I, Kurosa Y, Nakai O, Shindo S, Shinomiya K: Long-term results of the anterior floating method for cervical myelopathy caused by ossification of the posterior longitudinal ligament. *Spine* 2001;26:241-248.

94. Yamaura I, Kurosa Y, Matuoka T, Shindo S: Anterior floating method for cervical myelopathy caused by ossification of the posterior longitudinal ligament. *Clin Orthop Relat Res* 1999;359:27-34.

95. Yamazaki A, Homma T, Uchiyama S, Katsumi Y, Okumura H: Morphologic limitations of posterior decompression by midsagittal splitting method for myelopathy caused by ossification of the posterior longitudinal ligament in the cervical spine. *Spine* 1999;24:32-34.

96. Ishida Y, Ohmori K, Suzuki K, Inoue H: Analysis of dural configuration for evaluation of posterior decompression in cervical myelopathy. *Neurosurgery* 1999;44:91-95.

97. Iwasaki M, Okuda S, Miyauchi A, et al: Surgical strategy for cervical myelopathy due to ossification of the posterior longitudinal ligament: Part 1. Advantages of anterior decompression and fusion over laminoplasty. *Spine* 2007;32:647-653.

98. Iwasaki M, Okuda S, Miyauchi A, et al: Surgical strategy for cervical myelopathy due to ossification of the posterior longitudinal ligament: Part 2. Clinical results and limitations of laminoplasty. *Spine* 2007;32:654-660.

99. Hori T, Kawaguchi Y, Kimura T: How does the ossification area of the posterior longitudinal ligament thicken following cervical laminoplasty? *Spine* 2007;32:E551-E556.

100. Salvi FJ, Jones JC, Weigert BJ: The assessment of cervical myelopathy. *Spine J* 2006;6:182S-189S.

101. Humphreys SC, An HS, Eck JC, Coppes M, Lim TH, Estowski L: Oblique MRI as a useful adjunct in evaluation of cervical foraminal impingement. *J Spinal Disord* 1998;11:295-299.

102. Sasai K, Adachi T, Togano K, Wakabayashi E, Ohnari H, Iida H: Two-level disc herniation in the cervical and thoracic spine presenting with spastic paresis in the lower extremities without clinical symptoms or signs in the upper extremities. *Spine J* 2006;6:464-467.

103. Khan MH, Smith PN, Balzer JR, et al: Intraoperative somatosensory evoked potential monitoring during cervical spine corpectomy surgery: Experience with 508 cases. *Spine* 2006;31:E105-E113.

104. Ito T, Oyanagi K, Takahashi H, Takahashi HE, Ikuta F: Cervical spondylotic myelopathy: Clinicopathologic study on the progression pattern and thin myelinated fibers of the lesions of seven patients examined during complete autopsy. *Spine* 1996;21:827-833.

105. al-Mefty O, Harkey HL, Marawi I, et al: Experimental chronic compressive cervical myelopathy. *J Neurosurg* 1993;79:550-561.

106. Ohshio I, Hatayama A, Kaneda K, Takahara M, Nagashima K: Correlation between histopathologic features and magnetic resonance images of spinal cord lesions. *Spine* 1993;18:1140-1149.

107. Chen CJ, Lyu RK, Lee ST, Wong YC, Wang LJ: Intramedullary high signal intensity on T2-weighted MR images in cervical spondylotic myelopathy: Prediction of prognosis with type of intensity. *Radiology* 2001;221:789-794.

108. Yukawa Y, Kato F, Yoshihara H, Yanase M, Ito K: MR T2 image classification in cervical compression myelopathy. *Spine* 2007;32:1675-1678.

109. Mizuno J, Nakagawa H, Inoue T, Hashizume Y: Clinicopathological study of "snake-eye appearance" in compressive myelopathy of the cervical spinal cord. *J Neurosurg Spine* 2003;99:162-168.

110. Naderi S, Ozgen S, Pamir MN, Ozek MM, Erzen C: Cervical spondylotic myelopathy: Surgical results and factors affecting prognosis. *Neurosurgery* 1998;43:43-49.

111. Wada E, Yonenobu K, Suzuki S, Kanazawa A, Ochi T: Can intramedullary signal change on magnetic resonance imaging predict surgical outcome in cervical spondylotic myelopathy? *Spine* 1999;24:455-461.

112. Lee TT, Manzano GR, Green BA: Modified open-door cervical expansive laminoplasty for spondylotic myelopathy: Operative technique, outcome, and predictors of gait improvement. *J Neurosurg* 1997;86:64-68.

113. Yone K, Sakou T, Yanase M, Ijiri K: Preoperative and postoperative magnetic resonance image evaluations of the spinal cord in cervical myelopathy. *Spine* 1992;17:S388-S392.

114. Gregorius FK, Estrin T, Crandall PH: Cervical spondylotic radiculopathy and myelopathy: A long-term follow-up study. *Arch Neurol* 1976;33:618-625.

115. Baba H, Furusawa N, Imura S, Kawahara N, Tsuchiya H, Tomita K: Late radiographic findings after anterior cervical fusion for spondylotic myeloradiculopathy. *Spine* 1993;18:2167-2173.

116. Cannada LK, Scherping SC, Yoo JU, Jones PK, Emery SE: Pseudoarthrosis of the cervical spine: A comparison of radiographic diagnostic measures. *Spine* 2003;28:46-51.

117. Ploumis A, Mehbod A, Garvey T, Gilbert T, Transfeldt E, Wood K: Prospective assessment of cervical fusion status: Plain radiographs versus CT-scan. *Acta Orthop Belg* 2006;72: 342-346.

118. Phillips FM, Carlson G, Emery SE, Bohlmann HH: Anterior cervical pseudarthrosis: Natural history and treatment. *Spine* 1997;22:1585-1589.

119. Carreon L, Glassman SD, Campbell MJ: Treatment of anterior cervical pseudarthrosis: Posterior fusion versus anterior revision. *Spine J* 2006; 6:154-156.

Complications of Cervical Spine Surgery

Complications of Cervical Spine Surgery

The chapters in this section present an important overview of the potential complications of cervical spine surgery. Okubadejo and associates provide a comprehensive description of postoperative dysphonia and dysphagia, two of the most common complications following anterior cervical spine surgery. Rihn and associates discuss the thoroughly studied and widely debated topic of adjacent segment disease, which has received increased attention with the advent of cervical disk replacement. Devin and Kang review vertebral artery injury, one of the most dreaded and potentially devastating complications of cervical spine surgery. These chapters present information that is invaluable to surgeons who perform cervical spine surgery.

The chapter on postoperative dysphonia and dysphagia by Okubadejo and associates is unique in that it offers a comprehensive review of the anatomy and physiology of the normal processes of speaking and swallowing. This information is very helpful in understanding the pathophysiology of these postoperative complications. Dysphagia is the most common complication of anterior cervical spine surgery, occurring in 60% to 70% of patients in the early postoperative period. Fortunately, it is typically a transient phenomenon. Postoperative dysphagia is likely caused by a combination of traction of the superior and recurrent laryngeal nerves and retraction of the esophagus during anterior cervical spine surgery. There are some discrepancies in the literature regarding the contribution of certain factors to the frequency and severity of postoperative dysphagia, including the number of levels involved in the surgery, the duration of the surgery, the side of the approach (left versus right), the cervical level involved (upper versus lower cervical levels), the deflation and subsequent reinflation of the endotracheal cuff after retractor placement, the association with revision surgery, and the gender, age, and body mass index of the patient. Numerous prospective studies have examined dysphagia following anterior cervical spine surgery. The findings of these studies are summarized in the chapter.

Dysphonia, which is believed to be most frequently caused by traction of the recurrent laryngeal nerve during anterior cervical spine surgery, is a less common complication than dysphagia. Okubadejo and associates estimate that the frequency of this complication ranges from 0.07% to 11%. Risk factors for postoperative dysphonia are similar to those for dysphagia, most notably the side of the approach (right-sided versus left-sided) and the deflation of the endotracheal cuff after placement of retractors. Postoperative dysphonia usually improves on its own in the first 6 weeks to 3 months after surgery. If there is no improvement by 3 months, it is advisable for the patient to consult an otolaryngologist for an evaluation and possible treatment to improve vocal cord function.

Esophageal perforation is another possible complication of anterior spine surgery. This complication can lead to devastating outcomes including the development of mediastinitis or death. It can occur postoperatively, from erosive injury by an anterior cervical plate and/or screws, or intraoperatively, usually by unintended dissection during revision procedures. Esophageal perforation can usually be diagnosed intraoperatively by placing 60 mL of diluted methylene blue into an orogastric tube placed by the anesthesiologist. When performing this test, the tip of the orogastric tube should be in the esophagus just distal to the level of surgery. A finger is then placed within the wound and pressure is applied to the esophagus distal to the tip of the orogastric tube. The dye is then inserted by the anesthesiologist and the wound is inspected for dye. The diagnosis and management of esophageal perforation also is reviewed in this chapter.

The chapter by Rihn and associates discusses the topic of adjacent segment disease following cervical spine surgery. The widely quoted 1999 study by Hilibrand and associates, which is referenced in the chapter, reported a rate of adjacent segment disease of 2.9% per year, with a survivorship analysis showing that adjacent segment disease will develop in approximately 25% of patients by 10 years following anterior cervical diskectomy and fusion. There is continued debate as to whether adjacent segment disease develops as a result of the fusion or as a result of the natural history of disk degeneration. Biomechanical studies have reported mixed results regarding the motion and disk pressure adjacent to a cervical fusion, with some studies showing an increase and some showing no difference in these parameters following anterior cervical fusion. Well-designed, long-term clinical studies are needed. It is interesting, however, that Hilibrand and associates found a decreased incidence of adjacent segment disease in multilevel fusions compared with single-level fusions. Biomechanical studies suggest that the opposite finding should be true if the cause of adjacent segment disease is actually biomechanical in nature.

The issue of adjacent segment disease has led to the popularity of cervical disk replacement. The theory behind cervical disk replacement is that the device preserves biomechanical properties at the operated segment and prevents or slows the development of adjacent segment disease. Biomechanical studies support the theory that arthroplasty preserves motion and maintains normal intradiskal pressure at the adjacent segments but also show that it may increase the load of the facet joints at the operated segment. Clinically, it seems that equivalent outcomes regarding pain and function are achieved with anterior cervical diskectomy and fusion compared with cervical disk replacement. No significant difference in the rate of adjacent segment disease has been found based on available follow-up reports. Clinical studies with longer term follow-up will likely demonstrate whether cervical disk replacement significantly affects the rate of adjacent segment disease.

The chapter by Devin and Kang is a detailed and comprehensive review of iatrogenic vertebral artery injury during cervical spine surgery. This potentially devastating complication is a concern for all spine surgeons. The authors provide a description of the anatomy of the vertebral artery as it relates to both the subaxial and atlantoaxial cervical spine. An understanding of this anatomy is vitally important to the cervical spine surgeon. It is essential to recognize the potential for abnormal or anomalous vertebral artery anatomy. In every patient undergoing cervical spine surgery, the preoperative imaging studies, including CT and MRI scans, should be carefully reviewed for evidence of a vertebral artery anomaly. Identification of such an anomaly is the first step in avoiding this potentially lethal complication.

Devin and Kang explain that injury to the vertebral artery is relatively rare during anterior spine surgery, with a reported incidence ranging from 0.3% to 0.5%. The vertebral artery is more commonly injured during posterior surgery in the upper cervical spine, with a reported incidence of up to 8%. These injuries typically occur when instrumenting the C1 and/or C2 vertebrae. The management of an intraoperative vertebral artery injury can be challenging and varies depending on the location of the injury (upper versus subaxial cervical spine), the nature of the injury, and the surgical approach used (anterior versus posterior). A detailed flowchart illustrating the appropriate management of vertebral artery injury is included in the chapter.

Alexander R. Vaccaro, MD, PhD
Professor
Department of Orthopaedic Surgery
Thomas Jefferson University
The Rothman Institute
Philadelphia, Pennsylvania

Jeffrey A. Rihn, MD
Assistant Professor of Spine Surgery
Department of Orthopaedic Surgery
Thomas Jefferson University
The Rothman Institute
Philadelphia, Pennsylvania

Dr. Vaccaro or an immediate family member serves as a board member, owner, officer, or committee member of the American Spinal Injury Association, North American Spine Society, AO North America, Computational Biodynamics, Progressive Spinal Technology/Advanced Spinal Intellectual Properties, Location Based Intelligence, and the Scoliosis Research Society; has received royalties from Aesculap/B. Braun, Biomet, DePuy, Globus Medical, Lippincott, Elsevier, Medtronic Sofamor Danek, Stryker, Thieme, K2Spine, Stout Medical, and Progressive Spinal Technology/Applied Spinal Intellectual Properties; is a member of a speakers' bureau or has made paid presentations on behalf of Stryker, Medtronic Sofamor Danek, and DePuy Spine; serves as a paid consultant to or is an employee of Biomet, DePuy, Medtronic Sofamor Danek, Stryker, and Osteotech; has received research or institutional support from AO North America, DePuy, Medtronic Sofamor Danek, and Stryker; and owns stock or stock options in Globus Medical, Disc MotionTechnology, Progressive Spinal Technologies/Advanced Spinal Intellectual Properties, Computational Biodynamics, Stoud Medical, Paradigm Spine, K-2 Medical, Replication Medical, Spinology, Spine Medical, Orthovita, Vertiflex, Small Bone Technologies, NeuCore, Crosscurrent Syndicom, InVivo, Flagship Surgical, Pear Drive, Location Based Intelligence, Acumed, and Gamma Spine. Dr. Rihn or an immediate family member is a member of a speakers' bureau or has made paid presentations on behalf of Synthes and has received nonincome support (such as equipment or services), commercially derived honoraria, or other non–research-related funding (such as paid travel) from DePuy and Stryker.

32

Dysphonia, Dysphagia, and Esophageal Injuries After Anterior Cervical Spine Surgery

Gbolahan O. Okubadejo, MD
Justin B. Hohl, MD
William F. Donaldson, MD

Abstract

Anterior cervical spine surgery is commonly used by spine surgeons to treat numerous pathologic entities. The most common procedures involve decompression of the cervical spine through either diskectomy or corpectomy. Procedures that involve anterior dissection of the neck can lead to various complications, including dysphonia, dysphagia, and esophageal injuries.

Dysphonia and dysphagia are two complications that have been frequently reported following anterior cervical spine procedures. Dysphonia involves alteration in voice production, whereas dysphagia is defined as difficulty in swallowing foods and liquids. Reported frequencies of dysphagia in association with anterior cervical spine surgery range from 11% to 60%.[1-5] Dysphagia is usually transient, often resolving within 3 months. Moderate to severe dysphagia persists in 4% to 35% of patients.[1] Dysphonia may be seen at rates up to 60% in the early postoperative period.[4]

The most commonly cited cause of dysphonia and dysphagia is traction palsy involving the recurrent laryngeal nerve.[1] The recurrent laryngeal nerve is believed to be more vulnerable to injury during right-sided approaches because its course is more variable on the right than on the left side. Many authors have advocated the use of a left-sided approach to minimize the risk of this complication.[6] It is important to note that swallowing and voice difficulties also can occur with left-sided approaches, although at a lower rate.[2] Some studies have reported that female gender and surgery involving higher levels of the cervical spine (C2-C3) are risk factors for the development of dysphagia; however, these specific associations have not been universally observed.[3] Age, smoking status, duration of surgery, the number of levels operated on, the plating system used, previous anterior neck surgeries, and the presence of implant complications have been ruled out as causes of dysphagia.[3]

Anatomy of Swallowing

The mammalian pharynx and larynx are specialized to allow both food ingestion and respiration (Figure 1). The ability to close the respiratory tract from the alimentary tract requires complex layers of central neural control.[7] In the central nervous system, the swallowing center is located in the brainstem adjacent to the sensory and motor nuclei of the vagus nerve, near the area that controls respiration, blood pressure, temperature, and other functions. This swallowing center relays the glottic closure reflex, which closes the glottis in less than 25 ms (1/40 of a second). The fastest hand-eye reflex, in comparison, is one fourth that speed.[7]

The vagus nerve provides motor and sensory function to the palate, pharynx, esophagus, stomach, and respiratory tract. It exits the skull through the jugular foramen and travels adjacent to the internal and then common carotid artery, giving off several significant branches.[7] The superior laryngeal nerve branches off the vagus nerve high in the neck, bifurcating into the internal and external branches. Crucial in protecting against aspiration, the internal branch provides sensation to the supraglottic region and the hypopharynx. The external branch innervates the cricothyroid muscle, which tenses the vocal cord and aids in the ability to produce high notes.[7]

The recurrent laryngeal nerve also originates from the vagus nerve

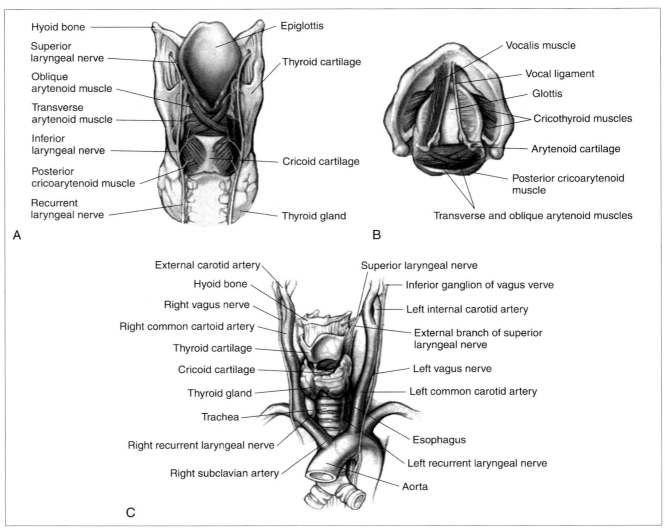

Figure 1   **A,** Normal anatomy of the anterior neck, depicting the critical structures associated with tracheoesophageal function. **B,** A close-up view of the vocal cords and associated muscles. **C,** Hyoid bone and thyroid and cricoid cartilage are often used by spine surgeons as superficial landmarks in determining spinal levels. Note the close relationship of the carotid artery and aorta to the anterior cervical spine and the relationship of the recurrent laryngeal nerves to these structures.

but follows a more circuitous route because of embryologic ascent of the pharyngeal structures. On the right side, the recurrent laryngeal nerve branches off the vagus nerve and loops around the right subclavian artery. It then crosses the anterolateral cervical spine in a circuitous cephalad path before entering the tracheoesophageal groove. The left recurrent laryngeal nerve originates where the vagus nerve crosses the

arch of the aorta, looping under the ligamentum arteriosum and traveling cephalad in the tracheoesophageal groove. In approximately 1% of patients, the right fourth branchial arch fails to develop into the right subclavian artery and the nerve does not loop around the artery (called the nonrecurrent recurrent laryngeal nerve). For this reason and also because the left recurrent laryngeal nerve lies more medial in the trache-

oesophageal groove, right-sided approaches may have a higher risk for recurrent laryngeal nerve injuries.[7]

The recurrent laryngeal nerves supply sensation to the glottic and subglottic regions. All of the intrinsic laryngeal muscles are supplied by the recurrent laryngeal nerve except the cricothyroid muscle, which is supplied by the vagus nerve. The recurrent laryngeal nerve notably innervates the posterior cricoarytenoid, the only muscle that abducts the vocal cords. Coordination of pharyngeal function during swallowing is orchestrated by the pharyngeal plexus, which consists of the glossopharyngeal nerve and the pharyngeal branch of the vagus nerve.[7]

The purpose of swallowing is to transport food from the mouth to the stomach in a safe manner. Swallowing has three phases: oral (under voluntary control) and pharyngeal and esophageal (under involuntary control). During the oral phase, the lips, tongue, mandible, palate, and cheeks act together to grind food so that the pharyngeal phase of swallowing can occur safely. This function is controlled largely by the cranial nerves, including the trigeminal, glossopharyngeal, facial, vagus, and hypoglossal nerves.

The pharyngeal phase consists of velopharyngeal closure (soft palate) to prevent reflux, closure of the larynx to prevent aspiration, contraction of the pharyngeal constrictor, elevation of the larynx and hyoid bone toward the base of the tongue, and relaxation of the contracted cricopharyngeus to allow food to pass into the esophagus. The pharyngeal phase is primarily mediated by the internal branch of the superior laryngeal nerve, with some help from the glossopharyngeal and recurrent laryngeal nerves (at the lower larynx level).[7]

The last phase of swallowing is the esophageal phase, which is under the involuntary control of the brainstem. The upper third of the esophagus consists of striated muscle, the middle third is made up of striated and smooth muscle, and the lower third consists entirely of smooth muscle. These layers of muscle propagate peristaltic waves that transfer food boluses into the

stomach. Prevention of aspiration is a key component of swallowing that is mediated by both basal and response mechanisms. The basal mechanisms include the vagally mediated upper and lower esophageal sphincters, which operate constantly. The response mechanisms are reflexes that include the esophagoglottal reflex, the pharyngoglottal closure reflex, the pharyngo-upper esophagus reflex, and the esophago-upper esophagus reflex. These reflexes act in response to mechanical stimulation of the pharynx or distension of the esophagus.[7] This complex interplay of nerves and reflexes allows the coordinated acts of breathing and swallowing. Although transient difficulty with breathing or swallowing sometimes occurs after cervical spine surgery, the objective is to minimize trauma to this orchestration of activities.

Dysphonia

When dysphonia or vocal cord injury occurs during anterior cervical spine surgery, it is often presumed to be secondary to injury to the recurrent laryngeal nerve. The incidence of recurrent laryngeal nerve injury after anterior cervical diskectomy is reported to be 0.07% to 11%.[3,8] Many potential risk factors have been proposed, including the surgical approach, primary versus revision surgery, the application of tension to the nerve with retraction, failure to deflate the endotracheal tube, and the length of the surgical procedure.

The most widely cited cause of vocal cord injury is traction injury to the recurrent laryngeal nerve. Numerous theories have been proposed to explain this phenomenon. In a widely cited retrospective study by Apfelbaum and associates,[9] the authors hypothesized that pressure

from the endotracheal tube when cervical retractors are in place results in recurrent laryngeal nerve compression. They found that the rate of temporary vocal cord paralysis was decreased from 6.4% to 1.69% by deflating the endotracheal tube cuff for 5 seconds after retractors were placed. This cuff deflation was believed to allow the endotracheal tube to recenter itself within the larynx, minimizing impingement on the vulnerable intralaryngeal segment of the recurrent laryngeal nerve (Figure 2). However, these findings were subsequently refuted by Audu and associates[6] in a randomized, prospective, double-blinded study. They reported a 3.2% occurrence of vocal fold paralysis, with no significant difference between patients who had endotracheal tube cuff deflation and those who did not. This study, however, found a significant difference between patients treated with a right-sided or left-sided approach, with frequencies of vocal cord paralysis of 27% and 0%, respectively.

In addition to the issue of cuff deflation to protect the recurrent laryngeal nerve, the side of the approach to the cervical spine also has been a source of debate. The recurrent laryngeal nerve travels in the tracheoesophageal groove and descends the neck in a different manner on the right side than on the left side of the neck. On the right side, the recurrent laryngeal nerve leaves the main trunk of the vagus nerve and passes anterior to and under the subclavian artery. It then ascends in the tracheoesophageal groove and often bifurcates before entering the larynx.[8] The right recurrent laryngeal nerve also is shorter and has a more oblique course than the left recurrent laryngeal nerve.[10] On the left side of the neck, the recurrent

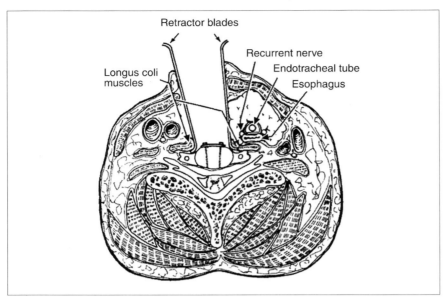

Figure 2 Cross-sectional anatomy of the neck showing the relationship of retractor placement to the remaining structures in the neck during anterior spinal surgery.

laryngeal nerve descends parallel to the carotid artery but then passes under and posterior to the aorta at the ligamentum arteriosum. The nerve then ascends in the tracheoesophageal groove more medial than on the right side, to lie under the lateral lobe of the thyroid gland.[8] The left recurrent laryngeal nerve has a more consistent course on the left side of the neck, travels within the tracheoesophageal groove, and does not drape around the subclavian artery.

This is believed to make a left-sided approach safer, but many surgeons prefer a right-sided approach because most surgeons are right handed and believe that approaching the neck from the right makes anterior cervical procedures easier. Other arguments in favor of a right-sided approach are that the thoracic duct and esophagus are at higher risk of injury with a left-sided approach because they both lie anatomically more toward the left. An argument in favor of a left-sided approach, in addition to the recurrent laryngeal nerve having a more consistent and gradual course, is the possibility of a right-sided nonrecurrent inferior laryngeal nerve. However, the reported frequency of this anomaly is less than 1%.[8,11-14] Kilburg and associates[15] compared right-sided and left-sided approaches retrospectively in 418 patients and did not find a significant difference in the frequency (1.8% and 2.1%, respectively) of recurrent laryngeal nerve palsy. There was no injury to either the esophagus or the thoracic duct with left-sided approaches.

Diagnosis
Suspicion of vocal cord paresis after surgery can be made by observing patients for symptoms such as dysphagia, hoarseness, or aspiration. The diagnosis can be confirmed by a laryngologist who can assess the patient's gag reflex and palatal movements to evaluate vagus nerve function.[14] A mirror examination followed by laryngoscopy with either a rigid or flexible endoscope can be used to directly examine the vocal cords. Asymmetric movement, vocal fold bowing, horizontal and vertical position of the vocal folds, and tilting of the posterior larynx are suggestive of vocal cord paresis. Videolaryngoendoscopy can be used to document the current function of the vocal cords and for comparison with future studies.[14]

Treatment
The treatment of patients with vocal cord paralysis depends on whether the pathology is unilateral or bilateral. After cervical spine surgery, unilateral vocal cord paresis is more common. The initial treatment should involve work with a speech language pathologist who can educate the patient about phonation and the specific abnormality.[14] Training includes head and neck muscle relaxation exercises, aerobic conditioning, abdominal and thoracic muscle strength and control exercises, and various voice exercises that build vocal strength. Patients who do not improve may require surgical treatment, which usually involves medialization or reinnervation. Medialization procedures include injection laryngoplasty or laryngeal framework surgery. Many materials have been used for injection, including polytetrafluoroethylene, Gelfoam, fat, and collagen. Polytetrafluoroethylene is no longer the most popular material because it is permanent, leads to a chronic granulomatous inflammatory response, and can migrate locally or to other parts of the body. Gelfoam can be used as a temporary measure, particularly when return of function is anticipated. Gelfoam generally is absorbed in 3 months. Fat also can be used and is resorbed partially within

3 to 4 months. Collagen can be obtained from allogeneic, autogenous, or bovine sources and may last up to 3 years. Collagen is known to soften scar tissue and improve the vibratory qualities of the vocal fold.[14]

A more permanent treatment for vocal cord paralysis is reinnervation using the ansa cervicalis, the phrenic nerve, preganglionic sympathetic neurons, the hypoglossal nerve, or nerve-muscle pedicles. The primary purpose of reinnervation is to prevent denervation atrophy of laryngeal muscles. Reinnervation is the most definitive treatment for vocal cord paralysis when other methods have failed.[14]

Dysphagia

Dysphagia is a manifestation of dysfunction associated with components of the swallowing mechanism. Various organic and nonorganic factors may be associated with dysphagia, and individual patient factors independent of anterior cervical spine surgery may put patients at risk for dysphagia.[4]

A study by Smith-Hammond and associates[2] showed preexisting dysphagia in patients before cervical spine surgery. A 3-year prospective cohort study of 83 patients compared the frequencies and risk factors associated with dysphagia after anterior cervical, posterior cervical, and posterior lumbar spine procedures. Patients had preoperative and postoperative swallowing evaluations. A significant increase in swallowing difficulties was reported in patients treated with anterior cervical procedures. Forty-seven percent of patients treated with anterior cervical surgery had dysphagia on postoperative videofluoroscopic swallowing evaluation compared with 21% of those treated with posterior cervical surgery. No patient who had

posterior lumbar surgery showed evidence of postoperative dysphagia. Being older than 60 years was the only significant risk factor for the development of dysphagia. Surgical level, instrumentation, surgical time, and comorbidities were not significant risk factors. However, it should be noted that none of the surgery on patients in this study was at the C2-C3 level. Of the patients treated with anterior cervical procedures who experienced dysphagia, 70% recovered within 2 months, whereas 23% required some level of compensatory swallowing behavior up to 10 months after surgery.

Bazaz and associates[3] conducted telephone interviews at 1, 2, 6, and 12 months postoperatively with 249 patients who had anterior cervical surgery and found that 50.2% experienced dysphagia immediately after surgery. By 6 months, only 4.8% of patients were experiencing moderate or severe dysphagia. The significant risk factor associated with dysphagia 1 and 2 months postoperatively was surgery at multiple disk levels; female gender was a significant factor in dysphagia 6 months postoperatively. The precise etiology of dysphagia in most patients was unknown; vocal cord paresis was identified in only 1.3% of the patients at 12 months.

Lee and associates[16] reported an overall frequency of dysphagia of 13.6% in 310 patients 2 years after anterior cervical surgery; however, only 0.3% had severe dysphagia. Risk factors for dysphagia included gender (women 18.3%, men 9.9%), revision surgery (27.7%, compared with 11.3% after primary surgery) and multilevel surgery (19.3%, compared with 9.7% for patients with two or fewer levels). Another study using objective modes of assessing dysphagia, including a modified bar-

ium swallow and videolaryngoendoscopy, supports the finding of an approximate 50% rate of dysphagia after anterior cervical procedures.[5] In addition to the risk factors already noted, soft-tissue swelling in the neck is believed to be a significant cause of postoperative dysphagia.[5]

Preexisting dysphagia before anterior cervical surgery also has been suggested as a cause of postoperative dysphagia. In one study, approximately 50% of patients had preoperative evidence of swallowing abnormalities, although none had any obvious underlying medical cause for dysphagia.[5] The authors speculated that a decrease in sensitivity of the pharyngeal and supraglottic area occurs with aging. Alternatively, cervical spondylosis may cause swallowing dysfunction by interfering with the preganglionic, sympathetic outflow or spinal afferents, thus interrupting the balance between the sympathetic and parasympathetic control mechanisms.

Rare occurrences of dysphagia beginning late after surgery without immediate postoperative observation of swallowing difficulty have been reported. Vanderveldt and Young[17] described a 29-year-old woman treated with C5 corpectomy and C4-5 and C5-6 diskectomies with cage and plate fixation who suddenly developed long-term recurrent dysphagia 2 months after surgery. Radiographs determined that the hardware was in appropriate position. An esophagram showed a segment of significant cervical esophageal stricture just anterior to the cervical hardware (Figure 3). The patient required multiple dilations to regain effective swallowing function. The authors emphasized the importance of postoperative assessment to ensure that patients recover fully from anterior cervical procedures.

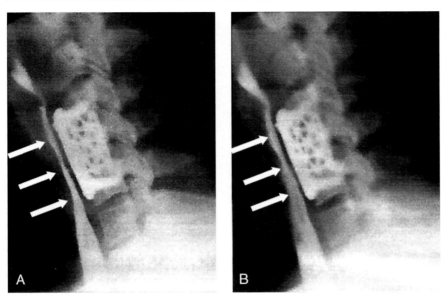

Figure 3 Strictures may result from the close relationship of anterior cervical implants to the remaining strictures in the neck. **A** and **B,** Progression of contrast through the esophagus. There is obvious constriction at the level of the implants.

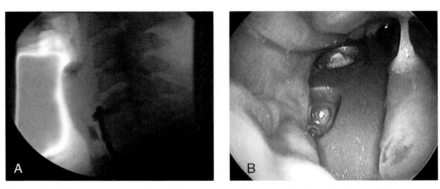

Figure 4 Plates may sometimes be seen eroding through the soft tissue. This is a rare occurrence but may occur spontaneously after implants have been in place for a long period of time. **A,** Radiograph of a plate that has eroded through the esophagus. There is no obvious evidence of erosion based on radiography. **B,** Intraoperative findings reveal erosion of the anterior cervical plate through the esophagus.

Treatment

Consultation with a speech pathologist is recommended for patients who experience postoperative dysphagia.[16] Videolaryngoendoscopy also may be indicated for evaluating the function of the vocal cords. Specific treatment depends on the cause of the dysphagia. For patients with unknown causes, observation is appropriate if the dysphagia is mild to moderate and there is a limited risk of aspiration. Patients with more severe dysphagia may be transiently limited from consuming solid foods until symptoms improve. A speech pathologist also may assist the patient with instruction in specific swallowing maneuvers.[17]

Patients with protracted dysphagia should first be treated with temporizing measures until a more definitive assessment of the prognosis has been established. The two main surgical options for patients with unilateral vocal fold paralysis are medialization and reinnervation as described for dysphonia. Patients with dysphagia also may require cricopharyngeal myotomy to eliminate or reduce symptoms.[17,18] Dilation of the esophagus can be done in patients with esophageal stricture.[17]

Esophageal Perforation

Esophageal perforation is a rare but potentially devastating complication of anterior cervical surgery. It has been reported to occur at a rate of 0.1% to 1.49% with cervical fractures.[19,20] Although it may occur during the surgical procedure, most reports of this injury are associated with instrumentation migration at varying time intervals after surgery. Perforation also can be caused by the erosion of anterior cervical implants through soft tissues in the neck (Figure 4). Most reports of esophageal perforation are case reports with causes including anterior cervical screw migration, extrusion into the gastrointestinal tract, esophageal injury with and without instrumentation, and oral extrusion.[19-26]

The most commonly described cause of esophageal perforation is instrumentation failure. Sahjpaul[21] described migration of anterior cervical instrumentation in a 58-year-old man who had C6 vertebrectomy and C5-C7 interbody fusion with a cage and an anterior cervical plate. Fever and recurrence of preoperative symptoms developed after surgery. A barium swallow showed an esophageal fistula caused by a migrated screw, which ultimately passed through the gastrointestinal tract. The site of leakage was confirmed with intraoperative injection of methylene blue. The esophageal perforation was repaired primarily, and the patient ultimately recovered with minimal residual deficit. The authors recommended using barium rather than diatrizoate meglumine and diatrizoate sodium because it is less likely to lead to a false-negative result.[21]

Fountas and associates[22] described a 70-year-old man who had anterior cervical decompression and fusion at C5-C6 with autologous bone graft and a dynamic plate using locking, expanding screws. Sixteen months after the procedure, the patient presented with severe dysphagia. Radiographs showed pulling out of the implanted plate and screws. During surgery to remove the instrumentation, one of the screws was not found in the cervical spine with the rest of the instrumentation. Using abdominal radiography, the screw was subsequently located in the right lower abdominal quadrant. The screw was removed endoscopically, and the patient was treated with antibiotics and restricted from oral intake for 4 days. He was subsequently discharged without symptoms on a soft mechanical diet. It is notable that the esophageal perforation associated with screw migration was not located or repaired, but the patient recovered uneventfully. This scenario suggests that slower migrations of instrumentation are less likely to lead to catastrophic clinical outcomes because lesions are chronic and evolve slowly.

Another study described a delayed esophageal injury without instrumentation failure in a patient treated with anterior surgical decompression with corpectomies from C3 to C5 and a structural fusion with a fibular allograft.[23] The patient's immediate postoperative course was complicated by a large

hematoma and dislodgement of the fibular graft, leading to airway compromise and complete quadriplegia. The hematoma was emergently evacuated, the graft was revised by extension of the corpectomies to include the C6 vertebral body, and the fusion was extended to C7. The new construct was built with a fibular strut graft and fixed with a cervical plate spanning C2-C7. The patient gradually improved in both motor and sensory function over a period of years but had remaining deficits. Two years after surgery, the patient had severe dysphagia along with recurrent episodes of pneumonia. Cervical esophagoscopy showed that the cervical plate had eroded through the esophagus 1 cm inferior to the postcricoid region. A large rent in the esophagus extended beyond the inferior screws in T1. The cervical plate was in good position with no evidence of slippage, fracture, or malalignment. The hardware was removed and the esophagus was repaired, with the closure reinforced with a sternocleidomastoid muscle flap. The authors hypothesized that chronic pressure necrosis by the cervical plate on the posterior retropharyngeal esophagus resulted in a controlled tear.

Esophageal perforation should be suspected when a patient has unexplained postoperative fever, dysphagia, or odynophagia; drainage of food, saliva, or air from the neck wound; unexplained tachycardia; or blood in the nasogastric tube.[20,21] Some patients also may have airway compromise.[21] A cervical spine radiograph may show prevertebral swelling, prevertebral air, or loose or missing instrumentation. If radiographs do not adequately show the instrumentation, advanced imaging studies such as CT or MRI should be used to confirm that there has

been no migration. Conventional imaging techniques should detect 77% of esophageal injuries.[23] Methylene blue injection through a nasogastric tube during surgery can help identify the site of leakage from the esophagus and assist in the repair.[21] Another study demonstrated that a nasogastric tube alone may not be adequate to identify a perforation.[27] The authors recommended using a distally placed Foley catheter in addition to the nasogastric tube for more accurate identification of esophageal perforations.

Esophageal perforation has been successfully treated with observation alone.[28] This is believed to be adequate management because of the relatively slow migration of instrumentation into the esophageal lumen, resulting in a process of localized and contained inflammation and scarring. In more acute occurrences of esophageal perforation, more direct treatment usually is warranted, including urgent revision with exploration and repair, esophageal diversion, and esophageal rest with antibiotic administration and wound drainage.[18] A sternocleidomastoid muscle flap often is used to reinforce primary repair.[29] When esophageal perforation is recognized early, patients may be successfully treated and recover without incident from this potentially fatal complication.

Summary

There are numerous causes of dysphagia, dysphonia, and esophageal perforation in association with anterior cervical spine surgery. Although iatrogenic causes are sometimes responsible, the most common etiologic factors are still unknown. The key to successful patient outcomes is prompt recognition and expedient treatment.

References

1. Yue WM, Brodner W, Highland TR: Persistent swallowing and voice problems after anterior cervical discectomy and fusion with allograft and plating: A 5- to 11-year follow-up study. *Eur Spine J* 2005;14:677-682.

2. Smith-Hammond CA, New KC, Pietrobon R, Curtis DJ, Scharver CH, Turner DA: Prospective analysis of incidence and risk factors of dysphagia in spine surgery patients: Comparison of anterior cervical, posterior cervical and lumbar procedures. *Spine* 2004;29:1441-1446.

3. Bazaz R, Lee MJ, Yoo JU: Incidence of dysphagia after anterior cervical spine surgery: A prospective study. *Spine* 2002;27:2453-2458.

4. Tervonen H, Niemela M, Lauir ER, et al: Dysphonia and dysphagia after anterior cervical decompression. *J Neurosurg Spine* 2007;7:124-130.

5. Frempong-Boadu A, Houten JK, Osborn B, et al: Swallowing and speech dysfunction in patients undergoing anterior cervical discectomy and fusion: A prospective, objective preoperative and postoperative assessment. *J Spinal Disord Tech* 2002;15:362-368.

6. Audu P, Artz G, Scheid S, et al: Recurrent laryngeal nerve palsy after anterior cervical spine surgery: The impact of endotracheal tube cuff deflation, reinflation and pressure adjustment. *Anesthesiology* 2006;105:898-901.

7. Carrau RL, Murry T: *Comprehensive Management of Swallowing Disorders.* San Diego, CA, Singular Publishing Group, 1999, pp 11-29.

8. Beutler WJ, Sweeney CA, Connolly PJ: Recurrent laryngeal nerve injury with anterior cervical spine surgery: Risk with laterality of surgical approach. *Spine* 2001;26:1337-1342.

9. Apfelbaum RI, Kriskovich MD, Haller JR: On the incidence, cause, and prevention of recurrent laryngeal nerve palsies during anterior cervical spine surgery. *Spine* 2000;25:2906-2912.

10. Jung A, Schramm J, Lehnerdt K, et al: Recurrent laryngeal nerve palsy during anterior cervical spine surgery: A prospective study. *J Neurosurg Spine* 2005;2:123-127.

11. Ebraheim NA, Lu J, Skie M, et al: Vulnerability of the recurrent laryngeal nerve in the anterior approach to the lower cervical spine. *Spine* 1997; 22:2664-2667.

12. Cannon CR: The anomaly of nonrecurrent laryngeal nerve: Identification and management. *Otolaryngol Head Neck Surg* 1999;120:769-771.

13. Henry JF, Audoffret J, Denizot A, Plan M: The nonrecurrent inferior laryngeal nerve: Review of 33 cases, including two on the left side. *Surgery* 1988;104:977-984.

14. Rubin AD, Sataloff RT: Vocal fold paresis and paralysis. *Otolaryngol Clin North Am* 2007;40:1109-1131.

15. Kilburg C, Sullivan HG, Mathiason MA: Effects of approach side during anterior cervical discectomy and fusion on the incidence of recurrent laryngeal nerve injury. *J Neurosurg Spine* 2006;4:273-277.

16. Lee MJ, Bazaz R, Furey C, Yoo J: Risk factors for dysphagia after anterior cervical spine surgery: A two-year prospective cohort study. *Spine J* 2007;7:141-147.

17. Vanderveldt HS, Young MF: The evaluation of dysphagia after anterior cervical spine surgery: A case report. *Dysphagia* 2003;18:301-304.

18. Stewart M, Johnston RA, Stewart I, Wilson JA: Swallowing performance following anterior cervical spine surgery. *Br J Neurosurg* 1995;9:605-609.

19. Patel NP, Walcott WP, Johnson JP, et al: Esophageal injury associated with anterior cervical spine surgery. *Surg Neurol* 2008;69:20-24.

20. Gaudinez RF, English GM, Gebhard JS, Brugman JL, Donaldson DH, Brown CW: Esophageal perforation after anterior cervical surgery. *J Spinal Disord* 2000;13:77-84.

21. Sahjpaul RL: Esophageal perforation from anterior cervical screw migration. *Surg Neurol* 2007;68:205-210.

22. Fountas KN, Kapsalaki EZ, Machinis T, Robinson JS: Extrusion of a screw into the gastrointestinal tract after anterior cervical spine plating. *J Spinal Disord Tech* 2006;19:199-203.

23. Witwer BP, Resnick DK: Delayed esophageal injury without instrumentation failure: Complication of anterior cervical instrumentation. *J Spinal Disord Tech* 2003;16:519-523.

24. Newhouse KE, Lindsey RW, Clark CR: Esophageal perforation following anterior cervical spine surgery. *Spine* 1989;14:1051-1053.

25. Geyer TE, Foy MA: Oral extrusion of a screw after anterior cervical spine plating. *Spine* 2001;26:1814-1816.

26. von Rahden BH, Stein HJ, Scherer MA: Late hypopharyngo-esophageal perforation after cervical spine surgery: Proposal of a therapeutic strategy. *Eur Spine J* 2005;14:880-886.

27. Taylor B, Patel AA, Okubadejo GO, Albert T, Riew KD: Detection of esophageal perforation using intra-esophageal dye injection. *J Spinal Disord Tech* 2006;19:191-193.

28. Pompili A, Canitano S, Caroli F, et al: Asymptomatic esophageal perforation caused by late screw migration after anterior cervical plating: Report of a case and review of the relevant medical literature. *Spine* 2002;27:E499-E502.

29. Navarro R, Javahery R, Eismont F, et al: The role of the sternocleidomastoid muscle flap for esophageal fistula repair in anterior cervical spine surgery. *Spine* 2005;30:E617-E622.

Adjacent Segment Disease After Cervical Spine Fusion

Jeffrey A. Rihn, MD
James Lawrence, MD
Charley Gates, MD
Eric Harris, MD
*Alan S. Hilibrand, MD

Abstract

Anterior cervical diskectomy and fusion is one of the most common cervical spine procedures. Although it is usually successful in relieving the symptoms of radiculopathy and myelopathy, the subsequent development of clinically significant disk disease at levels adjacent to the fusion is a matter of concern. Adjacent segment cervical disease occurs in approximately 3% of patients; the incidence is expected to increase to more than 25% of patients within the first 10 years after the index fusion procedure. The disease is well described in the literature, and significant basic science and clinical research has been conducted. Nonetheless, the cause of the disease is a matter of debate. A combination of factors probably contributes to its development, including the increased biomechanical stress placed on the disk space adjacent to a fusion and the natural history of cervical spondylosis in patients known to have such pathology. Clinical and biomechanical data are available to support each of these claims. Symptomatic disk disease adjacent to a cervical fusion is a significant clinical problem, and, therefore, motion-sparing technology has been developed to reduce its incidence. Two cervical disk replacement systems are currently approved by the US Food and Drug Administration for the treatment of symptomatic cervical spondylosis.

Adjacent segment disease of the cervical spine is among the most controversial topics in spinal surgery. Although the true definition of the disease is debated, in general the term refers to the development of radiculopathy or myelopathy referable to the level above or below a fused intervertebral segment. Adjacent segment degeneration is the preferred term for describing the degenerative appearance of the adjacent level as seen on imaging studies. In contrast, adjacent segment disease describes the development of symptoms attributable to pathology at the spinal level adjacent to that of a fusion. There is considerable debate as to whether adjacent segment disease develops after contiguous fusion, which theoretically alters the biomechanics at the adjacent levels of the cervical spine, or is wholly attributable to the natural history of cervical spondylosis in patients who are known to be susceptible to such pathology. Several biomechanical and clinical studies have contributed to the understanding of adjacent segment disease in the cervical spine. There is increasing interest in cervical disk replacement surgery, which may preserve motion and possibly prevent or delay the development of adjacent segment disease.

Normal Cervical Spine Biomechanics

Discussion of adjacent segment disease and motion-sparing technology

Alan S. Hilibrand, MD or the department with which he is affiliated has received research or institutional support from DePuy and Synthes and royalties from Biomet and Zimmer.

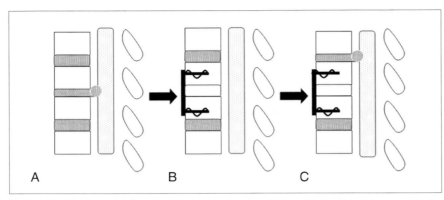

Figure 1   Schematic drawing depicting the development of adjacent segment disease after a single-level anterior cervical diskectomy and fusion. **A,** Cervical disk herniation. **B,** Anterior cervical diskectomy and fusion. **C,** Adjacent segment disease in the superior segment.

must be correlated with a thorough understanding of the anatomy and biomechanics of the normal subaxial cervical spine. Each cervical spine segment moves in six degrees of freedom, with translation and rotation about each orthogonal axis (flexion-extension, axial rotation, and lateral bending). Most biomechanical studies have focused on rotation about each axis. Panjabi and associates[1] performed load-deformation testing on human cadaver spine specimens. When a standard amount of load was increasingly applied to the cervical spine specimens, most of the flexion-extension and axial rotation occurred at the occiput-C1 and C1-2 levels. Lateral bending was more equally distributed among the cervical segments, from occiput-C1 downward to C6-C7; each segment had from 5° to 9° of lateral bending.[1] Comparison of the results of in vivo and in vitro studies reveals that 50% to 70% of flexion-extension and axial rotation is derived from the occiput-C1 and C1-C2 segments.[1,2] Each of the subaxial cervical spine segments have similar ranges of normal motion (6° to 10° of flexion-extension, 3° to 7° of rotation, and 5° to 9° of lateral bending).[1]

The term coupled motion refers to the concept that a cervical spine segment responds to a unidirectional load with more than one type of motion (rotation about and/or translation along one or more of the orthogonal axes). A considerable amount of coupled motion occurs in the subaxial cervical spine. Coupled axial rotation occurs in the same direction as an applied lateral-bending load, and coupled lateral bending occurs in the same direction as an applied axial rotation load.[1,3,4] With axial loading of the cervical spine, slight coupled extension and posterior-lateral translation occurs above the C4-C5 level.[1,2,4] Under the same loading conditions, coupled flexion and posterior-lateral translation occurs caudal to and at the C4-C5 level.[1,2,4] Therefore, with axial rotation the cervical vertebrae are loaded posteriorly above the C4-C5 level and anteriorly at and below the C4-C5 level.[1] In vitro biomechanical studies have also evaluated intradiskal pressure in the subaxial cervical spine. The mean intradiskal pressure in the subaxial

cervical spine in a neutral, resting position is approximately 30 psi.[5] In axial rotation, lateral bending, and flexion-extension at the C4-5 level, the intradiskal pressure increases to approximately 45, 50, and 150 psi, respectively.[6]

Studies of Adjacent Segment Disease
Biomechanical Studies
The pathogenesis of spondylosis adjacent to cervical spine fusion is not completely understood. It has been suggested that fusion alters the biomechanical conditions at adjacent segments, resulting in increased loading, excessive motion, and, ultimately, accelerated disk degeneration (Figure 1). Published data do not consistently support this belief.

Increased mechanical demands are known to adversely affect the disk by interfering with its normal nutritional supply, and impaired disk nutrition has been identified as the most significant cause of disk degeneration.[7] The disk lacks a true blood supply and depends on the diffusion of nutrients from peripheral blood vessels and vertebral end plates. Increased pressure within the disk is believed to inhibit diffusion of these nutrients and thereby leads to the accumulation of waste products, elevated lactate levels, decreased pH, and, ultimately, cell death. In addition, increased compressive forces over time unfavorably alter the extracellular matrix composition, increasing the presence of type I collagen while decreasing proteoglycans, chondroitin sulfate, and type II collagen.[8]

These changes also occur during the normal aging process. As the disk ages, its nutrition is impaired as the presence of fewer peripheral arteries and calcification of the cartilage end plates cause a reduction in vascular supply. Loss of viable cells, modification of matrix proteins, and fatigue failure of the matrix also occur. When disk degeneration appears, it can be difficult to discern whether the deleterious effects of normal aging or increased mechanical strain are responsible.

Several biomechanical studies have supported the belief that cervical fusion increases load and motion at adjacent levels, causing localized trauma and subsequent disk degeneration.[9-13] A finite element analysis of the cervical spine after fusion found increased internal stress at junctional segments.[11] Eck and associates[12] tested six cadaver specimens that were stabilized at T1 and loaded at C3 to 20° of flexion and 15° of extension before and after anterior cervical plating at C5-C6. After fusion, flexion caused intradiskal pressure to increase by 73% at the superior segment (C4-C5) and 43% at the inferior segment (C6-C7). Extension caused no significant difference in intradiskal pressure at either adjacent level. Segmental motion increased at both adjacent levels during both flexion and extension.

Park and associates[13] studied the effect of two-level anterior cervical diskectomy and fusion (ACDF) on the superior adjacent segment. Five cadaver specimens were stabilized at T1 and loaded at C3 to 15° flexion, 10° extension, and 10° lateral bending before and after simulated two-level ACDF at C5-C7. They found a significant increase in intradiskal pressure and segmental motion at the superior adjacent C4-C5 level and postulated that the increased pressure and hypermobility were accelerating normal degenerative changes at the adjacent vertebral levels.

Comparison of the results of this study of two-level simulated fusion with those of the study of single-level fusion by Eck and associates[12] suggests that the two-level procedure produces a substantially greater increase in intradiskal pressure at the superior segment than the single-level procedure. After single-level fusion at the C5-6 level, the pressure at the superior segment (C4-C5) increased by 73% during flexion and 5.7% during extension. After two-level fusion (C5-C7), the pressure at C4-C5 increased by 164% during flexion and 50% during extension.[13] These findings suggest that eliminating motion at a single level increases the loads applied to the adjacent levels, and this effect is magnified if levels of fusion are added.

Other biomechanical studies have not found a difference in intradiskal pressure and intervertebral motion following fusion.[14-16] Rao and associates[14] simulated fusion of the C5-C6 segment in seven human cadaver spines (C2-T1) and tested them in flexion, extension, lateral bending, and torsion with loads as great as 2.5 N/m. Intradiskal pressures and intervertebral motion at the adjacent levels were not significantly affected by the instrumented anterior fusion. These results suggest that the natural history of the disks may have a more significant effect on degeneration than the biomechanical effects of fusion.

Fuller and associates[15] studied the acute kinematic consequence of segmental fusion on the remaining open motion segments in cadaver cervical spines. Simulated one-, two-, and three-level fusions were followed by testing through a 30° range of sagittal plane rotation. Motion was recorded using three-dimensional stereophotogrammetry. No disproportionate increase in motion was found at the segments immediately adjacent to the fusion. Displacement-control testing was used to measure pressure and motion in adjacent segments, rather than load-control testing. The displacement-control loading paradigm assumes that patients attempt to achieve a range of motion while performing a specific activity rather than under the influence of load per se; it is considered by some to be a closer simulation of in vivo changes after spinal fusion than a load-controlled application of motion.[16]

The conflicting results of biomechanical studies may reflect the limited capacity of cadaver studies to accurately model the in vivo biomechanical conditions after fusion. The available studies tested cervical spines that were stabilized inferior to the C1-C2 articulation. At least 50% of flexion and extension occurs at the occipitoatlantal articulation, and 50% of rotation occurs at the atlantoaxial articulation. The exclusion of these articulations from the studies appears to be significant. Exclusion was necessary because of technical difficulties in fixation of the skull and upper cervical spine to a testing device, the application of load, and the recording of motion. Inclusion of these joints, which account for most of the motion in a patient's cervical spine, could have resulted in less motion being seen at segments adjacent to a fusion.

Most studies tested cadaver cervical spines through a particular range of motion and then repeated testing through the same range of motion after fusion of one, two, or three levels. Because the presurgical and postsurgical motions are the same and the contribution of the fused level is lost, it seems reasonable to assume that motion will increase in the adjacent segments as well as all other remaining segments; the concept is that the lost motion must go somewhere. However, the concept of "lost motion" may have limited application. In clinical practice, patients have been found to have increased motion after cervical spine fusion of as many as four levels.[17] Patients do not attempt to reproduce a predetermined range of motion after surgery; instead, they attempt to perform specific activities. To do so, they may use other joints or adapt their movements in other ways.

The results of biomechanical testing may be confounded by variations in the age and quality of the tested cadavers. The mechanical properties of the ligaments, disks, vertebrae, and other soft-tissue structures vary widely among cadaver specimens and are beyond the control of investigators.

In vivo biomechanical studies eliminate many limitations of a cadaver study. In a prospective in vivo study, Reitman and associates[18] evaluated changes in motion that occurred at the level cephalad to a cervical fusion by comparing measurements before and after ACDF in 21 patients who underwent a one-, two-, three- or four-level fusion. The researchers used fluoroscopy and a computer software system designed to accurately capture and quantify motion. Several intervertebral motions were measured: change in height of the anterior disk space, change in height of the posterior disk space, flexion, extension, and translation. At the level cephalad to the cervical fusion, no significant differences were found between any of the motions, as measured before surgery and at an average 13-month follow-up (range, 10 to 22 months). The researchers' conclusion was that cervical fusion does not affect motion at the adjacent segment in the first 1 to 2 years after surgery.

Despite significant research, it re-mains unclear whether long-term adjacent segment disease is the result of increased mechanical demands, the normal aging process, or a combination of these two factors. Patients with degenerative changes significant enough to warrant fusion may be predisposed to disk degeneration at other levels. However, the increased mechanical demands of the fusion may accelerate degenerative changes at the adjacent levels. More representative cadaver fusion models and more precise testing are needed to definitively assess the biomechanical consequences of cervical fusion.

Clinical Studies

Researchers vary in their definition and method of diagnosing adjacent segment disease, and this variation is important in assessing the literature. Adjacent segment degeneration can be identified on plain radiography, CT myelography, and MRI. In most patients, however, such a finding is not clinically relevant, as a large percentage of the asymptomatic general population is believed to have radiographically observable degenerative cervical disk disease. Boden and associates[19] obtained MRI studies of 63 individuals with no history of cervical disease symptoms and found that the intervertebral disk was narrowed or had degenerated at one or more cervical levels in 25% of those younger than 40 years and 60% of those older than 40 years. In contrast, the original description of adjacent segment disease was based on clinical observation of recurrent radiculopathy or myelopathy attributed to the cervical segment adjacent to a fusion (Figure 2).[20] Several studies have observed that the radiographic presence of adjacent segment degeneration after ACDF is not correlated with clinical outcome.[21-23] At a mean 27-month follow-up after ACDF, Dohler and associates[21] found that 14 of 21 patients (67%) had translation at the adjacent cervical segment. This radiographic finding was not correlated with persistent or recurrent pain.

Katsuura and associates[22] studied the effect of kyphotic alignment, which may be a predisposing factor for adjacent segment disease after ACDF. At an average 9.8-year follow-up, radiographic evidence of adjacent segment degeneration was found in 50% of 42 patients, of whom 77% had kyphotic alignment at the level of fusion. The researchers did not determine whether patients with a multilevel fusion were more likely to develop adjacent segment disease than patients with a single-level fusion. Neurologic status, the only outcome assessed in this study, was measured using the Japanese Orthopaedic Association score. There was a significant and lasting overall improvement in the postsurgical scores. However, comparison of the patients with and without adjacent segment disease revealed no significant difference between the groups in scores before or after surgery or at final follow-up. Goffin and associates[23] studied the long-term clinical and radiographic outcomes of 180 patients who underwent ACDF. The extent of adjacent disk degeneration was graded based on disk height and presence and osteophyte size, as determined from a lateral cervical radiograph. At an average 100.6-month follow-up, 92% of the patients had radiographic evidence of adjacent segment disk degeneration. The extent of adjacent disk degeneration and the time since surgery were positively correlated. The extent of adjacent disk degeneration and the number of fused cervi-

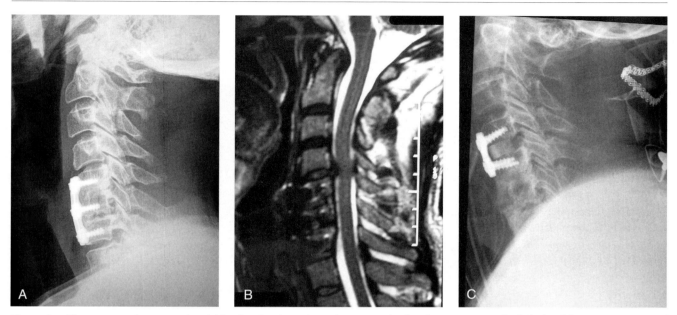

Figure 2 Three years after a two-level (C5-C6, C6-C7) ACDF, the patient had radiating pain in the left shoulder, symptomatic of cervical spondylosis adjacent to the fused segments. **A,** Lateral radiograph showing loss of disk height and posterior osteophyte formation at the C4-5 level. **B,** T2-weighted sagittal MRI study showing significant disk herniation with cord compression at the C4-5 level; a T2-weighted axial MRI study revealed that the disk herniation was left sided, with obliteration of the anterior cerebrospinal fluid and deformation of the spinal cord at this level. The patient's history or physical examination did not suggest myelopathy, although he had slight motor weakness in his left deltoid. After 3 months of unsuccessful nonsurgical treatment, the patient underwent removal of the index procedure instrumentation, followed by ACDF at the adjacent C4-5 level. **C,** Lateral cervical radiograph showing the revision ACDF.

cal levels were not significantly correlated. Clinical outcomes immediately after surgery and at long-term follow-up were assessed using the Odom score; for patients who were myelopathic at the time of surgery, the Nurick Scale was also used. No significant correlation was found between the extent of adjacent segment degeneration present on radiographs and the assessed clinical outcomes.

Several studies have evaluated the development of clinically significant, symptomatic adjacent segment disease after ACDF. Of these studies, one of the most frequently cited is that of Hilibrand and associates,[20] who defined adjacent segment disease as "the development of new radiculopathy or myelopathy referable to a motion segment adjacent to the site of a previous anterior arthrodesis of the cervical spine."[20] The clinical records and imaging studies of 374 patients who had a total of 409 anterior cervical fusion procedures for the treatment of radiculopathy or myelopathy caused by cervical spondylosis were retrospectively reviewed. A grading system from I to IV was devised based on radiography, MRI, and CT. The annual incidence of symptomatic adjacent segment disease after the initial procedure was found to be 2.9%. Survivorship analysis predicted that symptomatic adjacent segment disease would develop in more than 25% of the patients within 10 years of the anterior cervical fusion. The greatest risk occurred when the C5-C6 or C6-C7 segments were adjacent to a fusion (five times the risk to other cervical levels). The authors found that the risk of symptomatic adjacent segment disease after a multilevel fusion was significantly less than after a single-level fusion. This finding is contrary to the result expected if the biomechanical consequences of fusion were the only cause of adjacent segment disease. The authors suggested that the explanation lies in the fact that the motion segments at high risk of developing adjacent segment disease were fused during the initial multilevel procedure. Among the patients in whom adjacent segment disease developed, those with more extensive degeneration at the adjacent level before the initial fusion surgery were affected by symptomatic disease at the adjacent level sooner after the initial surgery. This finding supports the argument that decompression and fusion of the levels adjacent to the symptomatic level should be done during the index procedure if presurgical imaging studies reveal significant degeneration at the adjacent levels. Nonsurgical treatment was unsuccessful in approximately two thirds of the patients with symptomatic adjacent segment disease; these patients required repeat surgical treatment.[20]

The findings of other studies that evaluated the development of symptomatic adjacent segment disease after anterior cervical fusion were similar to those of Hilibrand and associates.[20,24,25] At an average 7.2-year follow-up, Yue and associates[24] studied the clinical and radiographic outcomes of 71 patients treated with ACDF. Radiographic evidence of adjacent segment degeneration was found in 73%, although only 17% required revision surgery for symptomatic disease. The number of levels fused during the index procedure was not related to the development of radiographic adjacent segment disease or the need for revision surgery for symptomatic disease. Ishihara and associates[25] studied the development of symptomatic adjacent segment disease in 112 patients at a minimum 2-year follow-up after ACDF. In the 19% of patients with symptomatic adjacent segment disease, 37% had unsuccessful nonsurgical treatment and required revision surgery. Survivorship analysis revealed a 16% rate of symptomatic adjacent segment disease 10 years after the index procedure and a 33% rate at 17 years. The patient's risk of symptomatic adjacent segment disease was increased if there was evidence of disk disease with compression of the dura at the adjacent level before the index procedure. The development of adjacent segment disease was not corre-

lated with the number of levels fused during the index procedure or cervical spine alignment before the index procedure.

Although adjacent segment disease traditionally has been discussed in the context of cervical fusion, some studies have examined the rate of disease after cervical laminoforaminotomy. If the biomechanical consequences of cervical fusion were the only factor in the development of adjacent segment disease, laminoforaminotomy would not increase the risk. In a prospective study, Herkowitz and associates[26] compared ACDF to treat soft disk herniation in 28 patients with posterior cervical laminoforaminotomy in 16 patients. After ACDF, 41% of the patients had radiographic evidence of adjacent segment degeneration at an average 4.5-year follow-up, compared with 50% of those who underwent posterior cervical laminoforaminotomy. Clarke and associates[27] studied the development of symptomatic same segment disease and adjacent segment disease after single-level posterior cervical laminoforaminotomy for the treatment of cervical radiculopathy in 303 patients. At an average 7.1-year follow-up, 3.3% had same segment disease, and 4.9% had symptomatic adjacent segment disease. Of those in whom symptomatic adjacent segment disease developed, 60% required revision surgery. Survivorship analysis revealed a 6.7% rate of symptomatic adjacent segment disease 10 years after the index procedure, with a 0.7% annual rate. Although this rate is lower than the rate reported after ACDF, it is higher than would be expected if the biomechanical effect of cervical fusion were the only contributing factor. This finding suggests that other factors, including the natural history of cervical disk disease, contribute to

the development of adjacent segment disease. This study had several limitations. It was a retrospective chart review that lacked a uniform method of data collection, did not include a review of imaging studies, and had limited follow-up for a significant percentage of study patients (12% had fewer than 10 days of follow-up, and 22% had fewer than 100 days).[27]

Motion-Sparing Devices

Total disk arthroplasty has been proposed for the treatment of primary spondylosis or radiculopathy, partly as a means of avoiding the development of disease at the segment adjacent to cervical fusion. Biomechanical factors adjacent to levels treated with cervical arthroplasty have been experimentally evaluated using laboratory methods and data from available clinical trials.[6,28-30] Motion and kinetics, intradiskal pressure, and radiographic changes have been assessed in a manner somewhat similar to the study of ACDF.[6,28-30] In vitro and in vivo biomechanical studies have examined the motion of the index segment and the adjacent segment to characterize motion patterns after ACDF and arthroplasty.[29-34] It also has been suggested that motion-sparing devices (cervical disk replacement systems) may be useful in treating disease adjacent to a cervical fusion. ProDisc-C Total Disc Replacement (Synthes, West Chester, PA) and Prestige Cervical Disc (Medtronic Sofamor Danek, Memphis, TN) are the two cervical disk replacement systems currently approved by the US Food and Drug Administration for treating symptomatic cervical spondylosis.

Intradiskal Pressure and Facet Loads

A current hypothesis for the development of adjacent segment disease suggests that increased intradiskal pressure results in accelerated degeneration. Dmitriev and associates[6] used a human cadaver model to compare intradiskal pressure and segmental kinematics in spine specimens that were intact or had undergone unplated ACDF, plated ACDF, or arthroplasty using a Bryan Cervical Disc (Medtronic Sofamor Danek). Similar intradiskal pressures at the adjacent segment were found in the intact spine and arthroplasty specimen groups under all loading modes (flexion-extension, axial rotation, and lateral bending); significantly higher intradiskal pressures were found in both ACDF specimen groups.[6] Chang and associates[28] performed a similar cadaver study that compared spine specimens that were intact or had undergone plated ACDF or arthroplasty using the ProDisc-C or Prestige prosthesis. Similar intradiskal pressures were found in the intact and arthroplasty specimen groups; significantly higher intradiskal pressures were found at the adjacent posterior anulus fibrosus in extension and the anterior anulus fibrosus in flexion in the ACDF specimens. Although no differences were found among the groups in facet joint forces in flexion, bending, and rotation, significant differences occurred in extension. The arthroplasty group had significantly greater facet forces in extension at the index level; the forces at the adjacent segment were similar to those in the intact group. The ACDF groups had decreased facet forces at the index segment and increased forces at the adjacent facets.[28] This study suggests that although arthroplasty may normalize intradiskal pressure and facet loads at the adjacent segment, it can place the facets at the index segment under greater load.

Biomechanical Studies of Motion

Numerous biomechanical studies have compared motion at the index and adjacent segments after ACDF and arthroplasty, using different cervical disk replacement devices. Although differences in motion pattern are to be expected at the index segment after ACDF or arthroplasty, differences at the adjacent segment may subject the disk to increased load and predispose it to earlier degeneration. The prosthetic device attempts to mimic the coupled motion of the cervical spine, and the device's design and method of constraint (constrained or semiconstrained) are important in determining the range and type of motion at the index and adjacent segments. In a series of cadaver biomechanical studies of the semiconstrained arthroplasty devices, DiAngelo and associates[29,30] found significantly increased motion at levels adjacent to cervical fusion, compared with those of intact specimens and those implanted with the Prestige and the ProDisc-C artificial disks. Chang and associates[28] similarly compared motion after ACDF and motion in intact specimens with motion after placement of a ProDisc-C or Prestige II artificial disk. After arthroplasty, increased range of motion was found at the index segment, and no change was found at the adjacent segment. After ACDF, significantly increased range of motion was found at the adjacent segment.

Clinical Studies of Motion

Clinical studies of cervical disk replacement systems have used various methods to compare motion outcomes after arthroplasty with those of ACDF. It has been postulated that the restoration of motion maintains or decreases motion at the

adjacent segment and therefore helps protect it from degeneration (Figure 3). Pickett and associates[31] evaluated motion using quantitative motion analysis in patients who underwent single-level or two-level arthroplasty using the unconstrained Bryan prosthesis. The device was found to achieve near-normal range of motion at 24-month follow-up (mean, 7.8° per segment). Using roentgen stereometric analysis, Nabhan and associates[32] found significantly better motion retention as late as 1 year after arthroplasty using the ProDisc-C device, compared with ACDF. Porchet and Metcalf,[33] in a prospective, randomized clinical trial comparing the Prestige device with autograft fusion, found no difference at 12-month follow-up between the two patient groups in adjacent segment motion related to the development of adjacent segment disease. Using flexion-extension radiographs, Wigfield and associates[34] found increased motion at adjacent levels in patients treated with autograft ACDF compared with patients treated with cervical arthroplasty using the Prestige device.

Radiographic Studies

Measurement of intradiskal pressure and examination of motion patterns are valuable tools for understanding the natural history of adjacent segment disease. However, radiographic and clinical assessment of adjacent segment disease is perhaps even more valuable. In a prospective, randomized comparison of autograft fusion (24 patients) with arthroplasty (22 patients) using the Bryan prosthesis, Hacker[35] found at 1-year follow-up that adjacent segment disease had developed in none of the patients after fusion and in one patient after arthroplasty. Mummaneni and associates[36] recently de-

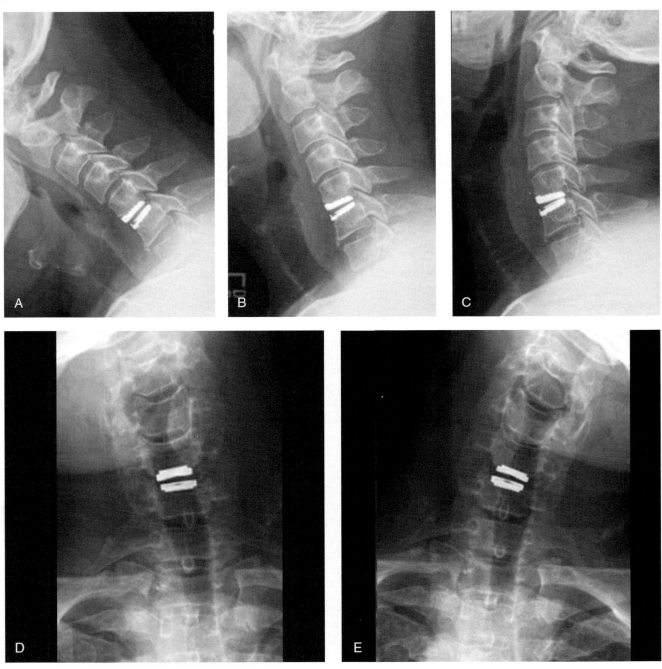

Figure 3 Radiographs taken 1 year after cervical disk arthroplasty at the C5-6 level using the PCM Artificial Cervical Disc (Cervitech, Rockaway, NJ). Lateral radiographs showing lateral flexion (**A**), neutral (**B**), and extension (**C**); the change in anterior and posterior disk height as well as the translation of C5 onto C6 can be seen by comparing the three radiographs. AP radiographs showing right bending (**D**) and left bending (**E**); the change in the right- and left-sided disk height relative to the direction of bending can be seen, and this preserved motion is believed to delay or prevent the development of adjacent segment disease.

scribed the results of a randomized multicenter study comparing 223 patients after arthroplasty using the Prestige ST prosthesis with 198 patients after ACDF using allograft and plating performed for symptomatic single-level degenerative disk disease. At 2-year follow-up, there was no significant difference between the patient groups in scores on the Medical Outcomes Study Short Form-36 Health Survey, the Neck Disability Index, or numeric rating scales for neck and arm pain. Of the patients treated with ACDF, 3.4% required a secondary procedure for adjacent segment disease, compared with 1.1% of patients treated with arthroplasty ($P = 0.0492$).

Although the natural history of adjacent segment disease is not well understood, considerable data suggest that fusion and arthroplasty lead to different biomechanical scenarios at the adjacent segment. Preclinical studies suggest that ACDF results in more compensatory motion and higher intradiskal pressures; studies of arthroplasty have found more normal values.[28-34] However, some data suggest that arthroplasty leads to higher facet loads at the index segment, which may accelerate same-segment disease while generally sparing the adjacent segment.[28] It is not yet known how these changes affect long-term outcomes. Fusion and arthroplasty may be best considered as complementary procedures, rather than competitors. Appropriate patient selection may prove to be the key issue in surgical intervention for adjacent segment disease.

Summary

Adjacent segment disease after cervical fusion surgery has been well described, although its cause remains controversial. In addition, there is dispute as to whether radiographic findings or symptoms should define clinically significant disease. Multiple factors, including altered biomechanical stresses and the natural history of cervical disk disease, probably contribute to the development of adjacent segment

disease. Available clinical data on cervical disk replacement are promising. The use of motion-sparing technology may decrease the incidence of adjacent segment disease. Longer-term follow-up of prospective, randomized studies comparing ACDF to cervical disk replacement should further contribute to our understanding of adjacent segment disease.

References

1. Panjabi MM, Crisco JJ, Vasavada A, et al: Mechanical properties of the human cervical spine as shown by three-dimensional load-displacement curves. *Spine* 2001;26:2692-2700.

2. Mimura M, Moriya H, Watanabe T, Takahashi K, Yamagata M, Tamaki T: Three-dimensional motion analysis of the cervical spine with special reference to the axial rotation. *Spine* 1989;14:1135-1139.

3. Ishii T, Mukai Y, Hosono N, et al: Kinematics of the cervical spine in lateral bending: In vivo three-dimensional analysis. *Spine* 2006;31: 155-160.

4. Ishii T, Mukai Y, Hosono N, et al: Kinematics of the subaxial cervical spine in rotation in vivo three-dimensional analysis. *Spine* 2004;29:2826-2831.

5. Menkowitz M, Stieber JR, Wenokor C, Cohen JD, Donald GD, Cresanti-Dakinis C: Intradiscal pressure monitoring in the cervical spine. *Pain Physician* 2005;8:163-166.

6. Dmitriev AE, Cunningham BW, Hu N, Sell G, Vigna F, McAfee PC: Adjacent level intradiscal pressure and segmental kinematics following a cervical total disc arthroplasty: An in vitro human cadaveric model. *Spine* 2005;30:1165-1172.

7. Buckwalter JA: Aging and degeneration of the human intervertebral disc. *Spine* 1995;20:1307-1314.

8. Hutton WC, Toribatake Y, Elmer WA, Ganey TM, Tomita K, Whitesides TE: The effect of compressive

force applied to the intervertebral disc in vivo: A study of proteoglycans and collagen. *Spine* 1998;23:2524-2537.

9. Schwab JS, Diangelo DJ, Foley KT: Motion compensation associated with single-level cervical fusion: Where does the lost motion go? *Spine* 2006;31:2439-2448.

10. Ragab AA, Escarcega AJ, Zdeblick TA: A quantitative analysis of strain at adjacent segments after segmental immobilization of the cervical spine. *J Spinal Disord Tech* 2006;19: 407-410.

11. Maiman DJ, Kumaresan S, Yoganandan N, Pintar FA: Biomechanical effect of anterior cervical spine fusion on adjacent segments. *Biomed Mater Eng* 1999;9:27-38.

12. Eck JC, Humphreys SC, Lim TH, et al: Biomechanical study on the effect of cervical spine fusion on adjacent-level intradiscal pressure and segmental motion. *Spine* 2002;27: 2431-2434.

13. Park DH, Ramakrishnan P, Cho TH, et al: Effect of lower two-level anterior cervical fusion on the superior adjacent level. *J Neurosurg Spine* 2007; 7:336-340.

14. Rao RD, Wang M, McGrady LM, Perlewitz TJ, David KS: Does anterior plating of the cervical spine predispose to adjacent segment changes? *Spine* 2005;30:2788-2792.

15. Fuller DA, Kirkpatrick JS, Emery SE, Wilber RG, Davy DT: A kinematic study of the cervical spine before and after segmental arthrodesis. *Spine* 1998;23:1649-1656.

16. Dekutoski MB, Schendel MJ, Ogilvie JW, Olsewski JM, Wallace LJ, Lewis JL: Comparison of in vivo and in vitro adjacent segment motion after lumbar fusion. *Spine* 1994;19:1745-1751.

17. Hilibrand AS, Balasubramanian K, Eichenbaum M, et al: The effect of anterior cervical fusion on neck motion. *Spine* 2006;31:1688-1692.

18. Reitman CA, Hipp JA, Nguyen L, Esses SI: Changes in segmental intervertebral motion adjacent to cervical

arthrodesis: A prospective study. *Spine* 2004;29:E221-E226.

19. Boden SD, McCowin PR, Davis DO, Dina TS, Mark AS, Wiesel S: Abnormal magnetic-resonance scans of the cervical spine in asymptomatic subjects: A prospective investigation. *J Bone Joint Surg Am* 1990;72:1178-1184.

20. Hilibrand AS, Carlson GD, Palumbo MA, Jones PK, Bohlman HH: Radiculopathy and myelopathy at segments adjacent to the site of a previous anterior cervical arthrodesis. *J Bone Joint Surg Am* 1999;81:519-528.

21. Dohler JR, Kahn MR, Hughes SP: Instability of the cervical spine after anterior interbody fusion: A study on its incidence and clinical significance in 21 patients. *Arch Orthop Trauma Surg* 1985;104:247-250.

22. Katsuura A, Hukuda S, Saruhashi Y, Mori K: Kyphotic malalignment after anterior cervical fusion is one of the factors promoting the degenerative process in adjacent intervertebral levels. *Eur Spine J* 2001;10:320-324.

23. Goffin J, Geusens E, Vantomme N, et al: Long-term follow-up after interbody fusion of the cervical spine. *J Spinal Disord Tech* 2004;17:79-85.

24. Yue WM, Brodner W, Highland TR: Long-term results after anterior cervical discectomy and fusion with allograft and plating: A 5- to 11-year radiologic and clinical follow-up study. *Spine* 2005;30:2138-2144.

25. Ishihara H, Kanamori M, Kawaguchi Y, Nakamura H, Kimura T: Adjacent segment disease after anterior cervical interbody fusion. *Spine J* 2004;4:624-628.

26. Herkowitz HN, Kurz LT, Overholt DP: Surgical management of cervical soft disc herniation: A comparison between the anterior and posterior approach. *Spine* 1990;15:1026-1030.

27. Clarke MJ, Ecker RD, Krauss WE, McClelland RL, Dekutoski MB: Same-segment and adjacent-segment disease following posterior cervical foraminotomy. *J Neurosurg Spine* 2007;6:5-9.

28. Chang UK, Kim DH, Lee MC, Willenberg R, Kim SH, Lim J: Changes in adjacent-level disc pressure and facet joint force after cervical arthroplasty compared with cervical discectomy and fusion. *J Neurosurg Spine* 2007;7:33-39.

29. DiAngelo DJ, Roberston JT, Metcalf NH, McVay BJ, Davis RC: Biomechanical testing of an artificial cervical joint and an anterior cervical plate. *J Spinal Disord Tech* 2003;16:314-323.

30. DiAngelo DJ, Foley KT, Morrow BR, et al: In vitro biomechanics of cervical disc arthroplasty with the ProDisc-C total disc implant. *Neurosurg Focus* 2004;17:E7.

31. Pickett GE, Rouleau JP, Duggal N: Kinematic analysis of the cervical spine following implantation of an artificial cervical disc. *Spine* 2005;30:1949-1954.

32. Nabhan A, Ahlhelm F, Shariat K, et al: The ProDisc-C prosthesis: Clinical and radiological experience 1 year after surgery. *Spine* 2007;32:1935-1941.

33. Porchet F, Metcalf NH: Clinical outcomes with the Prestige II cervical disc: Preliminary results from a prospective randomized clinical trial. *Neurosurg Focus* 2004;17:E6.

34. Wigfield C, Gill S, Nelson R, Langdon I, Metcalf N, Robertson J: Influence of an artificial cervical joint compared with fusion on adjacent-level motion in the treatment of degenerative cervical disc disease. *J Neurosurg* 2002;96(suppl 1):17-21.

35. Hacker RJ: Cervical disc arthroplasty: A controlled randomized prospective study with intermediate follow-up results. Invited submission from the Joint Section Meeting on Disorders of the Spine and Peripheral Nerves, March 2005. *J Neurosurg Spine* 2005;3:424-428.

36. Mummaneni PV, Burkus JK, Haid RW, Traynelis VC, Zdeblick TA: Clinical and radiographic analysis of cervical disc arthroplasty compared with allograft fusion: A randomized controlled clinical trial. *J Neurosurg Spine* 2007;6:198-209.

Vertebral Artery Injury in Cervical Spine Surgery

Clinton J. Devin, MD
James D. Kang, MD

Abstract

Vertebral artery injuries during cervical spine surgery are rare, with a reported incidence of 0.3% to 0.5%. The vertebral artery enters the vertebral foramen most commonly at C6 and courses from anterior and lateral to medial and posterior with respect to the vertebral body up to C3. The vertebral artery has a more variable course in the atlantoaxial region. Careful assessment on preoperative imaging will identify common anomalies and help avoid a vertebral artery injury. If a vertebral artery injury occurs, rapid action is required to prevent exsanguination or catastrophic neurologic injury. Every attempt should be made to repair the vertebral artery because the contralateral artery may not provide sufficient blood flow in this spondylotic population. If repair is not possible and contralateral circulation is deemed adequate, endovascular coiling or primary ligation should be performed. Tamponade should be avoided as the definitive treatment because of well-known complications.

The vertebral artery is infrequently injured during cervical spine surgery. The unique anatomy of the vertebral artery in the subaxial spine puts it at increased risk with anterior procedures, with a reported incidence of injury of 0.3% to 0.5%.[1,2] In contrast, injury to the atlantoaxial segment of the vertebral artery is more likely with posterior cervical procedures, occurring in up to 4.1% to 8.2%.[3-5] Because of the advent of new fixation methods and more extensive decompressions, it is imperative that surgeons have a thorough understanding of the vertebral artery anatomy and a treatment plan in place should an injury occur, so as to prevent irreversible neurologic injury.

Vertebral Artery in the Subaxial Cervical Spine

The vertebral artery is divided into four segments, from its origin at the subclavian artery to the point where it unites with the contralateral vertebral artery to form the basilar artery. The basilar artery, in turn, provides the posterior circulation of the brain, including the brainstem, occipital lobes, and the labyrinthine branches to the inner ear.[6] Ultimately, the posterior circulation communicates with the anterior circulation through the circle of Willis. This evolutionary redundancy in circulation allows for a portion of the system to sustain an injury without catastrophic effect. However, certain vascular anomalies and ath-erosclerosis can compromise collateral circulation, increasing the importance of repairing the injury. The vertebral artery has unique risks of injury during cervical spine surgery at each level.

The first (prevertebral) segment branches off the subclavian artery at the level of T1, ascending postero-superiorly between the anterior scalene and longus colli muscles. The vertebral artery passes just lateral and anterior to the transverse process of C7.[7] It typically enters at C6, but in a small percentage of patients, the first foramen that it enters is more cephalad or caudad to the C6 vertebral body—3.5% to 5.4% at C7, 6% at C5, 0.5% to 1.3% at C4, and 0.1% at C3.[8] In addition to various levels of entry, duplicate foramina are present in 7% and triplicate foramina or no foramina in 7%. If duplicate foramina exist at a given level, the vertebral artery is found in the medial foramen.[9]

The second (cervical) segment of the vertebral artery ascends from the transverse foramen of C6 to the atlas. The vertebral artery from C6 to C3 is most vulnerable during anterior cervical procedures. The overall dimensions of the transverse foramen decrease in size from C6 to C3.[10-14] The transverse foramen on the left side of the cervical spine typically is larger than on the right, correlating with the fact that the left vertebral artery is more commonly the dominant artery, providing a greater percentage of hind-brain blood flow.[2,9,15] The contents of the transverse foramen include a single artery, a sympathetic nervous plexus, and a venous plexus. The venous plexus lies medial to the artery within the foramen and often is the initial bleeding encountered on accidental entry into the foramen. Unlike the vertebral artery, this usually can be adequately controlled by tamponade with hemostatic agents such as an absorbable gelatin sponge soaked in thrombin.[9] Fibroligamentous tissue attaches the contents of the foramen to the uncinate process. This implies that the final lateral decompression of the uncus should be done with a curette or Kerrison punch to avoid tangling this fibroligamentous tissue around a burr and injuring the artery.[11,16]

The general course of the vertebral artery and its respective foramina from C6 to C3 is from anterior and lateral to medial and posterior with respect to the vertebral body. Vaccaro and associates[13] evaluated CT scans, noting the interforaminal distance (medial aspect of the left transverse foramen to the medial aspect of the right transverse foramen) and location of the transverse foramen relative to the posterior aspect of the vertebral body between C3 and C6. The average interforaminal distance was noted to increase from 25.90 ± 1.89 mm at C3 to 29.30 ± 2.70 mm at C6. The posterior border of the transverse foramen relative to the posterior border of the vertebral body was noted to increase from 2.16 ± 1.16 mm at C3 to 3.53 ± 1.56 mm at C6.[13] Similar values were reported in cadaver studies.[10,17] Because surgeons must rely on imaging studies for preoperative planning, Heary and associates[9] compared the interforaminal

distance measured with a caliper on cadaver specimens to the value obtained with a CT scan. The interforaminal distance on the gross specimens were consistently larger than the distances of these same specimens on a CT scan, indicating that the CT scan is a reliable means of determining a safe width of resection.[9] These data indicate that a corpectomy at C3 should be narrower than one at C7. In multilevel corpectomies, the area of resection should appear as a trapezoid, with the most cephalad vertebra being narrower than the caudad vertebra.

The interforaminal distance provides a maximal allowable width of resection, but this is much wider than is required to adequately decompress the spinal cord and exiting nerve root. However, performing too narrow a decompression has been shown to lead to poor outcomes in myelopathic patients.[18,19] The width of the spinal canal is relatively constant in the subaxial spine, measuring approximately 13 to 14.5 mm.[2,17] Adhering to this width of resection will provide sufficient decompression of the spinal cord itself but will leave the exiting nerve root inadequately decompressed. Many anatomic landmarks have been evaluated as intraoperative reference points for maintaining a safe distance from the vertebral artery, yet providing adequate lateral decompression. Smith and associates[2] recommended using the medial margin of the longus colli as a reference for lateral decompression. In anatomic studies, the distance from the medial margin of the longus colli to the transverse foramen was found to increase from C3 (9.0 ± 1.3 mm) to C6 (11.5 ± 1.0 mm).[20] Elevation of the longus colli should begin in the middle of the vertebral body, where it dips inward. This area of the body

is less likely to be affected by spondylosis, and the transverse process, which is located in the middle of the vertebral body, provides further protection to the vertebral artery.[11,21] Before the longus colli is elevated toward the desired uncovertebral joint, spondylotic spurs should be resected about the disk space with a Lexel rongeur. Elevation of the longus colli should proceed toward the uncovertebral joint with great care because of the proximity of the vertebral artery. The distance from the tip of the uncinate process to the nearby vertebral artery ranges from 0.8 to 1.6 mm.[21] Lateral dissection should cease once the uncovertebral joint can be seen curving upward and should not proceed all the way to the uncinate process. The distance from the medial margin of the longus colli to the vertebral artery is a helpful reference during dissection; however, once the retractors have been placed, it becomes less useful. Most surgeons use the uncovertebral joint as a reference for adequate lateral decompression. The distance between the medial margins of the uncovertebral joints at C3 is approximately 15 mm, and at C6 it is 19 mm. It is important to compare the width of the resection with something of known length, such as the surgeon's index fingertip. Decompressing up to the medial margin of the uncovertebral joint leaves approximately 5 mm of bone protecting the vertebral artery.[17] For a thorough foraminotomy, the osteophytes should be resected using a curette or Kerrison punch off the uncus in line with the exiting nerve root up to the medial edge of the pedicle. Adequate lateral decompression is further confirmed by the presence of epidural fat and veins surrounding the exiting nerve root. This is important to ensure a successful outcome, but it should be done with caution because the vertebral artery is within 1 to 6 mm of this lateral resection.[17] Using these anatomic landmarks will generally avoid a vertebral artery injury between C3 and C6, but anomalies in the course of the vertebral artery can lead to disastrous complications if not recognized preoperatively.

The vertebral artery and its respective foramina are well lateral to the medial edge of the uncovertebral joint; however, in a small percentage of patients, the artery takes a tortuous course, causing it to be medialized and in danger if the uncovertebral joint is used as the lateral extent of the decompression. Oga and associates[22] provided an interesting explanation as to the etiology of a tortuous vertebral artery in patients with spondylosis. They devised a grading system that described the course of the vertebral artery in relation to the uncovertebral joint and evaluated preoperative magnetic resonance angiograms in 22 patients undergoing anterior cervical decompression. There was a direct correlation between the degree of spondylosis and the amount of vertebral artery tortuosity. The vertebral artery is relatively fixed in the confines of the transverse foramen. As the disk space collapses, the vertebral artery loops inward. Osteophytes further alter the course of the vertebral artery. Over time, the pulsation of the vertebral artery against the vertebral body induces erosion and deformation of the foramen.[22] An extensive cadaver study of 888 vertebrae between C3 to C6, from the Hamann-Todd skeleton collection, was analyzed for the presence of a medialized transverse foramen.[23] In 2.7% of the specimens, the foramen was, on average, 0.14 mm medial to the uncovertebral joint. Interest-

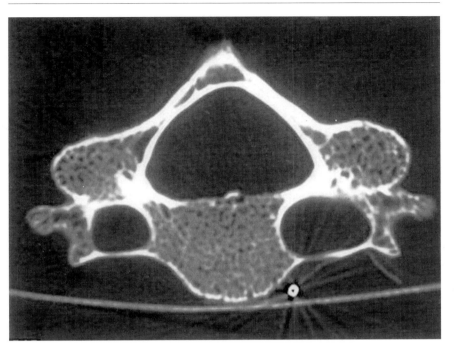

Figure 1 Axial CT scan of an abnormal cadaver specimen with the vertebral foramen extending medial to the uncovertebral joint. (Reproduced with permission from Curylo LJ, Mason HC, Bohlman HH, Yoo JU: Tortuous cource of the vertebral artery and anterior cervical decompression. *Spine* 2000;25:2860-2864.)

ingly, the medial displacement of the foramen occurred at the midbody level and returned to a more normal position at the uncovertebral joint (Figure 1). This in part explains why vertebral artery injuries are more common in corpectomies than in diskectomies.[23] Certain populations, such as patients with rheumatoid arthritis, are believed to have an even higher incidence of a tortuous vertebral artery caused by the progressive destruction of articular surfaces. There should be a heightened awareness and low tolerance for further imaging with a CT angiogram or magnetic resonance angiogram in this group of patients.[24] These studies stress the importance of carefully evaluating the preoperative images, noting the location of the vertebral artery in all patients undergoing anterior cervical decompression. If

there is suspicion of a tortuous vertebral artery, a CT angiogram or magnetic resonance angiogram will provide invaluable information. In the presence of a tortuous vertebral artery, a posterior decompressive procedure should be considered, if possible. If an anterior procedure is required because of focal kyphosis or significant retrovertebral disease, a hybrid anterior decompression should be performed in which a diskectomy is done above the vertebra with a tortuous artery and a corpectomy is done on the next caudal vertebra.[23]

Using a microscope for decompression with anterior approaches to the subaxial cervical spine provides multiple advantages, including improved lighting, equivalent view for the surgeon and assistant, and improved visualization of neurologic structures and potential sites of compression.[25] However, when using the microscope, the overall field of view can be lost, resulting in an asymmetric resection. In one study, a microscope was used in five of the six vertebral artery injuries that occurred.[26] To avoid loss of the overall field of view, most of the dissection should be done with loupes, elevating the longus colli as described previously so that both uncovertebral joints are visible. This provides definition of the true midline. At this point, the microscope is brought in and centered perpendicular to the level of interest so that the uncovertebral joints are at the periphery of the field of view. Proper orientation of the scope should be confirmed by stepping back and observing the angle of the scope relative to the wound. The orientation of the microscope should be periodically assessed throughout the remainder of the decompression, and the surgeon also should intermittently move the scope out of the way and look at the bony resection. Adhering to these safety checks avoids an asymmetric resection and potential vertebral artery injury.

Vertebral Artery in the Atlantoaxial Cervical Spine

The vertebral artery exits the C3 foramen and continues in a posteromedial ascent toward C2, where it makes an acute lateral bend just under the superior articular facet of the axis before exiting the C2 foramen at a 45° angle.[27] It then ascends vertically and slightly ventral to enter the C1 transverse foramen. The artery then turns sharply, taking on a horizontal and posterolateral course in the groove on the superior arch of the atlas. Approximately 1.5 cm lateral to the midline of the atlas, the vertebral artery ascends upward,

piercing the atlanto-occipital membrane and entering the cranial cavity. This region of the vertebral artery is the third segment, also termed the V3 segment. Previous forms of posterior fixation around the atlantoaxial region included some permutation of interspinous wiring, which had minimal risk of vertebral artery injury. However, there are multiple challenges with interspinous wiring, including lower fusion rates, the need for posterior elements, the risk of neurologic injury, and the requirement of prolonged halo immobilization.[28,29] This caused surgeons to seek alternative methods of atlantoaxial fixation. Although these newer techniques boast improved fusion rates and avoid halo immobilization, they pose an increased risk of vertebral artery injury. There can be significant heterogeneity in the course of the vertebral artery at the craniovertebral junction. There are intraosseous and extraosseous anomalies that have unique relevance to the different forms of spinal fixation. An increased incidence of vertebral artery anomalies has been demonstrated in those with bony anomalies of C1 or C2. Additionally, those with a bony anomaly also are more likely to have dominance of one of the vertebral arteries.[30,31] The bony anomalies can include os odontoideum, asymmetric diameter of the vertebral foramen at C1, or a congenital fusion, among others. These should always raise suspicion of a vertebral artery anomaly, and careful assessment of the course of the vertebral artery should be made on preoperative imaging. However, vertebral artery anomalies can exist in the absence of bony anomalies, essentially requiring that preoperative assessment of the vertebral artery course be made in all patients. This often can be accom-

plished using the soft-tissue windows in a CT scan with sagittal and coronal reconstructions, or alternatively magnetic resonance angiography or CT angiography if finer detail is required.

Atlantoaxial transarticular screws provide superior biomechanical properties and higher fusion rates and do not require postoperative halo immobilization, but have been reported to be the most dangerous form of fixation.[32,33] The reported rates of vertebral artery injury range from 4.1% to 8.2%.[3-5] Injury to the artery can occur because of a misguided trajectory, or the isthmus of C2 through which the screw is to pass is narrowed by a high-riding vertebral artery. A high-riding vertebral artery is one that courses too medial or dorsal within the isthmus of the axis, making the width or height of the isthmus too narrow to allow safe passage of a screw. Cadaver measurements and CT imaging of the C2 isthmus have demonstrated asymmetry of the right side versus the left in 41% to 100%.[4,34] Furthermore, the C2 isthmus has been found to be too narrow to accept a 3.5-mm screw on at least one side in 18% to 23%, and both sides were too narrow in 5% to 6% of those evaluated.[4,34-36] Based on these studies, it is imperative that preoperative CT angiography, with sagittal and coronal reconstructions, is obtained to determine if the isthmus will allow safe passage of a screw. This also provides a template to determine screw trajectory. The trajectory determined on the preoperative CT scan has been shown to accurately translate to the trajectory determined with intraoperative biplanar fluoroscopy.[37,38] Before screw placement, the atlantoaxial joint must be perfectly reduced. In one retrospective series of vertebral artery injuries during placement of transarticular screws, two thirds of the patients were reported to have an inadequately reduced C1-C2 joint. To capture the C1 lateral mass, the screw had taken on a flatter trajectory, causing it to violate the C2 isthmus inferiorly and injure the vertebral artery.[4] Once the C1-C2 joint is reduced and it has been determined that the isthmus is wide enough to allow safe passage of the screw, a 3.5-mm screw is inserted with the assistance of biplanar fluoroscopy. An aiming device improves the accuracy of C1-C2 screw placement but does not eliminate the risk of a misguided screw.[39,40] If it is determined preoperatively that one C2 isthmus is too small for a screw, then hybrid fixation with a unilateral transarticular screw and interspinous wiring has demonstrated successful fusion without the need for a halo.[41] Neo and associates[39] argued that bilateral placement of transarticular screws can be done despite a narrow C2 isthmus by using the proper starting point. They successfully placed bilateral screws in 54 consecutive patients using a trajectory that placed the screw in the most superior and medial aspect of the isthmus. In 7 of the 54 patients, the isthmus was believed to be too narrow for screw placement by other studies' standards; however, they had no complications.

In summary, C1-C2 screws pose a significant risk of injury to the vertebral artery. A thorough preoperative evaluation using CT angiography with sagittal reconstruction should be done to determine if the isthmus is wide enough for screw placement and, if so, the proper screw trajectory. Before screw placement, the C1-C2 joint must be perfectly reduced. Biplanar imaging is used to place the screw in the most

posterior and medial aspect of the isthmus on a trajectory determined by the CT scan. Contraindications to screw fixation include obesity that precludes adequate biplanar imaging, incomplete reduction of C1-C2, a C2 isthmus smaller than the screw being inserted, cervicothoracic kyphosis preventing the necessary trajectory, and fractures of the C1 lateral mass or C2 isthmus.

The dangers associated with transarticular fixation prompted the development of a biomechanically equivalent alternative. The advent of polyaxial screw systems renewed interest in segmental fixation of C1-C2. A screw-rod construct provides similar advantages as transarticular screws, including high fusion rates, no need for posterior elements, and no postoperative halo immobilization. Unique advantages of a screw-rod construct over transarticular screws include the ability to use the screws for an intraoperative reduction and to better integrate the fusion into a multilevel occipitocervical construct.[42] Biomechanically, unilateral segmental fixation with a screw-rod construct was found to be more stable than a unilateral transarticular screw. If the anatomy allows for bilateral fixation, then the two methods of fixation are essentially equivalent, with the screw-rod construct being slightly more stable in flexion/extension.[43]

Screw placement into C1 rather than C2 is very different, with anatomy dictating unique challenges at each level. Placement of C1 lateral mass screws begins with careful evaluation of preoperative imaging. A preoperative CT angiogram with sagittal and coronal reconstructions should be obtained to determine suitability for screw placement, trajectory, location of the vertebral and internal carotid artery, and screw length.[44] This also will help identify

vertebral artery anomalies that can occur in this region.

Hong and associates[31] analyzed CT angiography in 1,013 patients, carefully noting the course of the vertebral artery. The frequency of a persistent intersegmental artery was 4.6%, and the frequency of a fenestrated vertebral artery was 0.5%. The posterior inferior cerebellar artery originates between the atlas and axis, coursing into the spinal canal in 0.2%.[31] These anomalies are shown in Figure 2. All three of these anomalies have significant implications, given that they cross the insertion point for a C1 lateral mass screw, potentially causing significant hemorrhage or a stroke in the posterior inferior cerebellar artery distribution if not recognized. Once these anomalies have been ruled out on preoperative imaging, the surgeon can proceed with cautious dissection and exposure. The midline of the posterior arch is identified and dissection should proceed laterally up to approximately 1 to 1.5 cm from midline. Further dissection should proceed on the inferior aspect of the arch to avoid the vertebral artery, which is coursing in the groove on the superior aspect of the posterior arch. The medial wall of the C1 lateral mass can be palpated with a Penfield dissector. To avoid bleeding that can occur from the venous plexus surrounding the C2 nerve root, the tissue should be elevated in a subperiosteal manner, starting on the inferior aspect of the C1 arch and proceeding caudally until the inferior aspect of the lateral mass is visible. The Penfield dissector should be held in this position to protect the C2 nerve root. If bleeding from this epidural venous plexus occurs, it can be controlled through tamponade with an absorbable gelatin sponge soaked in thrombin and a

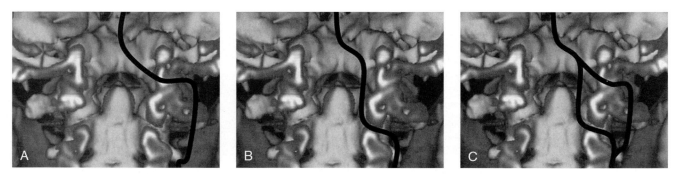

Figure 2   Schematics of the vertebral artery and its anomalies. **A,** Usual course of the vertebral artery (primary vertebral artery). **B,** Course of the first intersegmental artery (without persistence of the primary vertebral artery). **C,** Course of a fenestrated vertebral artery (with persistence of the primary and first intersegmental arteries). (Reproduced with permission from Takahashi T, Tominaga T, Hassan T, Yoshimoto T: Cervical cord compression with myelopathy caused by bilateral persistence of the first intersegmental arteries: Case report. *Neurosurgery* 2003;53:234-237.)

cottonoid.[45] Finding the ideal starting point can be challenging. Placing the screw too inferior can injure the C2 nerve root and lead to greater occipital neuralgia, whereas a superior starting point places the vertebral artery at risk. Cadaver measurements have shown that the average thickness of the posterior arch where the screw is placed ranges from 3.95 to 4.6 mm.[46,47] In females, the average thickness of the posterior arch somewhat thinner, at 3.5 mm.[48] A minimal thickness of 5 mm is believed to be necessary to safely place a screw in the posterior arch, which precludes the use of screws in most patients.[46] There is a particular anomaly termed ponticulus posticus, which is a bony arch that covers the vertebral artery on the posterior arch of the atlas. A cadaver study demonstrated a frequency of 15.9% in men and 8.1% in women.[46] An analysis of 464 consecutive lateral radiographs showed a prevalence of 15.5%.[49] The normal posterior arch of the atlas thins out laterally, whereas those with a ponticulus posticus demonstrate an arch that broadens laterally (Figure 3). In patients with this anomaly, the posterior arch appears much thicker than it

is; using this as a reference to place a screw can injure the underlying vertebral artery. To avoid injury to the vertebral artery, a modified method has been developed that uses a 2-mm burr to take down a small portion of the inferior aspect of posterior arch in line with the screw trajectory. This method provides more bony purchase for the screw and prevents a steep trajectory that can potentially impinge on the C2 nerve root. The entry point for the screw is 3 to 5 mm lateral to the medial aspect of the lateral mass, at the junction of the posterior arch and the lateral mass. The screw is angled 10° to 15° medial to avoid the vertebral artery laterally and the internal carotid artery on the anterior aspect of C1. It is also angled 10° to 15° cephalad to avoid entry into the C1-C2 joint. Intraoperative fluoroscopy in the lateral plane is recommended during placement of this screw. The screw head should be left posterior to the C1 arch.

Fixation of the axis can be obtained in the pars interarticularis or the pedicle. These terms have been used interchangeably, and there has been much confusion as to the true definition. The pars interarticularis

is defined as the portion of the C2 vertebra between the superior and inferior articular processes. The pedicle is the portion of bone beneath the superior facet and anteromedial to the transverse foramen.[50] The pars interarticularis starting point is 3 to 4 mm cephalad and lateral to the inferomedial aspect of the C2-C3 facet joint. The screw follows a similar trajectory to a transarticular screw, aiming cephalad and slightly medial. This places the screw in the superomedial aspect of the isthmus and farther away from the vertebral artery. The pedicle screw starting point is 5 to 6 mm cephalad and lateral to the inferomedial aspect of the C2-C3 facet joint. Palpation of the medial aspect of the pedicle provides the medial angulation, and the screw should be aimed cephalad approximately 20°. Because the pedicle screw and pars interarticularis screw pose similar risks to the vertebral artery, many surgeons argue that a pedicle screw is more advantageous because a much longer screw can be used.[45] Regardless of the fixation chosen, a preoperative CT angiogram should be carefully scrutinized for suitability of screw placement and tra-

Management of a Vertebral Artery Injury

Iatrogenic vertebral artery injury can result in exsanguination with hemodynamic instability and neurologic insult. The vertebral artery provides the dominant blood supply to the posterior circulation of the brain. Blood flow that is not compensated by the contralateral vertebral artery can lead to the development of lateral medullary infarction (Wallenberg syndrome, which is characterized by decreased sensation to pin prick on the ipsilateral face and contralateral limbs, nystagmus, ataxia, dysmetria in the ipsilateral limbs; and Horner syndrome on the ipsilateral side), cerebellar infarction, isolated cranial nerve palsies, quadriparesis, and hemiplegia.[52] The goal is to minimize hemorrhage and prevent neurologic insult. Direct repair, bypass, clean ligation, endovascular coiling, and tamponade can be used with differing degrees of success.

If a vertebral artery injury occurs during an anterior approach to the subaxial cervical spine, the surgeon should expediently carry out a predetermined treatment plan. The head should be returned to a neutral position because rotation and extension can impair blood flow in the contralateral vertebral artery.[53] Hemorrhage should be controlled by packing, and the anesthesiologist alerted so that perfusion pressure can be maintained and fluids or blood products can be given. The packing should be done with large pieces of hemostatic agents such as an absorbable gelatin sponge and a cottonoid, avoiding agents that can break apart into small pieces and embolize.[1] The patient should be hemodynamically stable before proceeding. At this point, an attempt should be made to repair the artery because the status of the contralater-

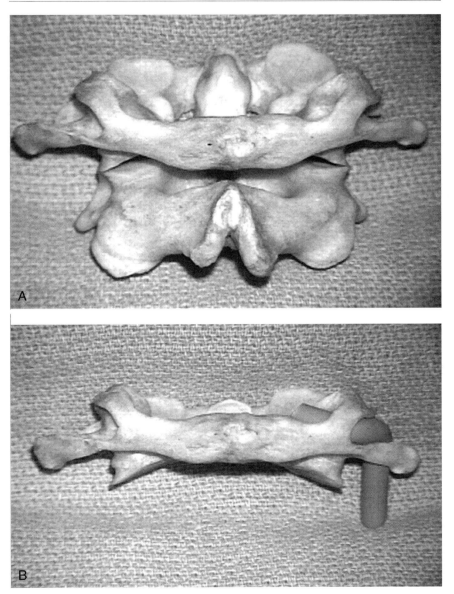

Figure 3 Posterior view of osseous specimens demonstrating a ponticulus posticus bilaterally **(A)** and revealing the vertebral artery coursing medially within the arcuate foramen and deep to the ponticulus posticus **(B)**. (Reproduced with permission from Young JP, Young PH, Ackermann MJ, Anderson PA, Riew KD: The ponticulus posticus: Implications for screw insertion into the first cervical lateral mass. *J Bone Joint Surg Am* 2005;87:2495-2498.)

jectory. There is a paucity of literature on the incidence of vertebral artery injury from pars interarticularis screws or pedicle screws. In a review of multiple studies, nearly 2,577 cervical pedicle screws from C2 to C7 were inserted with only one vertebral artery injury. The bleeding was managed by packing the hole with bone wax and not placing a screw. There were no postoperative complications and the patients did not have a neurologic deficit.[51]

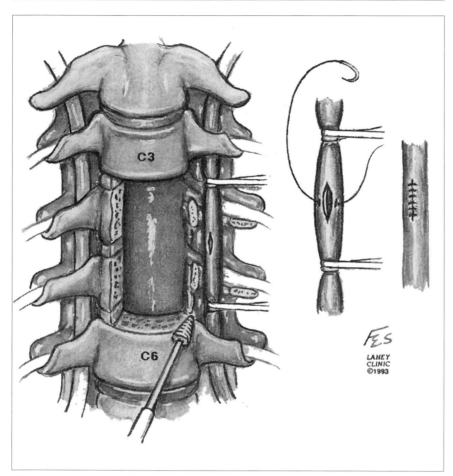

Figure 4 Schematic demonstrating primary repair of the vertebral artery. (Courtesy of Lahey Clinic, Burlington, MA.)

al artery is unknown and is more likely impaired in a spondylotic population. The artery should be exposed one level above and below the site of injury, with periosteal elevators retracting the longus colli muscles laterally over the transverse process. An alternative method of exposure is splitting the longus colli at the seventh cervical vertebra because the artery is not confined within a bony foramen at this level. The longus colli should be split in a longitudinal fashion, taking care to not injure the sympathetic chain, which is coursing in the fascia of the longus colli. The anterior aspect of the transverse foramen is then un-

roofed with a diamond-tipped burr or 2-mm Kerrison punch. This can result in bleeding from the venous plexus that surrounds the vertebral artery, which can easily be controlled with gentle packing of hemostatic agents. The artery can then be mobilized and the injury isolated. A temporary aneurysm clip is applied proximal to the laceration. If strong retrograde flow occurs, this provides some confidence that good collateral circulation exists; ligation or embolization can be considered if the initial attempt at repair fails. If the hemorrhage is controlled with this initial clip, collateral blood flow likely is poor, and the involved ver-

tebral artery is unilaterally dominant. The second aneurysm clip is applied distal to the site of injury. The laceration is primarily repaired with 7-0 Prolene (Ethicon, Sommerville, NJ). Before completion of the repair, the distal clip should be removed to allow back bleeding so as to prevent propagation of air or platelet emboli. Using this protocol, the average blood loss was 825 mL, and none of the three patients suffered neurologic deficit[1] (Figure 4). A postoperative CT angiogram or magnetic resonance angiogram should be obtained to assess the repair and identify any infarct. The patient should be admitted to the intensive care unit to closely monitor hemodynamics and quickly identify a neurologic deficit. Once the perioperative risk of an epidural hematoma decreases, an antiplatelet agent should be given. If a neurologic deficit occurs and imaging studies demonstrate an infarct, the stroke team should be consulted to determine the need for anticoagulation such as heparin. If primary repair is not possible, the adequacy of collateral circulation should ideally be assessed with intraoperative angiography. Endovascular stenting can be done at the time of the angiography.[54] If an endovascular team is not available, and there is not adequate backflow on clamping of the proximal portion of the vertebral artery, a vascular surgeon should be consulted intraoperatively to determine if a saphenous vein interposition graft or transposition grafting of the internal or external carotid artery might be possible.[55,56] If collateral circulation is adequate and repair is not possible, alternative treatments are available.

The injured vertebral artery should be treated with endovascular coiling or clean ligation proximal and distal to the site of injury if repair is not possible. Tamponade as a definitive treatment has led to multiple complications, including arteriovenous fistulas, pseudoaneurysm with delayed hemorrhage and airway obstruction, and significant blood loss.[2,57,58] Before ligation or endovascular coiling, it is critical to confirm adequate collateral circulation. The left vertebral artery is hypoplastic in 5.7% and absent in 1.8% of patients. The right vertebral artery is hypoplastic in 8.8% and absent in 3.1% of patients.[1] The reported frequency of ischemic complication from coiling or ligation of the vertebral artery ranges from 1.8% to 12%.[15,59,60] Smith and associates[2] reported that three of seven vertebral artery injuries treated with ligation sustained an infarct. This is higher than expected; however, in a spondylotic population, the frequency of atherosclerosis and a compromised circulation is higher than that seen in the trauma population, from which results of vertebral artery ligation have been reported.[12] Once there has been confirmation of collateral circulation, the vertebral artery should be ligated proximal and distal to the site of injury. If bleeding cannot be controlled without continuous tamponade, endovascular embolization can be done intraoperatively or soon thereafter. A CT angiogram or magnetic resonance angiogram should be obtained postoperatively to evaluate the ligation or coiling and assess for any infarct. The patient should be admitted to the intensive care unit for hemodynamic and neurologic monitoring (Figure 5).

Little information is available in the literature on the management of vertebral artery injuries in proximity to the atlantoaxial region.[61] If a vertebral artery injury occurs intraoper-

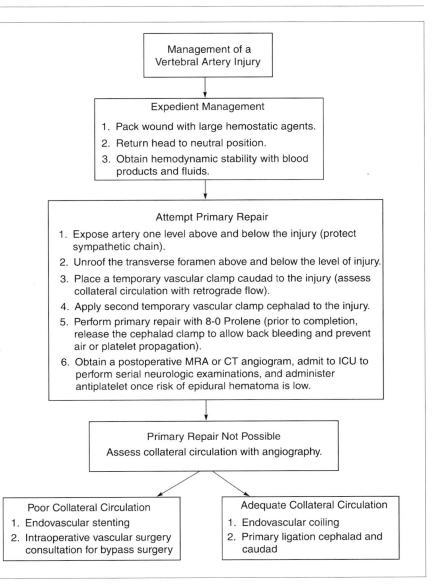

Figure 5 Algorithm for repair of the vertebral artery. MRA = magnetic resonance angiogram, ICU = intensive care unit.

atively, some surgeons suggest that the screw should quickly be placed to tamponade the bleeding. Others think that the screw should not be placed, and the hole should be covered with bone wax. The contralateral screw should not be attempted, and a more conventional method of fixation such as Brooks interspinous wiring should be used. The senior author has successfully treated an

injury in this region with endovascular embolization. If these methods are unsuccessful and a pseudoaneurysm or arteriovenous fistula develops, it is optimally approached anteriorly by a vascular team. The artery is ligated proximally just above the C2 nerve root and the distal aspect of the artery is transposed to surrounding arteries, if possible, or ligated.[52]

Summary

Every cervical spine surgeon should understand how to treat a vertebral artery injury but, more importantly, should know how to avoid a vertebral artery injury. The axial CT or MRI images should be carefully reviewed preoperatively for evidence of a tortuous vertebral artery. If these images suggest an anomaly, a magnetic resonance angiogram or CT angiogram should be obtained to better delineate the abnormality. For procedures about the atlantoaxial joint, these additional imaging studies should be obtained in all patients. This provides invaluable information on whether instrumentation is possible and the resultant trajectory to avoid vascular injury. Anterior approaches to the subaxial cervical spine begin by removing spondylotic spurs back to more normal anatomy and performing adequate dissection to expose the uncovertebral joints and define the lateral border of the decompression. Similarly, the bony anatomy in the atlantoaxial region should be well exposed to provide a reference for accurate screw placement. If a vertebral artery injury occurs in the subaxial cervical spine, repair of the injury should be attempted. If a primary repair is not possible and collateral circulation is inadequate, a transposition, grafting, or stenting is indicated. When collateral circulation is deemed adequate, a primary ligation or endovascular coiling should be done. Injuries in the atlantoaxial region should be treated by first resorting to an alternative means of instrumentation such as wiring or translaminar screws in C2. Endovascular embolization can be done, or the artery can be approached anteriorly and ligated.

References

1. Golfinos JG, Dickman CA, Zabramski JM, Sonntag VK, Spetzler RF: Repair of vertebral artery injury during anterior cervical decompression. *Spine* 1994;19:2552-2556.

2. Smith MD, Emery SE, Dudley A, Murray KJ, Leventhal M: Vertebral artery injury during anterior decompression of the cervical spine: A retrospective review of ten patients. *J Bone Joint Surg Br* 1993;75:410-415.

3. Dickman CA, Sonntag VK: C1-2 transarticular screw fixation for atlantoaxial arthrodesis. *Neurosurgery* 1999; 44:687-690.

4. Madawi AA, Casey AT, Solanki GA, Tuite G, Veres R, Crockard HA: Radiological and anatomical evaluation of the atlantoaxial transarticular screw fixation technique. *J Neurosurg* 1997; 86:961-968.

5. Wright NM, Lauryssen C: Vertebral artery injury in C1-2 transarticular fixation: Results of a survey of the AANS/CNS section on disorders of the spine and peripheral nerves: American Association of Neurological Surgeons/Congress of Neurological Surgeons. *J Neurosurg* 1998;88: 634-640.

6. Romanov VA, Miller LG, Gaevyi MD: Effect of vertebral nerve on circulation in the inner ear (cochlea). *Biull Eksp Biol Med* 1973;75:10-12.

7. Xu R, Ebraheim NA, Tang G, Stanescu S: Location of the vertebral artery in the cervicothoracic junction. *Am J Orthop* 2000;29:453-456.

8. Argenson G, Franke JP, Sylla S, Dintimille H, Papasion S, DiMarino V: The vertebral arteries (segments V1 and V2). *Anat Clin* 1980;2:29-41.

9. Heary RF, Albert TJ, Ludwig S, et al: Surgical anatomy of the vertebral arteries. *Spine* 1996;21:2074-2080.

10. Ebraheim NA, Lu J, Brown JA, Biyani A, Yeasting RA: Vulnerability of vertebral artery in anterolateral decompression for cervical spondylosis. *Clin Orthop Relat Res* 1996;322: 146-151.

11. Kawashima M, Tanriover N, Rhoton AL, Matsushima T: The transverse process, intertransverse space, and vertebral artery in anterior approaches to the lower cervical spine. *J Neurosurg* 2003;98:188-194.

12. Cagnie B, Barbaix E, Vinck E, D'Herde K, Cambier D: Extrinsic risk factors for compromised blood flow in the vertebral artery: Anatomical observations of the transverse foramina from C3 to C7. *Surg Radiol Anat* 2005;27:312-316.

13. Vaccaro AR, Ring D, Scuderi G, Garfin SR: Vertebral artery location in relation to the vertebral body as determined by two-dimensional computed tomography evaluation. *Spine* 1994;19:2637-2641.

14. Ebraheim NA, Reader D, Xu R, Yeasting RA: Location of the vertebral artery foramen on the anterior aspect of the lower cervical spine by computed tomography. *J Spinal Disord* 1997;10:304-307.

15. Shintani A, Zervas NT: Consequence of ligation of the vertebral artery. *J Neurosurg* 1972;36:447-450.

16. Ebraheim NA, Lu J, Haman SP, Yeasting RA: Anatomic basis of the anterior surgery on the cervical spine: Relationships between uncus-artery-root complex and vertebral artery injury. *Surg Radiol Anat* 1998;20: 389-392.

17. Oh SH, Perin NI, Cooper PR: Quantitative three-dimensional anatomy of the subaxial cervical spine: Implication for anterior spinal surgery. *Neurosurgery* 1996;38:1139-1144.

18. Yonenobu K, Okada K, Fuji T, Fujiwara K, Tamashita K, Ono K: Causes of neurologic deterioration following surgical treatment of cervical myelopathy. *Spine* 1986;11:818-823.

19. Ou Y, Lu J, Mi J, Cheng-li Zhang J, Li Y, Sheng N: Extensive anterior decompression for mixed cervical spondylosis: Resection of uncovertebral joints, neural and transverse foraminotomy, subtotal corpectomy, and fusion with strut graft. *Spine* 1994;19:2651-2656.

20. Lu J, Ebraheim NA, Georgiadis GM, Yang H, Yeasting RA: Anatomic considerations of the vertebral artery: Implications for anterior decompression of the cervical spine. *J Spinal Disord* 1998;11:233-236.

21. Pait TG, Killefer JA, Arnautovic KI: Surgical anatomy of the anterior cervical spine: The disc space, vertebral artery, and associated bony structures. *Neurosurgery* 1996;39:769-776.

22. Oga M, Yuge I, Terada K, Shimizu A, Sugioka Y: Tortuosity of the vertebral artery in patients with cervical spondylotic myelopathy: Risk factor for the vertebral artery injury during anterior cervical decompression. *Spine* 1996;21:1085-1089.

23. Curylo LJ, Mason HC, Bohlman HH, Yoo JU: Tortuous course of the vertebral artery and anterior cervical decompression. *Spine* 2000; 25:2860-2864.

24. Tumialan LM, Wippold FJ II, Morgan RA: Tortuous vertebral artery injury complicating anterior cervical spinal fusion in a symptomatic rheumatoid cervical spine. *Spine* 2004;29: E343-E348.

25. Spetzler RF, Roski RA, Selman WR: The microscope in anterior cervical spine surgery. *Clin Orthop Relat Res* 1982;168:17-23.

26. Burke JP, Gerszten PC, Welch WC: Iatrogenic vertebral artery injury during anterior cervical spine surgery. *Spine J* 2005;5:508-514.

27. Goel A, Gupta S: Vertebral artery injury with transarticular screws. *J Neurosurg* 1999;90:376-377.

28. Boden SD, Dodge LD, Bohlmann HH, Rechtine GR: Rheumatoid arthritis of the cervical spine: A long-term analysis with predictors of paralysis and recovery. *J Bone Joint Surg Am* 1993;75:1282-1297.

29. Farey ID, Nadkarni S, Smith N: Modified Gallie technique versus transarticular screw fixation in C1-C2 fusion. *Clin Orthop Relat Res* 1999;359: 126-135.

30. Yamazaki M, Koda M, Aromomi M, Hashimoto M, Masaki Y, Okawa A: Anomalous vertebral artery at the extraosseous and intraosseous regions of the craniovertebral junction: Analysis by three-dimensional computed tomography angiography. *Spine* 2005;30:2452-2457.

31. Hong JT, Lee SW, Son BC, Park CK: Anatomical variations of the bone and vascular structures around the posterior atlantal arch: Analysis by three-dimensional computed tomography angiography. San Francisco, CA, *Cervical Spine Research Society Meeting Proceedings*, 2007, pp 122-123.

32. Grob D, Crisco JJ III, Panjabi MM, Wang P, Dvorak J: Biomechanical evaluation of four different posterior atlantoaxial fixation techniques. *Spine* 1992;17:480-490.

33. Grob D, Jeanneret B, Aebi M, Markwalder TM: Atlanto-axial fusion with transarticular screw fixation. *J Bone Joint Surg Br* 1991;73:972-976.

34. Igarashi T, Kikuchi S, Sato K, Kayama S, Otani K: Anatomic study of the axis for surgical planning of transarticular screw fixation. *Clin Orthop Relat Res* 2003;408:162-166.

35. Nogueira-Barbosa MH, Defino HL: Multiplanar reconstructions of helical computed tomography in planning of atlanto-axial transarticular fixation. *Eur Spine J* 2005;14:493-500.

36. Paramore CG, Dickman CA, Sonntag VK: The anatomical suitability of the C1-2 complex for transarticular screw fixation. *J Neurosurg* 1996;85:221-224.

37. Liu J, Shafiq Q, Ebraheim NA, Karkare N, Asaad M, Woldenberg L, Yeasting RA: Value of intraoperative true lateral radiograph of C2 pedicle for C1-2 transarticular screw insertion. *Spine J* 2005;5:434-440.

38. Solanki GA, Crockard HA: Preoperative determination of safe superior transarticular screw trajectory through the lateral mass. *Spine* 1999; 24:1477-1482.

39. Neo M, Sakamoto T, Fujibayashi S, Nakamura T: A safe screw trajectory for atlantoaxial transarticular fixation achieved using an aiming device. *Spine* 2005;30:E236-E242.

40. Gebhard JS, Schimmer RC, Jeanneret B: Safety and accuracy of transarticular screw fixation C1-2 using an aiming device. *Spine* 1998;23:2185-2189.

41. Song GS, Theodore N, Dickman CA, Sonntag VK: Unilateral posterior atlantoaxial transarticular screw fixation. *J Neurosurg* 1997;87:851-855.

42. Harms J, Melcher RP: Posterior C1-C2 fusion with polyaxial screw and rod fixation. *Spine* 2001;26:2467-2471.

43. Kuroki H, Rengachary SS, Goel VK, Holekamp SA, Pitkanen V, Ebraheim NA: Biomechanical comparison of two stabilization techniques of the atlantoaxial joints: Transarticular screw fixation versus screw and rod fixation. *Neurosurgery* 2005;56:151-159.

44. Currier BL, Todd LT, Maus TP, Fisher DR, Yaszemski MJ: Anatomic relationship of the internal carotid artery of the C1 vertebrae: A case report of cervical reconstruction for chordoma and pilot study to assess the risk of screw fixation of the atlas. *Spine* 2003;28:E461-E467.

45. Sasso RC: C1 lateral screws and C2 pedicle/pars screws. *Instr Course Lect* 2007;56:311-317.

46. Lee MJ, Cassinelli E, Riew KD: The feasibility of inserting atlas lateral mass screws via the posterior arch. *Spine* 2006;31:2798-2801.

47. Tan M, Wang H, Wang Y, et al: Morphometric evaluation of screw fixation in atlas via posterior arch and lateral mass. *Spine* 2003;28:888-895.

48. Ebraheim NA, Xu R, Ahmad M, Heck B: The quantitative anatomy of the vertebral artery groove of the atlas and its relation to the posterior atlantoaxial approach. *Spine* 1998;23: 320-323.

49. Young JP, Young PH, Ackermann MJ, Anderson PA, Riew KD: The ponticulus posticus: Implications for screw insertion into the first cervical lateral mass. *J Bone Joint Surg Am* 2005;87:2495-2498.

50. Ebraheim NA, Fow J, Xu R, Yeasting RA: The location of the pedicle

and pars interarticularis in the axis. *Spine* 2001;26:E34-E37.

51. Abumi K, Shono Y, Ito M, Taneichi H, Kotani Y, Kaneda K: Complications of pedicle screw fixation in reconstructive surgery of the cervical spine. *Spine* 2000;25:962-969.

52. Golueke P, Sclafani S, Phillips T, Goldstein A, Scalea T, Duncan A: Vertebral artery injury: Diagnosis and management. *J Trauma* 1987;27:856-865.

53. Mitchell JA: Changes in vertebral artery blood flow following normal rotation of the cervical spine. *J Manipulative Physiol Ther* 2003;26:347-351.

54. Garcia Alzamora M, Rosahl SK, Lehmberg J, Klisch J: Life-threaening bleeding from a vertebral artery pseudoaneurysm after anterior cervical spine approach: Endovascular repair by a triple stent-in-stent method. *Neuroradiology* 2005;47:282-286.

55. Kieffer E, Praquin B, Chiche L, Koskas F, Bahinia A: Distal vertebral artery reconstruction: Long-term outcome. *J Vasc Surg* 2002;36:549-554.

56. Berguer R, Morasch MD, Kline RA: A review of 100 consecutive reconstructions of the distal vertebral artery for embolic and hemodynamic disease. *J Vasc Surg* 1998;27:852-859.

57. Cosgrove GR, Théron J: Vertebral arteriovenous fistula following anterior cervical spine surgery. *J Neurosurg* 1987;66:297-299.

58. de los Reyes RA, Moser FG, Sachs DP, Boehm FH: Direct repair of an extracranial vertebral artery pseudoaneurysm: Case report and review of the literature. *Neurosurgery* 1990;26:528-533.

59. Thomas GI, Anderson KN, Hain RF, Merendino KA: The significance of anomalous vertebral-basilar artery communications in operations on the heart and great vessels: An illustrative case with review of the literature. *Surgery* 1959;46:747-759.

60. Higashida RT, Halbach VV, Tsai FY, et al: Interventional neurovascular treatment of traumatic carotid and vertebral artery lesions: Results in 234 cases. *AJR Am J Roentgenol* 1989;153:577-582.

61. Neo M, Matsushita M, Iwashita Y, Yasuda T, Sakamoto T, Nakamura T: Atlantoaxial transarticular screw fixation for high riding vertebral artery. *Spine* 2003;28:666-670.

Index